DIURETICS: BASIC, PHARMACOLOGICAL, AND CLINICAL ASPECTS

DEVELOPMENTS IN NEPHROLOGY

Schück, O., ed.: Examination of the Kidney Function. 1981. ISBN 0–89838–565–2.

Strauss, J., ed.: Hypertension, Fluid-Electrolytes and Tubulopathies in Pediatric Nephrology. 1981. ISBN 90–247–2633–6.

Strauss, J., ed.: Neonatal Kidney and Fluid-Electrolytes. 1983. ISBN 0–89838–575–X.

Strauss, J., ed.: Acute Renal Disorders and Renal Emergencies. 1984. ISBN 0–89838–663–2.

Didio, L.J.A. and Motta, P.M., eds.: Basic, Clinical and Surgical Nephrology. 1985. ISBN 0–89838–698–5.

Friedman, E.A. and Peterson, C.M., eds: Diabetic Nephropathy: Strategy for Therapy. 1985. ISBN 0–89838–735–3.

Dzurik, R., Lichardus, B. and Guder, W., eds.: Kidney Metabolism and Function. 1985. ISBN 0–89838–749–3.

Strauss, J., ed: Homeostasis, Nephrotoxicity, and Renal Anomalies in the Newborn. 1986. ISBN 0–89838–766–3.

Oreopoulos, D.G., ed: Geriatric Nephrology. 1986. ISBN 0–89838–781–7.

Paganini, E.P., ed: Acute Continuous Renal Replacement Therapy. 1986. ISBN 0–89838–793–0.

Cheigh, J.S., Stenzel, K.H. and Rubin, A.L., eds.: Hypertension in Kidney Disease. 1986. ISBN 0–89838–797–3.

Deane, N. Wineman, R.J. and Bemis, J.A., eds.: Guide to Reprocessing of Hemodialyzers. 1987. ISBN 0–89838–798–1.

Ponticelli, C., Minetti, L. and D'Amico, G., eds.: Antiglobulins, Cryoglobulins and Glomerulonephritis. 1987. ISBN 0–89838–810–4.

Strauss, J., ed: Persistent Renal-Genitourinary Disorders. 1987. ISBN 0–89838–845–7.

Diuretics: Basic, Pharmacological, and Clinical Aspects

Proceedings of the International Meeting on Diuretics, Sorrento, Italy, May 26–30, 1986

edited by
V.E. Andreucci, M.D.
Antonio Dal Canton, M.D.
Department of Nephrology
University of Naples
Naples, Italy

Martinus Nijhoff Publishing
a member of the Kluwer Academic Publishers Group
Boston/Dordrecht/Lancaster

Distributors for North America:
Kluwer Academic Publishers
101 Philip Drive
Assinippi Park
Norwell, MA 02061, USA

Distributors for the UK and Ireland:
Kluwer Academic Publishers
MTP Press Limited
Falcon House, Queen Square
Lancaster, LA1 1RN, UNITED KINGDOM

Distributors for all other countries:
Kluwer Academic Publishers Group
Distribution Centre
Post Office Box 322
3300 AH Dordrecht, THE NETHERLANDS

Library of Congress Cataloging-in-Publication Data

International Meeting on Diuretics (1986 : Sorrento, Italy)
Diuretics : basic, pharmacological, and clinical aspects.

(Developments in nephrology)
Includes bibliographies.
1. Diuretics—Congresses. I. Andreucci, Vittorio E. II. Dal Canton, Antonio. III. Title. IV. Series.
[DNLM: 1. Diuretics—congresses. W1 DE998EB / QV 160 1614d 1986]
RM377.I58 1986 615'.761 87-7704
ISBN 0-89838-885-6

Printed in the United States of America

CONTENTS

IX. DIURETICS AND RENAL DISEASE.

X. DIURETICS IN CIRRHOSIS.

XI. DIURETICS AND STONE FORMATION.

XV. EFFECTS OF DIURETICS ON RENAL FUNCTION.

XVI. DIURETICS AND PROSTAGLANDINS.

CONTRIBUTING AUTHORS

Abitbol J.P.
Theraplix Lab.
Paris, France

Achhammer A.
Boehringer Mannheim GmbH
Tubingen, FRG

Adorati M.
Division of Nephrology, City Hospital
Udine, Italy

Ajello A.
Istituto di Clinica Medica
University of Messina
Messina, Italy

Alcazar J.M.
Service of Nephrology
1 Octubre Hospital
Madrid, Spain

Alfonso L.
Department of Nephrology and Dialysis "V.Fazzi" Hospital
Lecce, Italy

Alsina J.
Nephrology Department
Hospital de Bellvtige
Barcelona, Spain

Altomonte M.
Department of Nephrology Secund Faculty of Medicine
Naples, Italy

Ambrosioni E.
Cattedra e Servizio di Farmacologia Clinica, Policlinico S. Orsola
Universita' di Bologna
Bologna, Italy

Amenos A.M.
Hospital de Bellvtige
"Princeps d'Espanya"
Barcelona, Spain

Andreasen F.
Institute of Pharmacology
University of Aarhus
Aarhus, Denmark

Andreoli T.E.
Department of Internal Medicine
University of Texas
Medical School
Houston, USA

Andres E.
Nephrology Department
Hospital de Bellvtige
Barcelona, Spain

Andreucci V.E.
Department of Nephrology Secund Faculty of Medicine
Naples, Italy

Antonelli E.
Istituto di Cardiologia
Policlinico S. Orsola
Universita' di Bologna
Bologna, Italy

Antonello A.
Institute of Internal Medicine
Postgraduate School of Nephrology
University of Padua
Padua, Italy

Antonucci F.
Division of Nephrology, City Hospital
Udine, Italy

Aprile M.
Department of Nephrology and Dialysis, "V.Fazzi" Hospital
Lecce, Italy

Arzilli F.
Clinica Medica I, University of Pisa
Pisa, Italy

Asta N.
Institute of Clinical Medicine
Chair of Medical Therapy
University of Palermo
Palermo, Italy

Atherton J.C.
Manchester, Great Britain

Aucella F.
Department of Nephrology, Secund Faculty of Medicine
Naples, Italy

Backer A.
Division of Nephrology
Medizinische Poliklinik
University of Bonn
Bonn, FRG

Baczyk K.
Department of Nephrology
Academy of Medicine
Poznan, Poland

Baggio B.
Institute of Internal Medicine
Universita' of Padua
Padua, Italy

Bakhle D.S.
Division of Clinical Pharmacology
Grant Medical College
Bombay, India

Banderali G.
Hypertension Unit, Rho Hospital
Milan, Italy

Bandiani G.
Servizio di Nefrologia e Dialisi
Ospedale Civile S. Andrea
La Spezia, Italy

Bandiera F.
Cattedra di Patologia Medica II
University of Sassari
Sassari, Italy

Baranes J.
IHB Research Labs
Le Plessis, France

Barba G.
Institute of Internal Medicine and Metabolic Disease
Second Medical School
University of Naples
Naples, Italy

Barbagallo Sangiorgi G.
Institute of Internal Medicine and Geriatrics
University of Palermo
Palermo, Italy

Bardelli M.
Institute of Clinical Pathology
University of Trieste
Trieste, Italy

Bariety J.
Hopital Broussais
Paris, France

Bartoli E.
Institute of Medical Pathology
University of Sassari
Sassari, Italy

Bartolini A.
Department of Preclinical and Clinical Pharmacology
University of Florence
Florence, Italy

Baumelou A.
Hopital de la Pitie'
Paris, France

Bazzato G.
Department of Nephrology and Dialysis
Umberto I Hospital
Venice, Italy

Bech O.M.
Department of Pharmacology
University of Copenhagen
Copenhagen, Denmark

Beerman B.
Karolinska Institute
Huddinge Hospital
Huddinge, Sweden

Bellati G.
Department of Internal Medicine A
St. Anna's Hospital
Como, Italy

Bellini G.
Institute of Clinical Pathology
University of Trieste
Trieste, Italy

Beltrame G.
Department of Nephrology
University of Turin
Turin, Italy

Benazzi E.
Renal Unit, Ospedale Niguarda
Ca' Granda
Milan, Italy

Benetollo P.
Istituto di Medicina Interna
Universita' di Padova
Padova, Italy

Benos D.J.
Department of Physiology and
Biophysic
Birmingham, USA

Benzoni D.
Department of Physiology and Clinical
Pharmacology
Faculty of Pharmacy
Lyon, France

Besenfelder E.
Boehringer Mannheim GmbH
Mannheim, FRG

Bianchetti A.
Department of Anaesthesia
Ospedale Maggiore
Trieste, Italy

Bianchi C.
Cattedra di Nefrologia Medica
Universita' di Pisa
Pisa, Italy

Bianchi G.
Istituto Scienze Mediche Universita'
di Milano
Milan, Italy

Bichisao E.
Clinica Medica I, University of Pisa
Pisa, Italy

Bidea J.
Service de Nephrology
Hospital de Cruces
Bilbao, Spain

Biollaz M.
Ciba-Geigy Limited
Pharmaceutical Division
Basel, Switzerland

Bionda A.
Istituto di Clinica Medica II
Universita' di Pisa
Pisa, Italy

Bobinski H.
Department of Physiology
University of Manchester
Manchester, Great Britain

Boer W.H.
Department of Nephrology and
Hypertension, University Hospital
Utrecht, The Netherlands

Boero R.
Department of Nephrology
University of Turin
Turin, Italy

Boisson J.
Hopital Notre Dame de Bon Secours
Paris, France

Bonadio, M.
Cattedra di Nefrologia Medica
Universita' di Pisa
Pisa, Italy

Bonaduce D.
Institute of Internal Medicine
Second School of Medicine
University of Naples
Naples, Italy

Bonomini V.
Institute of Nephrology
S. Orsola University Hospital
Bologna, Italy

Borghi C.
Cattedra e Servizio di Farmacologia
Policlinico S. Orsola
Universita' di Bologna
Bologna, Italy

Borgnino C.
Medical Department, Bayer Italia
Milan, Italy

Borsatti A.
Institute of Internal Medicine
University of Padua
Padua, Italy

Boschetti E.
Istituto di Semeiotica Medica
Universita' di Perugia
Perugia, Italy

Boschi S.
Cattedra e Servizio di Farmacologia
Policlinico S. Orsola
Universita' di Bologna
Bologna, Italy

Branca G.
Institute of Medical Pathology
University of Sassari
Sassari, Italy

Braquet P.
IHB Research Labs
Le Plessis, France

Breglio R.
Institute of Internal Medicine
Second School of Medicine
University of Naples
Naples, Italy

Brennan F.
Department of Pharmacology
Smith Kline and French
Swedeland, USA

Brouard R.
Hopital de la Pitie'.
Paris, France

Brown W.
MRC Blood Pressure Unit
Western Infirmary
Glasgow, Great Britain

Brunel P.
Service de Nephrologie CHU
Amiens, France

Brunner G.
Department of Medicine
University of Hannover
Hannover, FRG

Brunner H.R.
Division of Hypertension
University Hospital
Lausanne, Switzerland

Bruno M.
Department of Nephrology
Mauriziano Umberto I Hospital
Turin, Italy

Brunori G.
Department of Nephrology
School of Medicine
University of Brescia
Brescia, Italy

Buemi M.
Institute of Internal Medicine
School of Medicine
University of Messina
Messina, Italy

Bugge J.F.
Institute for Exper. Med. Research
Oslo, Norway

Buhrle C.P.
Department of Pharmacology and Physiology
University of Heidelberg
Heidelberg, FRG

Calapristi I.
Istituto di Clinica Medica
University of Messina
Messina, Italy

Calo L.
Institute of Internal Medicine
Postgraduate School of Nephrology
University of Padova
Padua, Italy

Camaiora E.
Servizio di Nefrologia e Dialisi
Ospedale Civile S. Andrea
La Spezia, Italy

Campanacci L.
Institute of Clinical Pathology
University of Trieste
Trieste, Italy

Campieri C.
Institute of Nephrology
Orsola University Hospital
Bologna, Italy

Cannella G.
Department of Nephrology
Spedali Civili
Brescia, Italy

Canonico V.
Institute of Internal Medicine
Second School of Medicine
University of Naples
Naples, Italy

Cantaro S.
Institute of Internal Medicine
Postgraduate School of Medicine
University of Padua
Padua, Italy

Cantin M.
CRIM 110
Montreal, Quebec, Canada

Capel B.
Service de Physiologie
Universite' de Mons
Mons, Belgium

Cappello A.
Istituto di Clinica Medica
University of Messina
Messina, Italy

Capra C.
Clinica Medica
University of Verona Medical School
Policlinico
Verona, Italy

Capuana G.
Institute of Clinical Medicine
Chair of Medical Therapy
University of Palermo
Palermo, Italy

Carnovali M.
Hypertension Unit, Rho Hospital
Milan, Italy

Carosi M.
Medical Department, Bayer Italia
Milan, Italy

Carreras L.
Hospital de Bellvtige
"Princeps d'Espanya"
Barcelona, Spain

Carretta R.
Institute of Medical Pathology
University of Trieste
Trieste, Italy

Castelao A.M.
Nephrology Department
Hospital de Bellvtige
Barcelona. Spain

Castellano M.
Department of Social Sciences
Istituto Universitario Orientale
University of Naples
Naples, Italy

Castrignano R.
Istituto di Medicina Interna
Universita' di Padova
Padova, Italy

Cecconcello A.
Istituto di Medicina Interna
Universita' di Padova
Padova, Italy

Cervi V.
Istituto di Cardiologia
Policlinico S. Orsola
Universita' di Bologna
Bologna, Italy

Chabrier P.E.
IHB Research Labs.
Le Plessis, France

Chambrin P.Y.
Clinical Pharmacology
La Salpetriere Hospital
Paris, France

Chan J.C.M.
Medical College of Virginia
Richmond, USA

Chauveau P.
Department of Nephrology
Necker Hospital
Paris, France

Christensen J.H.
Institute of Pharmacology
University of Aarhus
Aarhus, Denmark

Christensen S.
Department of Pharmacology
University of Copenhagen
Copenhagen, Denmark

Churchill S.
Department of Physiology
Harvard Medical School
Boston, USA

Cianciaruso B.
Department of Nephrology Secund Faculty of Medicine
Naples, Italy

Cipolloni S.
Istituto di Semeiotica Medica
Universita' di Perugia
Perugia, Italy

Clari G.
Institute of Biological Chemistry
University of Verona
Verona, Italy

Clegg K.
Hypertension Division
Sepulveda VA Medical Center
Los Angeles, USA

Clerico A.
Hypertension Unit, Clinica Medica I
University of Pisa
Pisa, Italy

Cocco F.
Cattedra di Patologia Medica II
University of Sassari
Sassari, Italy

Cofelice E.
Department of Nephrology
Second Faculty of Medicine
University of Naples
Naples, Italy

Coli U.
Department of Nephrology and Dialysis
Umberto I Hospital
Venice-Mestre, Italy

Colina I.
Department of Medicine
University Clinic
University of Navarra
Pamplona, Spain

Colussi G.
Renal Division
Niguarda Ca' Granda Hospital
Milan, Italy

Cominotto R.
Instituto di Clinica Medica II
Universita' di Pisa
Pisa, Italy

Condorelli M.
Institute of Internal Medicine
Second School of Medicine
University of Naples
Naples, Italy

Conforti G.
Institute of Internal Medicine
Second School of Medicine
University of Naples
Naples, Italy

Conte G.
Department of Nephrology
Second Faculty of Medicine
Naples, Italy

Copercini B.
Division of Nephrology
Hospital of Cremona
Cremona, Italy

Coratelli P.
Institute of Nephrology
University of Bari
Bari, Italy

Corliano C.
Department of Nephrology and Dialysis "V.Fazzi" Hospital
Lecce, Italy

Cornejo J.C.
National University and Istituto Privado de Especialidades Medicas
Cordoba, Argentina

Cosby R.L.
Division of Renal Disease
University of Colorado
Health Sciences Center
Denver, Colorado USA

Costa F.V.
Cattedra e Servizio di Farmacologia Clinica
Policlinico S. Orsola
Universita' di Bologna
Bologna, Italy

Crepaldi G.
Istituto di Medicina Interna
Universita' di Padova
Padova, Italy

Crespi E.
Hypertension Unit, Rho Hospital
Milan, Italy

Cucchiara G.
University of Palermo
Palermo, Italy

Cuisinaud G.
Department of Nephrology and Clinical Pharmacology
Faculty of Pharmacy
Lyon, France

Cushen M.
Department of Medicine
Waterford Regional Hospital
Waterford, Ireland

D'Angelo A.
Istituto di Medicina Interna
Universita' di Padova
Padova, Italy

Dal Canton A.
Chair of Medical Nephrology
University of Sassari
Sassari, Italy

Dalla Volta S.
Cardiology Division
University of Padua
Padua, Italy

Davies D.L.
University Department of Medicine
Gardiner Institute
Western Infirmary
Glasgow, Scotland

De Blasi V.
Department of Nephrology and Dialysis ''V.Fazzi'' Hospital
Lecce, Italy

De Bold A.
Queen's University Department of Pathology
Kingston, Canada

De Donatis M.
Department of Preclinical and Clinical Pharmacology
University of Florence
Florence, Italy

De Ferrari M.E.
Renal Division, Niguarda Ca' Granda Hospital
Milan, Italy

De Gasparo M.
Ciba-Geigy Limited
Pharmaceutical Division
Basel, Switzerland

De Gasperi M.
Clinica Medica
University of Verona Medical School, Policlinico
Verona, Italy

De Mendoca M.
INSERM U7, Hopital Necker.
Paris, France

De Wardener H.E.
Research Laboratories Charing Cross
London, Great Britain

Deabate M.C.
Department of Nephrology
University of Turin
Turin, Italy

Degan M.
Clinica Medica
University of Verona Medical School, Policlinico
Verona, Italy

Degli Esposti D.
Istituto di Cardiologia
Policlinico S. Orsola
Universita' di Bologna
Bologna, Italy

Del Chicca A.
Istituto di Fisiologia Clinica, CNR
Universita' di Pisa
Pisa, Italy

Delaney E.
Department of Medicine
Waterford Regional Hospital
Waterford, Ireland

Dello Russo A.
Department of Nephrology
Second Faculty of Medicine
Naples, Italy

Delva P.
Clinica Medica, University of Verona Medical School, Policlinico
Verona, Italy

Deray G.
Hopital de la Pitie'.
Paris, France

Deschamps de Paillette E.
IHB Labs. Le Plessis-Robinson
Le Plessis, France

Dessi-Fulgheri P.
Cattedra di Patologia Medica II
University of Sassari
Sassari, Italy

Di Felice A.
Department of Nephrology and Dialysis
St. Orsola University Hospital
Bologna, Italy

Di Minno G.
Department of Internal Medicine
Clinica Medica II
University of Naples
Naples, Italy

Di Piazza R.
University of Palermo
Palermo, Italy

Di Sciacca A.
Chair of Systematic Medical Therapy
University of Palermo
Palermo, Italy

Di Stefano A.
Max Planck Institut fur Biophysik
Frankfurt, FRG

Diaz Teveiro R.
Division of Nephrology
University Clinic
University of Navarra
Pamplona, Spain

Dietl P.
Department of Physiology
University of Wurzburg Medical School
Wurzburg, FRG

Diez J.
Division of Nephrology
University Clinic
University of Navarra
Pamplona, Spain

Dimona G.
Chair of Medical Therapy
University of Bari
Bari, Italy

Distratis C.
Istituto di Clinica Medica II
Universita' di Pisa
Pisa, Italy

Divine' C.
Clinical Pharmacology
La Salpetriere Hospital
Paris, France

Donadio C.
Cattedra di Nefrologia Medica
Clinica Medica II
Universita' di Pisa
Pisa, Italy

Dorfler A.
Klinikum Bamberg, III Medicine
Bamberg, FRG

Dorhout Mees E.J.
Department of Nephrology and Hypertension
University Hospital
Utrecht, The Netherlands

Dorigo P.
Department of Pharmacology
University of Padua
Padua, Italy

Durand J.L.
Clinical Pharmacology
La Salpetriere Hospital
Paris, France

Durante F.
University of Palermo
Palermo, Italy

Dusing R.
Division of Nephrology
Medizinische Poliklinik
University of Bonn
Bonn, FRG

Dytko G.
Department of Pharmacology
Smith Kline and French Laboratories
Philadelphia, USA

Earley L.E.
Dept of Med., Univ. of Pennsylvania
School of Medicine
Philadelphia, USA

El Esper N.
Service de Nephrologie CHU Amiens
Amiens, France

Englert H.C.
Max Planck Institut fur Biophysik
Frankfurt, FRG

Enzmann G.
Division of Nephrology, City Hospital
Udine, Italy

Ernst E.
Hemorheology Research Laboratory
Clinic for Physical Medicine
University of Munich
Munich, FRG

Errasti P.
Division of Nephrology
University Clinic
University of Navarra
Pamplona, Spain

Esanu A.
IHB Research Labs
Le Plessis, France

Esposito C.
Department of Nephrology Secund Faculty of Medicine
Naples, Italy

Fabris A.
Cattedra e Divisione di Nefrologia Medica-Istituti Ospitalieri
Verona, Italy

Fabris B.
Institute of Clinical Phatology
University of Trieste
Trieste, Italy

Faedda R.
Institute of Medical Pathology
University of Sassari
Sassari, Italy

Fargetta C.
Istituto di Patologia Medica I
Universita' di Catania
Catania, Italy

Fasoli G.
Cardiology Division
University of Padua
Padua, Italy

Faucher C.
Hopital de la Pitie'
Paris, France

Fava A.
Istituto di Clinica Medica
University of Messina
Messina, Italy

Favazza A.
Division of Nephrology
City Hospital
Udine, Italy

Federico S.
Department of Nephrology
II Faculty of Medicine
University of Naples
Naples, Italy

Ferrandi M.
Farmitalia Carlo Erba Centro Ricerche
Milan, Italy

Ferrara L.A.
Institute of Internal Medicine and Metabolic Disease
Clinica Medica, Second Medical School
University of Naples
Naples, Italy

Ferrari P.
Farmitalia Carlo Erba Centro Ricerche
Milan, Italy

Ferrario R.G.
Farmitalia Carlo Erba Ricerche
Milan, Italy

Ferrau' O.
Cattedra di Patologia Medica III
University of Messina
Messina, Italy

Ferrer C.
National University and Istituto
Privado de Especialidade Medicas
Cordoba, Argentina

Ferry N.
Department of Physiology and Clinical
Pharmacology
Faculty of Pharmacy
Lyon, France

Fievet P.
Service de Nephrologie, CHU Amiens
Amiens, France

Fine L.G.
Div. of Nephrology, Dept. of Medicine
Center for Health Sciences
UCLA School of Medicine
Los Angeles, USA

Fiore C.E.
Istituto di Patologia Medica I
Universita' di Catania
Catania, Italy

Fischetti F.
Institute of Clinical Pathology
University of Trieste
Trieste, Italy

Fitzgerald G.R.
Department of Medicine
Waterford Regional Hospital
Waterford, Ireland

Fitzgerald M.G.
Department of Medicine
Waterford Regional Hospital
Waterford, Ireland

Fluckinger J.P.
Division of Hypertension
University Hospital
Lausanne, Switzerland

Forneris G.
Department of Nephrology
University of Turin
Torino, Italy

Foti R.
Istituto di Patologia Medica I
Universita' di Catania
Catania, Italy

Fournier A.
Queen's University
Department of Pathology
Kingston, Canada

Fracasso A.
Department of Nephrology and
Dialysis
Umberto I Hospital
Venice-Mestre, Italy

Frattarelli L.
Istituto di Clinica Medica II
Universita' di Pisa
Pisa, Italy

Fredj G.
Clinical Pharmacology
La Salpetriere Hospital
Paris, France

Freni, M.A.
Istituto di Clinica Medica
University of Messina
Messina, Italy

Frisina N.
Institute of Internal Medicine
School of Medicine
University of Messina
Messina, Italy

Frontini A.
University of Palermo
Palermo, Italy

Fruttero B.
Department of Nephrology
Mauriziano Umberto I Hospital
Turin, Italy

Fuchs B.
Department of Pharmacology
Rheinisch Westfalische
Technische Hochschule Schneebergweg
Aachen, FRG

Furuya M.
Department of Pharmacology
National Cardiovascular Center
Research Institute
Osaka, Japan

Fyhrquist F.
Unit of Clinical Physiology
The Minerva Institute
Foundation Institute for Medical
Research
Helsinki, Finland

Gaggiotti M.
Department of Nephrology
School of Medicine
University of Brescia
Brescia, Italy

Gagliardi R.
Medical Department, Bayer-Italy
Naples, Italy

Gaion R.M.
Department of Pharmacology
University of Padua
Padua, Italy

Galletti F.
Institute of Internal Medicine
and Metabolic Disease
Second Medical School
University of Naples
Naples, Italy

Galli A.
Department of Preclinical and
Clinical Pharmacology
University of Florence
Florence, Italy

Gambaro G.
Institute of Internal Medicine
University of Padua
Padua, Italy

Gammaro L.
Cattedra e Divisione di Nefrologia
Medica-Istituti Ospitalieri
Verona, Italy

Ganeval D.
Department of Nephrology
Necker Hospital
Paris, France

Garay R.
INSERM U 7, Hopital Necker
Paris, France

Gaschard J.
Hopital Notre Dame de Bon Secours
Paris, France

Gazzotti R.M.
Department of Nephrology
II Faculty of Medicine
University of Naples
Naples, Italy

Genard J.
Service de Physiologie
Universite' de Mons
Mons, Belgium

Genchi R.
Department of Nephrology and
Dialysis
Umberto I Hospital
Venice Mestre, Italy

Geoffroy J.
Department of Nephrology and
Clinical Nephrology
Faculty of Pharmacy
Lyon, France

Ghielmi S.
Clinical Chemistry
School of Medicine
University of Brescia
Brescia, Italy

Ghiringhelli P.
Division of Nephrology
Hospital of Cremona
Cremona, Italy

Giannattasio M.
Institute of Nephrology
University of Bari
Bari, Italy

Giannini S.
Istituto di Medicina Interna
Universita' di Padova
Padova, Italy

Gil-Vernet S.
Nephrology Department
Hospital de Bellvtige
Barcelona, Spain

Gilligan D.
Department of Medicine
Waterford Regional Hospital
Waterford, Ireland

Giorcelli G.
Dept. of Nephrology and Dialysis
Ospedale Mauriziano Umberto I
Turin, Italy

Giordano R.
Servizio di Nefrologia e Dialisi
Ospedale Civile
Martinafranca, Italy

Giovannetti R.
Clinica Medica I
University of Pisa
Pisa, Italy

Giraudo G.
Department of Nephrology
University of Turin
Turin, Italy

Giunta A.
Department of Nephrology
Second Faculty of Medicine
University of Naples
Naples, Italy

Glocke M.
Boehringer Mannheim GmbH
Mannheim, FRG

Glorioso N.
Cattedra di Patologia Medica II
University of Sassari
Sassari, Italy

Gnocchi E.
Nuclear Medicine Service
Hospital of Cremona
Cremona, Italy

Godino F.
Servizio di Nefrologia e Dialisi
Ospedale Civile
Martinafranca, Italy

Graziadei L.
Clinica Medica I
University of Pisa
Pisa, Italy

Greco G.
Istituto di Patologia Medica
Universita' di Catania
Catania, Italy

Green R.
Manchester, Great Britain

Greger R.
Max Planck Institut fur Biophysik
Frankfurt, FRG

Gregoire I.
Service de Nephrologie CHU
Amiens, France

Greven J.
Department of Pharmacology
Rheinisch Westfalische
Technische Hoschule Schneebergweg s/n
Aachen, FRG

Grichois M.L.
INSERM U7, Hopital Necker
Paris, France

Grino J.M.
Nephrology Department
Hospital de Bellvtige
Barcelona, Spain

Grippa G.
Department of Internal Medicine and Renal Unit
Piacenza, Italy

Grob J.
Ciba-Geigy Limited, Pharmaceutical Division
Basel, Switzerland

Gronhagen-Riska C.
Unit of Clinical Physiology
Minerva Foundation
Helsinki, Finland

Gropuzzo M.
Division of Nephrology
City Hospital
Udine, Italy

Grossi C.
Servizio di Nefrologia e Dialisi
Ospedale Civile
Martinafranca, Italy

Grzegorzewska A.
Department of Nephrology
Academy of Medicine
Poznan, Poland

Guarena C.
Department of Nephrology
University of Turin
Turin, Italy

Guerra A.
Istituto di Semeiotica Medica
Universita' di Parma
Parma, Italy

Guilmard C.
IHB Research Labs
Le Plessis, France

Guzzardi F.
Istituto di Patologia Medica I
Universita' di Catania
Catania, Italy

Hackenthal E.
Department of Pharmacology and Physiology
University of Heidelberg
Heidelberg, FRG

Hadj Aissa A.
Clinic of Nephrology
Hospital E. Herriot
Lyon, France

Haecker W.
Boehringer Mannheim GmbH
Tubingen, FRG

Haenni H.
Ciba-Geigy Limited
Pharmaceutical Division
Basel, Switzerland

Hajdu' D.
Department of Clinical Research
Hoechst AG Frankfurt
Frankfurt, FRG

Hammarlund-Udenaes M.
Department of Biopharmaceutics and Pharmacokinetics
University of Uppsala
Uppsala, Sweden

Hannaert P.
INSERM U7. Hopital Necker
Paris, France

Hartmann A.
Institute for Experimental Medical Research
University of Oslo
Ullevaal Hospital
Oslo, Norway

Hasenfuss G.
Medizinische-Universitatsklinik Freiburg/Breisgau
Freiburg, FRG

Hayashi Y.
Department of Pharmacology
National Cardiovascular Center Research Institute
Osaka, Japan

Hene' R.J.
Department of Nephrology and Hypertension
University Hospital
Utrecht, The Netherlands

Holthe M.R.
Institute for Experimental Research
University of Oslo
Ullevaal Hospital
Oslo, Norway

Hornych A.
INSERM U 28
Hopital Broussais
Paris, France

Huffman W.
Department of Chemistry
Smith Kline and French Laboratories
Philadelphia, USA

Iacone R.
Institute of Internal Medicine and Metabolic Disease
Second Medical School
University of Naples
Naples, Italy

Iandolo R.
Department of Nephrology
II Faculty of Medicine
University of Naples
Naples, Italy

Icardi G.P.
Dept. of Nephrology and Dialysis
Ospedale Mauriziano Umberto I
Torino, Italy

Ickrath O.
Department of Internal Medicine
University of Tubingen
Tubingen, FRG

Ideo G.
Department of Internal Medicine A
St' Anna's Hospital
Como, Italy

Iliopoulou A.
Department of Clinical Therapeutics
University of Athens
''Alexandra'' Hospital
Athens, Greece

Imai M.
Department of Pharmacology
National Cardiovascular Center Research Institute
Osaka, Japan

Imperatore P.
Department of Nephrology
Second Faculty of Medicine
Naples, Italy

Ingrassia A.
University of Palermo
Palermo, Italy

Joss U.
Ciba Geigy Limited
Pharmaceutical Division
Basel, Switzerland

Juin G.
INSERM U7
Hopital Necker
Paris, France

Juncos L.I.
National University and Istituto Privado de Especialidades Medicas
Cordoba, Argentina

Jungers P.
Department of Nephrology
Necker Hospital
Paris, France

Just H.
Medizinische-Universitatsklinik Freiburg/Breisgau
Freiburg, FRG

Kanai T.
Department of Pharmacology
National Cardiovascular Center Research Institute
Osaka, Japan

Kaufmann B.
Boehringer Mannheim GmbH
Mannheim, FRG

Kawamura N.
Department of Urology
Tokai University School of Medicine
Tokyo, Japan

Kennedy M.J.
Department of Medicine
Waterford Regional Hospital
Waterford, Ireland

Kenny A.
Department of Medicine
Waterford Regional Hospital
Waterford, Ireland

Kiil F.
Instit. for Exper. Medic. Research
University of Oslo Ullevaal Hospital
Oslo, Norway

Kinter L.B.
Department of Pharmacology
Smith Kline and French Laboratories
Swedeland, USA

Kipnowski J.
Division of Nephrology
Medizinische Poliklinik
University of Bonn
Bonn, FRG

Kirstein D.
LEO Pharmaceutical Products
Ballerup, Denmark

Knauf H.
Medizinische-Universitatsklinik
Freiburg/Breisgau
Freiburg, FRG

Kohno M.
Hypertension Division
Sepulveda VA Medical Center
Los Angeles, USA

Kontoyanis D.
Department of Clinical Therapeutics
University of Athens
''Alexandra'' Hospital
Athens, Greece

Kontoyanis S.
Department of Clinical Therapeutics
University of Athens
''Alexandra'' Hospital
Athens, Greece

Koomans H.A.
Department of Nephrology and Hypertension Unit
University Hospital
Utrecht, The Netherlands

Koseki C.
Department of Pharmacology
National Cardiovascular Center Research Institute
Osaka, Japan

Kraenhenbuhl C.
Ciba Geigy Limited
Pharmaceutical Division
Basel, Switzerland

Kramer H.J.
Division of Nephrology
Medizinische Poliklinik
University of Bonn
Bonn, FRG

Kramp R.
Service de Physiologie
Universite' de Mons
Mons, Belgium

Krueger B.
Medical Clinic, Univ. of Erlangen-Nuernberg
Erlangen, FRG

Kulkarni R.D.
Division of Clinical Pharmacology
Grant Medical College
Bombay, India

Labeeuw M.
Clinic of Nephrology
Hospital E. Herriot
Lyon, France

Lahn W.
Department of Clinical Research
Hoechst AG Frankfurt.
Frankfurt, FRG

Lampreabe I.
Service of Nephrology
Hospital de Cruces
Bilbao, Spain

Landini S.
Department of Nephrology and Dialysis
Umberto I Hospital
Venice-Mestre, Italy

Lang H.J.
Max Planck Institut fur Biophysik
Frankfurt, FRG

Lang R.E.
Department of Pharmacology and Physiology
University of Heidelberg
Heidelberg, FRG

Langberg H.
Institute for Experimental Research
University of Oslo
Ullevaal Hospital
Oslo, Norway

Leary W.P.
Department of Experimental and Clinical Pharmacology
University of Natal
Durban, South Africa

Lechi A.
Clinica Medica
University of Verona Medical School
Policlinico
Verona, Italy

Leksell L.G.
Karolinska Institutet
Stockholm, Sweden

Lenoir R.
Service de Physiologie
Universite' de Mons
Mons, Belgium

Leonardi C.
Istituto di Patologia Medica
Universita' di Catania
Catania, Italy

Leone M.A.
Chair of Medical Therapy
University of Bari
Bari, Italy

Leprini R.
Institute of Clinical Pathology
University of Trieste
Trieste, Italy

Licata G.
Institute of Clinical Medicine
Chair of Medical Therapy
University of Palermo
Palermo, Italy

Linari F.
Department of Nephrology
Mauriziano Umberto I Hospital
Turin, Italy

Liviano D'Arcangelo G.
Department of Nephrology and Dialysis
St. Orsola University Hospital
Bologna, Italy

Lo Greco P.
Clinical Chemistry Laboratory
City Hospital
Udine, Italy

Lorusso P.
Cattedra di Nefrologia Medica Clinica Medica II
Universita' di Pisa
Pisa, Italy

Loschiavo C.
Cattedra e Divisione di Nefrologia Medica-Istituti Ospitalieri
Verona, Italy

Loubaris T.
Department of Nephrology
Necker Hospital
Paris, France

Lunetta M.
Cattedra di Malattie del Ricambio
University of Catania
Catania, Italy

Lupo A.
Cattedra e Divisione di Nefrologia
Medica-Istituti Ospitalieri
Verona, Italy

Macri' I.
Institute of Internal Medicine
School of Medicine
University of Messina
Messina, Italy

Madeddu P.
Cattedra di Patologia Medica II
University of Sassari
Sassari, Italy

Maduell F.
Division of Nephrology
University Clinic
University of Navarra
Pamplona, Spain

Magnani B.
Istitutio di Cardiologia
Policlinico S. Orsola
Universita' di Bologna
Bologna, Italy

Maione S.
Department of Nephrology and
Internal Medicine
Second Faculty of Medicine, Naples
Naples, Italy

Maiorca R.
Dept. of Nephrology, School of
Medicine
Spedali Civili, University of Brescia
Brescia, Italy

Malatino L.S.
Istituto di Patologia Medica I
Universita' di Catania
Catania, Italy

Malberti F.
Renal Unit
Ospedale Maggiore Lodi
Lodi, Italy

Malmberg-Aiello P.
Department of Preclinical and Clinical
Pharmacology
University of Florence
Florence, Italy

Malvasi L.
Istituto di Medicina Interna
Universita' di Padova
Padova, Italy

Mancini M.
Institute of Internal Medicine and
Metabolic Disease
University of Naples
Naples, Italy

Mandel J.L.
Duke University Medical Center
Physiology Department
Durham, USA

Mann W.A.
Department of Pharmacology
Smith Kline and French Laboratories
Swedeland, USA

Maragno I.
Department of Pharmacology
University of Padua
Padua, Italy

Marangella M.
Department of Nephrology
Mauriziano Umberto I Hospital
Turin, Italy

Marchini F.
Institute of Internal Medicine
University of Padua
Padua, Italy

Marotta T.
Institute of Internal Medicine and Metabolic Disease
Clinica Medica Second Medical School
University of Naples
Naples, Italy

Martini C.
Department of Nephrology
Mauriziano Umberto I Hospital
Turin, Italy

Martorano G.
Department of Nephrology Secund Faculty of Medicine
Naples, Italy

Marzaro G.
Institute of Internal Medicine
Universita' of Padua
Padua, Italy

Maschio G.
Cattedra e Divisione di Nefrologia
Medica-Istituti Ospitalieri
Verona, Italy

Mastrangelo F.
Department of Nephrology and Dialysis "V.Fazzi" Hospital
Lecce, Italy

Mastranzo P.
Institute of Internal Medicine and Metabolic Disease, Clinica Medica
Second Medical School
University of Naples
Naples, Italy

Matrai A.
Hemorheology Research Laboratory
Clinic for Physical Medicine
University of Munich
Munich, FRG

Matsueda G.
Division of Hypertension
University Hospital
Lausanne, Switzerland

Matsushita K.
Department of Urology
Tokai University School of Medicine
Tokyo, Japan

Mauri J.M.
Nephrology Department
Hospital de Bellvtige
Barcelona, Spain

Mavrikakis M.
Department of Clinical Therapeutics
University of Athens
"Alexandra" Hospital
Athens, Greece

Mazzia G.
Institute of Nephrology
University of Bari
Bari, Italy

Mc Innes G.T.
University Department of Medicine Gardiner Institute
Western Infirmary
Glasgow, Scotland

Memoli B.
Department of Nephrology
II Faculty of Medicine
University of Naples
Naples, Italy

Menegazzi M.
Clinica Medica
University of Verona Medical School
Policlinico
Verona, Italy

Messa M.
Division of Nephrology
City Hospital
Udine, Italy

Messa P.
Division of Nephrology
City Hospital
Udine, Italy

Messina A.
Hemodialysis Service
I Institute of Surgical Clinic
University "La Sapienza"
Rome, Italy

Metsarinne K.
Unit of Clinical Physiology
The Minerva Foundation Institute for Medical Research
Helsinki, Finland

Millet J.A.
Research Laboratories Charing Cross
London, Great Britain

Minestrini C.
Istituto di Semeiotica Medica
Universita' di Perugia
Perugia, Italy

Minetti L.
Renal Division
Niguarda Ca'Granda Hospital
Milan, Italy

Mioni G.
Division of Nephrology
City Hospital
Udine, Italy

Mira G.
University of Palermo
Palermo, Italy

Miranda B.
Service of Nephrology
1 Octubre Hospital
Madrid, Spain

Missaglia A.
Hypertension Unit
Rho Hospital
Milan, Italy

Mistry C.J.
Division of Clinical Pharmacology
Grant Medical College
Bombay, India

Montanari A.
Istituto di Semeiotica Medica
Universita' di Parma
Parma, Italy

Montanari C.
Department of Cardiology
Istituti Clinici di Perfezionamento
Milan, Italy

Montanaro D.
Division of Nephrology
City Hospital
Udine, Italy

Montemurro N.
Servizio di Nefrologia e Dialisi
Ospedale Civile
Martinafranca, Italy

Montenegro J.
Service de Nephrology
Hospital de Cruces
Bilbao, Spain

Montinaro A.M.
Department of Nephrology and Dialysis
"V. Fazzi" Hospital.
Lecce, Italy

Morachiello P.
Department of Nephrology and Dialysis
Umberto I Hospital
Venice, Italy

Moran J.
Service de Nephrology
Hospital de Cruces
Bilbao, Spain

Morgano G.
Institute of Internal Medicine
Second School of Medicine
University of Naples
Naples, Italy

Moulopoulos S.
Department of Clinical Therapeutics
University of Athens
"Alexandra" Hospital
Athens, Greece

Muiesan S.
Institute of Clinical Pathology
University of Trieste
Trieste, Italy

Muniz R.
Service of Nephrology
Hospital de Cruces
Bilbao, Spain

Murphy J.
Department of Medicine
Waterford Regional Hospital
Waterford, Ireland

Mussi A.
Cattedra e Servizio di Farmacologia Clinica
Policlinico S. Orsola
Universita' di Bologna
Bologna, Italy

Mutschler E.
Pharmakologisches Institut fur Naturwissenschaftler der J.W. Goethe-Universitat
Frankfurt, FRG

Napoli M.
Department of Nephrology and Dialysis "V. Fazzi" Hospital.
Lecce, Italy

Nazaret C.
INSERM U7, Hopital Necker
Paris, France

Neri M.
Istituto di Clinica Medica II
Universita' di Pisa
Pisa, Italy

Neugebauer G.
Boehringer Mannheim GmbH
Mannheim, FRG

Nicolini M.A.
Servizio di Nefrologia e Dialisi
Ospedale Civile S. Andrea
La Spezia, Italy

Nieto J.
Service of Nephrology
1 Octubre Hospital
Madrid, Spain

Nord E.P.
Division of Nephrology
Department of Medicine
Center for Health Sciences
UCLA School of Medicine
Los Angeles, USA

Novarini A.
Istituto di Semeiotica Medica
Universita' di Parma
Parma, Italy

Nussberger J.
Division of Hypertension
University Hospital
Lausanne, Switzerland

Oberleithner H.
Department of Physiology
University Wurzburg Medical School
Wurzburg, FRG

Odlind B.
Department of Internal Medicine
University Hospital
Uppsala, Sweden

Ohnuma N.
Department of Pharmacology
National Cardiovascular Center Research Institute
Osaka, Japan

Oldrizzi L.
Cattedra e Divisione di Nefrologia Medica-Istituti Ospitalieri
Verona, Italy

Oppes M.
Cattedra di Patologia II
University of Sassari
Sassari, Italy

Orsoni G.
Department of Nephrology and Dialysis
St. Orsola University Hospital
Bologna, Italy

Ortalda V.
Cattedra e Divisione di Nefrologia Medica-Istituti Ospitalieri
Verona, Italy

Ortolani P.
Istituto di Cardiologia
Policlinico S. Orsola
University of Bologna
Bologna, Italy

Ostensen J.
Institute for Experimental Medical Research
University of Oslo
Ullevaal Hospital
Oslo, Norway

Pacchiano G.
Department of Nephrology
II Faculty of Medicine
University of Naples
Naples, Italy

Paganin L.
Division of Nephrology
City Hospital
Udine, Italy

Palestini M.
Hemodialysis Service
I Institute of Surgical Clinic
University "La Sapienza"
Rome, Italy

Palla R.
Istituto di Clinica Medica II
Universita' di Pisa
Pisa, Italy

Panichi V.
Istituto di Clinica Medica II
Universita' di Pisa
Pisa, Italy

Panozzo M.
Hypertension Unit
Rho Hospital
Milan, Italy

Papa A.
Department of Nephrology
II Faculty of Medicine
University of Naples
Naples, Italy

Parrinello G.
Institute of Clinical Medicine
Chair of Medical Therapy
University of Palermo
Palermo, Italy

Pasanisi F.
Institute of Internal Medicine and Metabolic Disease
Second Medical School
University of Naples
Naples, Italy

Passavanti G.
Institute of Nephrology
University of Bari
Bari, Italy

Patruno P.
Department of Nephrology and Dialysis,
"V. Fazzi" Hospital
Lecce, Italy

Pecchini F.
Division of Nephrology
Hospital of Cremona
Cremona, Italy

Pedrinelli R.
Hypertension Unit
I Clinica Medica
University of Pisa
Pisa, Italy

Penninckx R.
Service de Physiologie
Universite' de Mons
Mons, Belgium

Perotta U.
Servizio di Nefrologia e Dialisi
Ospedale Civile S. Andrea
La Spezia, Italy

Petersen J.S.
Department of Nephrology
University of Copenhagen
Copenhagen, Denmark

Petralito A.
Istituto di Patologia Medica I
University of Catania
Ospedale Garibaldi
Catania, Italy

Petretta M.
Institute of Internal Medicine
Second School of Medicine
University of Naples
Naples, Italy

Peverelli C.
Department of Internal Medicine A
St. Anna's Hospital
Como, Italy

Piccoli G.
Department of Nephrology
University of Turin
Turin, Italy

Pinto Pereira L.M.
Hoechst India Limited
Bombay, India

Ponti G.B.
Hypertension Unit
Rho Hospital
Milan, Italy

Portis T.
Hospital de Bellvitge
"Princeps d'Espanya"
Barcelona, Spain

Pozet N.
Nephrology Clinic
Hospital E.Herriot
Lyon, France

Pozzetti G.
Istituto di Clinica Medica II
Universita' di Pisa
Pisa, Italy

Prandini R.
Institute of Nephrology
S. Orsola University Hospital
Bologna, Italy

Predel H.G.
Division of Nephrology
Medizinische Poliklinik
University of Bonn
Bonn, FRG

Prieto J.
Department of Medicine
University Clinic
University of Navarra
Pamplona, Spain

Purroy A.
Division of Nephrology
University Clinic
University of Navarra
Pamplona, Spain

Quarello F.
Department of Nephrology
University of Turin
Turin, Italy

Quinzanini M.
Clinical Chemistry, School of Medicine
University of Brescia
Brescia, Italy

Quiroga J.
Department of Medicine
University Clinic
University of Navarra
Pamplona, Spain

Rama H.
Hospital de Bellvitge
"Princeps d'Espanya"
Barcelona, Spain

Ramjoue' H.P.
Ciba-Geigy Limited
Pharmaceutical Division
Basel, Switzerland

Rampino T.
Department of Nephrology
II Faculty of Medicine
University of Naples
Naples, Italy

Rappelli A.
Cattedra di Patologia Medica II
University of Sassari
Sassari, Italy

Reeves W.B.
Division of Nephrology
University of Texas Medical School
Houston, USA

Regnier S.
IHB Research Labs
Le Plessis, France

Reyes A.J.
Dept. de Investig. Cardiovascular
Fundacion Procardias
Montevideo, Uruguai

Riera J.
Hospital de Bellvtige
"Princeps d'Espanya"
Barcelona, Spain

Righetto F.
Department of Nephrology and Dialysis
Umberto I Hospital
Venice-Mestre, Italy

Risler T.
Department of Internal Medicine
University of Tubingen
Tubigen, FRG

Rizzelli S.
Department of Nephrology and Dialysis "V.Frazzi" Hospital
Lecce, Italy

Robertson J.I.S.
MRC Blood Pressure Unit
Western Infirmary
Glasgow, Great Britain

Rodella A.
Clinical Chemistry, School of Medicine
University of Brescia
Brescia, Italy

Rodico J.
Service of Nephrology
1 Octubre Hospital
Madrid, Spain

Rodrigue F.
IHB Research Labs.
Le Plessis, France

Rolando B.
Department of Nephrology
University of Turin
Turin, Italy

Romano C.
Division of Nephrology
Hospital of Cremona
Cremona, Italy

Romano G.
Department of Nephrology
II Faculty of Medicine
University of Naples
Naples, Italy

Rombola' G.
Renal Division
Niguarda Ca' Granda Hospital
Milan, Italy

Romero M.
Hospital de Bellvitge
"Princeps d'Espanya"
Barcelona, Spain

Rosati C.
Department of Nephrology
University of Turin
Turin, Italy

Roubert P.
IHB Research Labs.
Le Plessis, France

Rubattu S.
Cattedra di Patologia Medica II
Universita' di Sassari
Sassari, Italy

Rugiu C.
Cattedra e Divisione di Nefrologia Medica-Istituti Ospitalieri
Verona, Italy

Ruilope L.M.
Service of Nephrology
1 Octubre Hospital
Madrid, Spain

Russo D.
Department of Nephrology
Second Faculty of Medicine
Naples, Italy

Sabbatini M.
Department of Nephrology
II Faculty of Medicine
University of Naples
Naples, Italy

Salvati P.
Farmitalia Carlo Erba Centro Ricerche
Milan, Italy

Salvetti A.
Clinica Medica I
University of Pisa
Pisa, Italy

Sambhi M.P.
Hypertension Division
Department of Medicine
Sepulveda VA Medical Center
University of California at Los Angeles
Los Angeles, USA

Sani E.
Istituto di Semeiotica Medica
Universita' di Parma
Parma, Italy

Sanna M.
Istituto di Patologia Medica II
University of Sassari
Sassari, Italy

Santos F.
Section of Pediatric Nephrology
N.S. Covadonga Hospital
Oviedo, Spain

Saracho R.
Service de Nephrology
Hospital de Cruces
Bilbao, Spain

Sariban-Sohraby S.
Department of Medicine
Harvard Medical School
Boston, USA

Sarrias X.
Hospital de Bellvitge
"Princeps d'Espana"
Barcelona, Spain

Sassard J.
Department of Physiology and Clinical Pharmacology
Faculty of Pharmacy
Lyon, France

Satta A.
Institute of Medical Pathology
University of Sassari
Sassari, Italy

Scaglione R.
Institute of Clinical Medicine
Chair of Medical Therapy
University of Palermo
Palermo, Italy

Scanferla F.
Department of Nephrology and Dialysis
Umberto I Hospital
Venice Mestre, Italy

Scarpioni L.
Department of Internal Medicine and Renal Unit
Piacenza, Italy

Schafer G.E.
Medizinische Klinik III
Offenbach, FRG

Schena F.P.
Chair of Medical Therapy
University of Bari
Bari, Italy

Schenkel L.
Ciba-Geigy Limited
Pharmaceutical Division
Basel, Switzerland

Schiffl H.
Medizinische Klinik Innestadt der Universitat Munchen
Munchen, FRG

Schmidt W.
Med. Univ.-Poliklinik
Munster, FGR

Schram Stokke E.
Instit. for Exper. Research
Univ. of Oslo, Ullevaal Hospital
Oslo, Norway

Schrier R.
Division of Renal Disease
University of Colorado
Health Sciences Center
Denver, USA

Schulz W.
Klinikum Bamberg, III Medicine
Bamberg, FRG

Scognamiglio R.
Cardiology Division
University of Padua
Padua, Italy

Scolari M.P.
Department of Nephrology and Dialysis
St. Orsola University Hospital
Bologna, Italy

Scortecci A.
Istituto di Semeiotica Medica
Universita' di Perugia
Perugia, Italy

Sebastiani G.
Department of Nephrology
Mauriziano Umberto I Hospital
Turin, Italy

Sejersted O.M.
Institute for Experimental Research
University of Oslo
Ullevaal Hospital
Oslo, Norway

Senn N.
INSERM U 7, Hopital Necker
Paris, France

Serra G.
Istituto di Patologia Medica
Universita' di Sassari
Sassari, Italy

Sievert H.
Medizinische Klinik III
Offenbach, FRG

Sigrist G.
Department of Pharmacology
Rheinisch Westfalische
Thechnische Hochschule Schneebergweg s/n
Aachen, FRG

Sironi A.
Department of Internal Medicine A
St. Anna's Hospital
Como, Italy

Sjostrom P.
Department of Internal Medicine
Central County Hospital
Orebro, Sweden

Solomon L.
Manchester, Great Britain

Sonkodi S.
First Department of Internal Medicine
Szeged University Medical School
Szeged, Hungary

Spadaro A.
Istituto di Clinica Medica
University of Messina
Messina, Italy

Spahn H.
Pharmakolog. Instit. fur Naturwis.
der J.W. Goethe-Universitat
Frankfurt, FRG

Spanedda M.
Division of Internal Medicine
Ospedale di Ittiri
Sassari, Italy

Spannbrucker N.
Med. Univ.-Klinik
Bonn, FRG

Spieker C.
Med. Univ.-Poliklinik
Munster, FRG

Squadrito F.
Institute of Internal Medicine
School of Medicine
University of Messina
Messina, Italy

Stassen F.
Department of Molecular
Pharmacology
Smith Kline and French Laboratories
Philadelphia, USA

Stefoni S.
Institute of Nephrology
S. Orsola University Hospital
Bologna, Italy

Steiness E.
Department of Pharmacology
University of Copenhagen
Copenhagen, Denmark

Stekle B.
Division of Nephrology
Medizinische Poliklinik
University of Bonn
Bonn, FRG

Stelkens H.
Division of Nephrology
Medizinische Poliklinik
University of Bonn
Bonn, FRG

Strazzullo P.
Institute of Internal Medicine and
Metabolic Disease
Second Medical School
University of Naples
Naples, Italy

Surian M.
Renal Unit, Ospedale Maggiore Lodi
Lodi, Italy

Taddei S.
Clinica Medica I, University of Pisa
Pisa, Italy

Tamburino G.
Istituto di Patologia Medica I
Universita' di Catania
Catania, Italy

Tanikawa K.
Department of Urology
Tokai University School of Medicine
Tokyo, Japan

Tartagni F.
Istituto di Cardiologia
Policlinico S. Orsola
Universita' di Bologna
Bologna, Italy

Tedeschi C.
Institute of Internal Medicine
Second School of Medicine
University of Naples
Naples, Italy

Tenschert W.
Med. Univ.-Poliklinik
Munster, FRG

Terni A.
Institute of Nephrology
S. Orsola University Hospital
Bologna, Italy

Tessitore N.
Cattedra e Divisione di Nefrologia
Medica-Istituti Ospitalieri
Verona, Italy

Testa A.
Department of Nephrology
Secund Faculty of Medicine
Naples, Italy

Thiemann R.
Medical Clinical, University of
Erlangen-Nuernberg
Erlangen, FRG

Thievant P.
IHB Research Labs
Le Plessis, France

Thormann B.
Theraplix Lab.
Paris, France

Thurau K.
Department of Physiology
University of Munich
Munich, FRG

Tichy, B.
First Department of Internal Medicine
Szeged University Medical School
Szeged, Hungary

Tikkanen I.
Unit of Clinical Physiology
The Minerva Foundation
Institute for Medical Research
Helsinki, Finland

Tikkanen T.
Unit of Clin. Phys.
The Minerva Foundation
Institute for Medical Research
Helsinki, Finland

Torielli L.
Farmitalia Carlo Erba Centro Ricerche
Milan, Italy

Torras J.
Nephrology Department
Hospital de Bellvitge
Barcelona, Spain

Tottermann K.J.
Unit of Clinical Physiology
The Minerva Foundation
Institute for Medical Research
Helsinki, Finland

Tramonti G.
Cattedra di Nefrologia Medica
Centro Nefrologico
Clinica Medica II, Universita' di Pisa
Pisa, Italy

Trevisan M.
Institute of Internal Medicine and
Metabolic Disease
Second Medical School
University of Naples
Naples, Italy

Tricerri A.
Department of Nephrology
Mauriziano Umberto I Hospital
Turin, Italy

Troffa C.M.
Cattedra di Patologia Medica II
University of Sassari
Sassari, Italy

Turrini F.
Istituto di Patologia Medica
Universita' di Sassari
Sassari, Italy

Uccello F.
Department of Nephrology
II Faculty of Medicine
University of Naples
Naples, Italy

Vacha G.
Dept. of Nephrology and Dialysis
Ospedale Mauriziano Umberto I
Turin, Italy

Valentini E.
Department of Pharmacology
University of Padua
Padua, Italy

Vallo A.
Department of Pediatrics
Hospital de Cruces
Bilbao, Spain

Valvo E.
Cattedra e Divisione di Nefrologia
Medica-Istituti Ospitalieri
Verona, Italy

Vangelista A.
Institute of Nephrology
S. Orsola University Hospital
Bologna, Italy

Veniero P.
Department of Nephrology
II Faculty of Medicine
University of Naples
Naples, Italy

Verbeelen D.
Renal Unit, Department of Medicine
Academisch Ziekenhuis-Vrije
Universiteit Brussel
Brussel, Belgium

Vergani A.
Department of Cardiology
Istituti Clinici di Perfezionamento
Milan, Italy

Vetter H.
Med. Univ.-Poliklinik
Munster, FRG

Vianello A.
Institute of Internal Medicine
Postgraduate School
University of Padua
Padua, Italy

Viggiani N.
Chair of Medical Therapy
University of Bari
Bari, Italy

Viossat I.
IHB Research Labs.
Le Plessis, France

Von Bergmann K.
Department of Medicine
University of Bonn
Bonn, FRG

Von Moellendorff E.
Boehringer Mannheim GmbH
Mannheim, FRG

Waeber B.
Division of Hypertension
University Hospital
Lausanne, Switzerland

Wallin C.J.
Karolinska Institutet
Stockholm, Sweden

Walter U.
Mainz, FRG

Wang W.
Department of Physiology
University of Wurzburg Medical
School
Wurzburg, FRG

Wangemann P.
Max Planck Institut fur Biophysik
Frankfurt, FRG

Whitebread S.E.
Ciba Geigy Limited
Pharmaceutical Division
Basel, Switzerland

Wittner M.
Max Planck Institut fur Biophysik
Frankfurt, FRG

Yap L.
Division of Nephrology
University Clinic
University of Navarra
Pamplona, Spain

Yee B.
Division of Renal Disease
University of Colorado
Health Sciences Center
Denver, Colorado, USA

Zech P.Y.
Nephrology Clinic, Hospital E. Herriot
Lyon, France

Zidek W.
Med. Univ.-Poliklinik
Munster, FRG

Ziroyanis P.
Department of Clinical Therapeutics
University of Athens
"Alexandra" Hospital
Athens, Greece

PREFACE

The need for adequate means by which to improve urine output is very old. Even in the "Scuola Salernitana", the oldest medieval medical school in Western Europe, about 1000 years ago it was taught how to improve urine output. The list of known "diuretica" included herbs, plants, roots, vegetables, in particular asparagus, fennel and carrot.

The first diuretic drugs, however, were mercurial compounds. Thus, calomel, mercurous chloride, was initially used as a diuretic in the sixteenth century by Paracelsus, being one of the ingredients of the so-called "Guy's Hospital pill". But calomel had a cathartic effect so that it was replaced by organic mercurial compounds. These diuretics were clearly toxic. After the discovery of the carbonic anhydrase, in the early 1930s, and the introduction of sulfanilamide as a chemotherapeutic agent, it was observed that this drug was inhibiting carbonic anhydrase in vitro and urinary acidification in vivo thereby causing metabolic acidosis; urine output, however, appeared to increase. Subsequent studies led to the synthesis of more potent analogs, in particular acetazolamide. Studies on carbonic anhydrase inhibitors led to the synthesis of benzothiadiazides which disclosed much less inactivating action on carbonic anhydrase and much more diuretic effect through an inhibition of tubular transport of sodium and chloride. Chlorothiazide was the first member of this class of diuretics. Thiazides are still used in clinical practice.

The so-called "loop diuretics" represented a further very important step in the diuretic therapy, being very potent ("high-sealing") diuretics, effective also in condition of renal failure. The classic loop diuretic has been for many years furosemide. In recent years new diuretics have been synthesized, some of them as potent as or even more effective than furosemide. Muzolimine was among these.

Despite the efficacy of these diuretics, we are still looking for something better. With available diuretic agents, in fact, there are still some problems to be solved: the loss of potassium, the increase in serum uric acid, the hyperglycemia. Furthermore there are some conditions, such as in acute renal failure, in which even the potent available diuretics are unable to increase urine output. Hence the need for further studies as well as for discussion on the results of research performed all over the world.

In recent years, in addition to new traditional diuretic agents, we have observed new developments in studies concerning diuretic states which led to the discovery of endogenous natriuretic substances. Among these an atrial natriuretic factor has been isolated from cardiac atria and then even synthesized. This opens new views on the way to increase salt excretion. Meanwhile good results have been obtained with substances able to increase only water excretion (without salt); thus a new category of drugs has been created: the so called "aquaretics".

The Sorrento International Meeting on diuretics was therefore organized because we thought it was time to have most of the experts on diuretics from all over the world, sit down and discuss the chemical, pharmacological and clinical aspects of diuretic drugs, atrial natriuretic factors, and aquaretics. These are the Proceedings of this meeting. The Proceedings begin with a historical review on urine in the Middle Ages, and include lectures, workshops, symposia and communications on the physiology of traditional diuretics, their use in investigating renal function, and their applications in cardiology, hypertension, renal stone disease and renal failure; the endogenous natriuretic substances and their possible mode of action; and the aquaretics. The meeting was a great success. Speakers came from Europe, North and South America, and Japan. It was held under the official sponsorship of the International Society of Nephrology. Among the outstanding participants were Dr. Donald W. Seldin, President of the International Society of Nephrology; Prof. Klaus Thurau and Dr. Robert W. Schrier, respectively President elect and Treasurer of the International Society of Nephrology; and Dr. Thomas E. Andreoli, Editor of Kidney International.

We are grateful to all speakers and participants. Special thanks to our sponsors: Bayer AG, Bayropharm Italia, Boehringer Biochemia Robin, Boehringer Mannheim GmbH and Merck Sharp & Dohme. We are grateful also to contributors: Cyanamid International, Ciba-Geigy, Smith & Kline French and Squibb. Special thanks to Martinus Nijhoff Publishing for the excellent and rapid publication of these Proceedings.

ACKNOWLEDGMENTS

This book includes the proceedings of the International Meeting on Diuretics, held in Sorrento, May 26–30, 1986. The International Meeting on Diuretics has been sponsored by:
BAYER AG
BAYROPHARM ITALIA
BOEHRINGER BIOCHEMIA ROBIN
BOEHRINGER MANNHEIM GmbH
MERCK SHARP DOHME
Contributions have been given by:
Ciba-Geigy
Cyanamid International
Smith Kline French
Squibb

I. HISTORICAL REVIEW

DIURETICS IN THE SALERNITAN MEDICINE

A. DAL CANTON and M. CASTELLANO*

Department of Nephrology, 2nd Faculty of Medicine, and
*Department of Social Sciences, Istituto Universitario Orientale,
University of Naples.

THE MEDICAL SCHOOL OF SALERNO: PATHOPHYSIOLOGY OF URINE FORMATION.

In Middle Ages, Salerno -a small town in Southern Italy- was the site of a very important School of Medicine, the most important in Western World at those times. The teachers were called "Magistri" (Masters), and often came to hold the prestigious Chairs of Salerno from distant countries. Arabian Magistri were well accepted and gave a fundamental contribution to Salernitan knowledge. They, in fact, knew very well the important texts of the Classic Medicine that had been almost forgotten in Western countries after the fall of the Roman Empire. And, of course, they brought new ideas, original concepts specific of the Arabian medical culture. The Arabian influence accounts for the great importance of the Science of Urine (so-called Uroscopy) in the Salernitan School (1). An Arabian physician, Isaac Ebreus (9th century), in fact, was the first who gave a rationale to the diagnostic value of urine, by introducing into the Classic theory of urine formation the new concept that urine is the final receptacle of any Humor excess (2). To understand how revolutionary was this assumption one has to remind that the four Humors (Blood, Choler, Melancholy and Phlegm) were believed, in Classic Medicine, to be responsible for both the physical and psycological characters of any individual (3). A state of disease in any member of the body was thought to depend on the excessive accumulation of one of the Humors in that part of the body. Originally, Isaac claimed that urine drains, at least in part,this excess (1), the drainage resulting from a process of "digestion" that separates the "impurities" in the peripheral tissues. These impurities are then brought to the liver by the venous circulation, and in the liver another "digestion" strains the superfluous Humor into urine. Thus, urine examination can unreveal the excess of Humor responsible for the disease. The excess of Humor can be diagnosed in urine because it changes the physical qualities of urine. "Humid" Humors (Phlegm and Blood) increase the density of urine, while "dry" Humors (Melancholy and Choler) make urine light and clear. "Cold" Humors (Phlegm and Melancholy) decrease the color of urine giving it a white, pale yellow or green appearance. "Warm" Humors (Blood and Choler) increase the color of urine rendering it red, brown or black (2).

DIURETICS

Many manuscripts of the Salernitan School have been saved and most of them are lists of substances that were suggested to cure various disorders. Even at a rapid glance of these lists one is impressed with the great number of substances of vegetal, animal and mineral origin that were credited of being "diuretic" (4,5,6). This depends in part on the meaning of the word diuretic, more comprehensive at those times than today. Diuretic, in fact, was called any substance facilitating the diuresis; diuretics, therefore, were not only those increasing urinary volume, but also those able to dissolve stones or push out them, and those facilitating micturition in dysuric or stranguric patients.

<u>Vegetal Diuretics.</u>

Most of diuretics were of vegetal origin and consisted of quite common herbs that were either grown in the so-called "horti simplicium" (gardens of simple herbs, where simple has the meaning of "basic for therapeutic preparations") or collected in woods and the country. Wild herbs were considered to be better and stronger than those grown in the gardens. The active parts differed in different herbs (Table 1). In some herbs more than one part had diuretic properties, but the different parts were indicated for different disorders. Thus, for example, the seeds of wild parsley increased urine output, while its roots served to push out stones.

Table 1. ACTIVE PARTS OF VEGETAL DIURETICS.*

Leaves:	spica nardi (spikenard), cipressum(cypress), urtica(nettle), salvia(sage), siselos(a kind of cumin), ruta(rue), foeniculum(fennel), tragoselinum(a kind of parsley), calamentum (wood calaminth), rosmarinum(rosemary), laurum(laurel), nepeta(penniroyal).
Roots:	saxifraga(saxifrage), sambucum(elder), apium(wild parsley), vitis silvestris(wild vine), vitis alba(white vine), pastinaca(wild parsnip), valeriana(valerian), lupinum (lupin), althea(marshmallow), anethum(dill), cyparum(the greek bulb), asarum(wild spikenard), acorum(venerea herb), camaleonta alba(camaleonta), mirtum(mirtle), capparum(caper) rafanum(horseradish), bettonica(betonyc), allium(garlic), cepa(onion), rapa(turnip).
Bark:	populus(poplar), balsamum(balm), aloes(aloe), squilla(sea onion).
Flowers:	Schoene antus(squinanth), camomilla(camomille), caulum (caulyflower).
Fruits:	quercus(oak), capparum(caper), sebesten(a kind of plum), lentis(lentils), juniperus(juiniper), mandorla(almond).
Seeds:	cucurbita(pumpkin), anisum(anise), petrosillum(parsley), apium(wild parsley), scariola(cikory), spargus(asparagus), carvum(caraway), mentastrum(mint), sisamum(sesame), cuminum (cumin), rabarbarum(rhubarb), sambucum(elder), pinus(pine), basilicum(basil), rafanum(horseradish).

*The names of the plants are given in medieval latin and (in parenthesis) in 18th century english. The translation of latin names is the responsability of an english lady who handwrote the english names under the latin ones in a 16th century herbarium, in 1736.

Mineral Diuretics.

Iron and cupper were thought to give diuretic property to wine if immersed into it after having been heated to incandescence. Calomel (mercurous chloride) was used to increase urine output and can be considered the precursor of modern mercurial diuretics. Other mineral compounds were nitrum (potassium nitrate) and allumen (aluminum potassium sulphate), sulfur, lapislazuli and natural crystal, lithargirium (lead sand ?), and the so-called "spuma maris" ("sea foam", we have not been able to identify this mineral, perhaps a coral formation).

Animal Diuretics.

Urine of goat, bull, man. Blood of goat. Stool of vultur, goat, mouse, pigeon. Meat of deer (useful against stones). Powder of worms and cantharides (a kind of small green butterfly). Bile of cow and pig.

Unclassifiable Diuretics.

Snails were indicated to treat edema and ascites, by rubbing them alive on the edematous members and the abdominal wall. A very precious substance was the "mumia", because it could be found only in ancient Egyptian tombs. It consisted, in fact, of the bituminous oinment containing aloe and myrrh, used in the process of mummification, and to be active it had to be mixed with "humiditate corporis humani" (the humidity of human body). Physical means to increase urinary flow were to take a bath (modern physiology knows that this determines an expansion of central blood volume), and to expose the patient to cold, northern winds.

PREPARATIONS AND USE.

The preparation of a diuretic medication was a quite difficult matter. One, in fact, had to take into account first the quality of diuretic substance(s) to be used for the disease to be treated. Diuretic substances were divided in "warm", "cold", "humid" and "dry" (7). These qualities are the same that were attributed to the Humors, i.e. the fluids whose excess was thought to be the cause of the disease. Different diuretics were indicated, depending on the Humor in excess. Diuretic substances were often used in association, always holding in mind their qualities, either to avoid contradiction, or to eliminate (by using partially contrasting substances) an unwanted effect. Some preparations, however, consisted of a single herb; the Sea Onion (Scilla Maritima), for example, was indicated alone for hydropisic (edematous) patients. A potion was prepared by leaving the bulb into new fermenting wine for six months, then filtering before administration(4)(the Scilla contains an active principle whose cardiotonic efficay is well known; therefore, this potion may have been effective in increasing diuresis in patients with edema secondary to congestive heart failure). Other substances were mixed to form potions, syrups, decoctions, infusions, preserves, and dry pills. Wine, vinegar, and a mixture of vinegar with honey ("oximel") were the most used eccipients. Some medications were amazedly complex, especially those that were invented by famous Magistri. Thus, for example, the Pill of Magister Maurus, who was the author of an important book entitled "Rules on Urine" in the 12th century, consists of 51 different herbs and minerals. The Pill was said to be useful for "...paraliticis, epilepticis, melancolicis omnibus, cefalargicis, cancrosis, scabiosis, et de flegmate salso leprosis, artheticis, podagricis, quartanariis; conservant memoriam, surditatem expellunt, stomacum confortant et splen, omnes frigidos humores crudos, viscosos, venenosos... Deo Gratias." ("...those suffering from paralysis, epilepsia, any kind of melancholy, headache, cancer, scabies, retention of phlegm and salt, arthrosis, gout, malaria; the Pill preserves memory, cures deafness, is of benefit to the stomach and spleen, and all cold, not digested, viscous, poisoning humors...Thanks to God.)(8).

A special class of medications were the so-called "diuretica forinseca", the diuretics for external use. These medications were either applied on the skin or injected through the urethra, in the latter case mainly to solve stones. Urethral instillation, however, was sometimes indicated to provoke diuresis, as we know from the"Commentarium Magistri Bernardi" (Comments of Master Bernardus) "...oil of scarabs, or petroleum oil introduced through the penis quickly and effectively produce urine output." (7).

1. Pazzini A. Pagine di Storia della Scienza e della Tecnica. 10:1-13, 1958.
2. Fontana E. Il Libro delle Urine di Isacco l'Ebreo tradotto dall'Arabo in Latino da Costantino l'Africano. In: Scienza Veterum (Ed. G. Del Guerra) , Pisa, Casa Editrice Giardini, 1966.
3. Ludovico Dureto Segusiano (Interprete et Narratore): Hippocratis Magni Coacae, Lutetiae Parisiorum, Ioannes Meiat Editore, 1621
4. Serapione: De Simplicibus. In: De Re Medica, Vol. II, edited by Othone Brunselsio, Audlanus, pp. 29-195, 1531.
5. Tabulae Salerni. De Virtutibus et Operationibus Medicinarum. In: Collectio Salernitana (Ed. De Renzi S.), Napoli, 1859, vol. 5, pp. 235-237.
6. De Simplicium Virtutibus. In: Collectio Salernitana (Ed. De Renzi S.), Napoli, 1859, vol. 5, pp. 25-76.
7. Commentarium Magistri Bernardi Provincialis super Tabulae Salerni. In: Collectio Salernitana (Ed. De Renzi S.), Napoli, vol. 5, pp. 279-280.
8. Pillule Magistri Mauri probate. In: Collectio Salernitana (De Renzi S. Ed.), vol 3, 1854, pp. 51-52.

II. EFFECTS OF DIURETICS ON ION TRANSPORT

ION TRANSPORT AND METABOLISM IN RENAL CELLS

L.J. MANDEL

Department of Physiology, Duke University Medical Center, Durham, North Carolina, U.S.A.

INTRODUCTION

The relationship between active transport at the plasma membrane and respiration has been studied extensively in the kidney, because this organ utilizes a large percentage of energy for this dissipative process. In the kidney, the rate of respiration follows linearly the rate of active transport. Various approaches have explored the coupling between these two variables (1,2,3). One of the simplest models that attempts to explain this coupling is the one proposed by Whittam and coworkers (4,5) on the basis of their studies of Na-K-ATPase-mediated ion transport and respiration in kidney cortex and brain slices. In this model, schematically shown in Fig.1, an increase in active ion transport could cause an increase in the rate of ATP hydrolisis, which would be expected to elicit a decrease in the cellular concentration of ATP and an increase in the concentration of the ATP hydrolisis products, ADP and P_i. Such an increase in ADP and P_i concentration could serve as a cytoplasmic feedback signal resulting in an acceleration of the mitochondrial respiratory rate, as described for isolated mitochondria by Chance and Williams (6). The same feedback signal operating in reverse would be expected to reduce thr respiratory rate when the active transport rate decreased. The fast turnover of ATP in proximal tubules from the kidney

(5-8 sec) is responsible for the close coupling observed between active transport and oxidative metabolism in this tissue (1). We have used for a number of years a preparation of proximal tubules in suspension (7,8) to probe the effects of various perturbations on this close coupling. Particularly, we have studied the effects of amiloride and some of its analogues (9,10), and those of short-term anoxia (11) on this preparation. The present communication deals with the effects of anoxia on proximal tubules and contrasts these with recent results obtained in a preparation of thick ascending limb (TAL) tubules in suspension (12).

METHODS

The preparation of proximal and TAL tubules from the rabbit kidney as well as the methods for measuring oxigen consumption

Fig.1

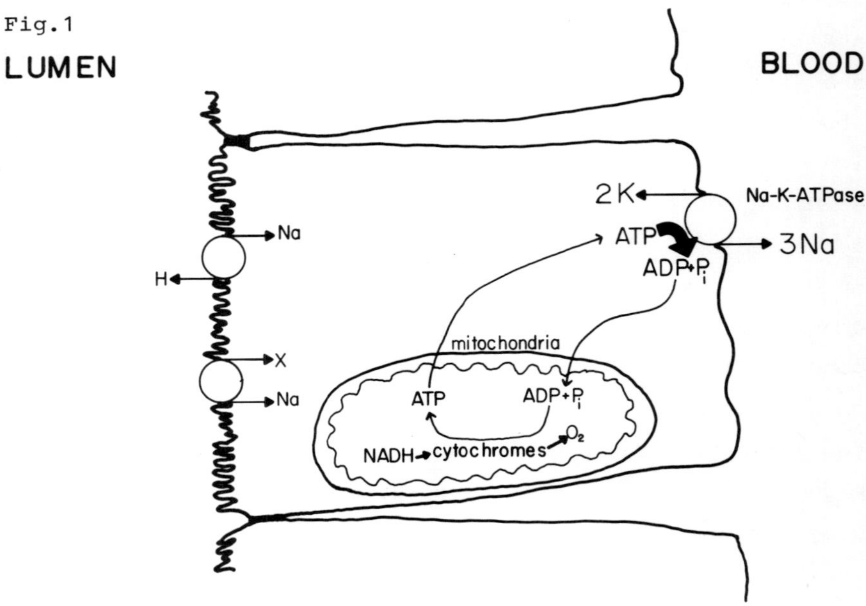

(QO_2) have been previously described in detail elsewhere (7,8,12). Several variables were measured to assess different aspects of cellular function. Normal feedback between oxidative metabolism and active transport was measured by use of the monovalent ionophore nystatin. Previous studies in our laboratory (13) have determined that the addition of nystatin to proximal tubules leads to a rapid increase in QO_2 caused by the entry of sodium from the extracellular medium and the consequent stimulation of Na-K-ATPase activity. The QO_2 obtained with nystatin addition has been shown to equal the mitochondrial state 3 respiratory rate under normal conditions (13). Therefore, the nystatin-stimulated QO_2 was used to measure the maximal rate of coupled respiration obtainable in the intact tubules before and after anoxia or hypoxia. Nystatin was added at a concentration of 160 ug/ml.

The integrity of the plasma membrane was assessed by measuring lactate deydrogenase (LDH) release from the cells (11). In addition, the cellular and extracellular levels of adenine nucleotides and their breakdown products were measured using high performance liquid chromatography (11). Each experiment was initiated with a 20-min preequilibration of the tubule suspension at 37°C in the normal NaCl solution bubbled with 95% O_2/5% CO_2. Anoxia or hypoxia was achieved in a specially designed chamber (11) and was maintained for 10, 20, 30, or 40 min. After each period of anoxia, the tubule suspension was reoxygenated for 20 min in a shaker bath under a 95 O_2/5% CO_2 atmosphere at 37°C. Samples were taken from the suspension at three times during each experiment immediately before anoxia, immediately after anoxia, and after reoxygenation. For each experiment, a tubule suspension was continuosly maintained in parallel under oxygenated conditions for the duration of the experiment. Samples were obtained from this suspension at the same times, and the same variables were measured and used as control values. Percent impairment of each function was calculated using the respective control value obtained at the same time for each experiment. For other experimental details, see ref. 11.

RESULTS AND DISCUSSION

Fig. 2 shows that the nystatin-stimulated QO_2 was progressively inhibited as the duration of anoxia was increased. Examination of the nystatin-stimulated rate immediately after reoxygenation showed a large degree of impairment even after 10 min of anoxia (Fig. 2A), linearly increasing to 63% impairment after 40 min of anoxia. 20 min of reoxygenation allowed a fairly good recovery of the tubules exposed to 10 and 20 min of reoxygenation (Fig. 2B). However, 30 and 40 min of anoxia

Fig. 2.

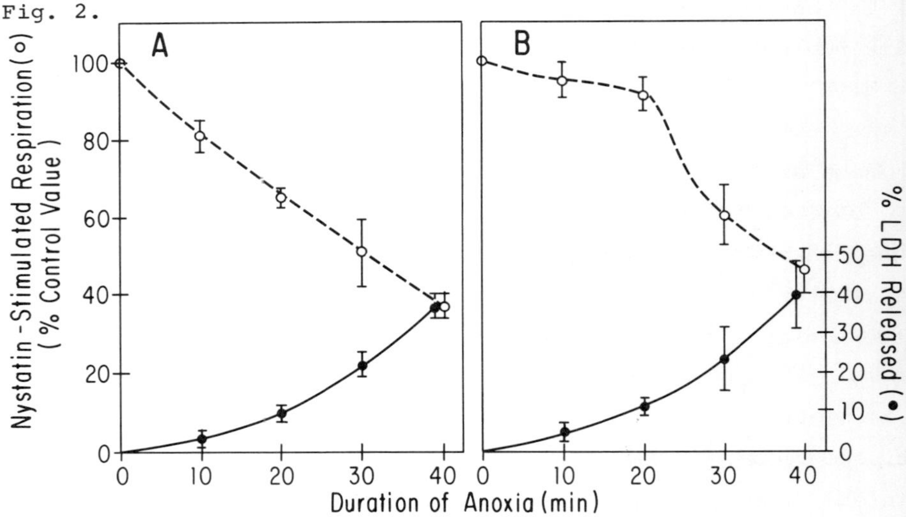

still eliceted 40% and 55% impairment, respectively, even after this period of reoxygenation.

The percentage of LDH released from the tubules increased with the duration of anoxia (Fig. 2A). The release was relatively small (<10%) when the duration of anoxia was 20 min or less, but increased rapidly with longer anoxia times. Most of this release occurred during anoxia, inasmuch as reoxygenation caused no further significant increase in %LDH released (Fig.2B).

Independent measurements of mitochondrial function (11) showed that up to 30 min of anoxia still retained close to normal respiratory capacity when sufficient ADP was provided to mitochondria. These results suggested that the decrease in nystatin-stimulated respiration was due to an impairment in the feedback signal schematically illustrated in Fig. 1, possibly due to a decrease in adenine nucleotide content. This possibility was investigated by measuring the adenine nucleotide content of the tubules as a function of time in anoxia, as shown in Fig. 3. The ATP level fell by more than 60% within the first 10 min, and continued to fall more slowly thereafter with time in anoxia. The ADP level remained approximately constant for the first 20 min, only decreasing after 30 min of anoxia. The AMP level at first increased rapidly, but also declined during longer anoxic times. The main breakdown product of adenine nucleotides in the tissue was hypoxantine (HX), which accumulated extracellularly as the duration of anoxia was increased, as also shown in Fig. 3. The total adenylate pool decreased with time in anoxia, being hydrolized mainly to HX.

Recovery from anoxia depended on the duration of anoxia. The tissue recovered completely from 20 min of anoxia after 40 min of recovery time. Most measured functional parameters returned to their original values, including the cellular ATP

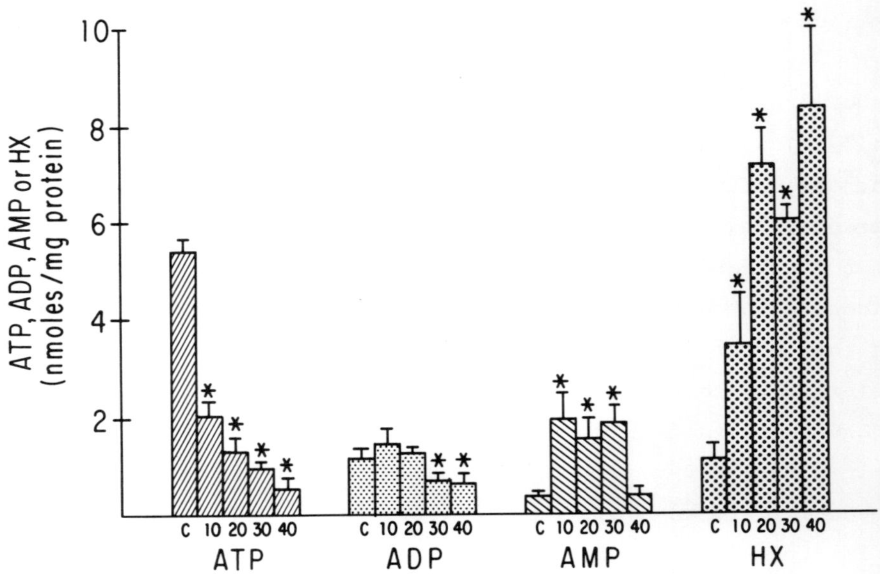

Fig. 3. C= control; 10, 20, 30, 40 are the times in minutes that the tubules were subjected to anoxia, respectively (n=4). * = Significantly different from control.

levels (14). However, after 40 min of anoxia and 20-40 min of reoxygenation there appeared to be irreversible inhibition of respiratory and transport functions (11). The ATP levels only returned to 25-50% of their original value and the HX levels remained elevated (14). This situation is similar to that encountered in vivo, where clamp-induced ischemia is reversible for periods of 20-30 min and irreversible after longer duration of ischemia (15-17).

Previous investigators have reported that addition of adenine nucleotides to perfusate ameliorated the effects of ischemic cellular injury (18,19). The effects of ATP addition were also tested in our preparation of proximal tubules.

Addition of a total of 1 mM Mg-ATP (magnesium chloride-treated ATP) during anoxia significantly improved functional recovery from 40 min of anoxia (11). In addition, cellular ATP levels returned to control values after 40 min of reoxygenation (14). Measurement of LDH release showed a significant decline <u>during</u> anoxia, as shown in Fig. 4, demonstrating a protective effect of the added ATP even during anoxia. This was not achieved through a change in cellular ATP levels during anoxia, since these remained unchanged in the presence of the added ATP (14).

Fig 4. *=Significantly different from control ($p<0.01$)

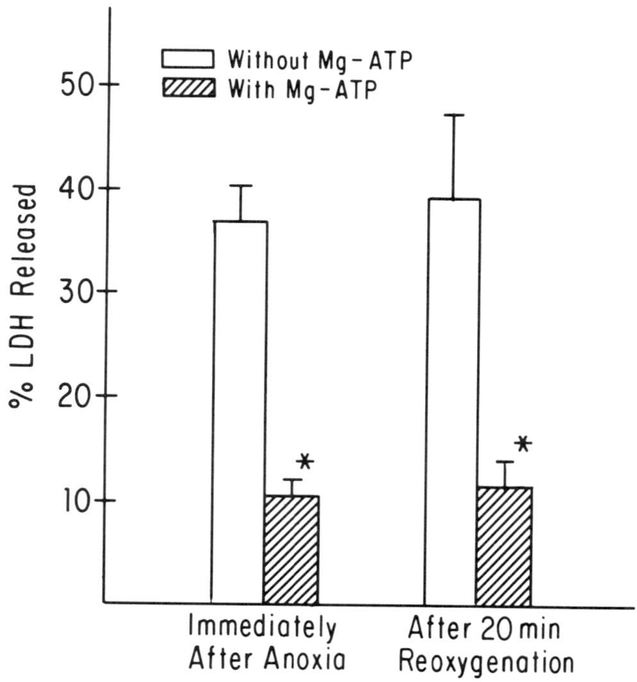

Added extracellular ATP was rapidly degraded to AMP and further hydrolytic products. Therefore, the protective effect was not likely to be directly through ATP but rather through one or more of its breakdown products, possibly AMP or adenosine (14).

From these results, it may be concluded that the protective action of exogenous ATP in proximal tubules occurs in two steps: 1) By inhibiting damage to the plasma membrane during anoxia, and 2) By providing precursors for adenine nucleotide synthesis during reoxigenation.

Recent experiments studying the effects of anoxia on a preparation of TAL tubules in suspension (20) provide an interesting contrast to the studies just described. Proximal tubules rely mainly on oxidative metabolism for their energy needs, having very low glycolitic capacity (1-3). It is not surprising, therefore, that anoxia causes such a rapid decrease in ATP levels in this tissue (Fig. 3). In contrast, the TAL has been shown to have a large glycolitic capacity (21,22) that can be activated by anoxia-like conditions (23). TAL tubules in suspension subjected to 10 min of anoxia retained 73% of their ATP levels as compared to 37% for proximal tubules (Fig. 3). Iodoacetate addition decreased the ATP levels by 57% in TAL during anoxia, indicating that glycolisis is an important pathway in suplying energy during anaerobiosis (20). This ability of the TAL suspension to withstand anoxia is consistent with its behavior in vivo, where it sustains little damage during short periods of ischemia (24).

In summary, results have been presented that analyze the separate effects of anoxia on transport and metabolic function, as well as the cellular feedback between these two variables. Loss of adeine nucleotide from the renal cells seems to play an important role in the irreversible damage caused by anoxia. Similar approaches have been taken to determine the effects of a few diuretics or prospective diuretics on metabolic and transport function (9,10).

ACKNOWLEDGEMENTS

The Author would like to thank the Organizers of the International Meeting on Diuretics for their kind invitation to attend this interesting meeting. The secretarial assistance of Mrs. J. Shelton was greatly appreciated. This work was supported by NIH Grant AM26816.

REFERENCES

1. Mandel L.J., Balaban R.S. Am. J. Physiol. 240:F357-F371, 1981.
2. Cohen J.J.,Kamm D.E. In: The Kidney (Eds B.M. Brenner and F.C. Rector)Philadelphia, W.B. Saunders Co., 1976, pp. 126-200.
3. Kinne R. In: Membrane Transport in Biology(Eds. G. Giebisch Tosteson H.H., D.C. Ussing). Berlin. Springer-Verlag, 1979, pp. 529-562.
4. Blond D.M., Whittam R. Biochem. J. 92:158-167, 1980.
5. Whittam R. Nature London. 191:603-604, 1961.
6. Chance B., Williams C.M. Adv. Enzymol. Relat. Areas Mol. Biol. 17:65-134, 1956.
7. Balaban R.S., Soltoff S., Storey J.L., Mandel L.J. Am. J. Physiol. 238:F50-F59, 1980.
8. Soltoff S.P., Mandel L.J. J. Gen. Physiol. 84:601-622,1984.
9. Soltoff S.P., Mandel L.J. Science 220:957-959, 1983.
10. Soltoff S.P., Mandel L.J. Am. J. Physiol. 250:C744-C747, 1986.
11. Takano T., Soltoff S.P.,Murdaugh S.? Mandel L.J. J. Clin. Inv. 76:2377-2384, 1985.
12. Chamberlin M.E., LeFurgey A., Mandel L.J. Am. J. Physiol. 247:F955-F964, 1984.
13. Harris S.I., Balaban R.S., Barrett L., Mandel L.J. J. Biol. Chem. 256:10319-10328, 1981.

14. Mandel L.J., Takano T., Soltoff S.P., Murdaugh S. J. Clin. Inv., submitted 1986.
15. Venkatachalam M.A., Bernard D.B., Donohoe J.F., Levinski N.G. Kidney Int. 21:583-591, 1982.
16. Trump B.F., Berezesky I.K., Cowley R.A. In: Pathophysiology of Shock, Anoxia and Ischemia. (Eds. Cowley R.A., Trump B.F.). William Wilkins, Baltimore. 6-46, 1982.
17. Johnston P.A., Remke H., Levinsky N.G. Am. J. Physiol. 246:F159-F166, 1984.
18. Siegel N.J., Glazier W.B., Chaudry I.H., Gaudio K.M., Lytton B., Baue A.E., Kashgarian M. Kidney Int. 17:338-349, 1980.
19. Gaudio K.M., Ardito T.A., Reilly H.F., Kashgarian M, Siegel N.J. Am. J. Pathol. 112:_38-346, 1983.
20. Chamberlin M.E., Mandel L.J. Am. J. Physiol. (Renal, Fluid and Electrolyte Physiol.), in press.
21. Guder W.G., Ross B.D. Kidney Int. 26:101-111, 1984.
22. Vandewalle A., Wirthensohn G., Heidrich H.G., Guder W.G. Am. J. Physiol. 240:F492-F500, 1981.
23. Bagnasco S., Good D., Balaban R., Burg M. Am. J. Physiol. 248:F522-F526, 1985.
24. Donohoe J.F., Venkatachalam M.A., Bernard D.B., Levinsky N.G. Kidney Int. 13:208-222, 1978.

HYDROGEN SECRETION REGULATED BY INTRACELLULAR MEMBRANE POTENTIAL: A HYPOTHESIS ON THE REGULATION OF RENAL ACIDIFICATION

H. OBERLEITHNER AND W. WANG

Department of Physiology, University Würzburg Medical School, Röntgenring 9, D-8700 Würzburg, FRG

ABSTRACT

The question was addressed whether the cell membrane potential could regulate net acid secretion in the kidney. Cells from the amphibian diluting segment were isolated and fused to giant cells. From the evaluation of the intracellular pH-recovery after an acute acid load we postulate an electroneutral Na^+/H^+ exchange and a rheogenic HCO_3^- transport system in the plasma membrane of these fused cells. Furosemide-induced hyperpolarization of the intracellular membrane potential acidifies the cell cytosol and the tubule fluid. Potassium-induced depolarization does the opposite. We conclude that the cell membrane potential regulates urinary acid secretion.

INTRODUCTION

In the proximal tubule and in the diluting segment of the kidney H^+ net secretion involves a luminal Na^+/H^+ exchange and a basolateral HCO_3^- transport system. The luminal Na^+/H^+ exchanger is electrically neutral and thus voltage-insensitive. However, recent experiments in renal brush-border vesicles demonstrated (1) that this transport system is regulated by the cytosolic pH, i.e. acidifying the cell interior activates the H^+ extrusion mechanism and vice versa. HCO_3^- ions, generated inside the cell by the carbonic-anhydrase catalyzed reaction from CO_2 and water cross the peritubular cell membrane as negatively charged anions (most likely coupled to Na^+ at a stoichiometry of $Na^+/HCO_3^-=1/3$; ref. 2, 3). Due to the rheogenicity of this transport system, the intracellular membrane potential should interfer with the net transfer of HCO_3^- across this cell barrier. The intracellular membrane potential, however, is altered at pathophysiological conditions. To test this hypothesis we chose an experimental model which allows intracellular pH (pH_i) measurements over long periods and in which the cell membrane potential can be hyperpolarized by furosemide or depolarized by hyperkalemia.

METHODS

Cells were isolated from the frog diluting segment and fused to giant cells (Fig 1, A and B). The isolation and fusion techniques were recently described (4).

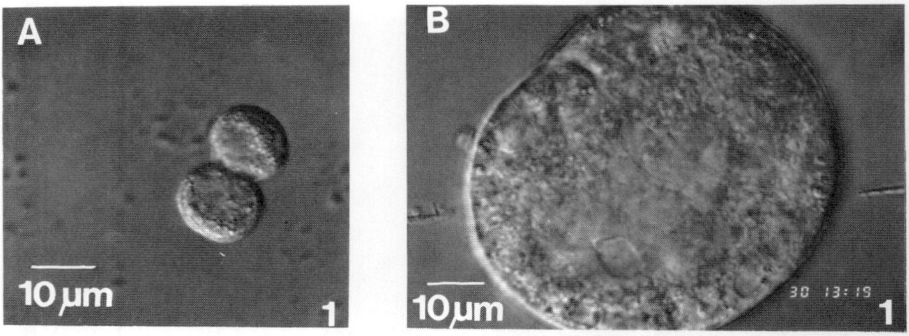

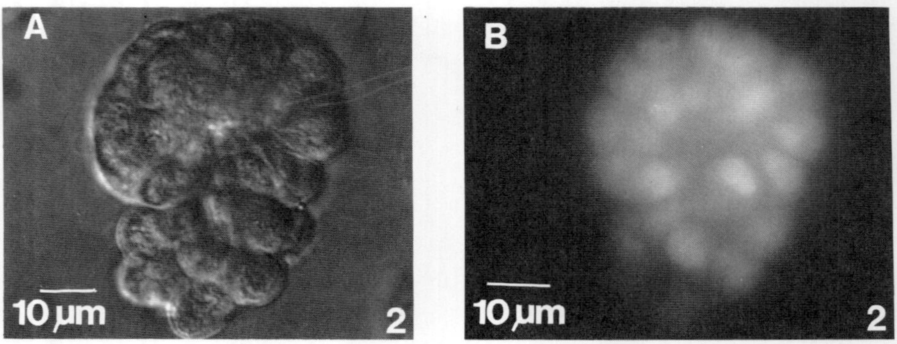

Fig. 1. A: Two renal tubule cells isolated from frog diluting segment. B: Fused "giant" cell.

Fig. 2. A: Fused renal epithelial cell (incomplete fusion).
B: Same cell but nuclei stained with the fluorescent dye acridine orange.

The giant cells were multinucleated (Fig. 2, A and B) and stable intracellular impalements could be performed for several hours using electrophysiological techniques. The giant cell was attached to the bottom of a perfusion chamber and superfused with amphibian Ringer solution composed of (mM): 87 NaCl, 3 KCl, 10 $NaHCO_3$, 1.5 $CaCl_2$, 1 $MgCl_2$, 5 glucose; gassed with 1% CO_2, pH 7.8. The giant cell was impaled by conventional and pH-sensitive microelectrodes (Fig. 3) to measure the cell membrane potential (V_m) and the transmembrane H^+ electrochemical potential (V_H). From these parameters pH_i can be calculated. The microelectrode techniques have been described in detail elsewhere (5). The cells were acid-loaded transiently by the so-called NH_4^+/NH_3-prepulse method (6) exposing the cells to the ammonia-buffer system (20 mM NaCl substituted by equivalent amounts of NH_4Cl) for 3 min. On removal of this buffer system from the bath solution, the cell cytosol acidifies transiently followed by a recovery phase (Fig. 4). The slope of the pH_i recovery is closely related to the activity and nature of the H^+ extrusion mechanism.

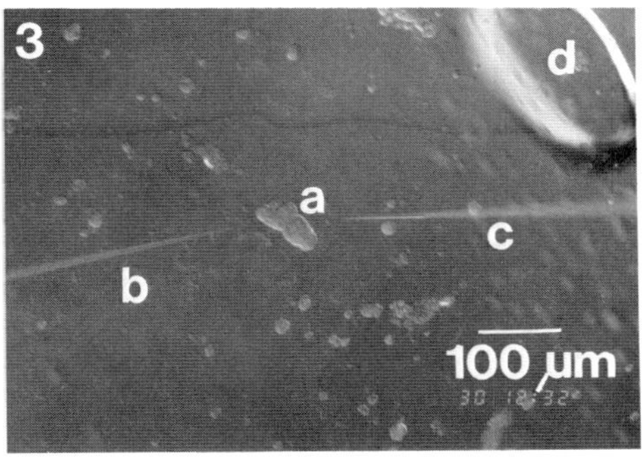

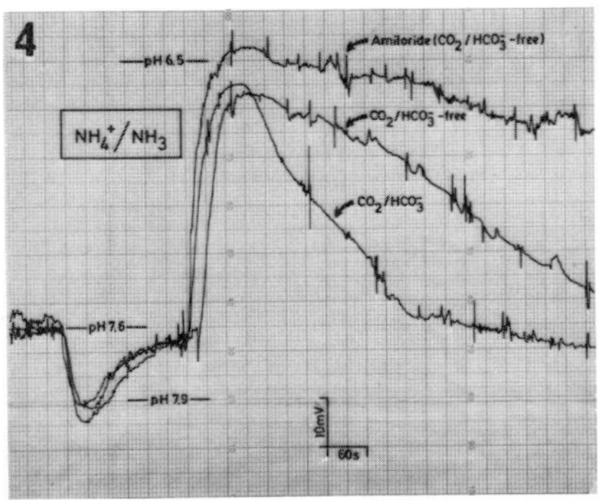

Fig. 3: a) Fused cell under study, b) conventional electrode, c) pH-sensitive electrode, d) superfusion pipette.
Fig. 4: Original records of the transmembrane H^+ gradients obtained from one giant cell.

RESULTS AND DISCUSSION

Fusion of single cells - isolated from intact renal tubules - to giant cells offers several major advantages to the electrophysiologist: The fused cells have diameters in the range of 100)m about 10 times the diameter of single cells (Fig. 1, A and B). Thus, with some luck, intracellular microelectrode measurements can be performed over hours (Fig. 3). The cells are multinucleated (Fig. 2, A and B) and, to our surprise, retain their original membrane properties (4). We have used this new experimental model to study the mechanism of pH_i regulation.

From previous studies we know that the amphibian as well as the mammalian diluting segment is capable for net H^+ secretion (5,7). Since the formation of H^+ ions in the cell cytosol was likely to result from the hydration of CO_2 (H^+ net secretion is inhibited by the carbonic-anhydrase inhibitor acetazolamide; unpublished observation) we postulated a HCO_3^- exit-step in the basolateral cell membrane. Fig. 4 shows an experiment which gives strong evidence for the existence of Na^+/H^+ exchange and for a HCO_3^- transport pathway. Exposing a giant cell to the ammonia buffer system leads to a transient alkalinization of pH_i due to titration of H^+ ions by NH_3 inside the cell. On removal of the ammonia buffer system from the extracellular fluid the cell interior acidifies. This is due to the fact that NH_3 leaves the cell and H^+ ions accumulate transiently. Fig. 4 shows that the pH_i recovery depends critically on at least two separate mechanisms: If the pH_i-recovery with CO_2/HCO_3^--free solution is used as a reference it becomes obvious that the inhibition of the Na^+/H^+ exchanger by amiloride (10^{-3} M) reduces pH_i-recovery (by a factor of 6) whereas substituting the HEPES buffer (10 mM) by equivalent amounts of the CO_2/HCO_3^- buffer system enhances pH_i recovery (by a factor of 5). This indicates strongly that H^+ are extruded by the Na^+/H^+ exchange system and at the same time H^+ are buffered by the uptake of HCO_3^-. The question arises by what mechanisms HCO_3^- could enter the cell. This was tested in an additional series of experiments in which extracellular HCO_3^- was rapidly increased from 10 to 20 mM (at constant pH). This maneouvre leads to a transient hyperpolarization of the cell membrane, typically for HCO_3^- transporting epithelia (2, 3). The voltage-change could be suppressed completely by stilbene-derivatives (unpublished observation). These findings, obtained from pH_i measurements in fused cells of the frog diluting segment are summarized in Fig. 5:

In addition to the Cl^- transport mechanisms (the luminal furosemide-sensitive cotransporter and the peritubular Cl^- conductance), the diluting segment is equipped with a luminal Na^+/H^+ exchanger, sensitive to amiloride and a peritubular HCO_3^- conductive pathway, sensitive to stilbene-derivatives.

Fig. 5: Cell model of the diluting segment.

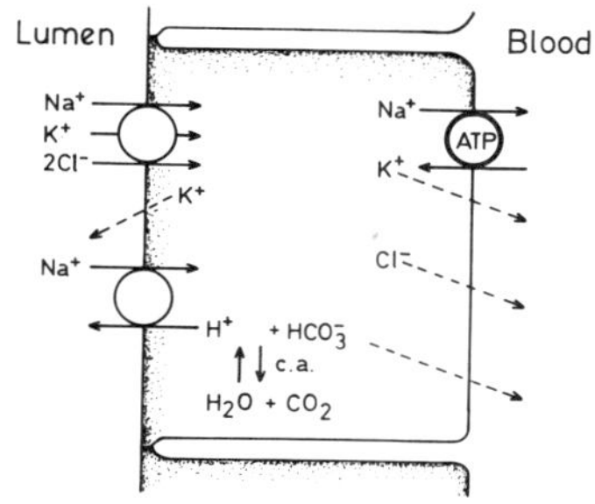

The peritubular efflux of HCO_3^- is rheogenic and thus must be voltage-sensitive. Two different maneouvers were used to test this hypothesis. First, we applied furosemide. This diuretic inhibits the luminal $Na^+/Cl^-/K^+$ cotransporter, decreases intracellular Cl^- and by this means hyperpolarizes the cell membrane potential (8,9). Fig. 6A documents that simultaneously with the hyperpolarization pH_i decreases. Recently, it was shown that an increase of H^+ at the cytosolic side of the cell membrane activates the Na^+/H^+ exchanger (1). This effect is thought to be independent of the existing transmembrane gradients for Na^+ or H^+ but to be rather a conformational change of the transport protein. Our experiments in the intact diluting segment support this view. The limiting luminal pH declines after addition of furosemide. Similar observations were made also in the mammalian kidney (7). In another set of experiments we depolarized the cell membrane by increasing extracellular K^+ from 3 to 15 mM. Indeed, the opposite occurs (Fig. 6B).

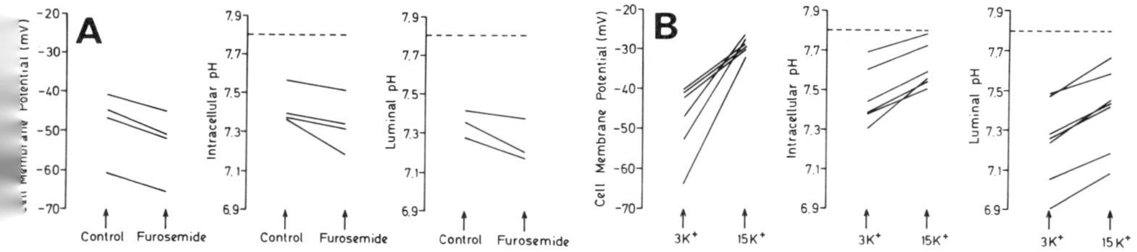

Fig. 6 A and B: Cell membrane potential and intracellular pH was measured in fused giant cells. Luminal pH was measured in intact diluting segments at zero net flux (lumen flow rate = zero). Dotted line corresponds to extracellular pH.

Concomitant with the cell membrane depolarization pH_i increases. In the intact tubule, luminal pH rises. This is consistent with the view that intracellular alkalinization inactivates the Na^+/H^+ exchanger. Then H^+ net secretion is switched off.

Loop diuretics as furosemide are known to enhance urinary acidification (10). The mechanisms described are consistent with this clinical finding. Hyperkalemia is known to be associated with systemic acidosis. At the level of the diluting segment, this can be explained by a lack of H^+ net secretion induced by K^+ induced depolarization of the renal epithelial cells. In conclusion we believe that the intracellular membrane potential plays an important role in the regulation of H^+ net secretion due to the fact that an electroneutral Na^+/H^+ exchanger operates in parallel with a rheogenic HCO_3^- transport system.

Acknowledgements: We thank Prof. Dr. S. Silbernagl for stimulating discussions during the course of the experiments. We thank Mrs. I. Ramoz and I. Schönberger for excellent secretarial assistance, Mrs. B. Schmidt for preparing the fused cells and Mrs. M. Schulze for doing the photographic work. This study was supported by the Deutsche Forschungsgemeinschaft (SFB 176-A6).

REFERENCES

1. Aronson, P.S., Nee, J. and Suhm, M.A. Nature, 299: 161-163, 1982.
2. Boron, W.F. and Boulpaep, E.L. J. Gen. Physiol. 81: 53-94, 1983.
3. Yoshitomi, K. and Frömter, E. Pflügers Arch. 405 (Suppl. 1): S121-S126, 1985.
4. Oberleithner, H., Schmidt, B. and Dietl, P. Proc. Natl. Acad. Sci. USA, 83: in press, 1986.
5. Oberleithner, H., Lang, F., Messner, G. and Wang, W. Pflügers Arch. 402: 272-280, 1984.
6. Boron, W.F. and Boulpaep, E.L. J. Gen. Physiol. 81: 29-52, 1983.
7. Good, D.W., Knepper, A. and Burg, M.B. Am. J. Physiol. 247 (Renal Fluid Electrolyte Physiol 16): F35-F44, 1984.
8. Greger, R. Physiol. Rev. 65: 761-797, 1985
9. Oberleithner, H., Guggino, W. and Giebisch, G. Am. J. Physiol. 242: F331-F339, 1982.
10. Hropot, M., Fowler, N., Karlmark, B. and Giebisch, G. Kidney International, 28: 477-489, 1985.

ISOLATION AND PURIFICATION OF THE AMILORIDE-SENSITIVE Na^+ CHANNEL FROM RENAL EPITHELIA

DALE J. BENOS and SARAH SARIBAN-SOHRABY

Department of Physiology and Biophysics, University of Alabama at Birmingham, Birmingham, Alabama USA and Department of Medicine, Harvard Medical School, Boston, Massachusetts USA

INTRODUCTION

The nature of alkali metal transport across biological membranes has been extensively investigated in recent years. This research encompasses perhaps the most central issue of physiology as well as reflecting the most primitive function of the cell membrane, namely, ion homeostasis. Most of our understanding of Na^+ transport across epithelial tissues has come from morphological and physiological studies of model systems such as the amphibian skin and urinary bladder preparations. The knowledge obtained from these studies has often been extrapolated to other less accessible epithelia such as the renal distal tubule and collecting duct. About 20 years ago, researchers at the pharmaceutical firm of Merck, Sharp and Dohme, synthesized a new K^+ sparing diuretic called amiloride. This drug is a very potent and specific inhibitor of Na^+ transport in a variety of cellular and epithelial transport systems ranging from human red blood cells to rat caudal epididymis, rabbit embryos to the body wall of annelid worms (1). Amiloride-sensitive Na^+ channels are found in Na^+ transporting tissues displaying high transepithelial electrical resistance (2). Although the electrophysiology of the channel has been widely studied, the molecular mechanisms underlying the Na^+ transport function as well as the primary structure of the channel are unknown.

The purpose of this paper is to describe the protocol for the purification of the amiloride binding protein which we believe is closely associated with Na^+ conducting unit because Na^+ transport function is maintained at each step of the purification. The extent of purification was followed by measuring the specific binding of tritiated methylbromoamiloride ($[H^3]$-CH_3BrA), an amiloride analogue that binds with high affinity to the Na^+ transport protein. This compound was synthesized by a reductive methylation reaction using bromoamiloride and CH_3I as starting material. As a result, a methyl group was transferred to a nitrogen on the acylguanidinium side chain of the parent molecule. This modification did not change the potency of the drug in that the half maximal inhibition of either short-circuit current in frog skin or $^{22}Na^+$ influx in cultured A6 cells was achieved at the same drug concentration as amiloride. When tritiated methyliodide was used in the reaction, we were able to synthesize a compound with a specific activity of around 1 to 2 Ci/mmole.

MATERIALS AND METHODS

The methods for cell culture, synthesis of $[^3H]$-CH_3BrA, and isolation, purification, and reconstitution of the epithelial amiloride-sensitive Na^+ channel can be found in references 3-6.

RESULTS AND DISCUSSION

The scheme for the initial step of the purification procedure we employed is shown in Figure 1 (5,6).

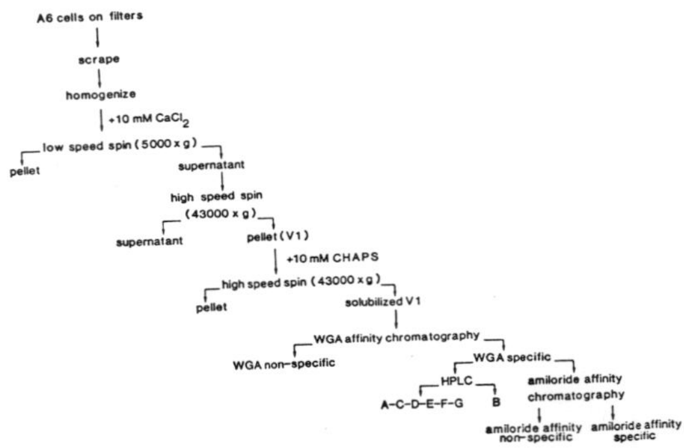

Figure 1. Purification scheme for the amiloride-binding protein from A6 cells. An identical procedure was used for bovine renal papilla.

Our starting material was either cultured A6 cells grown on filters or beef papilla. A6 cells are a continuous cultured cell line originating from toad kidney. The A6 cell line has Na^+ transport properties similar to naturally occurring, high resistance epithelia such as the frog skin, toad urinary bladder, or mammalian kidney collecting ducts including vasopressin and aldosterone responsiveness, and has thus proved to be a good model system with which to study apical Na^+ entry. Cells were cultured as confluent monolayers on porous supports so as to develop the characteristic property of amiloride inhibition of apical Na^+ entry (3). After the monolayers developed a stable transepithelial voltage of at least 10 mV, cells were scrapped off the filters and homogenized in a hypotonic medium containing 10 mm $CaCl_2$. After a series of differential centrifugations an enriched apical membrane fraction labelled V_1 was obtained. This fraction was enriched 10x in apical membrane markers, alkaline phosphatase and γ-glutamyl transpeptidase. This V_1 fraction was then exposed to the zwitterionic detergent CHAPS to yield a soluble protein fraction. We found that 10 mM CHAPS was the optimal concentration required to achieve maximal protein solubilization while recovering nearly all of the binding sites originally present in the V_1 fraction.

The number of specific binding sites was measured by incubating the samples with $[^3H]$-CH_3BrA on ice for 30 minutes in the presence or absence of a 1000-fold excess of unlabelled amiloride. The specific binding was calculated as the difference of total counts and non-displaceable counts. Non-specific binding represented about 40% of the total binding in the cell homogenate and decreased to less than 5% in the most purified samples. Specific binding of tritiated methylbromoamiloride was stable at room temperature for at least 3 hours. In contrast, the extent of binding was strongly dependent on the presence of exogenous phospholipids. In the soluble V_1 fraction the specific activity of binding was 25% of that of V_1 without addition of any exogenous phosphatidylcholine (PC). Addition of PC to a final concentration of 2 mM restored the binding activity to greater than 90% of the V_1 value. With a PC concentration of 2 mM, addition of CHAPS to a final detergent concentration of 50 mM resulted in almost complete loss of specific binding activity. This effect was reversed by increasing the concentration ratio of lipid to detergent to 1:10 and 1:5 indicating that the binding sites were not irreversibly denatured, but rather inactivated by the high detergent and/or low lipid concentration. To summarize, about 45% of the V_1 protein exposed to CHAPS was solubilized. The V_1 membrane fraction binding activity was enriched 9-10 times compared to the cell homogenate. Another 2-fold enrichment was achieved after detergent solubilization so that although we have lost about half the protein, the recovery of the total binding sites is complete.

The detergent soluble protein was reconstituted into phosphatidylcholine vesicles to insure that the conducting unit was still associated with the amiloride binding site. $^{22}Na^+$ uptake into the liposomes was measured against a large electrochemical Na^+ gradient that was set up by trapping Na^+ inside the liposomes and removing external Na^+ by passing the liposomes through Sephadex or Dowex columns as described by Garty and coworkers (7). Linear rates of $^{22}Na^+$ influx were observed for up to 15-30 s, and 92-95% of the influx was inhibited by 0.1 mM amiloride. Thus, we have a preparation of soluble proteins in which binding and transport activity are maintained.

We next subjected the soluble samples to affinity chromatography on wheat germ agglutinin (WGA) bound to agarose. This lectin retains glycoproteins with glucosamine and sialic acid residues and was chosen because most of the transport proteins thus far isolated have proven to be glycosylated proteins. Scatchard analysis of $[^3H]$-CH_3BrA binding data obtained after wheat germ chromatography shows that the apparent equilibrium dissociation constant (K_D) was 128 nM. In comparable experiments with V_1 protein, the K_D was 130 nm. These values of K_D are in excellent agreement with the inhibitory constant of amiloride in intact A6 cells, A6 V_1 membrane vesicles, and A6 single Na^+ channels incorporated into planar lipid bilayers. Similar values of K_D for the soluble and membrane bound receptor indicate that detergent solubilization did not alter the conformation of the amiloride binding site. The enrichment $[^3H]$-CH_3BrA binding activity after wheat germ chromatography for A6 cells and beef papilla was 148- and 115-fold compared to cell homogenate, respectively, with 50-100% recovery of total binding sites.

The next step in the purification was gel filtration using size exclusion high performance liquid chromatography (SEHPLC). Samples were loaded on a Dupont GF-250 HPLC column which has an effective exclusion limit around 670 kDa. When the crude cell homogenate was loaded onto the column, we obtained a whole range of molecular weights with poor discrimination between peaks. In the V_1 membrane fraction, a high molecular weight peak was clearly enhanced compared to other components. That peak, in fact, was contained in the void volume and thus corresponds to molecular weights greater than 670 kDa. After WGA chromatography, the SEHPLC separation was much better resolved with the high molecular weight fraction again in the void volume, and all other major peaks having molecular weights smaller than 21 kDa. The various fractions were collected separately from the SEHPLC column and assayed for specific $[^3H]$-CH_3BrA binding. The only fraction in which displaceable binding was measured was in the void peak and this was enriched > 2000-fold over homogenate. In preliminary experiments (Fig. 2) we have incorporated this SEHPLC peak into planar lipid bilayer membranes and have recorded single, amiloride-sensitive Na^+ channel activity. This result again demonstrates that at this stage of the purification, channel activity is co-purifying with binding activity.

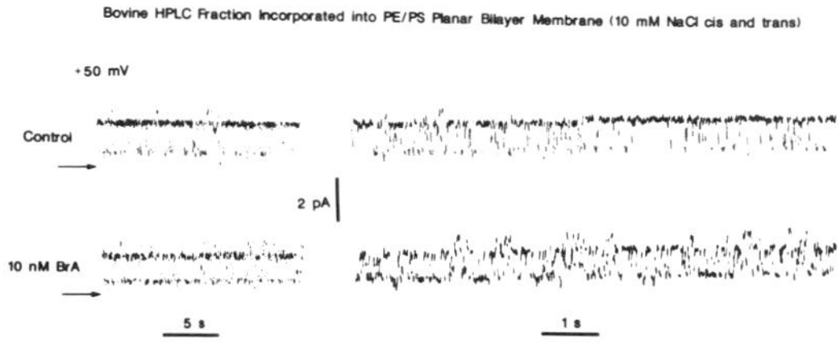

Figure 2. SEHPLC-purified bovine papillary Na^+ channels incorporated into planar, lipid bilayers. The bilayer was symmetrically bathed with a solution of 10 mM NaCl, 10 mM MOPS-Tris, pH 7.0. Symmetrical addition of 10 nM bromoamiloride (BrA) did not alter single Na^+ channel conductance (30 pS), but decreased the probability of the channel being in the open state from 0.85 to 0.56. Na^+ versus Cl^- selectivity of the channel was determined from dilution potential measurements. The channel was found to be perfectly Na^+-selective. See Ref. 8 for experimental details. The arrows indicate the zero current level.

In SEHPLC experiments where we lowered the ionic strength of the running buffer to 10 mM Na_2HPO_4, we were able to resolve this void peak into two components (Fig. 3). Separation of these components and measurements of specific binding activity indicated that only the lower molecular weight peak, i.e., around 700 kDa, displayed any specific binding. The enrichment and binding activity compared to homogenate was greater than 10,000-fold, and reached a final specific activity of 1300 pmoles/mg protein, assuming 1 amiloride molecule binds per protein molecule. The maximal theoretical binding activity for a protein of molecular weight 700,000 would be 1429 pmoles/mg. Therefore, we have achieved approximately 91% purification of this protein.

In summary, CHAPS solubilization of A6 or beef papilla apical membrane proteins was accomplished with maintenance of two important functions of high resistance epithelia: the amiloride binding and the Na^+ transport activity. Both functions were preserved at each step of the purification. Affinity chromatography on WGA followed by SEHPLC resulted in a more than 10,000-fold purification of the amiloride binding protein. The molecular weight of the native protein as determined by SEHPLC, is around 700,000 kDa. (This research was supported by NIH Grant AM37206. We thank D. Keeton, J. Parks, and E. Steadman for excellent technical help, and J. Tidwell for cheerful secretarial assistance).

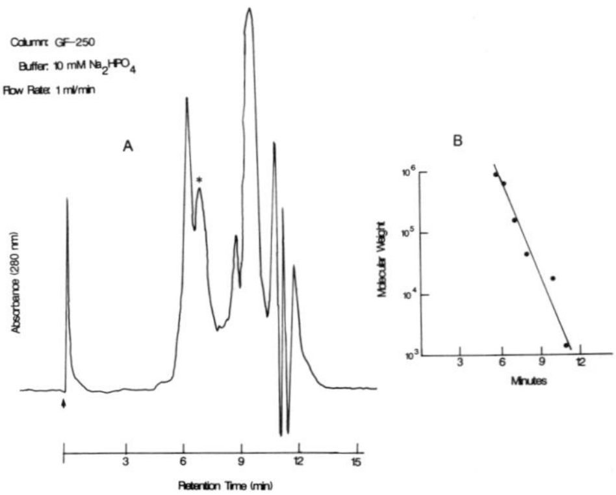

Figure 3. (A) SEHPLC elution pattern (Dowex GF-250 column) of bovine renal papilla WGA-eluted protein. The flow rate of elution was 1 ml/min, and the running buffer was 10 mM Na_2HPO_4, pH 7.0.
(B) Molecular weight versus retention time standard curve for the GF-250 column run under these conditions. Molecular weight markers included human IgM (900,000), thyroglobulin (670,000), gamma globulin (158,000), ovalbumin (44,000), myoglobin (17,000), and vitamin B-12 (1350).

REFERENCES

1. Benos, D.J. Am. J. Physiol. 242:C131-C145, 1982.
2. Sariban-Sohraby, S. and Benos, D.J. Am. J. Physiol. 250:C175-C190, 1986.
3. Sariban-Sohraby, S., Burg, M.B. and Turner, R.J. Am. J. Physiol. 245:C167-C171, 1983.
4. Lazorick, K., Miller, C., Sariban-Sohraby, S. and Benos, D.J. J. Membr. Biol. 86:69-77, 1985.
5. Sariban-Sohraby, S. and Benos, D.J. Biochemistry, in press, 1986.
6. Benos, D.J. and Sariban-Sohraby, S. (submitted).
7. Garty, H, Rudy, B. and Karlish, S.J.D. J. Biol. Chem. 258:13094-13099, 1983.
8. Sariban-Sohraby, S., Latorre, R., Burg, M. Olans, L. and Benos, D. Nature (Lond.) 308:80-82, 1984.

BLOCKERS OF ACTIVE TRANSPORT IN THE THICK ASCENDING LIMB OF THE LOOP OF HENLE

R. GREGER, P. WANGEMANN, M. WITTNER, A. DI STEFANO, H.J. LANG AND H.C. ENGLERT

Max-Planck-Institut für Biophysik, Kennedyalle 70, D 6000 Frankfurt, F R G and Chemie Pharmasynthese Hoechst AG, D 6230 Frankfurt, F R G

INTRODUCTION

Loop diuretics of the furosemide type are well known blockers of active NaCl reabsorption in the medullary and in the cortical thick ascending limb of the loop of Henle (1). They interact with one of the Cl^- binding sites of the $Na^+2Cl^-K^+$ carrier. Recently, we have developed a new class of substances which interferes with the Cl^- channels in the basolateral membrane of the same nephron segments and blocks the conductive transfer of Cl^- from the cell to the peritubule side (2,3). The same type of substance blocks chloride channels in a variety of other epithelia: colon (unpublished from the authors' laboratory), trachea (M. Welsh, personal communication), sweat duct (4), cortical collecting tubule (5), and rectal gland (6). Figure 1 indicates that both classes of substances, the loop diuretics of furosemide type and the chloride channel blockers, share some of their chemical structure, and that both compounds are similar to torasemide. Torasemide is a new diuretic interfering with the $Na^+2Cl^-K^+$ carrier and also, at about 100 times higher concentrations, with chloride channels (7). This compound, therefore, is an example of a compound that acts at both sites, the $Na^+2Cl^-K^+$ carrier, and the chloride channel. On the other hand, we have shown previously that compounds such as furosemide, piretanide, bumetanide do not interfere with chloride channels but do with the carrier, and, conversely, that diphenylamine-2-carboxylate does not interact with the $Na^+2Cl^-K^+$ carrier but does with chloride channels (1,2). The present study was designed to examine what modifications of loop diuretics of the furosemide type are necessary to produce chloride channel blockers, and, what modifications of chloride channel blockers could lead to blockers of the $Na^+2Cl^-K^+$ carrier. The results indicate that only minor modifications are sufficient to shift one type of compound to the other type.

MATERIALS AND METHODS

The technique of in vitro perfusion of isolated rabbit cortical thick ascending limb segments was used. The tubule segments were perfused with identical Ringers type solution on both sides. The equivalent short circuit current was measured as described previously (8). The compounds under study were added to the luminal or to the peritubular perfusate. For each substance a dose response curve was ob-

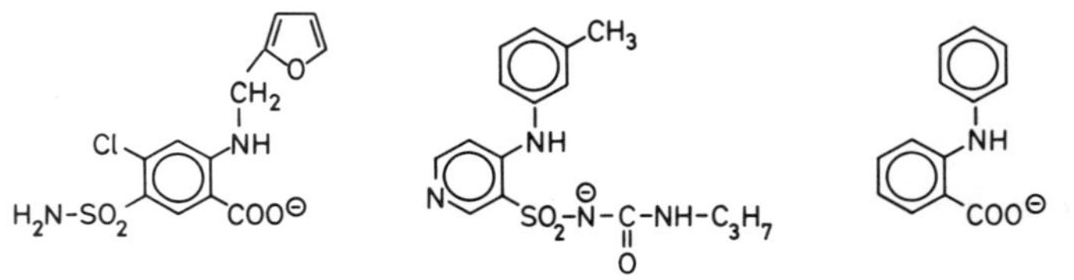

Fig.1: The chemical structure of furosemide. torasemide. and of diphenylamine-2-carboxylate. Note that all three compounds have in common the anionic site. the secondary amine. and an apolar site.

tained for at least 5 tubules for each concentration and application side (luminal/peritubular). The mean dose response curve was used to determine an IC_{50} value for the inhibition of the equivalent short circuit current from the peritubular (chloride channel) and from the luminal side ($Na^+2Cl^-K^+$ carrier). The compounds were obtained from standard sources or were synthetized as described previously (3). Data are presented as mean IC_{50} values.

RESULTS

Figure 2 shows data for derivatives of diphenylamine-2-carboxylate. Note that diphenylamine-2-carboxylate has no effect when added to the luminal perfusate. This substance is a specific blocker of chloride channels (2). Another derivative, closely related to diphenylamine-2-carboxylate. the thiophene compound #70 is an even stronger inhibitor of chloride channels. However. the pyridine analogue of diphenylamine-2-carboxylate (#85) has lost any effect from both epithelial sides. The 3`-trifluoromethyl substituted derivative triflocine. on the other hand. blocks the $Na^+2Cl^-K^+$ carrier from the luminal side but has no effect on chloride channels. This is an example where a chloride channel blocker is converted into a blocker of the $Na^+2Cl^-K^+$ carrier. The figure contains in addition an isomeric compound of triflocine. namely niflumate. This compound is inactive on the chloride channel and on the $Na^+Cl^-K^+$ carrier, but it is an inhibitor of the HCO_3^-/Cl^-exchange (band 3 protein) in red blood cells (9). It is worth mentioning that also diphenylamine-2-carboxylate is a weak inhibitor of the band 3 protein.

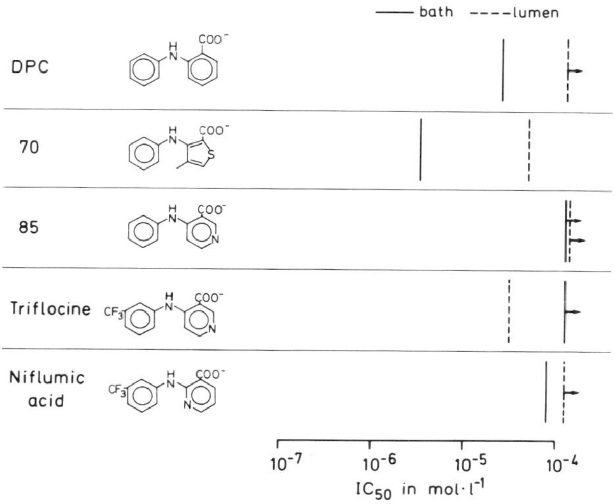

Fig.2: Effect of inhibitors in isolated perfused rabbit cortical thick ascending limb segments. The concentration of half maximal inhibition of the equivalent short circuit current (IC_{50}) is given for the inhibitor added to the luminal fluid (dashed line) or to the peritubular fluid (solid line). The arrows indicate that no effect was found at 10^{-4}mol/l. Higher concentrations were not tested.

Figure 3 shows another example where an inhibitor of chloride channels is converted into an inhibitor of the $Na^+Cl^-K^+$ carrier.

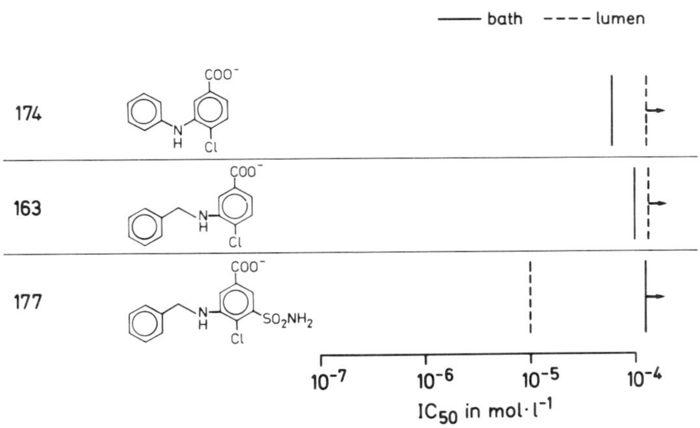

Fig.3: Explanations c.f. legend to figure 2.

The first compound shown in this figure is a chloride channel blocker (#174). A lengthening of the spacer between the two rings leads to some loss of the inhibtory potency on the chloride channel (#163). Now a sulfonamide group is introduced in meta positon and a strong inhibitor of the $Na^+2Cl^-K^+$ carrier is obtained. Note that this compound has some similarity to furosemide (Fig.1 and Fig.4).

Figure 4 gives an example in which a blocker of the $Na^+2Cl^-K^+$carrier was converted into a blocker of chloride channels.

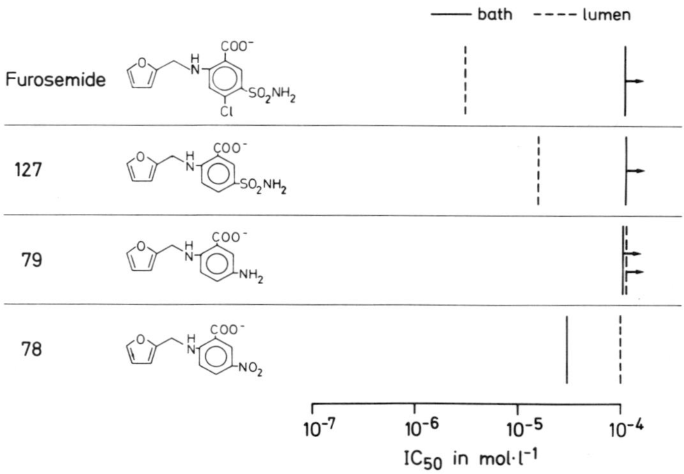

Fig.4: Explanations c.f. legend to figure 2.

Furosemide, as stated above, is a blocker of the $Na^+2Cl^-K^+$ carrier. Removal of the Cl-substitution in para position to the carboxylate group reduces the inhibitory potency (#127). Replacement of the sulfonamide group by an amino group destroyes the inhibitory activity (#79). If now the amino group is replaced by a nitro group (#78), we obtain an inhibitor of chloride channels with no activity on the $Na^+2Cl^-K^+$ carrier. We have made a comparable observation in an extensive series of torasemide derivatives. We were able to show that the replacement of the pyridino nitrogen by a NO_2 substituted carbon atom left almost untouched the ability of this compound to block chloride channels but abolished completely the ability to block the $Na^+2Cl^-K^+$ carrier (10).

Figure 5 is yet another example where a drug interacting with the $Na^+2Cl^-K^+$ carrier (piretanide) is converted into a blocker of chloride channels. Replacement of the phenoxy substitution (in para position to the carboxylate group) by Cl- abolishes any inhibitory activity (#149). Removal of the sulfonamide group generates a chloride channel blocker (#123). Removal of the chloride substitution abolishes any inhibitory potency.

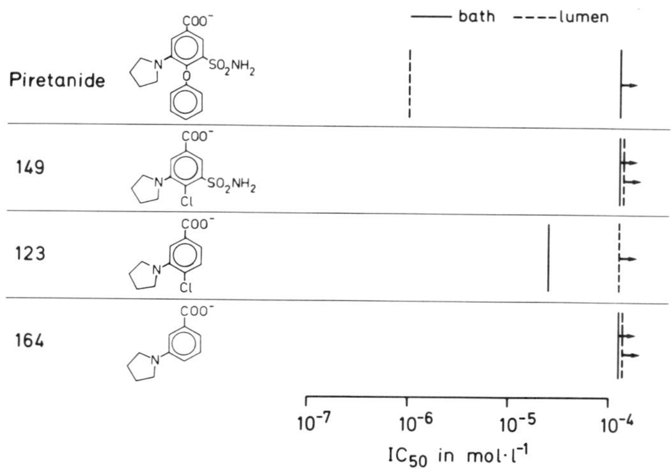

Fig.5: Explanations c.f. legend to figure 2.

DISCUSSION

The present study indicates that characteristic chloride channel blockers can be converted into blockers of the $Na^+2Cl^-K^+$ carrier, and that, conversely, blockers of this carrier system can be converted into blockers of chloride channel. A question that one might ask then is: what are the general properties of the two classes compounds, and what are the differences?

All compounds of this kind are weak acids with pK values between 4. and 6. Preferentially, these compounds are carboxylates. All compounds carry an amino nitrogen with a certain distance to the carboxylate group. The ortho- and meta- positioning between the two groups are active, larger distances are not tolerated. Both types of substances carry an apolar residue (phenyl moiety, furfuryl moiety etc.). The chloride channel blockers may or may not have a substituent on the "right" ring: a chloride substitution in para- position or a nitro substitution in meta- position. This moiety carries a partial negative charge. The blockers of the $Na^+2Cl^-K^+$ carrier possess an electronegative sulfonamide group in the same position. In general, the blockers of chloride channels are more hydrophobic than the blockers of the $Na^+2Cl^-K^+$ carrier.

Finally, it is worth mentioning that some blockers of the band 3 protein belong to the class of substances discussed in the present context (9) e.g. niflumate (fig.2) or flufenamate. It appears not unreasonable to predict that all three chloride transporting membrane proteins (the chloride channel, the $Na^+2Cl^-K^+$ carrier and the HCO_3^- carrier share in common some portion of the molecule, which then may explain the fact that very similar substances can inhibit any of the three membrane proteins, and that minor modifications of the molecules shifts one agent from one subclass to the other.

ACKNOWLEDGEMENTS
This work was supported by Deutsche Forschungsgemeinschaft Gre 480/6-5.

REFERENCES

1. Greger, R. Phys. Rev. 65: 760-797, 1985.
2. Di Stefano, A., Wittner, M., Schlatter, E., Lang, H.J., Englert, H.C. and Greger, R. Pflügers Arch. Suppl.1 405: 95-100, 1985.
3. Wangemann, P., Wittner, M., Di Stefano, A., Englert, H.C., Lang, H.J., Schlatter, E. and Greger, R. Pflügers Arch. in press 1986.
4 Bijman, J., Lang, H.J., Englert, H.C., Greger, R. and Frömter, E. Pflügers Arch. 405: R26, 1985.
5. Tago, K., Warden, D.H., Schuster, V., and Stokes J.B. Am. J. Physiol. Ren. Fluid and Electrolyte. in press 1986.
6. Greger, R. and Schlatter E. Pflügers Arch. 402 364-375, 1984.
7. Wittner, M., Schlatter, E., Delarge, J. and Greger, R.: Pflügers Arch. submitted 1986
8. Greger, R. and Schlatter, E. Pflügers Arch. 396: 315-324. 1983.
9. Cousin, J.L. and Motais, R. Biochim. Biophys. Acta 687: 147-155, 1982.
10.Wittner, M. Di Stefano, A., Wangemann, P., Delarge, J. Liegois, J.F. and , Greger, R. Pflügers Arch. submitted 1986.

THE USE OF AMILORIDE ANALOGS TO PROBE ADAPTATIONS OF THE PROXIMAL TUBULAR Na^+/H^+ ANTIPORTER IN RESPONSE TO A REDUCTION IN RENAL MASS

L.G. FINE and E.P. NORD

Division of Nephrology, Department of Medicine, Center for the Health Sciences, UCLA School of Medicine, Los Angeles, CA 90024, U.S.A.

One of the earliest manifestations of an acute reduction in renal mass is an elevation of the glomerular filtration rates of the remaining nephrons. Within 24 hrs of removing one kidney fluid reabsorption is increased in the proximal tubule, providing an effective mechanism for reclaiming the bulk of the increased filtered load of solutes and water. Since this enhanced tubular reabsorption can be demonstrated in vitro, it follows that the adaptation is intrinsic to the tubular epithelial cell and is not dependent upon extratubular factors (1).

The predominant sodium transport process in the proximal tubular brush border membrane is Na^+/H^+ exchange, an electroneutral process with a 1:1 stoichiometry and one which is inhibitable by amiloride and its analogs. In considering the nature of the adaptation of the luminal transport process which underlies the augmented fluid reabsorption of the remnant kidney proximal tubule we examined the following two possibilities: 1) that the brush border membrane surface area is increased per unit length of tubule, effectively increasing the number of antiporters in proportion to the increase in other membrane components or 2) that Na^+/H^+ specific activity is increased in a selective manner.

In experiments which quantitated the surface areas of luminal and basolateral membrane areas (2) we were surprised to find that the normal symmetry of these two membranes (i.e. approximately equal surface areas in the normal kidney) was disrupted in the remnant kidney. Quantitative histomorphometry showed that there was no increase in luminal membrane surface density (i.e. surface/volume ratio) whereas that of the basolateral membrane was increased. Despite this structural asymmetry, studies on isolated proximal tubular cells indicated that the number of ouabain-binding sites, an estimate of total Na^+-K^+-ATPase molecules, was increased in proportion to the overall increase in cell protein (Fig. 1). From these data we concluded that, although the proximal tubular cell hypertrophies in an asymmetrical fashion, it maintains a functional symmetry.

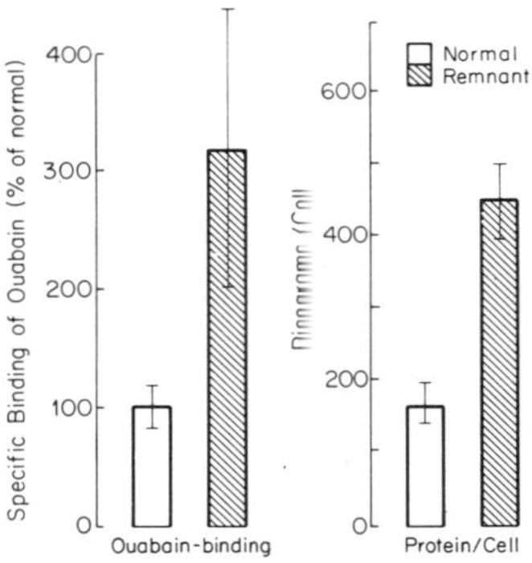

Fig. 1. A comparison between the increase in ouabain binding per cell (left panel) and protein per cell (right panel) in normal versus remnant kidney proximal tubular cells. The increase in ouabain-binding sites in the remnant kidney cells was roughly proportional to the increase in protein per cell. (Reprinted with permission from ref. 2).

We next examined whether the specific activity of Na^+/H^+ exchange is increased per unit of brush border membrane protein. Previous studies by Hruska et al in the dog had shown that Na-D glucose and Na-L proline cotransport processes were unchanged in the remnant kidney (3). As shown in Fig. 2, Na^+/H+ antiport was measured as amiloride-sensitive sodium uptake in isolated rabbit renal brush border membrane vesicles. The Jmax of the antiporter was increased by approximately 50% without a change in K_t, i.e. the affinity of the antiporter for Na^+ was unchanged. This adaptation was evident only when the transport process was studied under conditions of a pH gradient (pH_{in} 6.0/pH_{out} 7.5) as shown in Fig. 2A. In contrast, under pH equilibrium conditions ($pH_{in} = pH_{out} = 7.5$) Jmax was similar in sham-operated and remnant kidneys as shown in Fig. 2B. Similar observations were first made in the dog by Cohn et al (5) and in the rat by Harris et al (6), but in both instances the increase in Na^+/H^+ antiport activity was observed both under pH equilibrium and pH gradient conditions.

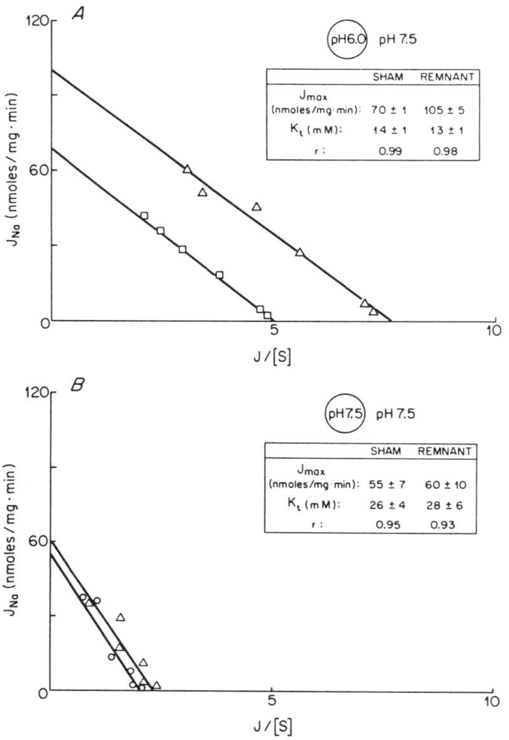

Fig. 2. Augustinsson-Eadie-Hofstee plots for Na^+ uptake by remnant kidney (△) and sham-operated kidney (□ and ○) membrane vesicles under pH gradient (pH 6.0_{in} vs. pH 7.5_{out}) (A) or pH equilibrium ($pH_{in} = pH_{out} = 7.5$) (B) conditions. Preequilibration of membrane vesicles was with 145 mM choline chloride, 5 mM KCl, 25 ug/ml valinomycin, and 7 mM Tris-14 mM MES buffered to pH 6.0 (A) or 8 mM Tris-12 mM HEPES at pH 7.5 (B). Incubation medium consisted of 0.5-20 mM NaCl, 5 mM KCl, 25 ug/ml valinomycin, and 11 mM Tris-9 mM HEPES buffered to pH 8.0 (A) or 8 mM Tris-12 mM HEPES at pH 7.5 (B). Isosmolarity was maintained by substitution of NaCl with choline chloride; 0.8 uCi of tracer-free ^{22}Na was added to incubation medium. Uptakes were performed at 2 sec. Data points represent amiloride-dependent component of total Na^+ flux. (Reprinted with permission from ref. 4).

Having demonstrated an increase in the maximal rate of Na^+/H^+ exchange, we sought an explanation for the adaptation by studying the dependence on internal and external pH of amiloride-sensitive Na^+ uptake by brush border membrane vesicles from uninephrectomized rabbits. Studies performed in collaboration with Vigue et al (7) are shown in Fig. 3.

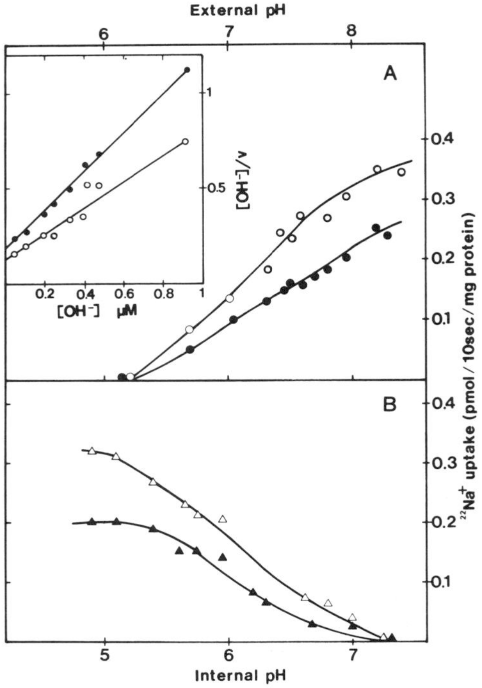

Fig. 3. Dependence on internal pH and external pH of the EPA-sensitive $^{22}Na^+$ uptake in normal and hypertrophied kidneys. Panel A: main panel, The external pH dependence of the rate of EPA-sensitive $^{22}Na^+$ uptake in brush border membranes prepared from normal (●) and hypertrophied kidneys (○). The internal pH was 6.2. Inset, Hanes-Woolf plot of the data presented in the main panel. Apparent pK was 7.25 in the two membrane preparations. Panel B, the internal pH dependence of the rate of EPA-sensitive ^{22}Na uptake in brush border membranes prepared from normal (▲) and hypertrophied kidneys (△). External pH was 7.2. (Reprinted with permission from ref. 7).

Although the rate of amiloride-sensitive Na^+ uptake was increased in the hypertrophied, uninephrectomized kidneys at each external and internal pH value, the sensitivity of the process was similar to that observed in sham-operated kidneys. The apparent pK of the external pH dependence was 7.25 and that for internal pH was 6.2 in both membrane preparations.

There remained two possible explanations for the increased Jmax of the remnant kidney: 1) the turnover number of individual antiporters is increased without an increase in antiport number or 2) the total number of antiporters, each with a normal turnover number, is increased. To study these possibilities we turned to the earlier observations of Vigne et al (8) who had examined the effects of a series of amiloride analogs on Na^+ uptake by rabbit brush border membrane vesicles. These workers found that substitution of the 5-amino group of amiloride yielded a hierarchy of affinities of the amiloride analogs for the antiporter with benzamil < amiloride < ethylpropylamiloride < ethylisopropylamiloride. Of interest, however, was the fact that the $K_{0.5}$ for kidney brush border membranes for each analog was higher than that described for other cell types, e.g. chick and rat myocardial cells, chick skeletal muscle cells.

To determine whether this apparent decrease in affinity of renal brush border membranes is an artifact related to the preparation of the vesicles or is an intrinsic property of the cell, we examined the sensitivity of isolated renal proximal tubular cells to various amiloride analogs (9). As shown in Fig. 4 the $K_{0.5}$ for ethylisopropylamiloride (EPA) was 2.9 uM. Since the incubation was performed at pH 6.1 and external H^+ is a competitive inhibitor of amiloride binding, the data were corrected for this pH effect yielding a $K_{0.5}$ of 0.3 uM for EPA. This value is one order of magnitude higher than the value for chick heart and skeletal muscle cells ($K_{0.5}$ = 0.03 - 0.05 uM) (cited in ref. 9). Thus there appears to be an inherent, decreased affinity of the renal Na^+/H^+ antiporter for amiloride analogs as compared with other cell systems.

Despite this lowered affinity Vigne et al were able to demonstrate specific binding of ^{3}H-ethylpropylamiloride (EPA) to solubilized rabbit brush border membrane vesicles with K_d of 70 nM (8). These studies had to be performed on a membrane preparation solubilized with 0.5% CHAPS since non-specific binding to the intact membrane vesicles was too high for accurate analysis. In these experiments on solubilized membranes, the bound ligand was separated from the free ligand on Sephadex G-50 columns pre-equilibrated with CHAPS.

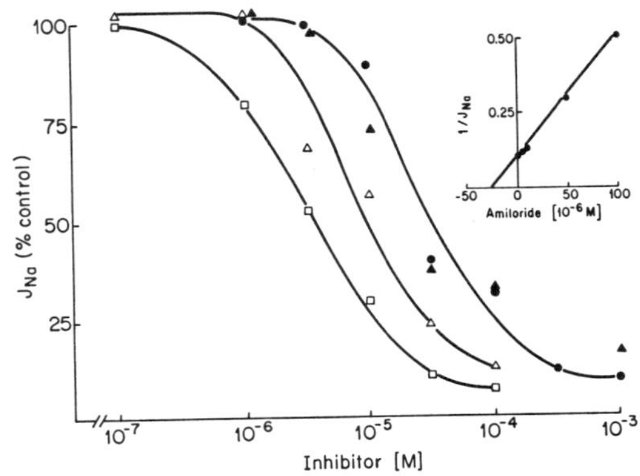

Fig. 4. Effect of amiloride analogs on rate of sodium uptake (J_{Na}). Preequilibration conditions for cells at pH 6.4 and composition of transport buffer (1 mM Na^+) are detailed in legend to Fig. 5. Uptakes performed at 10 sec were measured in presence of indicated concentrations of analog, which was added to transport buffer. Data presented for amiloride (closed circles) are means for 4 separate experiments and expressed as percentages of control. Control uptake value for 1 mM Na^+ (J_{Na}) was 9.55 ± 1.90 pmol.10^{-6} cells^{-1}.10 sec^{-1} (n=4). Data for amiloride analogs (DMA, closed triangles; MMPA, open triangles; and EIPA, squares) were repeated on at least 2 separate cell preparations. Inset: data replotted as $1/J_{Na}$ vs. amiloride concentration after correction of J_{Na} for amiloride-sensitive component of total sodium flux. (Reprinted with permission from ref. 9).

We next examined the binding properties of solubilized brush border membranes from hypertrophied kidneys of uninephrectomized rabbits using ^{3}H-EPA as a ligand as shown in Fig. 5 the binding characteristics of the hypertrophied kidneys were identical to control kidneys with the maximum number of binding sites for ^{3}H-EPA being 2.7 pmol/mg protein. The calculated turnover number at a maximal rate of Na^+ transport for the normal kidney is 2500 Na^+ ions/sec, a value which is comparable with the turnover number of Na^+-K^+-ATPase and 5000 times lower than that of the open form of the voltage-dependent Na^+ channel (7).

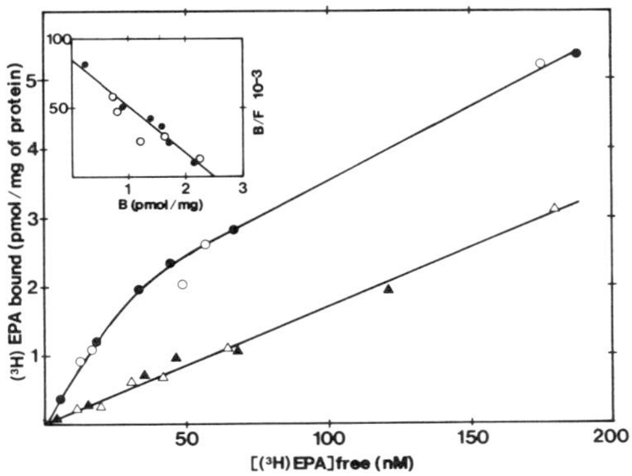

Fig. 5. Equilibrium [^{3}H]EPA binding to solubilized brush border membranes from normal and hypertrophied kidneys. Main panel, solubilized brush border membranes were incubated at 4°C for 120 min in the presence of increasing concentrations of [^{3}H]EPA in the presence (△,▲) or in the absence (○,●) of 0.1 mM unlabeled EPA at pH 8.35. Both the total binding component (○,●) and the nonspecific binding component (△,▲) are shown. ●, ▲, normal kidneys; ○, △, hypertrophied kidneys. Inset: Scatchard plot for specific [^{3}H]EPA binding to solubilized brush border membranes obtained from control (●) and hypertrophied kidneys (○). Control and hypertrophied kidneys were from the same rabbit. (Reprinted with permission from ref. 7).

While these data suggest that the proximal tubular cell adapts its Na^+/H^+ exchange activity by increasing the turnover number of a fixed number of antiporters rather than by inserting additional antiporte4s into the membrane, these conclusions may be premature and, in fact, misleading. It should be emphasized that the ^{3}H-EPA binding studies cited above were performed on a solubilized membrane preparation. Mircheff et al have pointed out that even purified brush border membranes can be further fractionated to yield at least one fraction with Na^+/H^+ antiport activity which does not copurify with maltase activity (10). If this represents a population of antiporters which is associated with, but not inserted into the membrane, the solubilization step could have included this non-transporting population which would have yielded a spuriously low turnover number in control kidneys. This could account for the apparent increase in turnover number in the hypertrophied kidneys. What is clearly needed is an assay system which permits a high percentage of specific binding to intact cells or membranes so that transport and ligand-binding can be performed in the same system. By blocking new protein synthesis it should become feasible to determine whether there exists a population of preformed antiporters which is shuttled in and out of the brush border membrane in response to the requirements for an increase or decrease in Na^+/H^+ exchange activity. In this regard the recent preliminary observations of Larsson and Tisher, which demonstrate a population of large apical endocytic vacuoles with an acidic interior lying below the brush border membrane, are intriguing (11).

REFERENCES

1. Fine, L.G. Kidney International 29: 619-634, 1986.
2. Salehmoghaddam, S., Bradley, T., Mikhail, N., Badie-Dezfooly, B., Nord, E.P., Trizna, W., Kheyfets, R. and Fine, L.G. Lab. Invest. 53 (4): 443, 1985.
3. Hruska, K., Klahr, S. and Hammerman, M. Am. J. Physiol. 242: F17-F22, 1982.
4. Nord, E.P., Hafezi, A., Kaunitz, J., Trizna, W. and Fine, L.G. Am. J. Physiol. 249: F90-F98, 1985.
5. Cohn, D.E., Hruska, K., Klahr, S. and Hammerman, M. Am. J. Physiol. 243: F293-F299, 1982.
6. Harris, R.C., Seifter J. and Brenner, B.M. J. Clin. Invest. 74: 1979-1987, 1986.
7. Vigne, P., Jean, T., Barbry, P., Frelin, C., Fine, L.G. and Lazdunski, M. J. Biol. Chem. 260: 14120-14125, 1985.
8. Vigne, P., Frelin, C., Audinot, M., Borsotto, M., Cragoe Jr., E.J. and Lazdunski, M. Embo. J. 3: 2647-2651, 1984.
9. Nord, E.P., Goldfarb, D., Mikhail, N., Moradeshagi, P., Hafezi, A., Vaystub, S., Cragoe Jr., E. and Fine, L.G. Am. J. Physiol. 250:F539-F550, 1986.
10. Mircheff, A.K., Ives, H.E., Yee, V.J. and Warnock, D.G. Am. J. Physiol. 246:F853-F858, 1984.
11. Larsson, L. and Tisher, CC. Clin. Res. 34: 698A, 1986.

RED BLOOD CELL Na^+-TRANSPORT, Na-K-ATPase AND PHOSPHATE ESTER METABOLISM IN ESSENTIAL HYPERTENSION

U. WALTER
Mainz, Elsa Brändströmstr. 21, West Germany

Introduction

Much evidence suggests that essential hypertension is partly due to an increase in the circulating concentration of an inhibitor of Na-K-ATPase by increasing vascular smooth muscle sodium concentration, thereby inducing changes that lead to a rise in peripheral vascular resistance. In essential hypertension, red blood cells (RBC) have been used as a model for cells in general to demonstrate the existence of this inhibitor. Findings on RBC Na^+ concentration, Na^+ transport and Na-K-ATPase, however, are controversial and may be attributed to different methodologies applied for measurements. The objective of the present study was to evaluate whether the conflicting data might depend on a variable removal of a Na-K-ATPase inhibiting factor due to different preparation procedures of the biological material prior to determination of biochemical parameters. Therefore, we measured intracellular concentrations of Na^+ and K^+ inorganic phosphate (P_i) ouabain-sensitive Na^+ transport, Na-K-cotransport, total and ouabain-sensitive p_i release of freshly drawn RBCs and finally Na-K-ATPase activity of haemolysed and dialysed RBCs and of haemoglobin-free RBC-membranes.

Materials and methods

a) *RBC Na^+ transport and intracellular electrolytes*
Total Na^+ efflux, ouabain-sensitive sodium efflux, furosemide-sensitive Na^+ efflux and the rate constants were measured in freshly drawn RBCs of 12 untreated men with essential hypertension and of 18 male normotensive controls after loading RBCs with $^{22}Na^+$ for 1 hr. Intracellular concentrations of electrolytes were determined in cells previously washed with isotonic Mg Cl_2 by flame photometry (1).

b) *RBC P_i release, intracellular Na^+, K^+ and P_i*
Total, ouabain-sensitive and ouabain-insensitive P_i release and RBC concentration of P_i was measured in freshly drawn RBCs previsously washed with an isotonic buffer solution in 14 untreated male hypertensive subjects and 21 male normotensive controls (2).

c) *ATPase activity*
Total ATPase activity and Na-K-ATPase activity were determined in haemolysed and dialysed RBCs and in haemoglobin-free RBC-membranes isolated by ultracentrifugation in 20 male untreated patients with essential hypertension and in 20 normotensive men (3).

Table 1. RBC Na^+ efflux and rate constants for Na^+ efflux (12 patients, 18 control subjects), RBC P_i release (14 patients, 21 control subjects), and ATPase activities of haemolysed and dialysed RBCs and of haemoglobin-free RBC membranes (20 patients, 20 control subjects) - results are mean ± SD.

Parameter	Normotensives	Hypertensives	p
Na^+ efflux,			
total (mmol/l RBC/hr)	2.39 ± 0.30	2.19 ± 0.32	NS
ouabain-sensitive (mmol/l RBC/hr)	1.77 ± 0.23	1.61 ± 0.24	NS
rate constant for ouab.-sens. (hr^{-1})	0.298 ± 0.029	0.263 ± 0.027	<0.005
furosemide-sensitive (mmol/l RBC/hr)	0.32 ± 0.10	0.28 ± 0.09	NS
rate constant for furos.-sens. (hr^{-1})	0.053 ± 0.014	0.044 ± 0.010	NS
intracellular [Na^+] (mmol/l RBC)	5.97 ± 0.66	6.11 ± 0.74	NS
P_i release			
total (mmol/l RBC/hr)	0.981 ± 0.142	1.063 ± 0.082	<0.05
ouabain-sensitive (mmol/l RBC/hr)	0.116 ± 0.022	0.080 ± 0.026	<0.001
furosemide-sensitive (mmol/l RBC/hr)	0.425 ± 0.066	0.507 ± 0.037	<0.001
intracellular [P_i] (mmol/l RBC)	0.59 ± 0.16	0.57 ± 0.13	NS
intracellular [Na^+] (mmol/l RBC)	5.99 ± 0.07	6.24 ± 0.78	NS
intracellular [K^+] (mmol/l RBC)	92.97 ± 4.52	90.82 ± 3.76	NS
ATPase, haemolysate			
total (μmol/l RBC/hr)	8.15 ± 0.89	8.88 ± 1.06	<0.05
ouabain-insensitive (μmol/l RBC/hr)	6.70 ± 0.77	7.97 ± 0.95	<0.001
Na-K-ATPase (μmol/l RBC/hr)	1.46 ± 0.26	0.91 ± 0.26	<0.001
ATPase, membranes			
total (μmol/mg membranes/hr)	0.235 ± 0.031	0.256 ± 0.019	<0.01
ouab.-insens. (μmol/mg membranes/hr)	0.157 ± 0.032	0.173 ± 0.016	NS
Na-K-ATPase (μmol/mg membranes/hr)	0.079 ± 0.020	0.083 ± 0.016	NS

Results

The intracellular concentrations of Na^+, K^+ and P_i were not different between normotensive and hypertensive subjects. The ratio of intracellular Na^+/K^+ concentrations, however, was increased in patients with hypertension (0.06867 ± 0.00849 vs. 0.06436 ± 0.0624, $p < 0.05$). RBC total Na^+ efflux, ouabain-sensitive Na^+ efflux and furosemide-sensitive Na^+ efflux (Na-K-cotransport) were not different between the two groups. The rate constant for ouabain-sensitive Na^+ efflux, however, was decreased in RBCs of essential hypertensive subjects.

RBC P_i release was linear for more than one hour and was almost twice as high as the intracellular level of P_i. Total P_i release was increased in RBCs of essential hypertensive subjects whereas ouabain-sensitive P_i release was decreased. Furosemide in a concentration of 1.0 mmol/l inhibited P_i release by an average of 50 % in both groups.

Total ATPase activity was increased in haemolysed and dialysed RBCs and in haemoglobin-free RBC-membranes of essential hypertensive patients. Na-K-ATPase activity was decreased in haemolysed RBCs of hypertensive patients but not in haemoglobin free membranes. Na-K-ATPase activity amounted to 10.3 ± 2.6 % and to 17.9 ± 2.6 % of total ATPase activity in haemolysate and to 32.4 ± 5.2 % and to 33.8 ± 7.9 % in haemoglobin free membranes in hypertensive and in normotensive subjects, respectively.

Discussion

Na-K-ATPase activity of haemolysed and dialysed RBCs was lower in patients with essential hypertension than in normotensive controls whereas in haemoglobin-free membranes, isolated by ultracentrifugation, Na-K-ATPase activites were almost the same to both groups. In haemolysed and dialysed cells Na-K-ATPase amounted to an average of 10 % of total ATPase activity in patients whereas in the normotensive subjects almost 18 % of ATPase was ouabain-sensitve. In haemoglobin-free erythrocyte membranes 33 % of ATPase activity was ouabain-sensitive in both groups. This observation probably is due to a non dialysable Na-K-ATPase inhibiting factor which is either tightly bound to the erythrocyte membrane or dissolved in the cytoplasm. Followig haemolysis with subsequent centrifugation this inhibitor is removed and thus differences in Na-K-ATPase activity demonstrable in haemolysed and dialysed erythrocytes are no longer apparent in haemoglobin-free membranes. The concentration of this inhibitor is increased in RBCs of patients with essential hypertension and is the cause for the decreased rate costant for ouabain-sensitive Na^+ efflux and for the decreased ouabain-sensitive RBC P_i release of freshly drawn RBCs of essential hypertensive patients.

References

1. Walter, U. Effect of ouabain and furosemide on erythrocyte sodium and phosphate transport. Clin. Pharmacol. Ther. 30: 709-717, 1981.

2. Walter, U. Erythrocyte phosphate release in essential hypertension. Hypertension 7: 430-437, 1985.

3. Walter, U. and Müller, S. Evidence for a Na-K-ATPase inhibition in erythrocytes of patients with essential hypertension. Europ. J. Clin. Invest. 15: 209-214.

CORRELATION BETWEEN BLOOD PRESSURE AND K^+ FLUXES IN ESSENTIAL HYPERTENSIVE PATIENTS TREATED FOR 2 YEARS WITH CICLETANINE.

R. GARAY, P. HANNAERT, C. NAZARET, E. DESCHAMPS DE PAILLETTE*, G. JUIN AND P. BRAQUET*.
INSERM U7. Hôpital Necker. Paris 75015. France
* IHB, Le Plessis-Robinson, France.

INTRODUCTION

Essential hypertension appears to result from a combination of genetic and environmental factors, of which an excess Na^+ intake is the most important (1). In the past ten years, the extensive investigation of Na^+ transport in erythrocytes from essential hypertensive patients revealed at least **four** different and **stable** Na^+ transport abnormalities (for details see ref. 2,3,4) :

(i) **[Leak (+)]** = increased passive entry of Na^+ in about 15 to 30% of human hypertensives (Leak (+) hypertensives).

(ii) **[Co (-)]** = decreased ability of the furosemide-sensitive Na^+,K^+ cotransport system to extrude a cell Na^+-load in about 30 to 40% of human hypertensives (Co (-) hypertensives).

(iii) **[Counter (+)]** = increased maximal rate of Na^+: Li^+ countertransport in about 20 to 40% of human hypertensives (Counter (+) hypertensives).

(iv) **[Pump (-)]** = decreased apparent affinity of the Na^+,K^+ pump for internal Na^+ in about 5-10% of human hypertensives.

Cicletanine is a new antihypertensive, slightly natriuretic drug which belongs to the family of furopyridines. Previous results <u>in vitro</u> showed that the main effect of cicletanine on ion transport was a stimulation of K^+ fluxes (5).

We investigated here whether the antihypertensive effect of cicletanine <u>in vivo</u> is correlated with : (i) the subgroup to which the hypertensive belongs and (ii) the stimulation of erythrocyte K^+ fluxes.

PATIENTS

Forty-six essential hypertensive patients (25 males, 21 females) aged from 30 to 70 years were treated for 2 years with 150 mg cicletanine/day. All patients remained untreated for at least 1 month before the study. Initial mean arterial pressure was 140 ± 6 mmHg (mean ± SD).

METHODS

At times (months): 0, 1, 4, 8, 12, 16, 20 and 24, venous blood was drawn in heparinized tubes and Na^+ and K^+ fluxes were measured in erythrocytes (see ref. 2, 3, 4, 5 for details). The patients were classified in different groups [Pump (-), Co (-), Counter (+) and Leak (+)], according to the membrane Na^+ transport pathway where a major and stable abnormality was found.

RESULTS

Table 1 shows the number of subjects which belong to each subgroup of hypertensives and their response to 1 year of antihypertensive treatment. Unfortunately, the number of studied subjects appears to be rather small in order to draw definitive conclusions. Nevertheless, it can be seen that Leak (+) hypertensives are more resistant to treatment than the other groups ($p < 0.05$). If Pump (-) and Co (-) hypertensives are included in a same group, they exhibited a more important decrease in blood pressure than the other hypertensives ($p < 0.02$).

Table 1.Mean blood pressure in different subgroups of hypertensives after 1 year of cicletanine treatment.

Subgroup	number of subjects	Mean blood pressure (mmHg)
Leak (+)	8	122.1 ± 6.8*
Co (-)	17	114.0 ± 7.3
Counter (+)	11	117.1 ± 7.5
Pump (-)	4	113.3 ± 7.1
non-identified	6	112.5 ± 2.8

Values in this Table are given as mean ± SD.
* $p < 0.05$.

Table 2 shows the effect of cicletanine-treatment on erythrocyte K^+ fluxes. It can be seen that they are significantly stimulated after 1 month of treatment. In addition, good correlations were obtained between stimulation of K^+ fluxes and antihypertensive response (for instance, K^+ fluxes vs mean blood pressure after 4 months of treatment exhibited $r : -0.52$; $p < 0.001$).

Table 2. Effect of cicletanine treatment on erythrocyte K^+ fluxes.

months of treatment	0	1	4	8	12	16	20	24
K^+ efflux*	9.2±1.1	9.8±1.4	11.2±1.7	12.8±2.6	12.6±2.3	13.6±2.4	11.3±1.7	11.4±2.1
p		<0.05	<0.001	<0.001	<0.001	<0.001	<0.001	<0.001

Values in this Table are given as mean ± SD.
* rate constant in $(h)^{-1} \times 10^3$.

DISCUSSION

Our results show that cicletanine is able to stimulate erythrocyte K^+ fluxes in vivo. This effect is strongly correlated with the antihypertensive efficiency of the compound.

Another factor determining the antihypertensive efficiency of cicletanine is the subgroup to which the hypertensive belongs. However, this factor appears to be of secondary importance. Further studies with higher number of subjects are required in order to draw definitive conclusions.

REFERENCES

1. Dahl, L.K. In : Hypertension. (Eds. J. Genest, E. Koiw and O. Kuchel), McGraw-Hill, New York, 1977, pp. 548-559.
2. Garay, R.P. and Nazaret, C. Cli. Sci. 69: 613-624, 1985.
3. Garay, R.P., Diez, J. and Braquet, P. In : The sodium pump. (Eds. I. Glynn and C. Ellory) The Company of Biologists Limited, Cambridge, UK, 1985, pp. 657-662.
4. Canessa, M., Spalvins, A., Adragna, N. and Falkner, B. Hypertension. 6: 344-351, 1984.
5. Garay, R., Nazaret, C., Diez, J., Etienne, A., Bourgain, R. Braquet, P. and Esanu, A. Bioch. Pharmacol. 33: 2013-2020, 1984

EFFECTS OF MUZOLIMINE ON CATION TRANSPORT IN HUMAN ERYTHROCYTES

A. MONTANARI, A. GUERRA, E. SANI and A. NOVARINI
Istituto di Semeiotica Medica, Università di Parma, Italy

The saluretic agent muzolimine (MZ) induces "in vivo" changes in urinary pattern similar to those observed with loop diuretics, as furosemide (FUR), bumetanide (BUM) or ethacrinic acid (ETHA) (1). These drugs inhibit NaK2Cl cotransport (COT) in both the luminal side of the thick ascending limb of Henle's loop (TAL) and in erythrocytes (RBC) (2). Thus, RBC may be an useful model to study the cellular effects of MZ (2). In this paper we studied RBC cation transport pathways in the presence of MZ.

MATERIALS AND METHODS

In order to measure the maximal rate of Na/K pump, COT and lithium-sodium countertransport (CT), washed RBC were loaded with nystatin (3) to contain 40-50 mmol/l Na, 40-50 K, 6-8 Li. Na effluxes were measured for 90 m' in 140 mM choline chloride (Ch) with 10 mM K, Ch 150 with 0.1 mM ouabain (OUAB) or Ch 150 with OUAB and 1 mM FUR. Li effluxes were measured in Ch 150 or in NaCl 150 mM. Na COT was also measured in the presence of equimolecular concentrations of MZ plus cysteine. Additional experiments were performed using nystatin-loaded RBC containing 70 mmol/l Li and 40 K; FUR sensitive Li efflux (LiCOT) from these RBC was measured in 100 mM Ch, 47 Na, 1.5 K, 2.0 Ca, 0.5 Mg and in a solution prepared by adding 1 volume of supernatant of human plasma deproteinized by boiling to 2 volumes of 150 mM Ch. Passive K permeability was tested in fresh RBC in 150 mM Ch with OUAB and FUR. Appropriate concentration of MZ or other diuretics were added when required. All solutions, including diluted plasma, were buffered to pH 7.4 with TRIS-HEPES 10 mM. PCV was 10% and osmolality was 295 mOsm/kg.

RESULTS

10^{-3} MZ had no effect on the RBC Na/K pump (6.6±0.6 mmol/lRBC·h^{-1} with MZ and 6.7±0.6 without MZ, n=6), LiNaCT (0.27±.03 vs 0.28±.03 mmol/lRBC·h^{-1}, n=5) nor on the passive K efflux (permeability constant .042±.004 h^{-1} with MZ, .036±.001 under control conditions and .097±.004 with 10^{-3} ETHA, n=5). In figure 1 we report the dose-response curve of MZ on NaCOT (n=7) and those of FUR, BUM and ETHA. Half-maximal inhibition of NaCOT by MZ was around $7 \cdot 10^{-4}$ M vs $7 \cdot 10^{-6}$ for FUR, $2 \cdot 10^{-7}$ for BUM and 10^{-4} for ETHA. MZ effect on COT was not enhanced by equimolecular cysteine: percent inhibition was 3±1 with 10^{-6} M MZ, 7±2 at 10^{-5} and 16±5 at 10^{-4} vs 2±1, 9±3 and 18±6 respectively with MZ plus cysteine (n=3). 10^{-4} M ETHA alone inhibited COT by 51±2% and by 99±4% when 10^{-4} M cysteine was added (n=3). LiCOT was inhibited to the same extent by MZ in NaCl-Ch medium (0.1±2% at 10^{-5} M; 40±3 at 10^{-4}; 52±5 at $5 \cdot 10^{-4}$) and in boiled plasma-Ch solution (3±1; 36±4; 53±6 respectively, n=3).

Figure 1: Dose-response curves of MZ, FUR, ETHA and BUM on NaK2Cl cotransport in human erythrocytes.

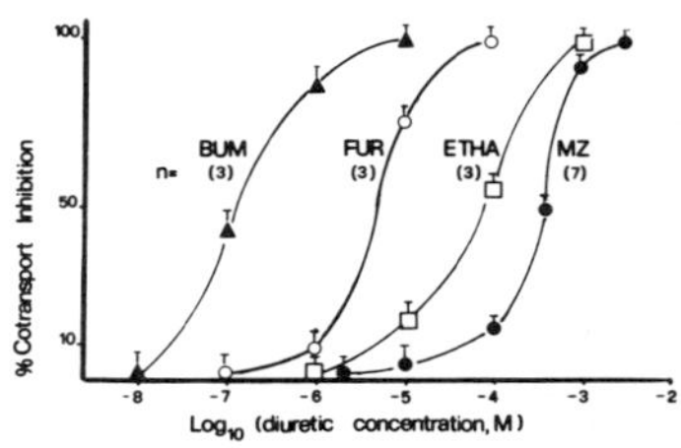

DISCUSSION

Little is known about cellular mechanisms of action of MZ (4). Despite its in vivo action similar to that displayed by loop diuretics, MZ has been found to be ineffective on NaK2Cl COT in isolated renal tubules when perfused with MZ into the tubular lumen (4). Previous findings in PCMBS-treated RBC have shown a MZ inhibition of COT only by 50% at 10^{-3} M (5). Under our experimental conditions 10^{-3} M MZ inhibits completely NaCOT; the half-maximal inhibition value of $7 \cdot 10^{-4}$ M shows a weak inhibitory potency of MZ on COT in comparison to other loop diuretics. In addition, unlike ETHA (2), no potentiation of the inhibition is observed with cysteine nor with any other "physiological" substance contained in boiled plasma. Finally, despite some chemical similarity with ETHA, MZ does not stimulate passive K efflux (6). The present study seems to rule out the possibility that the effect of MZ on NaK2ClCOT in TAL might be enhanced by some substance(s) physiologically present in the tubular fluid but not in perfusion media used in microperfusion experiments (4). The effect of MZ on RBC COT, being much weaker than that displayed by other loop diuretics, makes it difficult to conceive that an inhibition of COT in TAL under in vivo conditions might be involved in saluretic mechanisms of MZ. Thus, further investigations are needed in order to elucidate cellular effect of MZ in terms of cation transport.

REFERENCES

1. Berg K.J., Jørstad S., Tromsdal A., Pharmacotherapeutica 1: 319, 1976.
2. Ellory J.C., Stewart G.W., Br. J. Pharmac. 183: 75, 1982.
3. Canessa M., Bize I, J. Gen. Physiol. 8: 149, 1982.
4. Schlatter E., Greger R., Weidtke C., Pflügers Archiv. 396: 210, 1983.
5. Knorr A., Garthoff B., Ingedoh A., De Mendonça M., Z. Cardiol. 74: suppl. 2, 175, 1975.
6. Garay R.P., Nazaret C., Diez J., Etienne A., Bourgain R., Braquet P., Esanu A., Biochemical Pharmacology 33: 2013, 1984.

EFFECTS OF XIPAMIDE ON TRANSMEMBRANARY POTASSIUM MOVEMENTS AND PROSTACYCLIN PRODUCTION.

J.DIEZ,I.COLINA,J.QUIROGA,R.DIAZ-TEJEIRO,L.YAP,F.MADUELL,P.ERRASTI,A.PURROY,J.PRIETO.

Division of Nephrology & Department of Medicine,University Clinic,University of Navarra,Pamplona,Spain.

INTRODUCTION

Several observations suggest a possible interaction between ion transport mechanisms and the arachidonic acid cascade in the natriuretic and in the antihypertensive effects of diuretics(1).Moreover,several studies have established that some diuretic drugs may act on the arachidonic acid cascade(2).In fact,it has been recently reported that the modification of K^+ transmembrane gradient by some diuretic drugs may stimulate the generation of prostacyclin,PGI_2,(3).Xipamide,X,is a sulfonamide type drug with diuretic and antihypertensive effects but whose mechanism of action remains unknown(4).We,thus,have investigated whether X does modify transmembranary K^+ movements and PGI_2 production.

METHODS

K^+ fluxes were measured in fresh human red cells following a previously published method(5).Briefly,fresh washed red cells were suspended in Mg^{2+}-sucrose medium containing ouabain and bumetanide.External K^+ concentrations were measured at 0 time and after 0.5 and 1 hr incubation at 37°C.K^+ efflux was obtained by the difference in K^+ concentration divided by the final hematocrit and the incubation time.

Rings from aorta of Wistar rats were incubated at 37°C for 30 min and the amount of the stable derivative of PGI_2,6-keto-$PGF_{1\alpha}$,released into the medium was measured by direct radioimmunoassay according to a previously published method(6).

RESULTS

Figure 1 shows that X stimulates ouabain and bumetanide resistant K^+ efflux in human red cells.The maximal stimulattory effect being approximately of 70%.Half maximal stimulation is observed at concentrations of

X ranging between 5 x 10^{-4} and 7.5 x 10^{-4}M.

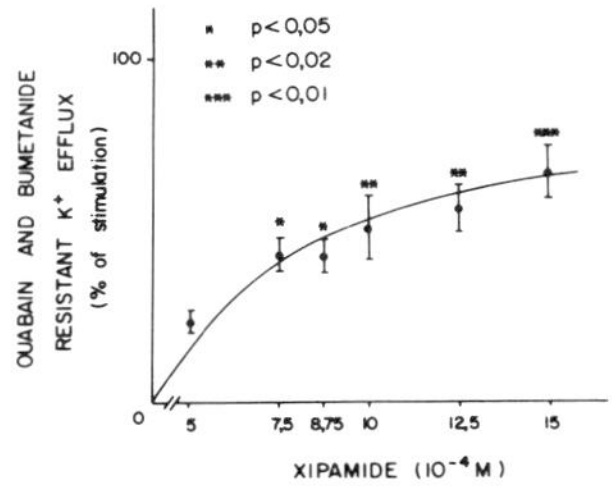

Figure 1:Dose-response curve of the effect of X on ouabain and bumetanide resistant K^+ efflux in human red cells.(Values are represented as MEANS$\pm$SEM of 12 experiments).

In additional experiments we have observed that the stimulated K^+ fluxes are also resistant to quinine.Moreover,the replacement of Cl^- by $NO_3^=$ ions in the Mg^{2+}-sucrose medium does not change the effect of X on K^+ fluxes.

Figure 2 shows that the amount of 6-keto-$PGF_{1\alpha}$ released into the medium is higher in tubes containing X 10^{-3}M as compared to control tubes containing only TRIS-HCl 50 mM pH:7.4 and vehicle,(35$\pm$5 vs 21$\pm$2.5,ng 6-keto-$PGF_{1\alpha}$/mg protein).In addition,it can be observed that the release of 6-keto-$PGF_{1\alpha}$ is not furtherly enhanced by adding Ca^{2+} 1 mM to the incubation medium containing X 10^{-3}M.

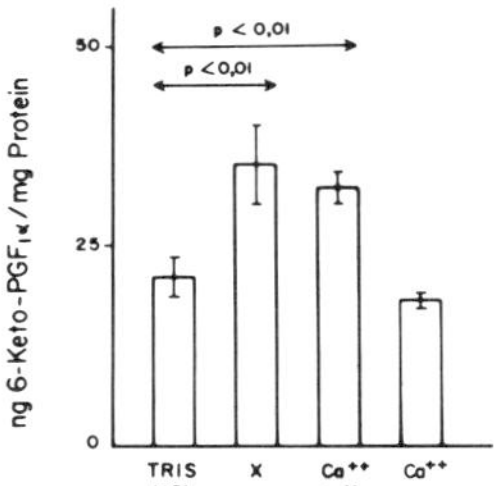

Figure 2:The effect of X on 6-keto-$PGF_{1\alpha}$ release by aortas from Wistar rats.(Values are represented as MEANS$\pm$SEM of 6 experiments).

DISCUSSION

X stimulates K^+ efflux across human red cell membrane.The stimulated K^+ efflux does not appear to be mediated by the Na^+,K^+-pump,the Na^+,K^+-cotransport,the Ca^{2+}-dependent K^+ permeability or by a Cl^--dependent K^+ carrier.Although non conclusive,these observations would suggest that X may stimulate a K^+ carrier present in human red cell membrane and non identified.On the other hand,our observations indicate that,"in vitro",X may stimulate PGI_2 production by the vascular wall,this effect being not dependent on the presence of extracellular Ca^{2+}.Thus,it appears that X does not activate phospholipase Ca^{2+}-dependent enzymes(7).Some authors have suggested that membrane hyperpolarization might activate synthesizing enzymes and/or inhibit degrading enzymes of the arachidonic acid cascade(3, 8).Since an increased K^+ efflux is mainly responsible for the hyperpolarization in several kind of cells,we suggest that this mechanism might be involved in the stimulation of PGI_2 synthesis by X.In turn,PGI_2 could mediate natriuretic and vasodilatatory effects of the drug.

ACKNOWLEDGMENTS

The authors are indebted to C.Miqueo,E.Elizalde and C.Wilhemi by their thecnical assistance.

REFERENCES

1. Dunn M.J.In:Renal Endocrinology.(Ed.:M.J.Dunn).Williams & Wilkins.Baltimore.1983.pp. 1-74.
2. Frolich P.,Filep P.,Kroemer H. et al.In:Diuretics.(Ed.:J.B.Puschett). Elsevier.New York.1984.pp. 415-418.
3. Braquet P.,Deby C.,Garay R. et al.Lancet 1:1218-1219,1983.
4. Prichard B.N.C.,Brogden R.N.Drugs 30:313-332,1985.
5. Garay R.,Nazaret C.,Díez J. et al.Biochem.Pharmacol.33:2013-2020,1984
6. Díez J.,Colina I.,Guarner F. et al.Clin.Sci.66:621-624,1984.
7. Erman A.,Raz A.Biochem.J.182:821-825,1979.
8. Poincelot B.,Russo-Marie F.In:Prostaglandins and membrane ion transport.(Ed.:P.Braquet).Raven Press.New York.pp. 67-73.

LACK OF EVIDENCE FOR Na/K ATPase INHIBITION AS A CAUSE OF LOW RENIN HUMAN HYPERTENSION

R.PEDRINELLI,*A.CLERICO,L.GRAZIADEI,S.TADDEI,°M.DEL CHICCA,A.SALVETTI
Hypertension Unit,I Clinica Medica,*Patologia Medica & °Istituto di Fisiologia Clinica,CNR,University of Pisa,56100 PISA,ITALY

INTRODUCTION

A circulating Na/K ATPase(sodium pump)inhibiting factor might cause hypertension in man.Furthermore,more recent evidence suggests that suppressed peripheral PRA values might be a marker for the presence of that factor in human hypertension(for a review see 1).We designed this study to further assess that possibility.Our specific aims were to evaluate whether biochemical or functional indices of Na/K ATPase inhibition are present in low renin human hypertension,either in primary aldosteronism (PA)or in the so called low renin essential hypertension(LREH).As controls,normal renin essential hypertensives(NREH) were taken.

MATERIAL AND METHODS

Three groups of age and sex matched patients (n=7 per group)took part to the study.The subjects with PA had bilateral adrenal hyperplasia as assessed through standard methods;low and normal renin, mild moderate essential uncomplicated hypertensives were classified according to their renin sodium index(2).The patients had been screened during a previous admission to the Clinic and then recruited for the present study after giving their informed consent to it.All medications were discontinued three weeks prior to the admission to the Clinic.Blood pressure was higher than 140/90 mm Hg at that time.A constant sodium and potassium chloride intake (80- 100 and 60 - 80 mMol/die respectively)was maintained throughout the study.Plasma samples for the measurement of a digoxin-like substance in plasma (3),as well as for PRA,Norepinephrine (NE),aldosterone and potassium(10 a.m.,standing position),were obtained after four or five days of admission.That same day,the effect of ouabain on forearm blood flow(strain gauge plethysmography) was studied (4).After a 20 min period of saline infusion,ouabain infusion was started at two sequential infusion rates (20 min each), .36 and .72 µg/min/100 ml forearm tissue (water displacement method)through a polyethylene cannula inserted into the left brachial artery under local anesthesia,and connected through stopcocks to a pressure transducer for systemic mean blood pressure and to an infusion pump for intraarterial drug administration.Forearm vascular resistances (FVR)values were derived accordingly.Non parametric tests were used for statistical analysis.

RESULTS

At the time of the study,all patients had reached a constant sodium excretion rate.As expected,patients with PA had higher plasma aldosterone and lower potassium than the two other groups.No statistical differences in PRA values were present between PA (.05 ±.01)and LREH(.17±.03);both groups differed from NREH(1.7±.4 ng AngioI/ml/hr) in this regard.Otherwise,no significant differences were present in the remaining set of variables(see method section)but mean arterial pressure,which was lower in NREH (106.4±5.) ,as compared with LREH (130.6±7.4) ,but not PA(112.1±5.1 mmHg).

Plasma DLS levels did not differ among the three groups of patients(Fig 1).No correlation was found between plasma DLS and potassium ,aldosterone and NE,either in the whole sample or in each separate subgroup of patients.

During ouabain ,FVR increased doserelatedly and plateaued during the first 5-10 minutes of infusionin in each patient,without changes in contralateral values or systemic arterial pressure.

No significant differences in the FVR response to ouabain were found among the three groups of patients(Fig 2).

Fig 1:Plasma DLS levels: distribution in the three groups of patients.

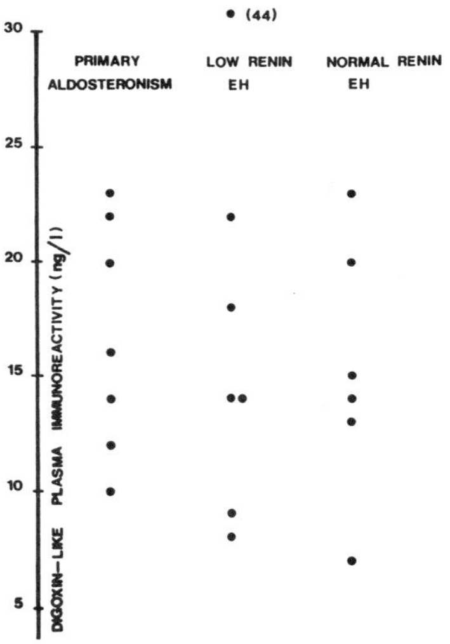

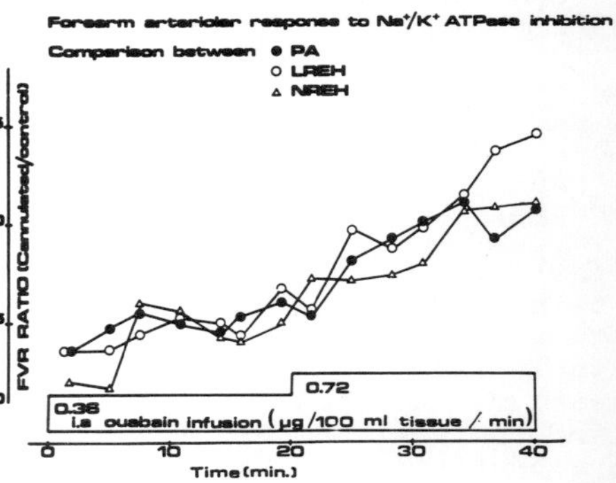

Fig 2:Comparison of the effect of ouabain infused into the brachial artery on FVR(expressed as the ratio of the infused to the contralateral forearm)

DISCUSSION

In our experimental conditions,we were unable to put in evidence any difference in DLS concentration among our three groups of patients,matched for age and sex and stratified according to their renin (and aldosterone) levels.Furthermore,no correlation was present between DLS and either PRA,aldosterone or NE levels,a finding at variance with data from other laboratories(5).Thus, hypertensive patients with suppressed PRA values,when compared with normal renin hypertensive controls, do not seem to be characterized by higher levels of a circulating sodium pump inhibitor,at least to the extent that the plasma DLS measured in our assay represent it.

As a next index of sodium pump suppression,we took the vasoconstrictor effect of ouabain on forearm arterioles as a physiologically relevant indicator of the basal sodium pump activity,an assumption validated by previous human studies(6).However even in this regard,no difference in the response to ouabain was present among our three selected groups of hypertensive patients.This finding is at variance with the assumption of a reduced pharmacological effect of ouabain in low renin hypertension,if greater amounts of a circulating digitalis like factor decreased the number of available receptors for ouabain itself at the vascular level.

Overall our data are not consistent with the hypothesis that human low renin hypertension might be causally associated with an endogenous sodium pump inhibitor.

REFERENCES

1.Haddy FJ,Pamnani MB J Cardiovasc Pharmacol 6:S71 S74,1984
2.Salvetti A,Pedrinelli R,Magagna A,Poli L,Sassano P,Arzilli F Nephron,26:189 194,1980
3.Balzan S,Clerico A,Del Chicca MG,Montali U,Ghione S Clin Chem 30:450 451,1984
4.Pedrinelli R,Taddei S,Graziadei L,Salvetti A Hypertension,in press
5.Hamlyn J,Levinson P,Ringel R,Levin P,Hamilton B,Blaustein M,Kowarski A,Fed Proc 44:2782 2788,1985
6.Robinson B,Phillips R,Wilson P,Chiodini P J Hypertension 1:165 169,1983

CANRENONE PREVENTS Na,K PUMP INHIBITION INDUCED BY VOLUME EXPANSION IN NORMAL SUBJECTS

R. BOERO, C. GUARENA, F. QUARELLO, C. ROSATI, B. ROLANDO, M.C. DEABATE, G. PICCOLI.

Cattedra di Nefrologia Medica dell'Universtità di Torino (Prof. A. Vercellone). Divisioni di Nefrologia e Dialisi. Ospedale S. Giovanni Battista. Torino, Italy.

INTRODUCTION

Canrenone is the main active metabolite of the diuretic and antihypertensive drugs spironolactone and K-canrenoate [1], and competes with aldosterone for a common cytosolic receptor in distal and collecting tubules of the nephron [2].

It has recently been demonstrated that canrenone *in vitro* may directly interphere with Na,K pump, acting as a partial agonist at the digitalis receptor site [3,4]. Moreover Garay et al. [4] showed that canrenone is able to restimulate the Na,K pump of human erythrocytes (RBC) blocked by high concentrations of ouabain. A large body of evidence supports the hypothesis that volume expansion elicits in mammals the release of a circulating "ouabain-like" Na,K pump inhibitor [5]; in a previous study we have observed an RBC Na,K pump inhibition after a saline infusion in normal subjects [6].

In this study we have evaluated the effects of canrenone administration on RBC sodium transport during an acute extracellular volume expansion in normal subjects.

SUBJECTS AND METHODS

Seven normal subjects (3 males, 4 females), mean age 30 yr (range 23-41 yr) were studied. They received an intravenous infusion of 2 litres of saline (0.9% NaCl) over 3 hr, beginning at 09.00 hr. Saline infusion was repeated after at least 2 wk, with oral administration of a single dose of canrenone (Phanurane, Théraplix, 150 mg). Blood was drawn before and after saline infusion for evaluation of sodium transport in fresh RBC.

Measurements of intracellular Na concentration, ouabain-sensitive (Na,K pump), bumetanide-sensitive (Na,K cotransport), Li-stimulated (Na,Li countertransport) outward Na fluxes and ouabain- and bumetanide- resistant (passive membrane leak) Na and K fluxes were made using the Garay's method, as previously reported [6]. Statistical analysis was carried out with the Wilcoxon matched pairs test. Data are expressed as mean values ± SEM.

RESULTS

Main results are reported in Tab. I and in Fig. 1. No effect of extracellular volume expansion, with and without canrenone, was observed on intracellular Na concentration, Na,Li countertransport and passive Na and K permeability (data not shown).

	CONTROL		CANRENONE	
	Pre	Post	Pre	Post
Na,K Pump	2172±107	1769±67*	2092±131	2042±125
	Δ% -18.1±2.2		Δ% -2.2±1.4**	
Na,K Cotransport	222±33	182±29*	183±23	135±19*
	Δ% -18.5±3		Δ% -26.7±2**	

Tab. I. Effects of volume expansion with and without canrenone on RBC Na,K pump and Na,K cotransport. *p<0.01 vs pre. **p<0.01 vs control.

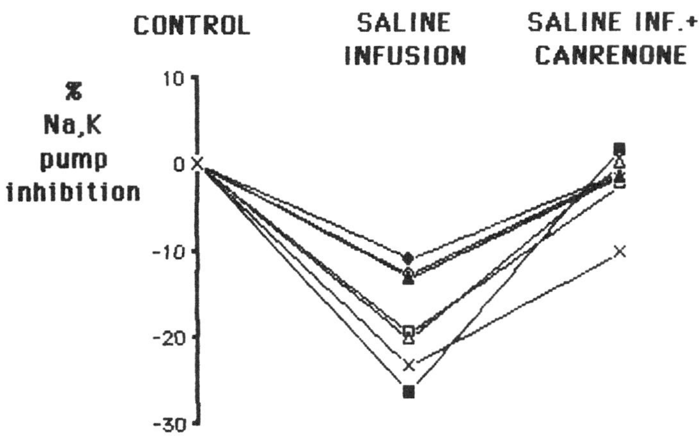

Fig. 1. Percent changes from baseline of RBC Na,K pump after volume expansion with and without canrenone. Individual values are shown.

DISCUSSION

The study of transmembrane sodium fluxes in erythrocytes during volume expansion provides a model to investigate the role of endogenous factors modulating the activity of these transport systems. In a previous study we have observed an RBC Na,K pump and Na,K cotransport inhibition after a saline infusion in normal subjects [6].

The present study confirms these results and suggests that administration of a single dose of 150 mg canrenone may prevent the inhibition of RBC Na,K pump due to acute volume expansion. In contrast, no protective effect of canrenone administration was seen as regards Na,K cotransport: indeed this transport system is significantly more inhibited by volume expansion in the presence of canrenone. This phenomenon is difficult to interpret, but suggests the existence of a distinct humoral control on Na,K cotransport, since canrenone does not interfere *in vitro* vith this transport system [7]. The specificity of the effect for Na,K pump and the analogy of our results with those reported *in vitro* [3,4] suggest that the protective effect of canrenone on Na,K pump is due to a competition with an endogenous ouabain-like factor. Interestingly, it has been shown that chronic administration of K-canrenoate to essential hypertensive patients, who may have high plasma levels of a circulating ouabain-like pump inhibitor [8], increases RBC Na,K pump activity [7,9].

Protection of Na,K pump against endogenous, other than exogenous, inhibitors seems then to be a pharmacological effect of canrenone, and may partly explain its antihypertensive activity.

REFERENCES

1. Sadée, W., Dagcioglu, M., Schroder, R. J. Pharmacol. Exp. Ther. 185: 686-695, 1973.
2. Marver, D., Kokko, J.P. Min. Electrolyte Metab. 9: 1-18, 1983.
3. Finotti, P., Palatini, P. J. Pharmacol. Exp. Ther. 217: 784-790, 1981.
4. Garay, R.P., Diez, J., Nazaret, C., Dagher, G., Abitbol, J.P. Arch. Pharmacol. 329: 311-315, 1985.
5. Buckalew, V., Gruber, K. In: The Kidney in Liver disease (Ed. M. Epstein). Elsevier Biomedical, New York 1983, pp 479-499.
6. Boero, R., Quarello, F., Guarena, C., Rosati, C., Piccoli, G. Clin. Sci. 69: 709-712, 1985.
7. Bianchi, G., Niutta, E., Tripodi M.G., Pati C., Cusi, D., Barlassina, C. Atti Convegno su: Ruolo del canrenoato di potassio nelle malattie cardiovascolari. Milano 1/3/1985. S.P.A. Milano, pp: 63-75.
8. De Wardener, H.E., MacGregor, G.A. In: Hypertension (Eds. J. Genest, O. Kuchel, P. Hamet, M. Cantin). McGraw Hill, New York 1983, pp. 84-95.
9. Pati, G., Niutta, E., Tripodi, M.G., Barlassina, C., Cusi, D., Bianchi, G. In: Atti XXVI Congresso Nazionale SIN (Eds. F. Mastrangelo, S. Rizzelli, V. De Blasi, L. Alfonso, D. Brancaccio) Wichtig, Milano 1985, pp. 247-250.

EFFECT OF THIAZIDES AND AMILORIDE ON THE PHOSPHORYLATION STATUS OF THE RED CELL MEMBRANE ANION CARRIER

B. BAGGIO, G. MARZARO, G. GAMBARO, F. MARCHINI, A. BORSATTI, G. CLARI*

Institute of Internal Medicine, University of Padova, Policlinico Universitario, 35100 Padova, Italia and Institute of Biological Chemistry, University of Verona*.

INTRODUCTION

We have recently reported an enhanced red blood cell (RBC) oxalate self-exchange in idiopathic calcium-oxalate nephrolithiasis (1,2) which seems to be linked to an anomalous phosphorylation of band 3 protein (the anion carrier) in RBC ghosts (3). We have also shown that the RBC anomaly can be corrected "in vivo" by the administration of hydrochlorothiazide (HCT) and amiloride (A) (2). Aim of the present study was the search of a bound between these drugs and band 3 phosphorylation.

MATERIAL AND METHODS

In three different sets of experiments on RBC from stone-former patients with abnormal oxalate flux rate (1), we studied 1)the effect of HCT (500 µM) and of A (150 µM) on the oxalate self-exchange in RBC, determined as previously reported (2); 2)the effect of increasing concentrations of HCT (from 150 to 600 µM) and of A (from 100 to 400 µM) on the endogenous phosphorylation of ghost membrane protein as previously described (3).

RESULTS AND DISCUSSION

The "in vitro" effects on RBC oxalate self-exchange exerted by HCT and A are shown in Fig.1. Both drugs appear to markedly lower oxalate flux rate.

Fig. 2 shows that band 3 phosphorylation is inhibited by

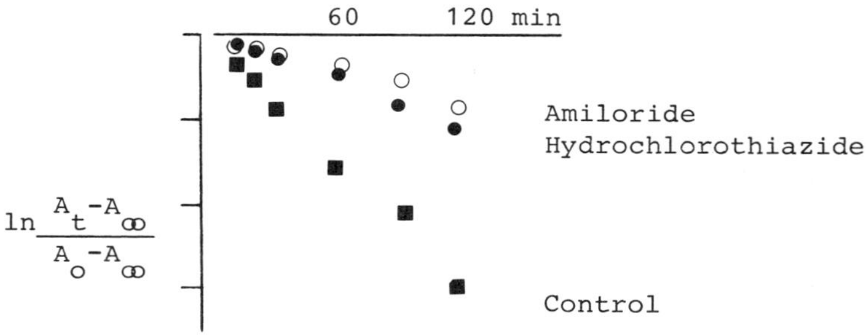

Fig. 1.

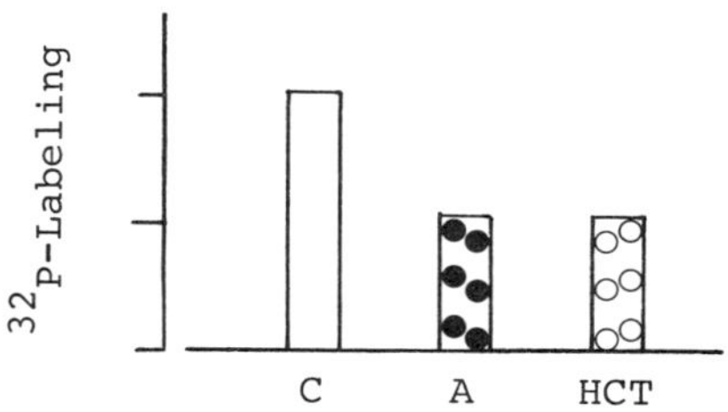

Fig. 2.

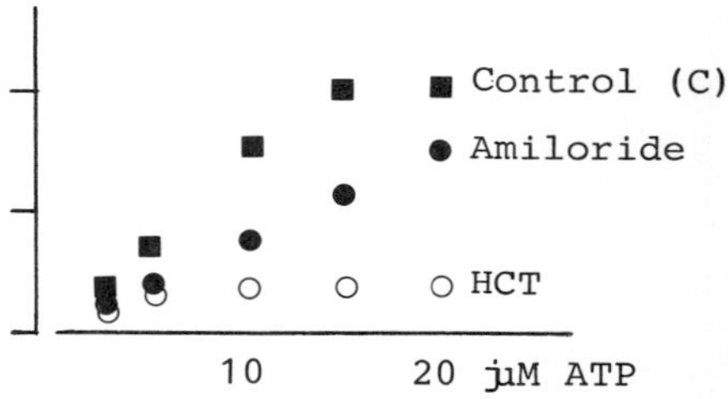

Fig. 3.

the two drugs. However, while A inhibition can be reversed by the addition of ATP, this does not happen for HCT (Fig. 3). So, though both drugs appear able to lower band 3 phosphorylation, the mechanism by which this action takes place looks different. In fact, A most seemingly acts by competing with ATP for the same catalytic binding site of the protein kinase responsible of band 3 phosphorylation (4). On the contrary, since HCT effect is not reversed by ATP addition, the most likely explanation is either a direct binding to the protein kinase phosphorylating band 3, or to band 3 protein itself in such a way to restrain its phosphorylation.

To summarize, this study shows that both A and HCT interfere with band 3 phosphorylation, although in different ways. This finding, besides explaining the effect exerted by these two diuretics on oxalate self-exchange, offers a further understanding of the mechanism of action of these substances on electrolyte metabolism.

REFERENCES

1. Baggio, B., Gambaro, G., Marchini, F., Cicerello, E., Borsatti, A. Lancet ii: 12-13, 1984.
2. Baggio, B., Gambaro, G., Marchini, F., Cicerello, E., Tenconi, R., Clementi, M., Borsatti, A. New Engl. J. Med. 314: 599-604, 1986.
3. Baggio, B., Clari, G., Marzaro, G., Gambaro, G., Borsatti, A., Moret, V. IRCS Med. Sc. 14: 368-369, 1986.
4. Holland, R., Woodgett, J.R., Hardie, D.G. FEBS Lett. 154: 269-273, 1983.

IN VITRO EFFECTS OF d(+) AND l(-) OZOLINONE ON SODIUM AND POTASSIUM FLUXES IN HUMAN ERYTHROCYTES

C. GUARENA, R. BOERO, C. ROSATI, G. FORNERIS, G. BELTRAME, F. QUARELLO, G. PICCOLI

Cattedra di Nefrologia Medica dell'Università di Torino (Prof. A. Vercellone).
Divisioni di Nefrologia e Dialisi dell'Ospedale Maggiore di S. Giovanni Battista. Torino. Italy.

INTRODUCTION

Several observations suggest that diuretic drugs may decrease renal Na reabsorption by direct inhibition of Na transport carrier in different segments of the nephron [1,2]. Ouabain inhibits basolateral sodium reabsorption, which is catalyzed by the Na,K pump; loop diuretics, like furosemide and bumetanide, cause natriuresis by inhibition of the Na,K,Cl cotransport system, which is located in the luminal side of Henle's loop cells.

Human erythrocytes (RBC) have been used for studying the cellular action of various diuretic drugs [3,4]: sodium movements across human RBC membranes are mediated by several transport systems, which are qualitatively similar to those present in renal tubular cells [4]. The ouabain-sensitive Na,K ATPase is the main mechanism maintaining the Na and K electrochemical gradients across RBC membranes against the passive Na and K diffusion. At least two additional transport systems, ouabain-insensitive, have been described in human RBC: a furosemide- (and bumetanide-) sensitive one to one Na,K cotransport system, which catalyzes a simultaneus efflux of both Na and K and a phloretin-sensitive Na,Na exchange, which can be detected by using Li as a tracer and is thus called Na,Li countertransport [4].

Etozolin is a diuretic and antihypertensive drug recently available in Italy (Elkapin, Knoll S.p.A.). The drug is a racemic mixture of two enantiomers; after oral administration both undergo liver metabolization in d+ and l-ozolinone, which are clinically active. Only the l-enantiomers show diuretic and natriuretic properties, while both optical isomers have vasodilating activity [5].

We thus decided to investigate whether the diuretic and vascular effects of d+ and l-ozolinone involve the Na and K transport systems, as studied in human RBC, to elucidate the underlying molecular mechanism.

METHODS

Simultaneous measurements of ouabain sensitive (Na,K pump), bumetanide-sensitive (Na,K cotransport), Li-stimulated (Na,Li countertransport), outward Na fluxes and ouabain- and bumetanide-resistant (passive permeability) Na and K efflux, were made in fresh erythrocytes by the method of Garay et al. [4], as previously reported [6]. D+ and l- ozolinone, dissolved in dimethylsulfoxid, were added to the incubation media in order to obtain the following final concentrations: 10^{-6}, 10^{-5}, 10^{-4}, 10^{-3} M.

RESULTS

Neither d+ nor l- ozolinone exert any significant effect on Na efflux mediated by Na,K pump, Na,Li countertransport and passive membrane leak (data not shown). The effects on Na,K cotrasport and passive K permeability are reported in Tab. I and in Figg. 1,2.

Drug Conc. (M)	Bumetanide-sensitive Na efflux		Quabain- and bumetanide- resistant K efflux	
	(µmol/l RBC/h)			
	l- ozolinone	d+ozolinone	l-ozolinone	d+ozolinone
CONTROL	190±27	209±22	781±59	843±101
10^{-6}	160±21	204±23	821±51	817±86
10^{-5}	131±21	192±22	1030±149	849±98
10^{-4}	121±17	190±24	908±111	827±89
10^{-3}	56±12	168±18	900±103	826±88

Tab.I Effects of d+ and l-ozolinone on Na,K cotransport and passive K permeability in human RBC. Values are expressed as mean±SEM of five experiments.

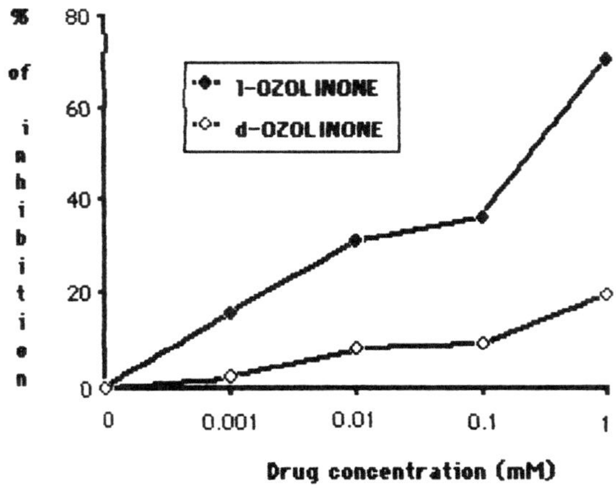

Fig. 1. Inhibition by d+ and l- ozolinone of Na efflux mediated by Na,K cotransport in human *RBC*.

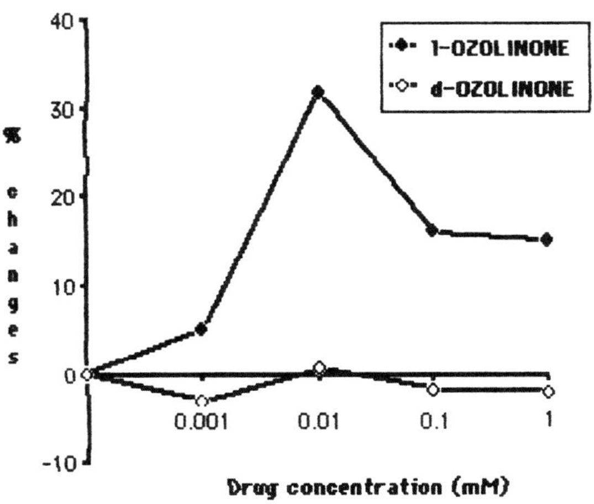

Fig. 2. Effects of d+ and l- ozolinone on passive K efflux in human RBC.

DISCUSSION

Our data show that *in vitro* l-ozolinone inhibits erythrocyte Na transport mediated by the Na,K cotransport, while the d+ isomer is only a weak inhibitor at the same concentrations (Tab. I, Fig. 1). Interestingly *in vivo* the l-enantiomer shows a much more pronounced natriuretic and diuretic effect [5].

Loop diuretic drugs of various classes, like furosemide, bumetanide, tienilic acid and ethacrynic acid have a common inhibitory effect on RBC Na,K cotransport system, which is similar to that located in the luminal side of Henle's loop cells; taken together these observations confirm, in agreement with micropuncture studies [7], that the loop of Henle is the site of action of ozolinone.

We have observed also a peculiar effect of l-ozolinone on passive membrane K leak. Like some diuretic/antihypertensive drugs (tienilic acid, l-indacrinone and furopyridines) [3,4], l-ozolinone increases K permeability (Tab. I, Fig. 2). Ozolinone, like indacrinone and some furopyridines, presents a stereospecificity with respect to the K stimulating effect: interestingly the l-series of these drugs have a much more pronounced diuretic effect than d+isomers. It has been suggested that changes in membrane potential due to the increase of K permeability may stimulate the secretion of natriuretic and vasodilating agents like prostacyclin [8]. Moreover membrane hyperpolarization in vascular smooth muscle cells due to K leak may lead to a reduction of vascular tone, thus explaining in part the direct vasodilating activity of l-ozolinone.

D+ozolinone, which has been found to be vasodilating and antihypertensive, but not natriuretic, does not significantly interfere with Na and K fluxes in red cells; its mechanism of action seems to involve other unknown mechanisms, and deserves further studies.

REFERENCES

1. Doucet, A. In: Actualités Nephrologiques Hôp. Necker, Flammarion Paris, 1984, pp. 7-64.
2. Burg, M.B. Kidney Int. 22: 454-464, 1982.
3. Cusi, D., Garay, R.P. Molec. Pharm. 19: 438-443, 1981.
4. Garay, R.P., Nazaret, C., Diez, J., Etienne, A., Bourgain, R., Braquet, P., Esanu, A. Bioch. Pharm. 33: 2013-2020, 1984.
5. Greven, J., Defrain, W., Glaser, K., et al. Europ. J. Physiol. 384: 57-68, 1980.
6. Boero, R., Quarello, F., Guarena, C., Rosati, C., Piccoli, G. Clin. Sci. 69: 709-712, 1985.
7. Greven, J. Heindereick, O. Arzneimittelforschung 27: 1755-1757, 1977.
8. Braquet, P., Deby, C., Garay, R.P., Larrue, J., Bourgain, R. Lancet i: 1218-1219, 1983.

III. EFFECTS OF DIURETICS ON TUBULAR TRANSPORT

THE EFFECTS OF DIURETICS ON SALT TRANSPORT IN RENAL DILUTING SEGMENTS

W. B. REEVES AND T. E. ANDREOLI

Department of Internal Medicine, University of Texas Medical School, Houston, Texas, USA 77225

The purpose of this paper is to communicate recent work from our laboratory pertaining to the mechanism of the ADH-induced increase in salt absorption in the medullary thick ascending limb of Henle's loop (mTALH) of mice. The specialized transport properties of the thick ascending limb of Henle's loop enable this segment of the nephron to dissociate salt and water absorption. Sodium chloride absorption by the cortical and medullary thick ascending limb is responsible for urinary dilution, since these segments are water-impermeable, as well as urinary concentration by creating a hypertonic medullary interstitium. The primary site of action of the "loop" diuretics, the TALH absorbs roughly 15% of the filtered sodium load.

It is well established that, in the mouse medullary TALH, antidiuretic hormone (ADH) increases the rate of net salt absorption and the spontaneous transepithelial voltage V_e (1). The hormone also increases the transepithelial electrical conductance, G_e, by increasing exclusively the transcellular electrical conductance, G_c; the hormone does not affect the paracellular conductance, G_s (2). Finally, ADH depolarizes the basolateral cell membrane voltage V_{bl} and to a lesser extent, the apical membrane voltage (3).

The studies reported here examined the factors responsible for the ADH-dependent increase in the transcellular conductance. In order to consider the mechanism for ADH action it is pertinent to review certain of the ionic conductance characteristics of the mTALH. The apical membranes are predominantly K^+ selective and these apical K^+ channels can be inhibited reversibly with luminal barium (2). Using the combination of zero luminal K^+ and 20 mM Ba^{++}, which produces almost complete blockade of the apical K^+ conductance, the cellular conductance is found to be approximately 40-50% of the total transepithelial conductance (4). The basolateral membrane contains the $(Na^+ + K^+)$-ATPase, a K^+ conductance, and a Cl^- conductance (5).

The mechanism of salt absorption in the TALH has been reviewed extensively elsewhere (8). Briefly, NaCl absorption begins with the electroneutral entry of Na^+, K^+ and Cl^- across the apical cell membrane by way of the $Na^+:K^+:2Cl^-$ cotransporter. This cotransport process is inhibited by the loop diuretics. It appears that the electrochemical gradient for Na^+ across the apical membrane is sufficient to drive the movement of K^+ and Cl^- into the cell. Thus Cl^- was found to be above its electrochemical equilibrium in the rabbit cTALH during transport, but fell to equilibrium when transport was inhibited by furosemide (24). Sodium is pumped out of the cell across the basolateral membrane by the $(Na^+ + K^+)$-ATPase. This step serves two purposes; first, it drives sodium efflux and hence maintains the gradient for sodium entry apically, and second, by keeping the cell hyperpolarized with respect to Cl^-, maintains the driving force for conductive Cl^- efflux across the basolateral membrane. The K^+ which enters via the $Na^+:K^+:2Cl^-$ transporter recycles into the lumen through the apical K^+ channels. A role for this K^+ conductance in NaCl absorption is indicated by the observation that luminal Ba^{++} can inhibit net Cl^- absorption, presumably by depolarizing the cell and reducing conductive Cl^- exit across the basolateral membrane (2,3). Furthermore, the cell to lumen K^+ movement allows for sodium absorption through the sodium-selective paracellular pathway such that 50% of transepithelial sodium absorption proceeds through the paracellular pathway (8).

We previously proposed that ADH increases apical $Na^+:K^+:2Cl^-$ entry into the mTALH cell and, as a consequence, produces a secondary rise in the basolateral membrane Cl^- conductance. We recently have conducted experiments designed to evaluate further this hypothesis (6). The rationale for these experiments is as follows. The transcellular conductance was measured in the presence and absence of ADH in the same tubule. Paired observations on the effects of bath Cl^- deletion on G_c permitted us to assess the effects of ADH on the magnitude of the change in G_c when bath Cl^- was removed (ΔG_c^{Cl}). Since luminal furosemide abolishes apical membrane salt entry, we also measured, in paired experiments, the interplay of bath ADH and/or luminal furosemide in modulating G_c and ΔG_c^{Cl}. We reasoned that if the primary action of ADH were to increase apical membrane $Na^+:K^+:2Cl^-$ entry, then furosemide should prevent the ADH-induced conductance changes. If, however, ADH had some direct effect on basolateral membrane conductance then these conductance changes should persist in the presence of furosemide. Furthermore, furosemide, by increasing the basolateral membrane resistance should allow changes in the basolateral resistance to be detected more reliably by transepithelial measurements.

Table I presents the results of a series of paired experiments on 26 tubules to evaluate quantitatively the effects of ADH on G_e, G_c and G_s. As found previously, the ADH-dependent increase in G_e is referable entirely to an increase in G_c.

Table II presents the results of paired experiments in which the effects of ADH and furosemide, individually and in combination, on G_c were determined. Without furosemide, ADH produced a 33% increase in G_c; the G_c and ΔG_c values being almost identical to those in Table I. However, in the presence of furosemide, G_c was decreased and ADH produced no significant change in G_c.

The effect of bath Cl^- deletion on G_c is presented in Table III. For convenience only the change in G_c produced by bath Cl^- deletion is tabulated (ΔG_c^{Cl}). ΔG_c^{Cl} was determined in each tubule under each of the four conditions listed in the table, thus, each tubule served as its own control. These data indicate clearly: that either with or without ADH furosemide reduced ΔG_c^{Cl}; that the furosemide-dependent fall in ΔG_c^{Cl} was nearly three-fold greater with ADH than without ADH; and that when luminal furosemide was present, ADH did not affect significantly ΔG_c^{Cl} (6).

When taken together, the transepithelial conductance data provide a set of congruent results consistent with the view that the ADH-dependent increase in G_c depends on an increased rate of apical membrane $Na^+:K^+:2Cl^-$ entry. This conclusion derives largely from an analysis of the interplay between ADH and furosemide in modulating transcellular ionic conductances.

Without luminal furosemide, ADH increases both the transcellular conductance G_c (Table I) and the R_a/R_{bl} ratio (2,3); thus the ADH-dependent increase in G_c involves an increase in the conductance of basolateral membranes. Moreover, without furosemide, the hormone-dependent increase in V_e occurs because V_{bl}, the basolateral membrane voltage, is depolarized to a greater extent than V_a, the apical membrane voltage. However, when luminal furosemide is present, ADH produces no detectable increase in G_c (Table II); the R_a/R_{bl} ratio is about 0.5-0.6, and unaffected by ADH; and V_a and V_{bl} are hyperpolarized to the same extent, so that V_e is virtually zero with or without ADH (3).

Thus when furosemide is used to block hormone-dependent increases in the rate of apical $Na^+:K^+:2Cl^-$ entry - which must attend hormone-dependent increases in the rate of net salt absorption - there is no ADH-dependent increase in G_c. Put differently, these data are consistent with the view that ADH increases the functional number of apical membrane $Na^+:K^+:2Cl^-$ cotransport units, and that G_c rises because the attendant changes in intracellular ionic activities result in a depolarization of V_{bl} and an increase in basolateral conductance (2,6). More specifically, it is plausible to argue that the latter increases because the ADH-dependent increase in apical $Na^+:K^+:2Cl^-$ units raises intracellular Cl^- activity, and thus depolarizes V_{bl}. According to this view, basolateral conductance rises because of a voltage-dependent rise in the Cl^- conductance of basolateral membranes (6).

In this regard, removal of bath Cl^- produces a striking reduction in G_c, and this reduction is considerably greater with ADH than without ADH; in other words, ADH increases basolateral Cl^- conductance (Table III). However, this ADH-dependent increase in basal Cl^- conductance is blocked by luminal furosemide. Moreover, by using the change in G_c which occurs with bath Cl^- removal in combination with R_a/R_{bl} data, it has been possible to estimate the effects of ADH and furosemide on intracellular Cl^- activity (6). Those calculations indicate that, without furosemide, ADH increases intracellular Cl^- activity from 16.3 mM to 25 mM; and that with furosemide, intracellular Cl^- is approximately 10.3 mM with or without ADH. These calculations are therefore congruent with the view that an ADH-dependent rise in intracellular Cl^- activity depolarizes V_{bl}, and thus produces a voltage-dependent increase in basolateral membrane conductance (6). Thus, basolateral Cl^- channels in the mTALH may have properties analogous to Goldman rectifiers.

According to this proposal, the primary effect of ADH on mTALH segments, by way of the second messenger cAMP (7,8) is to increase net Cl^- absorption by increasing apical membrane $Na^+:K^+:2Cl^-$ admittance. Such an apical membrane admittance effect for ADH in the mTALH is analogous to that of ADH in other epithelia: in mammalian cortical collecting tubules and in amphibian epithelia, ADH or cAMP increases the functional number of apical membrane water (9,10), Na^+ (11) and K^+ channels (12). In these latter ADH-sensitive epithelia, the hormone also increases the rate of fusion of sub-apical membrane vacuoles into apical intra-membranous aggregates (13,14). Finally, in primary cultures of chick kidney cells, Guggino et al. (15) have found that ADH increases the Ba^{++}-sensitive K^+ conductance of apical plasma membranes. There are also ADH-independent epithelia that are, in part, mirror images of the mTALH: they contain apical Cl^- channels and basolateral $Na^+:K^+:2Cl^-$ cotransport units. In such ADH-independent epithelia, such as the shark rectal gland (16,17), canine trachea (18,19), mammalian colon (20,21), corneal epithelium (22) and the Necturus gall bladder (23), cyclic nucleotides such as cAMP increase apical membrane Cl^- conductance (17,18,23). In other words, in these ADH-insensitive epithelia, cAMP also alters apical solute permeation.

TABLE I. THE EFFECTS OF ADH ON ELECTRICAL CONDUCTANCE

ADH	G_e	G_c	G_s	V_e
-	103.7 ± 6.0	45.1 ± 3.3	58.6 ± 4.7	5.6 ± 0.4
+	121.3 ± 8.3	60.2 ± 5.0	61.0 ± 5.1	9.9 ± 0.5
Δ	17.6 ± 3.6	15.1 ± 3.0	2.4 ± 1.8	4.2 ± 0.4
	($p < 0.001$)	($p < 0.001$)	(n.s.)	($p < 0.0001$)

(n = 26)

ADH, when present, was added to the bathing solutions at a final concentration of 10 μU/ml. G_e and V_e were measured with luminal 5 mM K^+ and zero Ba^{++}, and G_s was the conductance with 20 mM Ba^{++}, zero K^+. G_c was calculated as $(G_e - G_s)$. Data from Ref. 6.

TABLE II. EFFECTS OF ADH AND FUROSEMIDE ON G_c

	G_c (mS cm^{-2})		
Furosemide	-ADH	+ADH	Δ
-	44.5 ± 5.6	58.9 ± 8.9	14.3 ± 5.5 ($p < 0.02$)
+	36.5 ± 4.4	41.5 ± 6.4	5.0 ± 4.3 (n.s.)
Δ	8.0 ± 2.6	17.4 ± 3.2	
	($p < 0.01$)	($p < 0.001$)	

(n = 11)

Paired measurements of G_c were carried out in each tubule under each of four experimental conditions. ADH and furosemide, where indicated, were present at concentrations of 10 μU/ml of bathing solution and 10^{-4} M/l luminal solution, respectively. Data from Ref. 6.

TABLE III. EFFECTS OF FUROSEMIDE AND ADH ON ΔG_c^{Cl}

	ΔG_c^{Cl} (mS cm^{-2})		
Furosemide	-ADH	+ADH	Δ
-	19.2 ± 1.9	29.6 ± 4.3	10.4 ± 4.9 ($p < 0.05$)
+	11.8 ± 3.5	10.1 ± 2.1	1.7 ± 4.5 (n.s.)
Δ	7.4 ± 3.4	19.5 ± 5.0	
	($p < 0.05$)	($p < 0.01$)	

(n = 6)

The fall in transcellular conductance which occurred when bath Cl^- was removed is termed ΔG_c^{Cl} and was measured in each tubule for each of the four experimental conditions. Data from Ref. 6.

REFERENCES

1. Hebert, S. C., Culpepper, R. M. and Andreoli, T. E. Am. J. Physiol. 241:F412-F431, 1981.
2. Hebert, S. C., Friedman, P. A. and Andreoli, T. E. J. Memb. Biol. 80:201-219, 1984.
3. Hebert, S. C. and Andreoli, T. E. J. Memb. Biol. 80:221-233, 1984.
4. Hebert, S. C. and Andreoli, T. E. J. Gen. Physiol. 87:567-590, 1986.
5. Greger, R. and Schlatter, E. Pflügers Arch. 396:325-334, 1983.
6. Molony, D. A., Reeves, W. B., Hebert, S. C. and Andreoli, T. E. Am. J. Physiol. In press, 1986.
7. Culpepper, R. M. and Andreoli, T. E. Am. J. Physiol. 247:F784-F792, 1984.
8. Hebert, S. C. and Andreoli, T. E. Am. J. Physiol. 246:F745-F756, 1984.
9. Hebert, S. C. and Andreoli, T. E. Am. J. Physiol. 238:F470-F480, 1980.
10. Hays, R. M. and Franki, N. J. Memb. Biol. 2:263-276, 1970.
11. Li, H-Y. S., Palmer, L. G., Edelman, I. S. and Lindemann, B. J. Memb. Biol. 64:77-89, 1982.
12. Schafer, J. A. and Troutman. S. L. Kidney Internat. 27:320A, 1985.
13. Hays, R. M., Gourguet, J. and Chevalier, J. Proc. Am. Soc. Nephrol. p. 149A, 1981.
14. Wade, J. B., Statson, D. L. and Lewis S. A. Ann. N.Y. Acad. Sci. 372:106-117, 1981.
15. Guggino, S. E., Suarez-Isla, B. A., Guggino, W. B. and Sacktor, B. Am. J. Physiol. 249:F448-F455, 1985.
16. Greger, R., Schlatter, E. Pflügers Arch. 402:63-75, 1984.
17. Greger, R., Schlatter, E. and Gogelein, H. Pflügers Arch. 403:446-448, 1985.
18. Frizzell, R. A., Welsh, M. J. and Smith, P. L. Ann. N.Y. Acad. Sci. 372:558-569, 1981.
19. Shorofsky, S. R., Field, M. and Fozzard, H. A. J. Memb. Biol. 72:105-115, 1983.
20. Cartwright, C. A., McRoberts, J. A., Mandel, K. G. and Dharmsathaphorn, K. J. Clin. Invest. 76:1837-1842, 1985.
21. Dharmsathaphorn, K., Mandel, K. G., Masui, H. and McRoberts, J. A. J. Clin. Invest. 75:462-471, 1985.
22. Reinach, P. S. Curr. Eye Res. 4:462-471, 1985.
23. Petersen, K.-U. and Reuss, L. J. Gen. Physiol. 81:705-729, 1983.
24. Greger, R., Oberleithner, H., Schlatter, E., Cassola, A. C. and Weidtke, C. Pflügers Arch. 399:20-34, 1983.

ESTIMATION OF FREE WATER BACK DIFFUSION DURING WATER DIURESIS IN MAN USING LITHIUM CLEARANCE AND FUROSEMIDE EFFECT: SOME UNRESOLVED QUESTIONS

E.J. DORHOUT MEES, W.H. BOER, H.A. KOOMANS
Dept. of Nephrology and Hypertension, University Hospital, Catharijnesingel 101, 3511 GV, Utrecht, The Netherlands

INTRODUCTION

The only way to localize tubular action of diuretics in man is by clearance techniques. The clearance of solute-free water (CH_2O) is used to estimate NaCl reabsorption in the Loop of Henle and distal tubule. It is however well known that maximal CH_2O underestimates distal NaCl reabsorption because a substantial fraction of generated free water disappears by back diffusion (BD), even in the absence of ADH (1). Bartoli cs (2) have proposed to analyze tubular functions and BD using the effects of furosemide (F) based on the assumption that F: a) completely blocks NaCl reabsorption in the Loop of Henle, but not elsewhere, b) completely abolishes osmotic gradients in the medulla, and thus eliminates BD. Consequently, maximal urine flow during F measures distal delivery, and the fact that without F less urine is produced is due to BD. The proximal reabsorption (Rprox) can be calculated from distal delivery and filtration rate.

Recently, lithium clearance (CLi)has been proposed as a quantitative marker of proximal reabsorption (3). This notion is based on the following assumptions which are mainly supported by one micropuncture study (4): Lithium is reabsorbed in the proximal tubule (PT) at the same rate as sodium and water, but is not transported beyond the PT. Thus C_{Li} indicates fluid delivery to the distal tubule and the difference with flow rate represents BD of solute free water. Conversely, Rprox is given by lithium reabsorption. The present study was undertaken to test these two ("furosemide" and "lithium") hypotheses.

RESULTS

Five healthy males were studied during maximal water diuresis in the morning while recumbent. Clearances were calculated for each subject as the means of three 20 min. periods before and after furosemide 50 mg i.v.. The night before, 400 mg Li_2CO_3 was taken.

During the control period fractional lithium clearance (FCLi) exceeded fractional urine flow by 19% (table I). This amount must have diffused back if FCLi indicates fluid delivery out of the PT. After F fractional urine flow increased to 35%. If the F hypothesis is right, the increase (21 %) is due to abolishment of BD. Thus the estimates of the two methods agree fairly well. However after F there was a large increase in CLi, and the difference between CLi and urine flow remained. Thus according to the Li concept, there was no decrease in BD after F.

Table I. Some renal functional parameters before (c) and after (f) furosemide during maximal water diuresis.

	GFR ml/min	FENa %	FCH_2O %	Fvol %	FCLi %	F(Cli-vol) (=BD, %)
c	123 ± 4	1.4 ± 0.3	11.8 ± 0.8	14 ± 1	33 ± 0.8	19
f	140 ± 6	25.7 ± 1.9	7.9 ± 1.6	35 ± 3	56 ± 5.2	21

GFR = inuline clearance, F = fractional, ENa = sodium excretion, CH_2O = maximal free water clearance, CLi = lithium clearance, BD = back diffusion.

To analyze the F action further, we looked at other "proximal markers". Consistent increases in the clearances of calcium, phosphate and uric acid were observed and, as shown in table II, fractional reabsorption of all these substances decreased markedly.

Table II Fractional reabsorption (FR) rates of ultrafiltrable calcium (Ca), phosphate (Pi) and uric acid (ua) before (c) and after (f) furosemide.

	FRCa %	FRPi %	FRua %	FRLi %
c	99.4 ± 0.1	91.2 ± 0.2	91.5 ± 1.0	67 ± 0.8
f	92.0 ± 0.8	75.3 ± 1.7	85.9 ± 1.5	44 ± 5.2
Δ (%) fractional clearance	+++	+ 180%	+ 66%	+ 69%

DISCUSSION

The present study shows that BD of water during maximal ADH suppression assessed with two independent methods is about 20 % of filtration rate and Rprox is about 65 % in agreement with micropuncture studies (1). However, the fact that Li clearance was markedly increased by F can be explained either by a proximal action of F or by a change in Li kinetics beyond the PT. Thus both assumptions (a)"Li is an quantitative marker for proximal fluid reabsorption" and (b)"F acts only on Loop of Henle" cannot be true at the same time. In table III we calculated the changes in Li, NaCl and water transport that would result from both hypotheses.

Table III Consequences of both hypotheses (A) and (B) for furosemide induced changes (→) in "proximal" and "distal" fractional reabsorption (FR) of Li, NaCl and H_2O, based on observed urinary changes. Non-electrolyte osmoles have been neglected. FE = fractional excretion.

	(A) lithium transp.prox.		(B) furosemide only "distal"		
	FR prox %	FR dist %	FR prox %	FR dist %	FE %
Li	67→44	0→0	44→44	23→0	33→56
NaCl	67→44	32→31	65→65	24→10	1→25
H_2O	67→44	19→21	65→65	21→0	14→35

(A) If Li is only transported in the PT, the 23% increase in Li excretion after F would mean an equal increase in NaCl delivery to the distal tubule. This would account for nearly the whole F-induced increase in excretion. Thus "distal" NaCl reabsorption, generation and BD of free water would hardly change, and the inhibitory action of furosemide on Henle's Loop would only be expressed by a percent decrease in reabsorption (from 97 to 55% decrease in NaCl reabsorption and from 58 to 37% for water BD).

(B) When F acts only on Henle's Loop, the increased Li excretion of 23% must be due to blocking of Li transport at that site, implying that only 44% is reabsorbed proximally. This contrasts with micropuncture data (4). Moreover, the majority of micropuncture studies (5) have shown an inhibitory action of F on the PT. Our finding that clearances of other proximal markers are increased by F also favours this concept. Uric acid in particular, which is probably not transported beyond the proximal tubule, showed a percent increase of fractional clearance, which approached that of lithium (table II)

In sum our findings are not compatible with prevailing concepts of F action and Li handling at the same time. Complete acceptance of either hypothesis would lead to rather unlikely consequences. Probably, F has an important action on the PT, but also affects Li transport taking place in Henle's loop.

REFERENCES

1. Roy, D.R., and Jamison, R.J. Ch. 38 The Kidney. Raven press N.Y. 1985.
2. Carmine, Z., Bartoli, E., Curatela G. and Maggiore, G. Nephron 31:140-148, 1982.
3. Thomsen, K., Holstein Rathlou, N.H., and Leyssac, P.P. Am. J. Physiol. 241: F348-F355, 1981.
4. Hayslett, J.P., and Kashgarian, M. Pflügers Arch. 380: 159-163, 1979.
5. Seely, J.F. and Dirks, J.A., Kidney Int. 11: 1-8, 1977.

EFFECT OF OUABAIN AND ACETAZOLAMIDE ON PROXIMAL TUBULAR TRANSPORT IN DOGS.

E.S. STOKKE, J. ØSTENSEN AND F. KIIL

Institute for Experimental Medical Research, Ullevål Hospital, 0407 OSLO 4, Norway

Local application of ouabain in high doses may stop all tubular electrolyte transport. Ouabain administered in vivo in a dose inhibiting 80% of renal Na/K-ATPase activity, reduces transcellular NaCl reabsorption by 40-50% (1). A similar response is obtained by ethacrynic acid (3 mg/kg bwt) which selectively inhibits transcellular NaCl reabsorption without affecting bicarbonate and phosphate reabsorption (2). The purpose of the present study in volume-expanded, anesthetized dogs was to examine if ouabain during continuous ethacrynic acid infusion exerts any effect on lactate, phosphate and bicarbonate reabsorption. These anions are transported together with sodium mainly in the proximal tubules. In one series of experiments, acetazolamide, a potent inhibitor of $NaHCO_3$ reabsorption and associated NaCl reabsorption in the proximal tubules (3), was administered after ouabain. In a second series the order of administration was reversed. In all ten dogs plasma concentrations of lactate, phosphate and bicarbonate were raised to 9 $\pm$2, 2.4 $\pm$0.3 and 31 $\pm$1 mM respectively. Plasma pH was kept at pH 7.46 $\pm$0.03 and glomerular filtration rate (GFR) was varied by altering the renal arterial perfusion pressure.

Intrarenal infusion of ouabain (120 nmol/kg bwt) reduced at control GFR lactate reabsorption from 412 $\pm$86 to 291 $\pm$51 µmol/min (27%), phosphate reabsorption from 75 $\pm$18 to 43 $\pm$14 µmol/min (45%) and did not reduce bicarbonate reabsorption significantly, but reduced NaCl reabsorption by 21% and water reabsorption by 15%.

Acetazolamide (100 mg/kg bwt) reduced lactate reabsorption slightly more then ouabain (32%) whether administered before or after ouabain (Fig. 1). Phosphate reabsorption was reduced even more (54%). Acetazolamide exerted an additional effect after ouabain so that 74% of phosphate reabsorption was inhibited. Acetazolamide inhibited bicarbonate reabsorption by 55% and the associated NaCl and water reabsorption by 44% and 43% respectively.

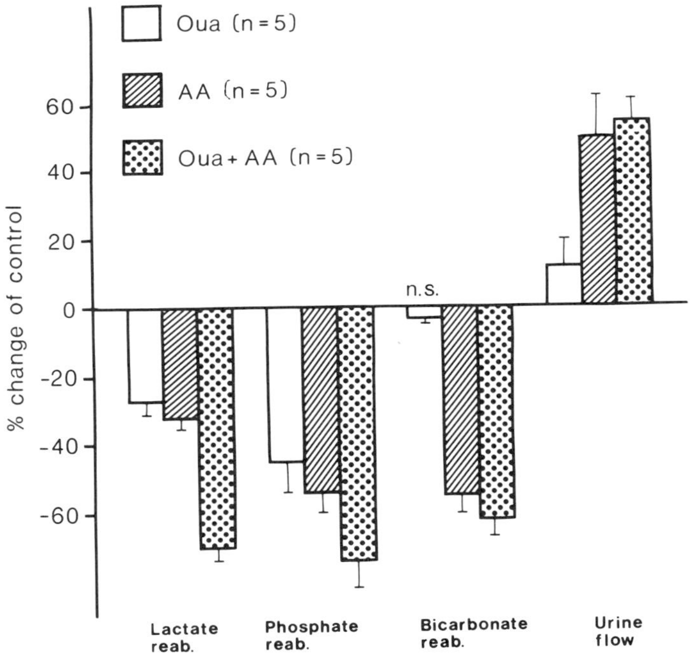

Fig. 1. Effect of ouabain and acetazolamide.

Thus, ouabain and acetazolamide, administrated in doses that are almost equipotent inhibitors of lactate and phosphate reabsorption, exert different effects on bicarbonate reabsorption. Although not inhibiting bicarbonate reabsorption, ouabain slightly, but significantly reduced the NaCl and water reabsorption remaining during continuous administration of ethacrynic acid. This response differs from that obtained in experiments in which the plasma concentration of phosphate and lactate were not elevated (4). It is possible that unreabsorbed salts of phosphate and lactate exert an osmotic effect and thus inhibit paracellular reabsorption of NaCl and water. Without lactate loading, acetazolamide seems to exert no inhibitory effect on lactate reabsorption (5).

REFERENCES

1. Sejersted, O.M., Mathisen, Ø. and Kiil, F. Am. J. Physiol. 232:F152-F158, 1977.
2. Steen, P.A., Hartmann, A. and Kiil, F. J. Pharmacol. Exp. Ther. 219:505-509, 1981.
3. Mathisen, Ø., Monclair, T., Holdaas, H. and Kiil, F. Scand. J. clin. Lab. Invest. 38:7-17, 1978.
4. Hartmann, A., Holdaas, H., Steen, P.A. and Kiil, F. Acta Physiol. Scand. 120:257-264, 1984.
5. Ullrich, K.J., Rumrich, G. and Kloss, S. Pflugers Arch. 395:212-219, 1982.

VOLTAGE-DRIVEN CALCIUM REABSORPTION IN DILUTING SEGMENT: INHIBITION BY FUROSEMIDE BUT NOT BY CALCIUM ANTAGONISTS

P. DIETL, H. OBERLEITHNER

Department of Physiology, University of Würzburg Medical School, Röntgenring 9, D-8700 Würzburg, FRG

ABSTRACT

The mechanisms of the calciuretic effect of furosemide was investigated in the diluting segment with electrophysiological methods. Furosemide completely inhibited Ca-reabsorption and reduced transepithelial voltage to zero. Ca-reabsorption revealed a linear voltage dependence. Nifedipine failed to block a transcellular route of Ca-reabsorption. From these data we conclude that Ca-reabsorption occurs paracellularly and furosemide reduces its electrical driving force.

INTRODUCTION

Using electrophysiological methods the cellular mechanism of Ca-reabsorption was studied in the diluting segment of the isolated perfused frog kidney which is a well established model of the mammalian thick ascending limb of Henle. The reabsorption process of NaCl creates a lumen positive transepithelial electrical potential difference (1,2) which therefore, is also called an active transport potential. Thus, reabsorption of Ca as a positive ion could occur simply by paracellular diffusion driven by the lumen positive transepithelial potential (3). It could also involve a transcellular process, such as a passive luminal Ca entry and an active basolateral Ca extrusion via Na/Ca-exchange or Ca-ATPase (4). The question was addressed whether furosemide exerts its calciuretic effect: a) directly by interacting with a putative transcellular Ca-reabsorption process, b) indirectly by eliminating NaCl reabsorption, and thus, diminishing the transepithelial potential difference. The former should also be affected by Ca-antagonists applied luminally, as Ca-channels should provide luminal Ca-entry into cells. This was examined using the drug nifedipine (5).

MATERIAL AND METHODS

Preparation

The right kidney of rana pipiens was removed and peritubular perfusion provided by inserting a catheter into the caudal vein. The lumen of a diluting segment was perfused via a glass pipette. Luminal and peritubular compartment were independently perfused with the following solution (mmol/l): NaCl 97, $CaCl_2$ 1.5, $MgCl_2$ 1, KCl 3, HEPES 3; pH 7.8.

Electrophysiological measurements.

A conventional and a Ca-sensitive microelectrode was inserted into the perfused lumen. Then the luminal perfusion was stopped. From the initial potential changes, luminal Ca activity changes and Ca net reabsorption (pmol. cm^{-2}. s^{-1}) were calculated. The limiting luminal Ca activity (luminal perfusion rate = zero) was compared to a peritubular Ca activity of 0.92 mmol/l. Paired measurements of Ca reabsorption and Ca activity were performed before and after addition of 5.10^{-5} mol/l furosemide and 10^{-4} mol/l nifedipine, respectively. Statistical significance was examined using paired t-test ($P<0.05$).

RESULTS

In a first set of experiments the ability of the segment to reabsorb Ca^{2+} and the inhibitory effect of furosemide were examined. Fig. 1 shows that under control conditions luminal Ca activity is almost half that of peritubular Ca^{2+} activity, whereas furosemide completely extincts this transepithelial gradient. Since we know that furosemide blocks NaCl reabsorption and reduces the transepithelial potential difference to zero, it was tested whether Ca reabsorption depends on transepithelial voltage. Therefore, we measured Ca net fluxes while generating various transepithelial diffusion potentials (by partial substitution of NaCl with impermeable ions). Fig. 2 clearly expresses a linear relationship between reabsorption and transepithelial potential. This phenomenon strongly suggests that: a) Ca movement occurs through the paracellular shunt-pathway. b) furosemide exerts its inhibitory effect by reducing the transepithelial voltage.

To exclude a putative transcellular pathway for Ca reabsorption, the Ca-antagonist nifedipine was applied to block luminal Ca entry into cells via Ca channels. Even at high concentrations (10^{-5} to 10^{-4} mol/l) nifedipine does not reduce Ca reabsorption. This indicates that the transcellular transport of Ca is unlikely.

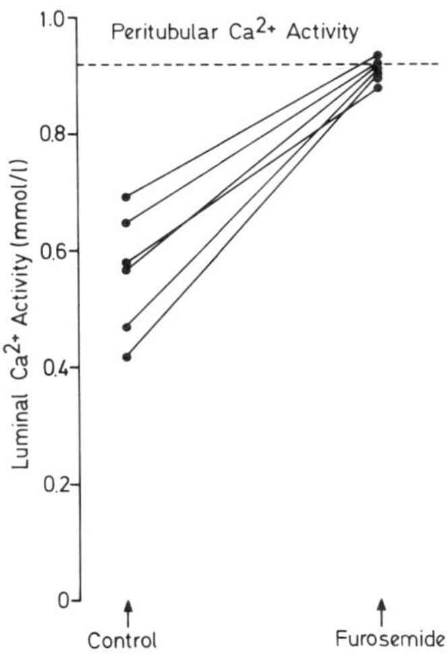

1

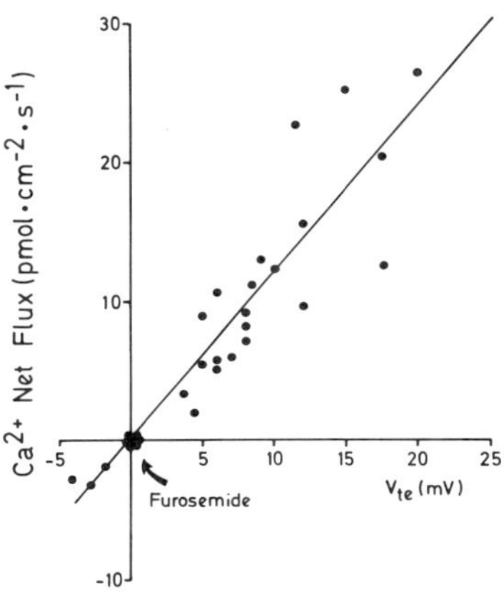

2

Fig. 1. Luminal Ca-activity measured at static head (luminal flow rate = zero). Concentration of furosemide = 5.10^{-5} mol/l.
Fig. 2. Ca-net flux at various transepithelial voltages (V_{te}). Positive = Ca^{2+} net reabsorption, negative = Ca $^{2+}$ net secretion.

Conclusions: Furosemide-induced inhibiton of NaCl reabsorption and of Ca reabsorption are linked: Inhibition of NaCl reabsorption (the primary event) eliminates transepithelial voltage; this in turn abolishes Ca^{2+} reabsorption (the secondary event).

Acknowledgement: This study was supported by DFG (SFB 176-A6).

REFERENCES
1. Greger, R. Physiol. Rev. 65 (3): 761-797, 1984.
2. Oberleithner, H., Guggino, W., Giebisch, G. Am. J. Physiol. 242: F331-F339, 1982.
3. Bourdeau, J.E., Burg, M.B. Am. J. Physiol. 5: F357-F364, 1979.
4. Imai, M. Pflügers Arch. 374: 255-263, 1978.
5. Fleckenstein, A. Ann. Rev. Pharmacol. Toxicol. 17: 149-166, 1977.

RELATIONSHIP BETWEEN Na,K-ATPase ACTIVITY AND TRANSCELLULAR NaCl REABSORPTION IN DOG KIDNEYS.

F. KIIL, A. HARTMANN, H. LANGBERG, O.M. SEJERSTED AND M. REE HOLTHE.

Institute for Experimental Medical Research, University of Oslo, Ullevaal Hospital, Oslo, Norway.

Ouabain inhibits Na,K-ATPase in all tubular cells, but is nevertheless a poor natriuretic agent. In hydropenic dogs only a slight natriuretic effect is found even after inhibiting more than 80% of Na,K-ATPase (1,2). It is possible that volume-expanded dogs respond differently, as illustrated in Fig 1.

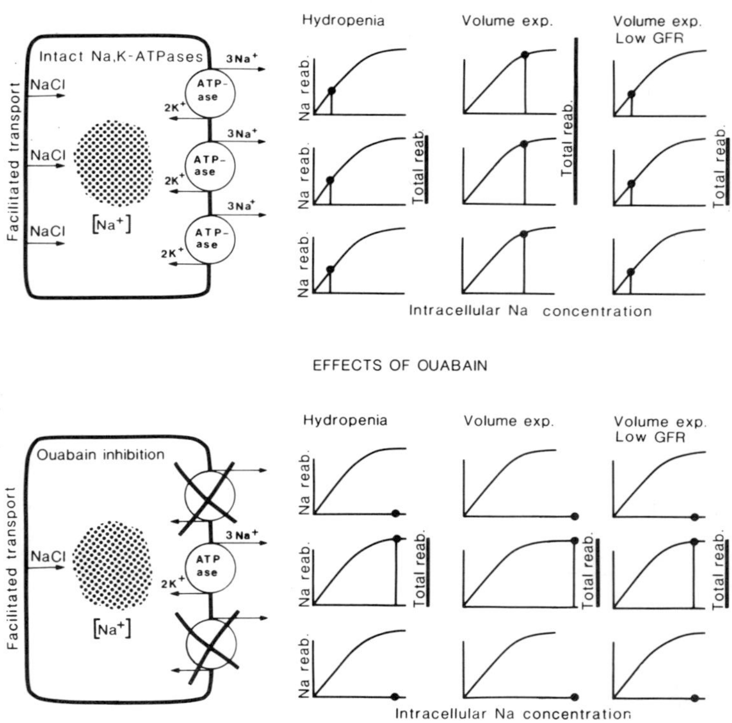

Fig 1. Schematic drawing of Na,K-ATPase kinetics.

When NaCl concentration is raised in the tubular fluid along the thick ascending limb, intracellular NaCl may approach concentrations which almost saturate Na,K-ATPase-mediated transport of sodium across the basolateral cell-membrane. Ouabain injected in a dose that blocks sodium transport in some Na,K-ATPase molecules, would by raising intracellular sodium concentration increase the turnover of the remaining intact Na,K-ATPases. In hydropenic dogs the natriuretic effect would be small because of this compensatory rise.

On the other hand, in volume-expanded dogs the transport capacity would be exceeded and even a small dose of ouabain might exert a natriuretic effect. After a large dose of ouabain the transcellular NaCl reabsorption would remain constant until the NaCl delivery to the distal nephron is greatly reduced. By applying various doses of ouabain to volume-expanded dogs, transcellular NaCl reabsorption would be inhibited in proportion to the intrarenal ouabain binding and in proportion to the reduction in Na,K-ATPase activity.

To examine these predictions clearance titrations were performed on anesthetized dogs. By administering acetazolamide (100 mg/kg b.wt.) prior to intrarenal injection of ouabain, $NaHCO_3$ reabsorption and associated proximal tubular NaCl reabsorption are greatly reduced and remain constant during mechanical reduction of glomerular filtration rate (GFR) (3).

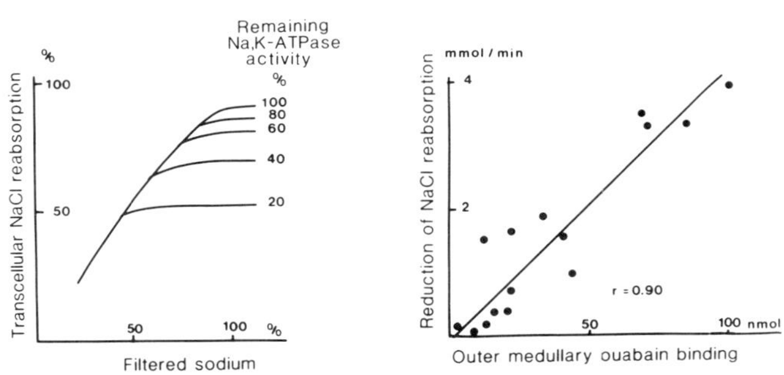

Fig 2. Effects of ouabain.

Fig 2, left panel shows that the inhibitory effect of ouabain on NaCl reabsorption increased as Na,K-ATPase activity was reduced. The remaining reabsorption stayed constant during reduction in GFR until the control relationship (100% Na,K-ATPase activity) between reabsorbed and filtered sodium was reached. After applying the highest dose of ouabain (120 nmol/kg b.wt.) NaCl reabsorption was reduced by 40-50% and stayed constant until GFR was reduced by about 50%. Fig 2 right panel shows that the reduction in NaCl reabsorption was correlated ($r = 0.90$) to ouabain bound to the outer medulla. Details are presented elsewhere (3).

We conclude:

1. Ouabain is a poor natriuretic agent until the transport capacity of the remaining intact Na,K-ATPases is exceeded.
2. In volume-expanded dogs receiving acetazolamide Na,K-ATPase transport rate is close to saturation and even a small dose of ouabain inhibits reabsorption of NaCl.
3. Under this condition the reduction in transcellular NaCl reabsorption is directly correlated ($r = 0.90$) to renal ouabain binding and inversely correlated to the renal Na,K-ATPase activity remaining after various doses of ouabain.
4. The transcellular NaCl reabsorption remaining after inhibiting 80% of Na,K-ATPase stays constant during mechanical reduction of GFR by 50% in volume-expanded dogs. At lower NaCl delivery from the proximal tubules ouabain exerts no natriuretic effect.

REFERENCES

1. Martinez-Maldonado, M., Allen, J.C., Inagaki, C., Tsaparas, N and Schwartz, A. J. Clin. Invest 51: 2544-2551, 1972.
2. Brady, J.M. and Neckay, B.R. J. Pharmacol. Exp. Ther. 190: 346-351, 1974.
3. Kiil, F., Hartmann, A., Langberg, H., Sejersted, O.M. and M. Ree Holthe, J. Pharmacol. Exp. Ther. In press.

DOSE DEPENDENCE OF INHIBITION OF PROXIMAL TUBULAR SODIUM REABSORPTION BY FUROSEMIDE IN CONSCIOUS RATS.

S. CHRISTENSEN, J. S. PETERSEN, E. STEINESS AND F. ANDREASEN*

Department of Pharmacology, University of Copenhagen, DK-2100 Copenhagen, and *Department of Pharmacology, University of Aarhus, DK-8000 Aarhus, Denmark.

INTRODUCTION

The loop diuretic furosemide (*Fur) exerts its major diuretic effect by inhibiting NaCl reabsorption in the thick ascending limb of Henle. However, many studies have suggested an additional effect of Fur on proximal tubular Na reabsorption, in particular when care was taken to minimize changes in renal hemodynamics due to diuretic-induced volume contraction (1). Very little is known about the dose dependence of the proximal effect of Fur, so this was investigated by clearance technique in conscious rats, using the renal lithium clearance as a measure for the delivery of Na out of the proximal tubule (2).

MATERIALS AND METHODS

Clearance experiments were performed in 35 conscious female 200 g Wistar rats restrained in plastic cylinders with catheters in the jugular vein and the bladder. Prior to experiments 0.5 mmol/kg LiCl was given orally. Urine was collected every 10-20 min and blood was taken from the tail tip every 40 min. Saline + ^{3}H-inulin was infused by 1.5 ml/hr throughout experiments.After a 1½ hr equilibration period and a 1 hr control period Fur (0.1 to 480 mg/kg; n=5 for each dose) was injected i.v. over 1 min, and clearance parameters were determined for another 2 hrs without replacement of volume losses. Electrolytes were determined by atomic absorption spectrometry, inulin by liquid scintillation counting and Fur by high performance liquid chromatography.

Assuming that C_{Li} equals the delivery of Na from the proximal tubule (2) the proximal fractional sodium excretion can be defined as:

---

*Abbreviations: Fur = furosemide; GFR = glomerular filtration rate; C = clearance; U = urine concentration; V = urine volume; FE = fractional excretion

$$FE_{Na\ prox} = C_{Li}/C_{In}$$

and the distal fractional sodium excretion as:

$$FE_{Na\ dist} = C_{Na}/C_{Li}$$

All presented data are mean values $\pm$ SE.

RESULTS

Fig. 1 indicates the time profiles for Fur excretion after i.v. bolus injection of different doses. Maximal excretion rates were always observed within 10 min after Fur administration. The excretion of Fur - and thus the delivery of drug to its tubular site of action - was not saturated within a dose range covering more than 3 decades.

Fig. 2 shows the time course for urinary sodium excretion after 3 different doses of furosemide. Maximal natriuretic response occurred within 10 min after injection, and both the peak value and the duration of natriuresis was increased with the dose of furosemide.

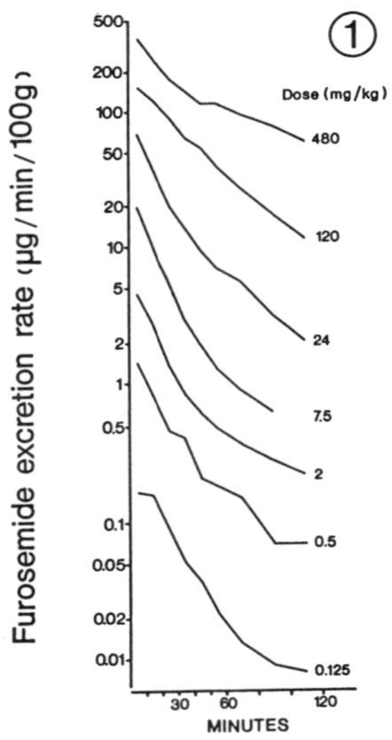

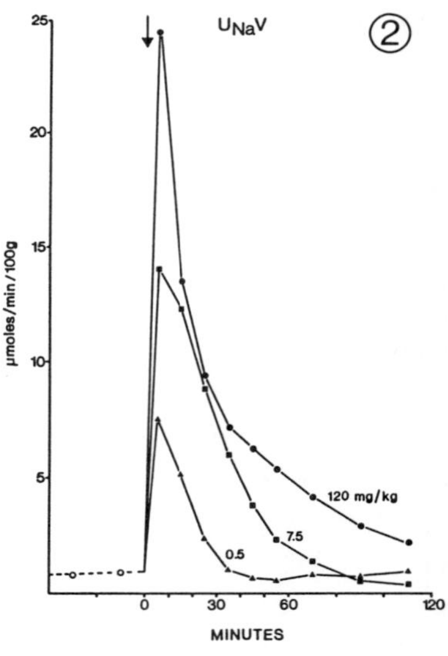

Fig. 3 indicates the changes in GFR after different doses of Fur. The GFR was not significantly changed during the first 10 min period where the peak response occurred, but fell abruptly after 10-20 min. The initial fall in GFR was largely independent of the dose of Fur.

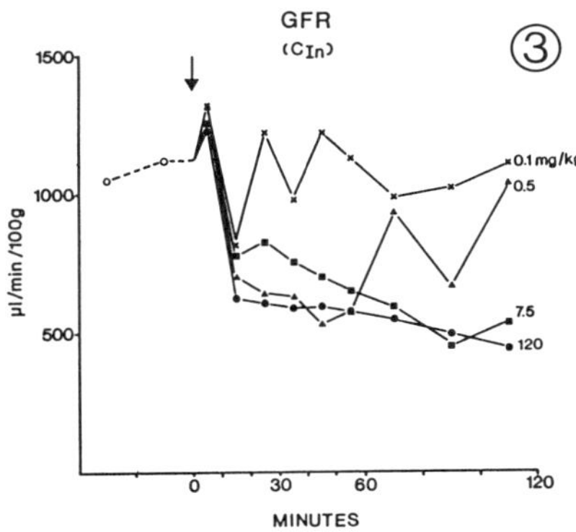

Figs. 4-8 show log dose response curves where the maximal changes in each parameter were plotted against the corresponding peak values for Fur excretion rate.

Urine flow (fig. 4) and total sodium excretion (fig. 5) increased rectilinearly with the log Fur excretion rate with only little tendency to saturation at the highest dose level (480 mg/kg) which was limited by the solubility of furosemide.

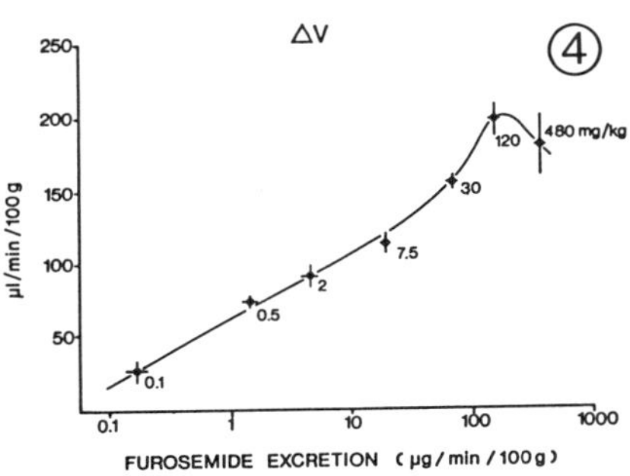

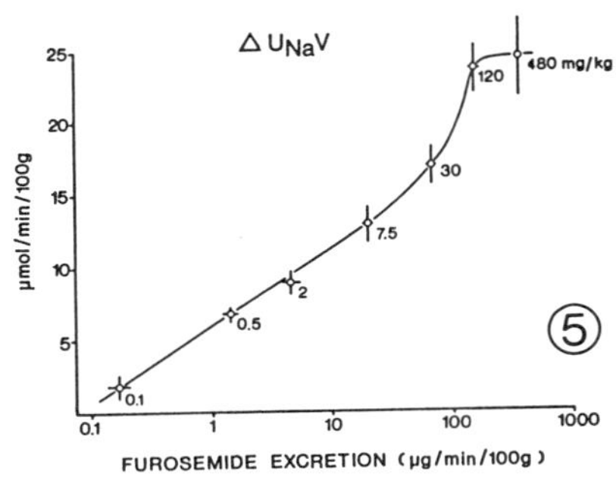

Fig. 6 shows the dose response curve for changes in fractional sodium excretion, indicating the inhibition of whole nephron sodium reabsorption. FE_{Na} was less than 20% after the highest dose of Fur, which according to the shape of the curve was submaximal.

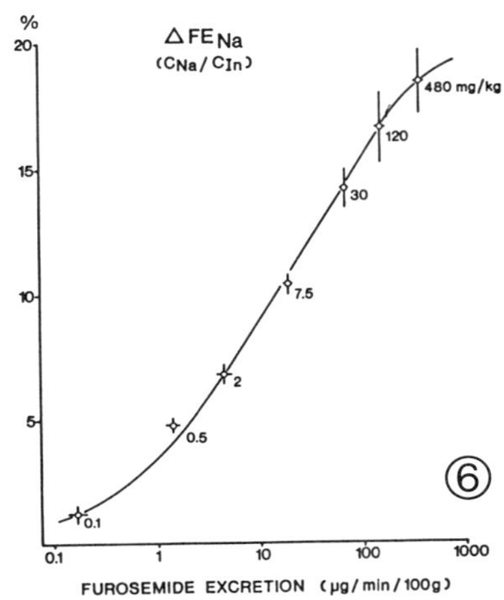

Fig. 7 shows the dose response curve for $FE_{Na\ prox}$, supposed to be an index for the fractional escape of Na ions from the proximal tubule. The curve suggests that proximal Na reabsorption was inhibited dose-dependently at low rates of Fur excretion whereas at higher rates there was no further inhibition. Maximal proximal effect was achieved with doses above 5 mg/kg and associated with excretion rates above 10 µg/min/100g.

Fig. 8 shows the dose-response curve for changes in $FE_{Na\ dist}$, which is the fraction of distally delivered Na ions being excreted in the urine. Within the dose range investigated there was no maximum for the effect of Fur on distal Na reabsorption.

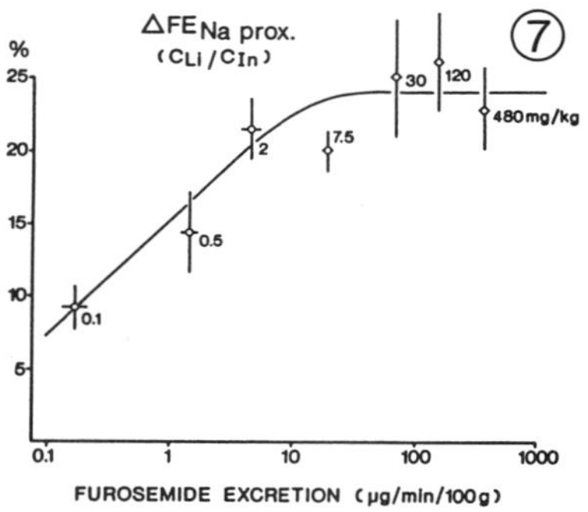

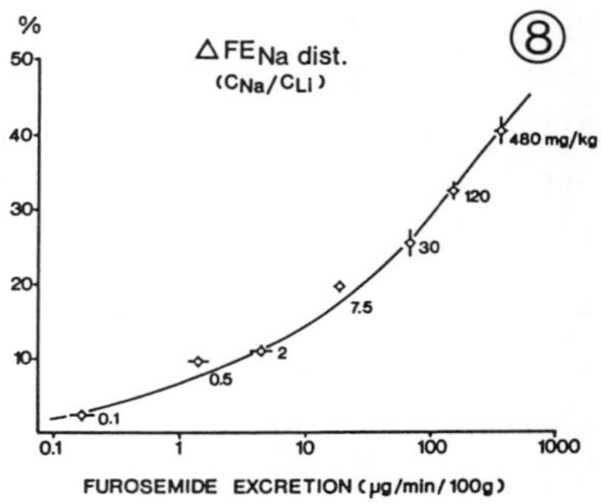

COMMENT

The interpretation of these results is based on the assumption that under Fur diuresis C_{Li} reflects the delivery of Na ions to the distal nephron (2; unpublished results). The findings may be summarized:

- The peak natriuretic response of Fur in conscious rats has a wide dose-dependence and is due to inhibition of Na reabsorption in the proximal tubule as well as in the distal nephron.
- Maximal inhibition of proximal tubular Na reabsorption is produced by relatively low doses of Fur (5 mg/kg ~ excr.rate 10 µg/min/100g).
- Within a dose range up to 480 mg/kg there is no maximum for the inhibition of distal tubular Na reabsorption.
- These findings are in variance with the general assumption that the proximal effect of Fur is only observed after high doses (1,3).

REFERENCES

1. Seely, J.F., Dirks, J.H. Kidney Int. 11: 1-8, 1977.
2. Thomsen, K. Nephron 37: 217-223, 1984.
3. Goldberg, M. In: Handbook of Physiology, Sect. 8: Renal Physiology (Eds. J. Orloff, R.W. Berliner and S.R. Geiger) Waverly Press, Baltimore 1973, pp. 1003-1031.

MODIFICATION IN RENAL HANDLING OF PHOSPHATE INDUCED BY HYDROCHLOROTHIAZIDE (HCTZ) AND AMILORIDE (A)

A.D'ANGELO,*A.FABRIS, L.MALVASI, S.GIANNINI, R.CASTRIGNANO, A.CECCONELLO, P.BENETOLLO, G.CREPALDI

Istituto di Medicina Interna, Università di Padova
*Istituto di Nefrologia Medica, Università di Verona

INTRODUCTION

Hydrochlorothiazide (HCTZ) has long been known as an effective hypocalciuric agent (1-3). When associated with amiloride,which has been shown to have hypocalciuric effect similar to that of thiazide (4),it may effectively reduce urine calcium excretion at dosages which are lower than those required by the single administration of each drug (5). For these reasons the combination of HCTZ and A has been widely used in patients with recurrent calcium nephrolithiasis (RCN). However,the mechanisms by which HCTZ and A act on the renal tubules are far from being clearly established and it is not known whether this drug combination may affect transport system other than those for sodium and calcium.

PATIENTS, METHODS AND RESULTS

The renal tubular transport of phosphate was investigated both in basal and after i.v. phosphate infusion in 10 patients with RCN and hypercalciuria,before and after administration of HCTZ and A,in 7 patients with primary hyperparathyroidism and RCN before and after parathyroidectomy and in 10 normal subjects.

In patients with idiopathic RCN basal calcium excretion averaged 332.7 ± 42.1 mg/day and it fell to 207.5±40.6 mg/day after 15 months of treatment with HCTZ,50 mg/day,and A,5mg/day. All patients had normal renal function. Mean urinary PO4 excretion was 918.9±126.4 mg/day before and 688.5±209.1 mg/day after treatment. Serum phosphate levels were 2.9±0.3 and 3.3±0.6 mg/dl,respectively.

An i.v.infusion of 3,430 mg of phosphate was performed before and 15 months after treatment. The TmPO4/GFR was below normal range before (2.2 ± 0.4 mg/100 ml) and rose to 2.7 ± 0.5 after treatment (t=3.61;p 0.01). Accordingly, the percent excretion of infused PO4 during the test time fell from 31 to 21% after treatment and serum PO4 peak from 11.5 ± 1.9 to 10.1 ± 0.9 mg/dl after treatment.

In patients with primary hyperparathyroidism (HPTH) and RCN,urine calcium and PO4 excretions fell from 304.2 ± 66 and 968.1 ± 118 mg/day,respectively,before,to 51.6 ± 16.7 and 346.8 ± 44 mg/day two weeks after surgery. Serum PO4 changed from 2.6 ± 0.5 to 4.1 ± 1.6. The TmPO4/GFR rose from 1.8 ± 0.2 mg/100 ml before to 5.1 ± 0.6 mg/100 ml two weeks after parathyroidectomy (PTX). Accordingly,the respective figures in percent excretions of infused PO4 were 25% and 18% (t=6.16;p 0.001). Serum PO4 peak rose from 10.4 ± 1.9 to 15.3 ± 2.3 mg/dl. The peak increase in serum PO4 during infusion in thiazide-treated patients was significantly lower than that recorded before treatment. On the contrary,after PTX the peak increase in serum PO4 was much higher than that recorded before surgery. The phosphate area was significantly reduced in patients with idiopathic RCN after treatment (Fig.1) whereas no change was observed in those with HPTH and RCN after surgery (Fig.2).

COMMENT

Our study shows that the combination of HCTZ and A, beside its well known hypocalciuric effect,may result in a significant reduction of the renal clearance of phosphate. In fact,urine phosphate excretion was reduced after treatment,and the Tm-regulated reabsorption of phosphate was increased after long term treatment with this drug combination.

However,the relatively large reduction in the percent excretion of infused phosphate was not apparently fully explained by the slight,though significant,increase in TmPO4/GFR.

On the other hand, the peak rise in serum phosphate during infusion was smaller after treatment than before and,accordingly,the phosphate area was decreased by this drug administration.

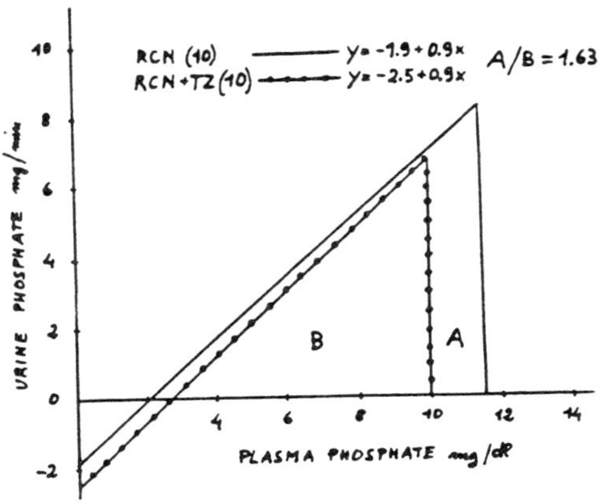

Fig. 1.

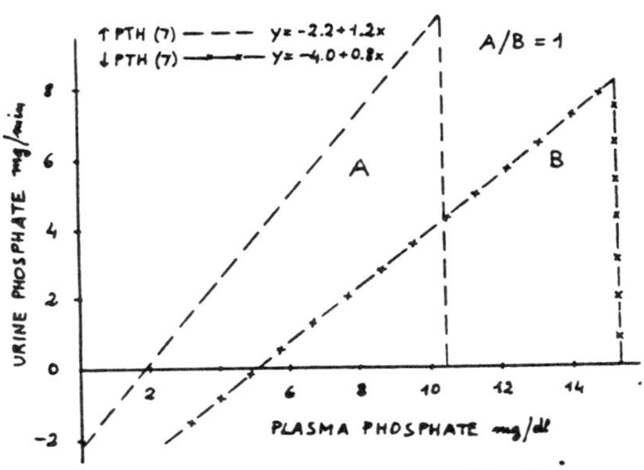

Fig. 2.

Conversely, in patients with HPTH,the phosphate area before and after surgery did not change despite significant modifications in both TmPO4/GFR and percent excretion of infused PO4. This is explained by the higher serum PO4 levels achieved with i.v. infusion after surgery. The less evident peak increase in serum PO4 observed in RCN patients after thiazide suggests a better utilization of PO4,possibly at bone level. The effects of thiazide on bone turnover are not fully understood,but the long-term administration of this drug has been shown to increase the mineral content of bone, at least in hypertensive patients (6).

REFERENCES

1. Coe, F.L. Ann. Intern. Med. 87: 404-410, 1977.
2. Yendt, R., Cohanim, M. Kidney Intern. 13: 397-409, 1978.
3. Pak, C.Y.C., Peters, P., Hurt, G., Kadesky, M., Fine, M., Reisman, D., Splan, F., Caramela, C., Freeman, A., Britton, F., Sakhaee, K., Breslau, N.A. Am. J. Med. 71: 615-622, 1981.
4. Costanzo, L.S., Weiner, I.M. Am. J. Physiol. 230: 67-73, 1976.
5. Maschio, G., Tessitore, N., D'Angelo, A., Fabris, A., Pagano, F., Tasca, A., Graziani, G., Aroldi, A., Surian, M., Colussi, G., Mandressi, A., Trinchieri, A., Rocco, F., Ponticelli, C., Minetti, L. Am. J. Med. 71: 623-626, 1981.
6. Wasnich, R.D., Benfante, R.J., Yano, K., Heilbrun, L., Vogel, T.M. New Engl. J. Med. 309: 344-347, 1983.

IV. PHARMACOKINETICS

INFLUENCE OF RENAL FAILURE ON THE PHARMACOKINETICS OF CICLETANINE.

P. JUNGERS, C. DIVINE*, J.L. DURAND*, P.Y. CHAMBRIN*, Ph. CHAUVEAU, T. LOUBARIS, D. GANEVAL, G. FREDJ*.

Departments of Nephrology, Necker Hospital and of *Clinical Pharmacology, La Salpêtrière Hospital, Paris, France.

INTRODUCTION

Cicletanine chlorhydrate (C) is the first of the furopyridines, a new class of antihypertensives. At low therapeutic doses C reduces peripheral vascular resistance and increases arterial compliance. At higher doses, a natriuretic effect is added. C exerts its antihypertensive action through vascular H1 and H3 receptors antagonism and increased prostacyclin release.

Pharmacokinetic studies of C in healthy volunteers have shown a mixed elimination, both hepatic and renal, with a mean elimination half-life of about 8 hours. As high blood pressure often is associated with impaired renal function, the aim of the present study was to investigate the absorption, distribution and elimination characteristics of C in patients with various degrees of chronic renal failure, by comparison with subjects having normal renal function.

MATERIALS AND METHODS

Patients

The study was performed in 12 healthy adult controls (aged 18 to 50) with normal renal function, i.e., creatinine clearance (Ccr) of at least 100 ml/mn/1.73 m2, and in 18 patients (aged 18 to 65) with chronic renal failure (RF). The latter were divided into 3 groups of 6 patients, according to the level of Ccr : mild RF (group I), Ccr (51-80); moderate RF (group II), Ccr 21-50, and severe RF (group III), Ccr 5-20 ml/mn/1.73 m2. All volunteered to participate and gave informed consent.

Study protocol

Patients received a single oral dose of 200 mg in the fasting state. Blood samples were collected pre-dosing and at 15,30,45,60, 90 min, and 2, 3, 4,6,8, 10, 24 and 48 hours post dosing (with additional samples at the 4th and 7th day in RF patients). Urine was collected 24 hours pre-dosing and 0-3, 3-8, 8-24 and 24-48 hours post-dosing (with additional samples

48-96, and 96-144 hrs in RF patients). Plasma and urine concentrations were assayed by high performance liquid chromatography, the sensitivity of the method being 50 ng/ml. Urinary conjugates were assayed after enzymatic hydrolysis with Helix Pomatia. Protein binding was determined by ultrafiltration method. Plasma time-concentration curves of free C were analyzed using a two-compartments open model with linear absorption and biexponential elimination.

RESULTS

Mean ($\pm$ 1 SEM) values for Ccr, plasma creatinine concentration (Pcr) and for pharmacokinetic parameters in the control group and in the three RF groups are shown in Table 1.

Table 1. Pharmacokinetic parameters (mean $\pm$ 1 SEM):

Parameters	control group	RF patient groups I mild	II moderate	III severe
Ccr (ml/min)	114 $\pm$ 4.5	59.1 $\pm$ 2.7	35.3 $\pm$ 3.1	11.3 $\pm$ 1.1
Pcr (μmol/L)	99 $\pm$ 5	190 $\pm$ 12	268 $\pm$ 35	640 $\pm$ 67
Tmax (hr)	0.65$\pm$0.09	0.83 $\pm$ 0.14	1.38 $\pm$ 0.53	2.1 $\pm$ 1.1*
Cmax (μg/ml)	9.2 $\pm$ 0.8	5.7 $\pm$ 0.9*	6.2 $\pm$ 1.3*	4.6 $\pm$ 0.9*
DV (l)	36.9$\pm$5.6	175 $\pm$ 39*	258 $\pm$ 84	205 $\pm$ 49*
CT (l/hr)	4.7 $\pm$0.5	7.0 $\pm$ 1.4	8.8 $\pm$ 3.3	1.8 $\pm$ 0.4*
T1/2 (hr)	5.6 $\pm$0.5	23 $\pm$ 7*	29. $\pm$ 7*	121 $\pm$ 41*
AUC (μg/ml.hr)	49 $\pm$ 5	45 $\pm$ 20	46 $\pm$ 17	92 $\pm$ 17*
Protein binding (%)	91 $\pm$ 1	86 $\pm$ 5	70 $\pm$ 11*	70 $\pm$ 8*

RF vs controls (Wilcoxon test) * $p < 0.05$)

A slower absorption (increased Tmax) and lower peak values (decreased Cmas) were observed in all RF patient groups when compared to healthy controls.

Distribution volume (DV) was markedly increased, especially in groups II and III, in parallel with a three-fold increase in the free fraction of the drug in the same groups. Total plasma clearance (CT) was significantly reduced in group III only, whereas apparent plasma elimination half-life (T1/2) was significantly increased in all groups, especially in group III more than ten-fold increase was observed. However, due to concomitant reduction in C max, AUC was unchanged in groups I and II by comparison with the control group, whereas a two-fold increase in AUC was observed in group III.

Total 0-48 hour urinary excretion accounted for 38 $\pm$ 4 % of the ingested dose in controls, 32 $\pm$ 8 % in groups I and II and 20 $\pm$ 4 % in group III. Despite the increase in plasma free fraction, urinary excretion of unchanged C did not substantially rise in RF groups (1.7 % of ingested dose vs 0.4 % in controls).

DISCUSSION AND CONCLUSIONS

In patients with mild or moderate renal failure, no major alteration in the pharmacokinetics of C are observed by comparison with subjects having normal renal function, because the opposite effects of decreased Cmax and increased T1/2 result in unchanged AUC and thus unchanged bioavailability of the drug.

By contrast, severe renal insufficiency markedly alters the pharmacokinetics of C. In patients with Ccr less than 20 ml/mn (group III), and in some group II patients with Ccr between 20 to 30 ml/mn as well, distribution volume and unbound fraction of the drug were greatly increased, whereas C max and total clearance were markedly decreased, resulting in a more than ten-fold increase in T1/2 and in a twofold increase in AUC.

In conclusion, bioavailability and probably metabolism of Cicletanine are greatly altered in patients with severe renal failure, whereas mild or moderate reduction in renal function does not significantly modify the bioavailability of the drug. Thus, the use of Cicletanine should be recommended only in patients having a creatinine clearance above 30 ml/min.

PHARMACOKINETICS AND -DYNAMICS OF PIRETANIDE IN CHRONIC RENAL FAILURE

A. Dörfler, W. Schulz, Klinikum Bamberg, III. Med., W. Lahn, D. Hajdù,
Dep for Clin. Research, Hoechst AG Frankfurt.

INTRODUCTION

Piretanide is a new high ceiling diuretic, acting like furosemide on the loop of Henle. In this study we examined piretanide pharmacokinetics as well as its diuretic, natriuretic and kaliuretic effectiveness in patients with different stage renal failure.

PATIENTS AND METHODS

Patients

Twelve patients with chronic renal failure were included in the study, divided into two groups. Group I consisted of 5 patients with a serumcreatinine of less than 4 mg% or a creatinineclearance of more than 20 ml/min. Group II consisted of 7 patients with a serumcreatinine of more than 8 mg% or a creatinineclearance of less than 10 ml/min. The age of the patients ranged between 20 and 48 years in group I and between 37 and 61 years in group II.

Piretanide administration

In the pre-treatment period of day 1 baseline values of diuresis and sodium and potassium excretion in urine were obtained.
On day 2, 60 mg piretanide were given intravenously during 30 min by an infusion pump. Days 3 and 4 were the wash-out period. On day 5, 60 mg piretanide were given orally as tablets after an overnight fasting period.
Safety parameters were obtained for each patient before the study, consisting of ECG, audiometry, serum electrolytes, renal retention values, liver enzymes, lipids, uric acid, blood glucose and blood count. Safety parameters were measured again 24 h after each piretanide administration.
Following piretanide administration blood samples were collected at 20 min intervals during the first 2 h, then at hourly intervals for a further 4 h. Urine was collected in hourly fractions for 6 hours after administration,

then in 12-hourly fractions for a further 36 h.

Assay methods

Piretanide in serum and urine was measured by a radioimmunoassay.

Statistical analysis

Results were expressed as means ± SD and were compared using Students t-test ($p < 0,05$).

RESULTS

Pharmacokinetics

Serum halflife of piretanide increased in patients with renal failure as compared with normal subjects (1), but there was no difference between the two groups with different stage renal failure. There was no difference in the elimination rate constant between the two groups. Total clearance of piretanide was the same in both groups. Metabolic clearance increased slightly in group II. Renal clearance decreased significantly ($p < 0,01$) with decreasing renal function in group II. Thus whereas in group I the recovery of unchanged piretanide in urine was 27% and 22% of the administered dose after intravenous and oral administration respectively, in group II only 3% of the administered dose was recovered following both intravenous and oral administration of Piretanide. In fig. 1, serum concentrations of piretanide are shown. The time courses of piretanide concentrations were very similar in both groups after intravenous and after oral administration. In both groups and after both administration routes, serum piretanide concentrations had fallen below the limit of detection 24 h after medication.

Pharmacodynamics

Maximal diuresis as well as sodium and potassium excretion were found during the first hour after intravenous administration and during the second hour after oral administration of piretanide in both groups. Pretreatment values were reached 12 hours after medication in group I and 24 hours after medication in group II. In fig. 2, changes in urine volume, sodium and potassium excretion are shown relative to pretreatment values. The 24 h urine volume was more than doubled in group I and nearly doubled in group II. Natriuresis was also more than doubled in group I. In group II, the increase of natriuresis was 80% after intravenous administration, but more than doubled after oral administration. The excretion of potassium increased in group I by 60% after both administration routes, in group II by 50% after intravenous administration and 80% after oral administration. On days 3 and 4 a decrease of diuresis, sodium and potassium excretion was seen in group I. This rebound phenomenon was very marked for natriuresis and was still apparent on days 4 and 6, the day after oral administration. In group II, the rebound effect was very small and was only seen for natriuresis. The excretion of potassium was increased on all treatment days compared to the pretreatment values.

Safety

No clinically relevant changes in safety parameters were observed during this study in any patient.

CONCLUSIONS

Compared to normal subjects serum half-life of piretanide increases three fold in patients with renal failure. This value is not affected by the stage of renal failure. Renal clearance of piretanide decreases with decreasing renal function, whereas metabolic clearance shows a slight compensatory increase. Even in high stage renal failure, piretanide produces a strong increase in diuresis and natriuresis. The duration of these effects is dependant on the stage of renal failure. The effect of piretanide on kaliuresis is lower than on diuresis and natriuresis.

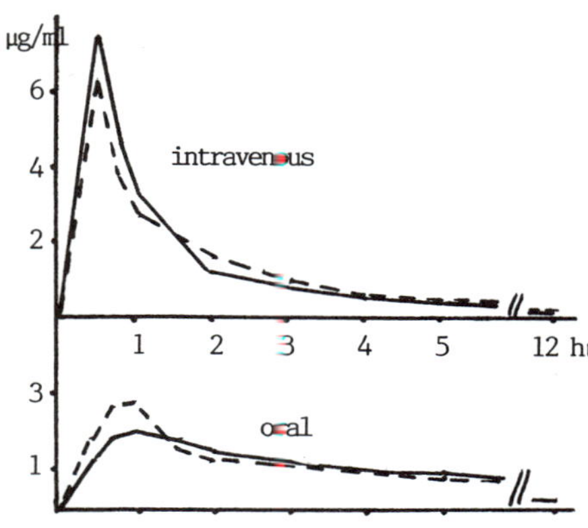

Fig.1: Serumconcentrations of piretanide
Group I: —— Group II: - - -

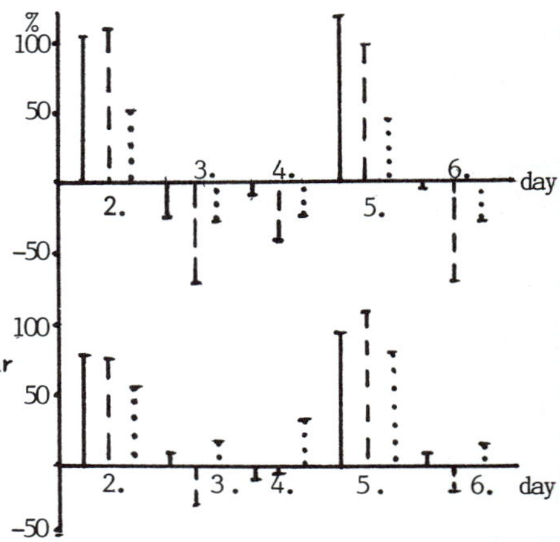

Fig.2: Changes in diuresis (——), Natriuresis (- - -) and kaliuresis (· · ·) relative to pretreatment values.

REFERENCES

1. Lawrence, J.R., Ansari, A.F., Elliott, H.L., Sumner, D.J., Brunton, G.F. Clin. Pharmacol. Ther. Vol 23, 5, 558-565, 1978

CHANGES IN FUROSEMIDE PHARMACOKINETICS INDUCED BY DEHYDRATION

Per Sjöström[1], Bo Odlind[2], Björn Beermann[3] and Margareta Hammarlund-Udenaes[2].

Department of Internal Medicine, Central County Hospital, Örebro[1], University Hospital, Uppsala[2] and Huddinge[3], Sweden.

INTRODUCTION

Furosemide (F) is active from the luminal side of the thick ascending loop of Henle (1, 2). Changes in its renal clearance (C_r) should therefore influence the diuretic response. F has a C_r of around 100 ml/min and a somewhat lower nonrenal clearance (3). Binding of F to plasma albumin is very high (98 to 99 %; ref.3), and the major part of its C_r is due to active tubular secretion by the organic acid transport system (2). This communication concerns changes in F pharmacokinetics, particularly factors behind reduced renal delivery of F as seen during dehydration.

MATERIALS AND METHODS

Eight healthy male volunteers were given a bolus dose (10 mg) followed by a constant infusion (8 mg/hr) of F during 5 hours. After two hours of dehydration without fluid replacement, the subjects were rapidly rehydrated and kept in isovolemia by intravenous saline and water orally. The study periods were the last hour of dehydration (dehydrated state, DS) and hour 4 and 5 (rehydrated state, RS). Clearances of inulin, PAH and F were determined in 30 minutes periods. F was determined with HPLC (4).

RESULTS AND DISCUSSION

The table shows mean values (S.D.) and significant differences (t-test for paired samples; *** = $p < 0.001$, ** = $p < 0.01$).

	DS		RS	
C_{Inulin}	92 (14)	***	109 (14)	ml/min * 1.73 m^2
C_{PAH}	402 (160)	**	622 (199)	"
C_{F}, renal	71 (17)	***	109 (27)	"
C_{F}, nonrenal	65 (15)	n.s.	65 (21)	"
U_F*V	66 (11)	**	79 (15)	µg/min * 1.73 m^2
P_F	1.0 (0.2)	***	0.8 (0.2)	µg/ml
$P_{albumin}$	48.2 (1.4)	***	40.4 (1.5)	g/l

In DS the subjects had lost 1.7+/-0.3 kg and the plasma volume had dropped 14+/-4 % according to plasma albumin. In RS body weight and plasma volume were equal to starting values.

The change in C_r of F followed the same pattern as that of inulin and PAH . The change in GFR can not explain the increase in C_r of F, since only 1 - 2 % of plasma F is filtered freely. However, since there is avid tubular secretion of F the changes in renal plasma flow should influence the tubular secretion rate. Unchanged renal extraction of F (C_F/C_{PAH}) of about 20 % speeks in favour of that.

It is of interest that the tubular secretion of F in the isolated perfused rat kidney has been shown to be restricted by protein binding (5). In a similar model Hall and Rowland (6) found a linear relationship between unbound fraction of F (fu) and its C_r. The conditions were, however, far from physiological (filtration fraction = 0.02 and F extraction 0.005). In clearance studies in nephrotic patients (7, 8, 9) there was no significant increase in C_r of F in spite of an increased fu. That means, that the nephrotic kidney has a decreased C_r of unbound F.

Our study gives an opportunity to discuss the consequences of changed proteinbinding to the tubular secretion of F in healthy kidneys.

A drop in plasma albumin causes an increased fu. In fact rehydration decreased not only the plasma albumin but also the filtration fraction (from 0.26 to 0.20), which means that plasma albumin at the site of secretion changed from 65.1 (48.2/0.74) to 50.5 (40.4/0.80) g/l.

The binding of F to albumin is assumed to obey the law of mass action. As the molar concentration of F in our study was low (2.5 µM) compared to albumin (700 µM) only the strongest binding site had importance (cf. 10). Therefore, it can be estimated, that the change in fu will be inversely proportional to that of albumin*, and that rehydration increased fu 19 % and 29 % in pre- and postglomerular blood, respectively.

C_r of F is related to fu, SC_{uf} and GFR**. Thus, C_r should have increased in proportion to the change in fu, if the other variables had

----

*) $F + A \rightleftharpoons FA$ (A=albumin); $[F]*[A]/[FA]=K$; $r=[F]/[FA]$; $r=K/[A]$; $r_1/r_2=[A_2]/[A_1]$. r approximates fu, when fu < 0.05.

**) Secretory clearance of F: $SC_F=C_F-fu*GFR$;
Secretory clearance of unbound F: $SC_{uf}=SC_F/fu$;
Consequently: $C_F=fu*(SC_{uf}+GFR)$.

been unchanged, which they were not (cf. ref. 6).

From our data and the estimated increase in fu (29%) the change in unbound secretory clearance can be calculated. That value increased 19 % from DS to RS, probably due to changed renal blood distribution and flow. There may be differences in F extraction among different nephron populations. The secretory surface may increase with the blood flow.

A change in the reabsorption of F should affect its clearance, but as the pK_a of F is 3.9, significant tubular reabsorption is unlikely to occur at tubular urinary pH values.

The rise in fu after rehydration also increased the volume of distribution and decreased the plasma F level. Initially this diminished the increase in F excretion rate (determined by the C_r and the plasma level). However, it was still significantly higher in RS compared to DS.

The pharmacokinetic consequences of dehydration can be summarized by looking at the fraction of a given dose excreted unchanged in the urine (determined by the renal/total clearance fraction), which in our study increased from 52 % in DS to 63 % in RS. At the same time the urine flow increased from 9.5 to 23.2 ml/min. Therefore changes in the renal sensitivity to F are more important than changes in the pharmacokinetics of the drug in determining the diuretic response in a dehydrated state.

ACKNOWLEDGMENTS

Dumex Ltd., Copenhagen, Denmark is acknowledged for financial support. We thank Mrs Lillemor Ek for skillfull technical assistance and Miss Lena Schneider for the F analysis.

REFERENCES

1. Burg MB. Kidney Int 9:189-197, 1976.
2. Odlind B, Beermann B. Clin Pharmacol Ther 27:784-790, 1980.
3. Andreasen F, Kjeldahl Christensen C, Kjaer Jacobsen F, Jansen J, Mogensen CE, Lederballe Pedersen O. Eur J Clin Invest 12:247-255, 1982.
4. Hammarlund MM, Paalzow LK. Biopharm & Drug Dispos 3:345-359, 1982.
5. Bowman RH. Am J Physiol 229:93-98, 1975.
6. Hall S, Rowland M. J Pharmacol Exp Ther 223:263-268, 1985.
7. Rane A , Villeneuve JP, Stone WJ, Nies AS, Wilkinson GR, Branch RA. Clin Pharmacol Ther 24:199-207, 1978.
8. Keller E et al. Clin Pharmacol Ther 32:442-449, 1982.
9. Smith E et al. J Pharm Sci 74:603-607, 1985.
10. Andreasen F, Jakobsen P. Acta Pharmacol et Toxicol 35:49-57, 1974.

PHARMACOKINETICS OF TORASEMIDE IN MAN

E v MOELLENDORFF E BESENFELDER B KAUFMANN G NEUGEBAUER
BOEHRINGER MANNHEIM GMBH D - 6800 MANNHEIM Federal Republic of Germany

INTRODUCTION

Torasemide (1-isopropyl-3-[4-(3-methyl-phenylamino)pyridine]-3-sulfonyl urea) is a new potent loop diuretic. Its profile of action is similar to that of furosemide, but it is characterized by a longer elimination half-life and thus a longer duration of action (1). The purpose of this study was to investigate the pharmacokinetics, bioavailability, and dose linearity of the kinetics of torasemide after administration of a standard-release tablet form.

MATERIAL AND METHODS

9 healthy male volunteers (age 19 - 44 years, weight: 67 - 109 kg, height: 168 - 184 cm) received in a three-way cross over-study in random order the following doses: 20 mg torasemide i.v. (1 hour-infusion), 20 mg or 40 mg torasemide p.o. The washout phase between administrations was one week. Torasemide was measured in plasma and urine up to 24 hr.

Heparinized blood samples were centrifuged immediately after collection. Plasma and urine aliquots were kept frozen at $-20^{o}C$ until analyzed. After extraction torasemide was determined by HPLC under gradient elution conditions and photometric detection. The detection limit in plasma and urine was 40 ng/ml, the assay variability was 8.5 %.

Kinetic evaluation was performed in conventional manner (AUC by trapezoidal rule, λ_z by the log-linear regression procedure). Since only in a minor part of the subjects torasemide could be detected in the 24 hr plasma samples, for the sake of uniformity λ_z was calculated by ommitting the 24 hr values. Kinetic data are expressed as medians and range or quantiles.

RESULTS (see Table 1)

The concentration maxima are reached at about 1 hour. Concentration maximum and AUC increase twofold after 40 mg torasemide in comparison to the 20 mg-dose. The elimination half-life is about 3 (p.o.) to 4 (i.v.) hours which corresponds well with the half lives in urine. The mean residence time is about 3 hours. The total clearance is about 40 ml/min, the distribution volume 16 l. The amounts excreted unchanged in the urine are 25 % (i.v.) and 20 % (p.o.) in 24 hours, the renal clearance is 10 ml/min. The bioavailability can be calculated for the two oral doses as 76 and 81 % from the plasma-AUC's and as 89 and 82 % from the amounts excreted in the urine.

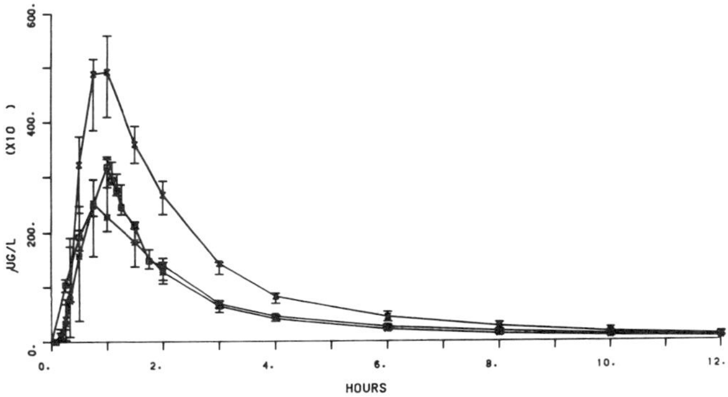

Fig 1 Plasma concentrations of torasemide (Median values, 25 % and 75 % quantiles) [] 20 mg i.v. * 20 mg p.o. x 40 mg p.o.

	C_{max} [/ug/l]	t_{max} [hr]	$AUC_{0-\infty}$ [/ugxhr/l]	$t_{1/2}$ [hr]	MRT* [hr]	Cl [ml/min]
20 mg i.v.	3178 (2743-3809)	1.00 (1.00-1.08)	8143 (5905-9341)	3.80 (2.52-5.95)	2.83 (2.47-3.97)	40.94 (36-56)
20 mg p.o.	2722 (1188-4077)	1.00 (0.33-2.00)	6292 (3776-8867)	3.16 (2.00-4.07)	2.80 (2.14-3.62)	--- ---
40 mg p.o.	5106 (3592-6083)	1.00 (0.50-1.50)	13197 (8803-14892)	3.03 (2.12-3.79)	2.89 (2.41-3.28)	--- ---

* MRT = mean residence time

	V_z [l]	F plasma [%]	Cl_R [ml/min]	$t_{1/2}$urine [hr]	Ae_{0-24hr} [%]	F urine [%]
20 mg i.v.	15.52 (9.07-20.98)	100	9.28 (8.81-13.40)	3.18 (2.64-3.56)	24.82 (17.68-29.44)	100
20 mg p.o.	--- ---	76 (58-107)	(n=7) 10.35 (6.69-15.97)	(n=7) 2.99 (2.18-4.11)	(n=7)20.57 (16.00-28.00)	89 (56-123)
40 mg p.o.	--- ---	81 (54-106)	10.46 (8.11-13.58)	3.28 (2.40-3.86)	21.35 (14.10-25.14)	82 (62-109)

Table 1 Pharmacokinetic parameters of torasemide (Median values and range)

CONCLUSIONS

The absorption of torasemide is fast and nearly complete. Plasma and urine elimination half-lives of 3-4 hr indicate long diuretic action. Torasemide exhibits dose-linear kinetics. The distribution volume of torasemide corresponds to the extracellular space. Renal clearance contributes only 25 % to the overall low systemic clearance.

REFERENCE

1. Lesne M, Clerckx-Braun F, Duhoux P, Ypersèle de Strihou Ch van, Int J Clin Pharmacol Ther Tox 20: 382 - 387 (1982)

FUROSEMIDE BLUNTS HYDROCHLOROTHIAZIDE (HCT) EFFECT.

R.FAEDDA, G.F.BRANCA, G.SERRA, A.SATTA, E.BARTOLI.

Istituto di Patologia Medica, Università di Sassari, Viale San Pietro 12 - 07100 Sassari, Italy.

INTRODUCTION

Our mathematical calculations for CH_2O fractionization allow us to calculate transport by the different segments of the nephron (1,2). A possible objection to the validity of this method could be brought by the pharmacological action of furosemide (F). By increasing the Na and Cl concentration in the thiazide-sensitive segment, the diuretic would indeed stimulate reabsorption, causing a spurious elevation in CH_2O-DT. The purpose of the present study is to verify this phenomenon by measuring the CH_2O-DT with our method before and after inhibiting the reabsorption in the thiazide-sensitive tract with HCT (3). If in fact the CH_2O-DT inhibition were greater when HCT is administered after F, this data could prove the hypothesis of a spuriously high value created by the large saline delivery induced by the loop diuretic.

MATERIALS AND METHODS

The experiment was carried out on 12 healthy subjects, 25 to 55 years old. All the patients were subjected to maximal water diuresis, as previously described (4). At the peak of diuresis, two consecutive clearance periods, lasting 10 minutes, were performed and the maintenance infusion (hypotonic solution) regulated according to the urinary flow. Urines was collected by a catheter inserted at the beginning of the test and kept in place for its duration. The distal block was obtained in 6 patients by administering at first furosemide (50 mg i.v.) and, once the clearances were performed, by injecting hydrochlorothiazide (50 mg i.v.). The time sequence was inverted in the remaining 6 subjects of the study. Osmolality and electrolytes were measured on urine and plasma samples. Urinary flow and GFR were calculated. Cosm, CH_2O, CH_2O-HL,

CH_2O-DT, CH_2O-BD were calculated and expressed in fractions of GFR x 100.

RESULTS

The results are reported in the following table:

Table 1. Effect of HCT giver either before or after furosemide.

	B		HCT		F	B		F	HCT
$\bar{V}$	15.5±0.8		16.9±1.9	*	34.0±2.2	15.7±1.1	*	30.7±3.2	31.7±4.0
Cosm	2.0±0.1	*	7.5±0.8	*	29.4±2.4	4.2±0.6	*	26.2±2.1	27.0±3.4
CH20	12.6±0.8	*	9.4±1.2	*	4.6±0.4	11.5±1.1	*	4.4±1.1	4.5±0.8
FENa	2.6±0.7	*	9.8±0.6	*	43.7±4.1	2.1±0.6	*	25.4±3.2	27.8±5.1

The table shows the results obtained during Baseline (B), and then during the subsequent injection of HCT and F. In the left hand side HCT preceded, while in the right side of the table it followed F. Means ± SE are reported. The flow data are in ml min^{-1} GFR^{-1} 100. $\bar{V}$=urine flow rate; Cosm=osmolar clearance; CH20=free-water clearance; FENa=fractional sodium clearance. The asterisks indicate the presence of statistical significance between adjeacent values.

The data show that both the fractional reabsorption of Na and the Cosm increased significantly more when HCT was administered before furosemide, and HCT caused a reduction of CH_2O only before F. The calculations of the fractional transportation of Na along the various segments of the nephron were not dissimilar: CH_2O-BD was 18.5±4.2 vs 14.7±8.5; CH_2O-HL 23.3±3.1 vs 21.8±2.3; CH_2O-DT 7.8±1.3 vs 4.4±0.9 ($P>0.5$ for all), confirming the validity of our calculation method.

DISCUSSION

Our calculation method of the distal sodium transportation, based on the known pharmacological properties of F, yields reproduceable data capable to pinpoint reabsorption defects in several clinical conditions (2,5,6). Perhaps the most important objection to this method stems from the fact that the first tract of the diluting segment of the distal tubule could compensate in part the inhibited transport in the loop. Therefore, CH_2O-DT could increase during furosemide, owing to the large rise in early distal Na concentration and gradient. If this were correct, the ratio of CH_2O-DT to CH_2O-HL calculated with the present technique, would be higher than that truly occurring, even though the calculation of CH_2O-T would remain unaffected. The results obtained by administering HCT before and after furosemide have surprisingly proved the opposite, that is that the diuretic efficacy of HCT is significantly reduced when this is administered after furosemide. It's possible that the high intraluminal sodium gradient following the Na load induced by F blunts the HCT action. For instance, the high chloride concentration could compete with HCT for receptor binding. Alternatively, Furosemide could compete with HCT for proximal secretion and partially inhibit it when given before the distal acting drug. While the present data do not disclose the reasons for the observed blunting of HCT effect by the preceding administration of furosemide, they do confirm the validity of our new technique and calculations. To the best of our knowledge there is no significant and detectable compensation of furosemide effect by the early distal tubule and there is no detectable spurious elevation of CH_2O-DT caused by the technique itself.

REFERENCES

1. Berliner,R.W., Levinsky,N.G., Davidson,D.G., Eden,M. Am.J.Med. 27: 730-744, 1958.
2. Bartoli,E., Satta,A., Faedda,R., Olmeo,N.A., Soggia,G., Branca,G.F. J.Clin. Pharmacol. 23: 56-64,1983.
3. Earley,L.E., Martino,J.A., Friedler,R.M. J.Clin.Invest. 45: 1668-1684,1966.
4. Bartoli,E., Arras,S., Faedda,R., Soggia,G., Satta,A., Olmeo,N.A. J.Clin. Pharmacol. 20: 452-458,1980.
5. Zoccali,C., Bartoli,E., Curatola,G., Maggiore,G. Nephron 32: 140-148,1982.
6. Satta,A., Faedda,R., Olmeo,N.A., Soggia,G., Branca,G.F., Bartoli,E. Renal Physiol. 7: 283-292,1984.

INFLUENCE OF RENAL INSUFFICIENCY ON THE PHARMACOKINETICS AND THE RENAL EFFECTS OF CICLETANINE

J. GOEFFROY, N. FERRY, N. POZET*, G. CUISINAUD, D. BENZONI, P.Y. ZECH* and J. SASSARD

Department of Physiology and Clinical Pharmacology, UA CNRS 606, Faculty of Pharmacy ; *Nephrology Clinic, Hôpital E. Herriot, Lyon France

INTRODUCTION

Cicletanide is a new antihypertensive agent with diuretic properties which have been postulated to rely partly upon the stimulation of the renal synthesis of prostacycline (1-2). In the present work, the kinetics as well as the effects of a single oral dose of cicletanine on the urinary excretion of electrolytes and of the metabolites of prostacycline and thromboxane A_2 were determined in patients with varying degrees of renal function.

MATERIALS & METHODS

Patients

After informed consent, 6 healthy volunteers (Group I), 9 patients with mild renal insufficiency (Group II) and 10 with severe renal impairment (Group III) were included in that study.

Protocol

Each overnight fasted subject received a single oral dose of 300 mg of cicletanine at 8 hr am. The first standardized meal was allowed at 12 hr. Plasma and urinary concentrations of cicletanine were measured using our previously described HPLC technique (3). Urinary 6 keto Prostaglandin $F_1\alpha$ (6KPGF$_1\alpha$) and thromboxane B_2 (TxB_2) the major stable metabolites of prostacycline and thromboxane A_2 respectively were measured by specific radioimmunoassays developed in the laboratory (4, 5).

The following model-independant parameters were calculated : maximum concentration (Cmax, µg/ml) ; time to reach (tmax, hr) ; apparent elimination half-life ((1/2, hr) ; aera under the curve (AUC 0-72, $\mu g.hr.ml^{-1}$) renal clearance (ClR, ml/min) and cumulative urinary excretion (CUE, mg). Results are expressed as mean ± SEM and statistical analysis used the Wilcoxon signed test.

RESULTS

Pharmacokinetics (see fig 1 and table 1)

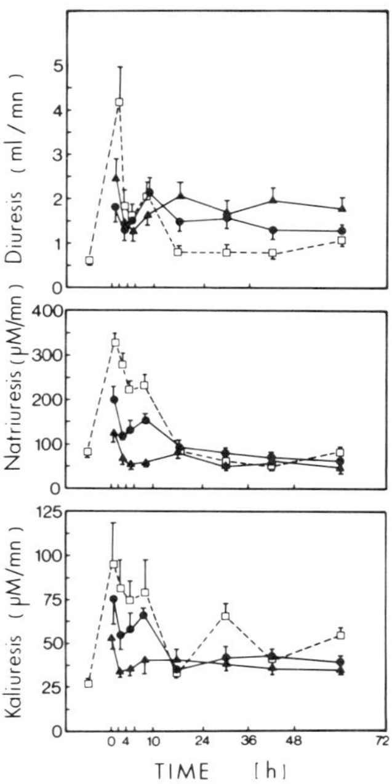

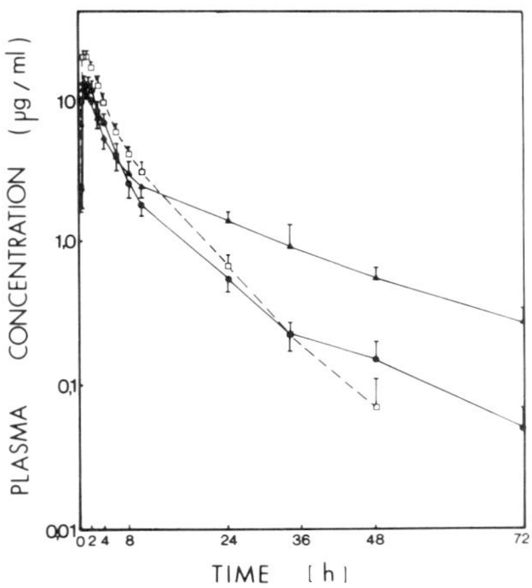

Fig 1 : Evolution with time of the plasma concentrations of cicletanine, of the diuresis and of the urinary excretion of Na+ and K+ in 6 healthy volunteers (□—□), 9 patients with mild (●—●) and 10 with severe renal insufficiency (▲—▲) having received at time 0 a single oral dose of 300mg of cicletanine.

Table 1. Glomerular filtration rate (GFR) and pharmacokinetics parameters of cicletanine in the 3 groups of patients studied. For abbreviations see text. (* $p < 0.05$; ** $p < 0.01$ vs Group I)

	GFR ml/min	Cmax μg/ml	tmax hr	t1/2 hr	AUC 0-72 $\mu g.hr.ml^{-1}$	ClR ml/min	CUE mg
G I	123 ± 9	20 ± 2	1.3 ± 0.1	7.4 ± 0.6	115 ± 19	0.42 ± 0.07	2.5 ± 0.4
G II	66 ± 9	14 ± 2 *	1.3 ± 0.2	12.4 ± 2.3	81 ± 13	0.65 ± 0.14	2.5 ± 0.4
G III	16 ± 2	13 ± 2**	0.95 ± 0.2	31 ± 8**	109 ± 15	0.19 ± 0.1*	1.1 ± 0.4*

In healthy volunteers, orally given cicletanine was rapidly and regularly absorbed. Its elimination half-life established between 5.8 and 9.9 hr. Mild renal insufficiency did not significantly alter the pharmacokinetics of cicletanine, excepted for a decrease in Cmax. Severe renal impairment was associated with an increase in its elimination half-life due to lowered renal clearance and cumulative urinary excretion. Positive relationships were found between the creatinine clearance and the renal clearance ($r = 0.72$, $n = 25$, $p < 0.001$) or the cumulative urinary excretion ($r = 0.73$, $n = 25$, $p < 0.001$) of cicletanine.

Electrolytes excretion (see fig. 1)

In healthy volunteers, a single oral dose of cicletanine induced a rapid and marked increase in the water (x 2), Na^+ (x 3 to 5) and K^+ (x 2) urinary excretion which lasted for 6 to 10 hr. Mild and, even more severe renal impairment reduced the drug effect on diuresis and natriuresis, while kaliuresis was less affected.

Urinary excretion of 6KPGF1α and TxB2

Renal insufficiency was associated with a significant decrease in the urinary excretion of $6KPGF_1\alpha$ (Group I : 14.2 ± 2 ; Group II : 8.9 ± 1 ; Group III : 5.5 ± 0.9 ng/hr) and TxB_2 (Group I : 3.3 ± 0.5 ; Group II : 2.4 ± 0.2 ; Group III : 1.6 ± 0.2 ng/hr). These values were found to be extremely stable and they were not influenced by the administration of cicletanine.

CONCLUSION

In conclusion the present work demonstrates that in patients with severe renal insufficiency the pharmacokinetics of cicletanine are significantly altered and its effects on the urinary excretion of water and electrolytes are decreased. In addition, it was shown that its pharmacological properties are unlikely to be related to major changes in the renal prostaglandins synthesis.

REFERENCES

1. Dorian, B., Larrue, J., Defundis, F.V., Salari, H., Borgeat, P. and Braquet, P. Biochem. Pharmacol. 33: 2265-2269, 1984.
2. Guinot, P. and Frolich, J.C. Arzneim. Forsch. 35: 1714-1716, 1985.
3. Cuisinaud, G., Terrier, M., Ferry, N. and Sassard J. J. Chromatogr. 341: 97-104, 1985.
4. Benzoni, D., Vincent, M., Cuisinaud, G. and Sassard J. Clin. Chem. Acta 126: 283-289, 1982.
5. Geoffroy, J. Benzoni, D. and Sassard J. Prostagland. Leuk. Med. 18: 393-399, 1985.

ACKNOWLEDGEMENTS

The helpful comments of Dr Tarrade and the financial support of IPSEN-BEAUFOUR laboratories are gratefully acknowledged.

A COMPARISON BETWEEN TORASEMIDE AND FUROSEMIDE EFFECTS AFTER APPLICATION UPON ONE KIDNEY OR AFTER I.V. INJECTION IN THE RAT

J. GENARD, R. PENNINCKX, B. CAPEL, R. LENOIR and R. KRAMP

Service de Physiologie, Université de Mons, B-7000 Mons, Belgium

INTRODUCTION

Torasemide, 1-isopropyl-3-{[4-(3'-methyl-phenylamino)-pyridine]-3-sulfonyl}urea, is a novel diuretic belonging to a new chemical series derived from 4-anilino-3-pyridine-sulfonylurea.

In the present study, the diuretic activity of torasemide and furosemide was compared using different modes of treatment, i.e. application upon the renal capsule, upon the renal cortex following decapsulation, or after i.v. injection.

METHODS AND CALCULATIONS

Anesthetized male Wistar rats weighing between 240 and 320 g were prepared as previously described with the left kidney exposed through an abdominal incision and each ureter catheterised (1). A solution of 5 % mannitol in isotonic saline was infused in order to maintain a control urine flow rate of approximately 40 ul/min/kidney.

Test-solutions were prepared as 200 ul of isotonic saline containing either placebo (time-control rats), torasemide (from 10^{-6} to 10^{-2} M) or furosemide (from 10^{-5} to 5.10^{-3} M). Following baseline determinations of urine flow ($\dot{V}$) and ion ($U_{Na}.\dot{V}$, $U_{Cl}.\dot{V}$, $U_{K}.\dot{V}$) excretion rates (control period), a test-solution was either applied upon the left renal capsule (A.L.R.C.), i.v. injected (I.V.) or applied upon the left decapsulated kidney (D). Urine was then rapidly and serially collected from the left and the right kidney (experimental period).

Net effects of the diuretics were calculated separately for the left and the right kidney by substracting the effects due to the mannitol infusion as well as the average of baseline measurements from urine flow and electrolyte excretion rates determined in each urine sample collected during the experimental period. The results are presented as peak and cumulated (15, 30 and 60 min after start of treatment) effects. Statistical significance was evaluated by variance and Student paired and unpaired t-tests, as appropriate.

RESULTS

General.

Experiments were satisfactorily carried out in 97 rats. No marked differences in baseline determinations of $\dot{V}$, $U_{Na}.\dot{V}$, $U_{Cl}.\dot{V}$ and $U_K.\dot{V}$ were found between the different animal groups. In 8 time-control experiments, $\dot{V}$ did change little from baseline measurements during the time course of experimentation. To the converse, as expected, $U_{Na}.\dot{V}$ and $U_{Cl}.\dot{V}$ progressively increased whereas $U_K.\dot{V}$ decreased.

Torasemide and furosemide treatment

Overall effects. Statistical significant changes from time-control experiments were found after left renal capsular applications of 10^{-3} M torasemide and 5.10^{-4} M furosemide and after i.v. injections of 10^{-4} M torasemide and 10^{-4} M furosemide. The effect of torasemide (~ 60 min) was somewhat longer than the effect of furosemide (~ 40 min). The peak diuretic response occurred sooner with furosemide treatment (~ 6 min) than with torasemide treatment (~ 12 min).

Peak effects and cumulated outputs. Peak effects (highest excretion rates in a timed urine collection) and cumulated outputs (15, 30 and 60 min after start of treatment) from the left and the right kidneys were calculated. Table 1 presents a comparison of diuretic potency for salient results upon diuresis and sodium excretion from the left kidney. Results from the right kidney were almost similar.

	T.		F.	T.		F.
		$\dot{V}$			$U_{Na}.\dot{V}$	
peak						
A.L.R.C.	10^{-2} M	$\ll$	5.10^{-3} M	10^{-2} M	$\ll$	5.10^{-3} M
I.V.	10^{-3} M	$\approx$	5.10^{-3} M	10^{-3} M	$\approx$	5.10^{-3} M
cumulated (60 min)						
A.L.R.C.	10^{-2} M	$\approx$	5.10^{-3} M	10^{-2} M	$\approx$	5.10^{-3} M
I.V.	10^{-3} M	$\approx$	5.10^{-3} M	10^{-3} M	$\approx$	5.10^{-3} M

No marked differences between left and right kidneys were found.
T = torasemide ; F = furosemide.

Following 10^{-3} M torasemide applications upon the left decapsulated kidney, peak effects and cumulated outputs were markedly enhanced (100 to 200 %) as compared to torasemide applications upon the left renal capsule. To the converse, cumulated outputs unexpectedly decreased (-20 to -70 %) following 10^{-3} M furosemide applications upon the left decapsulated kidney as compared to furosemide applications upon the left renal capsule.

COMMENTS

The results demonstrate differences between torasemide and furosemide related to the mode of treatment. The renal capsule is a barrier to torasemide since its transfer to the tubular site(s) of action seems to be impaired. Indeed, the effects of torasemide were markedly less pronounced after capsular application than after direct application upon the renal cortex or i.v. injection. To the converse, the renal capsule is greatly permeable to furosemide. Indeed, the effects of furosemide at equal concentrations were almost similar after application upon the renal capsule and after i.v. injection. Interestingly, cumulated outputs (30 and 60 min) were markedly reduced when furosemide was directly applied upon the renal cortex.

The results of cumulated outputs, 60 min after start of treatment, further demonstrate that torasemide is more potent than furosemide after i.v. injection or when directly applied upon the renal cortex although peak effects always occurred sooner after furosemide than after torasemide treatment.

REFERENCES

1. Kramp, R.A. and Lenoir, R. Distal permeability to urate and effects of benzofuran derivatives in the rat kidney. Am. J. Physiol. 228, n° 3:875-883, 1975.

V. ENDOGENOUS NATRIURETIC FACTORS

RECEPTOR BINDING SITES OF ATRIAL NATRIURETIC FACTOR IN BOVINE BRAIN MICROVESSELS

P.E. CHABRIER, P. ROUBERT, I. VIOSSAT, F. RODRIGUE, M. CANTIN* and P. BRAQUET.

IHB Research Labs, 17 avenue Descartes F92350 Le Plessis Robinson FRANCE.

*CRIM 110, avenue des Pins Ouest, MONTREAL, Québec CANADA H2 W 1R7.

INTRODUCTION

Atrial natriuretic factors (ANFs) have been isolated from secretory like granules present in the myocytes of mammalian atria. These peptides modulate blood pressure homeostasis, aldosterone production and extracellular fluid volume by acting as a circulating hormone (1,2). They possess potent vasorelaxant properties which are associated with ANFs binding to specific receptors in vascular tissues (3,4). Moreover, they counteract in many respects the action of Ang II. On the basis of evidence that ANF acts directly on vascular endothelium and since Ang II binding sites have been recently described in brain microvessels (5), we hypothetized that ANF receptors can also be present in brain microvessels. To test this hypothesis, radioreceptor binding of ^{125}I-labeled ANF (^{125}I-ANF) on pure and homogenous preparation of bovine brain microvessels was used.

MATERIALS AND METHODS

Isolation of bovine brain microvessels

Brain microvessels were isolated according to the method of GOLDSTEIN et al. (6) with some sligh modifications. All the procedures were carried out at 4° C. Briefly, after removal of the meninges by dissection, pieces of gray matter were scrapped from the surface of the cerebral cortex and gently homogenized in Ringer's solution containing 1 % B.S.A. The homogenate was passed through nylon sieves of graded porosity, centrifuged at 800 g for 10 min and then subjected 3 times to albumin flotation in 30 % BSA. The resulting pellets containing brain microvessels were filtrated on glass beads and rinced extensively with Ringer's buffer. The microvessels were washed 3 times by dispersion and centrifugation in cold buffer used for binding assay. Purity and homogenity of the microvessels preparation were assessed by phase contrast microscopy and by measurement of alkaline phosphatase and γ-glutamyl transpeptidase activities.

Binding assay of ANF.

Homogenate of brain microvessels were prepared in TRIS - Hcl buffer (pH = 7.4, 50 mM) containing 0.4 % BSA, bacitracin (0,02 %) and PMSF (0,5 mg/l) - ^{125} I-ANF (rat ANF [Ser 99 - Tyr 126] ; 28 AA, AMERSHAM) binding to microvessels was performed at 20°C ; specific binding was determined in the presence of 10^{-6} M of unlabeled ANF (rat ANF [Ser 99 - Tyr 126], 28 A.A, Novabiochem, switzerland). At the end of the 30 min of incubation, bound ^{125}I-ANF was separated from free ^{125}I-ANF by filtration through wathman GF/C glass fiber filters (WATHMAN). The filters were counted in a LKB γ-counter.

RESULTS

Bovine brain microvessels preparations, assessed by phase contrast microscopy, appeared free of identifiable neuronal and glial elements (Fig. 1). These microvessels consist mostly of capillaries less than 20 µM of diameter. In the present preparations, biochemical assay of alkaline phosphatase and γ-glutamyl transpeptidase which are though to be localized in small blood vessels in the central nervous system indicated that these enzymes were enriched 24 and 27 fold respectively when compared to the brain homogenate.

Preparation of microvessels was subjected to radioreceptor assay using ^{125}I-ANF. The results of a typical experiment with saturability of binding is shown in Fig. 2. Concentration of ^{125}I-ANF ranged from 10^{-11} M to 2.10^{-10} M. The Kd value and the maximum binding (B max) calculated by scatchard analysis were 1.72 10^{-10} M and 52,4 fmole/mg prot respectively. The reversibility of specific ANF binding to microvessels was shown by displacing ^{125}I-ANF binding by unlabeled ANF with a ki value for native ANF of 10^{-10} M. In comparison, no significant inhibition of binding of ^{125}I-ANF was observed with 10^{-6} M of Ang II, Met-enkephalin and Insulin.

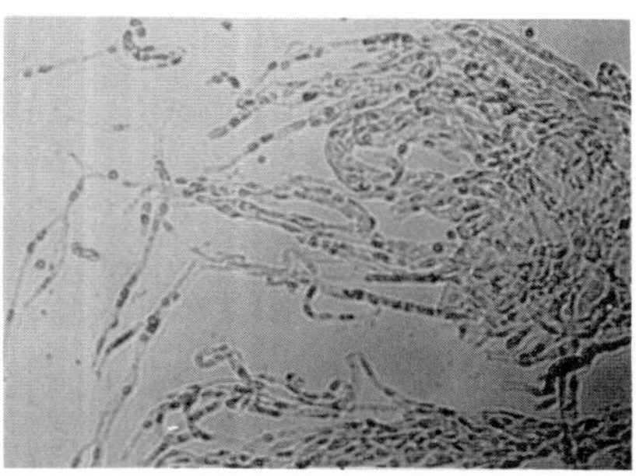

Fig. 1 : Brain microvessels (x400)

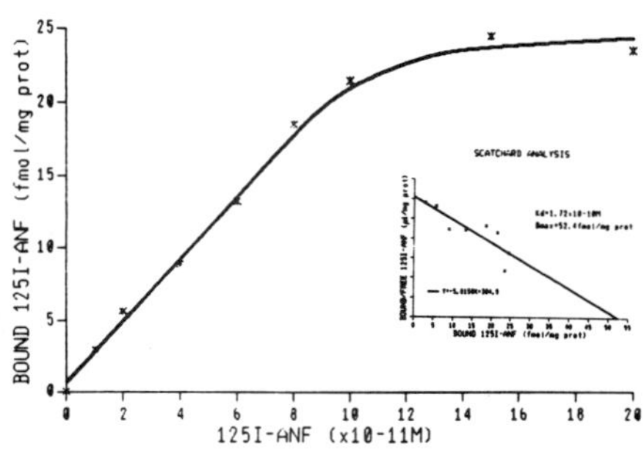

Fig. 2 : Specific binding of ^{125}I-ANF and Scatchard plots.

In an other set of experiments concerning association and dissociation rate of ^{125}I-ANF at 4°C it was observed that the peptide displayed a rate of association with a half life of 5 min and an apparent steady state after 30 min. Reversibility was also demonstrated by dissociation by 10^{-6} M of native ANF.

The specific binding of ^{125}I-ANF to bovine brain microvessels in the present study, fulfills many criteria for ANF binding sites. This binding is reversible, saturable and of high affinity. It could correspond well to a biological receptor of ANF since preliminary results show that ANF (10^{-8} M) elevates the level of cGMP on brain microvessels by 50 %. On the other hand, a recent study (7) in Montreal indicates clearly binding sites in all brain vascular beds in rat brain. Presently, there is no evidence for a physiological role of ANF in the regulation of the cerebral vasculature. This demonstration of ANF binding sites on brain microvessels constitutes a presumptive evidence for a physiological effect of ANF on the brain microcirculation.

REFERENCES

1. Needleman, P., Adma, S.P., Cole, B.R., Currie, M.G., Celler, D.M., Michener, M.L., Saper, C.B., Schwartz, D. and Standaert, D. 6 - Hypertension 7:469-482, 1985.
2. Cantin, M. and Genest, J. Endocrine Review 6:107-127, 1985.
3. Napier, M.A., Vandlen, R.L., Albers-Schönberg, G, Nutt, R.F., Brady, S., Lyle, T., Winguist, R., Faison, E.P., Heinel, L.A. and Blaine, Proc. Natl. Acad. Sci USA, E.H., 81:5946-5950, 1984.
4. Hirata, Y., Tomito, M., Yoshini, H. and Ikeda, M. Biochem. Biochem. Biophys. Res. Commun. 125:561-568, 1984.
5. Speth, R.C. and Harik, S.I. Proc. Natl. Acad. Sci USA 82:6340-6343, 1985.
6. Goldstein, G.W., Wolinsky, J.S., Csejtey, J. and Diamond, I. J. of Jeurochm 25:715-717, 1975.
7. Bianchi, C.,Gutkoskā , J., Thibault, G., Garcia, R., Genest, J. and Cantin, M. Abst. FASEB 512, April 21-26, 1985.

INTRARENAL LOCALIZATION AND PHOTOAFFINITY LABELING OF RECEPTORS FOR α-RAT ATRIAL NATRIURETIC POLYPEPTIDE

C. KOSEKI, Y. HAYASHI, M. FURUYA, Y. KANAI, N. OHNUMA, and M. IMAI

Department of Pharmacology, National Cardiovascular Center Research Institute, Osaka 565, and Department of Clinical Pharmacology, Suntory Institute for Biomedical Research, Osaka 618, Japan

INTRODUCTION

Although it has been well established that atrial natriuretic polypeptide (ANP) causes natriuresis by directly acting on the kidney, the detailed intrarenal distribution and characterization of ANP receptors are unknown. We examined intrarenal localization of receptors for α-rat ANP (α-rANP) in the rat kidney by *in vivo* (1) or *in vitro* (2) autoradiography, using ^{125}I-labeled ligand. In order to identify the receptors for α-rANP, [^{125}I]α-rANP was directly cross-linked to its receptors in isolated glomerulus, inner medullary collecting tubule (IMCT) rich fraction, adrenel gland, and aorta by direct UV-photoaffinity labeling (3). The purpose of this communication is to summarize the results of these recently reported studies.

MATERIALS AND METHODS

Male Sprague-Dawley rats weighing 200-250g were used for the experiments.

In vivo autoradiography

After 10^{-11}moles of [^{125}I]α-rANP (specific activity; 0.4-0.6 mCi/μg) with or without an excess of unlabeled α-rANP was injected into the aorta, the kidneys were immediately washed and removed. Frozen sections, or semithin or ultrathin sections were prepared for autoradiography.

In vitro Autoradiography

Frozen sections or microdissected IMCT were incubated with the ligand (4×10^{-10}M) with or without an excess of unlabeled α-rANP (4×10^{-6}M) for 10 min at 4°C, washed, dried, and apposed to X-ray filmes or nuclear track emulsion.

Binding Assay

Isolated glomerulus and IMCT rich fraction were incubated with the ligand. Apparent binding affinity (Kd) and receptor density (R) were obtained from their specific binding.

Photoaffinity labeling

After the binding assay, the samples were irradiated by UV lamp for 30min at 4°C. The photoaffinity labeled ligand-receptor complex was applied to sodium dodecyl sulfate (SDS)-polyacrylamide gel electrophoresis under the reduced condition, and the autoradiography was done to visualize the bands.

RESULTS AND DISCUSSION

The *in vivo* autoradiography was conducted to show the bining sites of a ligand under physiological conditions (1). The autoradiogram of cryostat sections of the kidneys which had been injected with $[^{125}I]\alpha$-rANP showed that the ligand predominantly bound to the glomerulus and the vasa recta of the outer medulla (1). Much less dense grains were distributed on the cortex,inner medulla, and renal pelvis. When an excess of unlabeled ligand was administerd two minutes before the injection of the labeled ligand, the density of grains was diminished in all sites, except in the cortical area other than glomeruli. High resolution autoradiograms of nuclear track emulsion-coated semithin sections revealed that the binding sites were distributed on the glomerular network, the arterial vasa recta of the vascular bundle in the outer medulla, and the vasa recta in the inner medulla. There were no bindings on the Bowman's capsule, afferent and efferent arterioles, or juxtaglomerular apparatus. The electron microscopic autoradiogram of the glomerulus showed that 65% of silver grains were distributed on the footprocess of the podocyte (Fig.1), suggesting that the action on podocytes may somehow be related with an increase in GFR by ANP.

In the *in vitro* autoradiography, much more dense grains than those in the *in vivo* one were observed in the inner medulla and renal pelvis as reported previously (2), in addition to the dense binding on the glomerulus. When the collecting tubules microdissected from the inner medulla were incubated with $[^{125}I]\alpha$-rANP with or without an excess unlabeled α-rANP, the specific binding was observed in this nephron segment. In this series of experiments, dense non-specific binding on the outer stripe of the outer medulla was observed.

The binding assay was done by using the isolated glomerulus and the IMCT rich fraction, which prepared by a sieving method and by a fractionation method with a Percoll density gradient, respectively. The specific binding was equilibrated after 10 min at 4°C. Scatchard analysis showed that apparent Kd and R in the former and later were Kd=3.2 and 21×10^{-9}M, and R=320 and 420

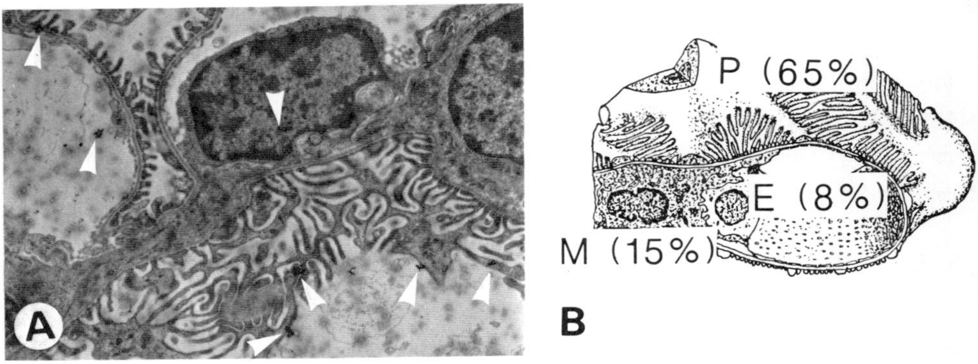

Fig.1 Intraglomerular localization of α-rANP by the electron microscopic autoradiography. (A) Silver grains(arrow heads) are mainly distributed on podocytes. (B) A schematic illustration of percent distribution of silver grains on endothelial cells(E), mesangial cells(M) and podocytes(P).

fmol/mg protein, respectively.

The autoradiogram of the photoaffinity labeled [^{125}]α-rANP-receptor complex showed the band of 65,000 daltons in the glomerulus and IMCT rich fraction(3). This band was displaceable with unlabeled α-rANP in a dose-dependent manner and not with 4×10^{-6}M angiotensin II. When the densitogram of this band was analysed quantitatively by the peak area, the inhibitory effect by unlabeled α-rANP was well consistent with that in the displacement assay using the isolated glomeruli. On the other hand, in the homogenates of the adrenal gland and the aorta, the cross-linked ligand receptor complex was observed as the band of 140,000 daltons, which displaced with an excess of unlabeled α-rANP. These data suggested that there are two different molecular species for α-rANP receptors depending on tissues.

REFERENCES

1. Koseki, C., Kanai, Y., Hayashi, Y., Ohnuma, N., and Imai, M. Japan. J. Pharmacol. *in press*
2. Koseki, C., Hayashi, Y., Torikai, S., Furuya, M., Ohnuma, N., and Imai, M. Am. J. Physiol. 250 (Renal Fluid Electrolite Physiol. 19): F210-F216, 1986
3. Koseki, C., Hayashi, Y., Ohnuma, N., and Imai, M. Biochem. Biophys. Res. Commun. 136: 200-207, 1986

ATRIAL NATRIURETIC PEPTIDE RAISE HEMATOCRIT IN CONSCIOUS NEPHRECTOMIZED RATS

J.P. FLUCKIGER, B. WAEBER, G. MATSUEDA, J. NUSSBERGER, H.R. BRUNNER
Division of Hypertension, University Hospital, Lausanne, Switzerland

INTRODUCTION

In 1981, De Bold and coworkers demonstrated that extracts originating from rat cardiac atria exert a diuretic and natriuretic effect when injected into rats. They also described a concomitant rise in hematocrit (1). It now appears that the rise in hematocrit induced by atrial natriuretic peptide (ANP) contained in atrial extracts cannot be fully explained by renal losses of water and electrolytes (2,3). In addition, preliminary in vitro studies carried out in our laboratory have shown that ANP does not modify hematocrit by increasing erytrocyte volume.

We recently hypothesized that the ANP-induced rise in hematocrit is due to an escape of fluid out of the vascular compartment (3). The aim of this study was to assess whether prostaglandins are involved in the hematocrit response to ANP.

MATERIALS AND METHODS

Male Wistar rats weighing 240 to 270 g were cannulated under ether anesthesia with a PE-50 catheter in the right femoral artery and vein and had their two kidneys removed. The rats were then allowed to recover for 120 min before starting the experiment. They were infused for 30 min with atriopeptin III (1 µg/min i.v.) 15 min after administration of a bolus-dose of either indomethacin (5 mg i.v., Group I, n=8) or its vehicle (Group II, n=5). In each rat, hematocrit was measured before and after the 30 min infusion. Atriopeptin II is an atrial natriuretic peptide of 24 amino-acids with the sequence of rat-ANP and has been synthetized as described previously (4). Data were evaluated by a one-way analysis of variance and a Student's paired t-test where appropriate. Results are reported as means ± SEM.

RESULTS

The 30 min infusion of atriopeptin III reduced mean blood pressure from 126 ± 6 to 114 ± 6 mmHg ($p < 0.01$) in rats pretreated with the vehicle of indomethacin (Figure 1). Acute inhibition of cyclo-oxygenase with indomethacin increased significantly mean blood pressure and did not blunt the blood pressure lowering effect of atriopeptin III. In rats given indomethacin mean blood pressure fell from 141 ± 3 to 122 ± 4 mmHg ($p < 0.001$) during infusion of the peptide.

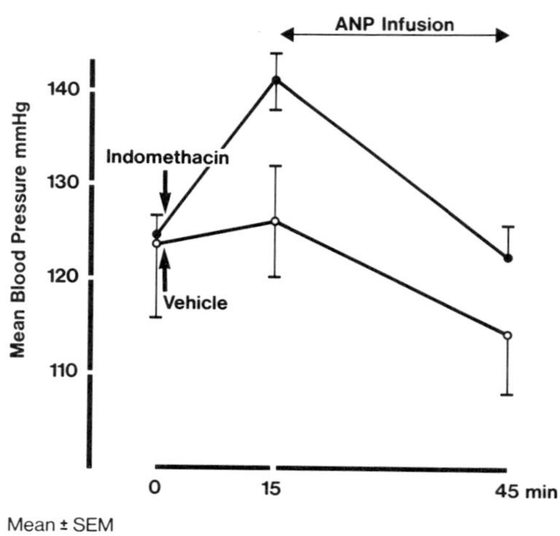

Figure 2 illustrates the effect of atriopeptin III on hematocrit in the 2 groups of nephrectomized rats. In control rats, hematocrit rose from 44 ± 1 to 47 ± 1 % ($p < 0.01$) during the course of the experiment. The magnitude of the hematocrit increase was similar in rats pretreated with indomethacin (from 43 ± 1 to 46 ± 1 %, $p < 0.01$).

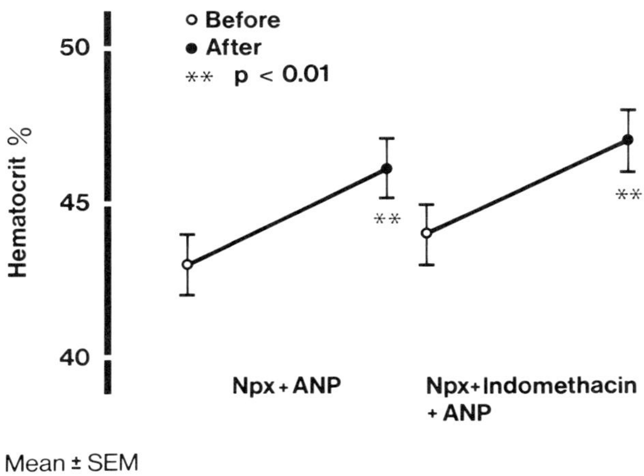

These data indicate that the presence of intact kidneys is not a prerequisite for the action of ANP on hematocrit, suggesting that these peptides shift volume out of the intravascular compartment. They also show that the ANP-induced increase in hematocrit is not influenced by acute blockade of prostaglandin synthesis.

REFERENCES

1. De Bold, A.J., Borenstein, H.B., Veres, A.T., and Sonnenberg, H. Life Sci. 28: 89-94, 1981.
2. Biollaz, J., Nussberger, J., Waeber, B., and Brunner, H.R. J. of Hypert. 1986 (In press).
3. Flückiger, J.P., Waeber, B., Matsueda, G., Nussberger, J., Brunner, H.R. Am. J. Physiol. 1986 (In press).
4. Waeber, B., Matsueda, G. Aubert, J.F., Nussberger J. and Brunner, H.R. Eur. J. Pharmacol. 1986 (In press).

TUBULAR EFFECTS OF ATRIAL EXTRACT AND OF ATRIOPEPTIN III IN CONSCIOUS RATS

H. J. KRAMER, J. KIPNOWSKI, B. STEKLE, A. BÄCKER, H. STELKENS, H. G. PREDEL, R. DÜSING

Division of Nephrology, Medizinische Poliklinik, University of Bonn, W-Germany

INTRODUCTION

The exact mechanisms underlying the diuretic and natriuretic effects of the newly discovered atrial natriuretic peptides (ANP) are still unknown. Hemodynamic effects, such as an increase in total renal plasma flow (RPF) or in medullary and papillary flow may contribute to its diuretic and natriuretic actions. In addition, a rise in glomerular filtration rate (GFR) by atrial extracts (AE) or synthetic ANP may lead to an increased tubular load of fluid and sodium (for ref. see (1)). However, since the diuretic and natriuretic effects may occur in the absence of changes in RPF or in GFR, a tubular action of ANP was postulated. The present study was therefore undertaken to investigate a potential tubular action as well as the sites of action of crude AE and of synthetic rat atriopeptin III (AP III; 24 amino acids) in conscious rats.

MATERIALS AND METHODS

Studies were performed in 24 conscious female Sprague-Dawley rats weighing 200 to 260 g which were fed a normal rat chow diet. The animals were anesthetized with methohexital (50 mg/kg body weight i.p.) and polyethylene catheters were inserted into the jugular vein (PE 50) and transabdominally into the urinary bladder (PE 90). During a 2-hour period for recovery from surgery and anesthesia, they were infused with 0.45% saline at a rate of 33 to 62 µl/min. Thereafter, all animals were given a priming dose of para-aminohippurate (PAH) followed by a continuous infusion of 0.45% saline containing PAH at an infusion rate to maintain a constant body weight throughout the experiments. After an equilibrium period of 60 min, during which urine was collected at 15 min intervals, six 2-min control urine collection periods were started. Subsequently, 1.0 ml of AE and of rat AP III, respectively, were infused over a 1-minute period and ten 2-min urine collection periods followed. At the end of the experiments the animals were anesthetized and blood was drawn from the abdominal aorta.

Atrial extracts were prepared as previously described (2) from tissue weighing approximately 300 mg. Synthetic rat AP III was provided as a kind gift by Drs. W. Bartmann and H. Hropot, Hoechst AG, Frankfurt, W-Germany. AP III was dissolved in 1.0 ml of the above infusion solution to result in doses of 40 ng, 1 µg, and 20 µg infused per 100 g body weight.

Endogenous creatinine clearance and the clearance (C) of PAH were used as estimates of GFR and of RPF, respectively. C_{PO_4} was used as a marker of proximal tubular function. Delivery of fluid and chloride beyond the proximal tubule to the distal diluting segments (DD = distal delivery) and distal fractional chloride absorption (DFA_{Cl}) were calculated as $DD = (C_{H_2O} + C_{Cl})/GFR \times 100$ and $DFA_{Cl} = C_{H_2O}/(C_{H_2O} + C_{Cl})$, respectively.

Statistical analysis was performed with a paired Student-t test and results are expressed as means ± S.E.M.

RESULTS

After infusion of AE or AP III a maximum diuresis of up to 10-fold that of control urine flow rate (V) was observed, whereas sodium excretion increased to maximum values of up to 50 times baseline sodium excretion. The maximum effects lasted only for two minutes and after 10 to 14 minutes the diuretic and natriuretic effects of AE and AP III had disappeared. After infusion of AE GFR increased by approximately 60%, C_{Na} and C_{Cl} more than 15-fold and C_{PO_4} and C_K more than 3-fold.

Infusion of 40 ng AP III per 100 g B.W. resulted in a rise in C_{PAH} by 32%, in V by 121%, and in C_{Cl} by 205%, whereas GFR, C_{Na}, C_{PO_4}, and C_K were unaltered. The higher doses of 1 and 20 µg/100 g B.W. resulted in a rise in GFR and in concomitant dose-dependent increases in C_{Na} and C_{Cl} (Fig. 1), and in V, C_{PO_4}, and C_K.

After infusion of AE DD rose approximately 3-fold from 2.4 ± 0.2 to 7.2 ± 1.0 µl/min per 100 µl GFR as did C_{PO_4}. C_{H_2O} increased from 56 ± 5 to 209 ± 25 µl/min. DFA_{Cl} decreased significantly from 0.94 ± 0.03 to 0.80 ± 0.07 ($p < 0.05$). Similarly, AP III at a dose of 1 µg/100 g B.W. resulted in a more than 3-fold rise in DD from 2.7 ± 0.1 to 8.9 ± 2.1 µl/min per 100 µl GFR in parallel to the almost 4-fold rise in C_{PO_4}. DFA_{Cl} decreased from 0.87 ± 0.03 to 0.54 ± 0.07 ($p < 0.01$). The lower dose of AP III (40 ng /100 g B.W.), which had no effect on C_{PO_4}, resulted in a slightly more than 2-fold rise in DD to 6.0 ± 0.1 µl/min per 100 µl GFR and a decrease in DFA_{Cl} to 0.81 ± 0.04 (n.s.) (Fig. 2).

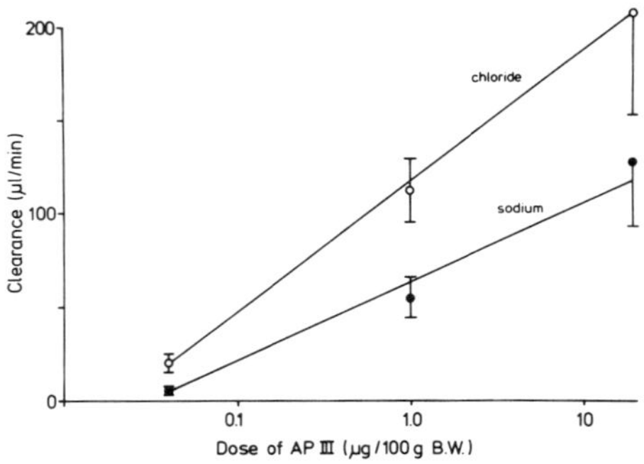

Fig. 1. Dose-dependent rise in the clearance of Na and Cl after injection of AP III.

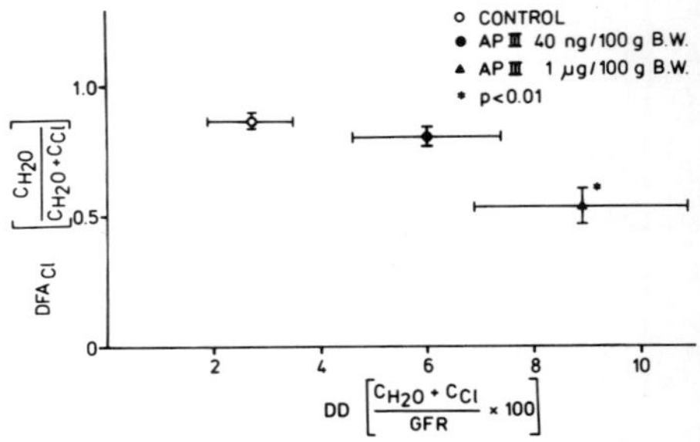

Fig. 2. Dose-dependent changes in DD and DFA_{Cl} after i.v. injection of AP III (Reproduced with permission from ref. 2).

DISCUSSION

In the present study AE and AP III increased RPF in all groups of animals. Low dose of AP III significantly increased V and C_{Cl}, whereas GFR, C_{Na}, C_{PO_4}, and C_K remained unaltered. The marked natriuresis at high doses of ANP was associated with a rise in GFR and in absolute and fractional C_{PO_4} as well as an increase in DD and C_K. AE and AP III (1 µg/100 g B.W.) decreased DFA_{Cl} from 0.94 and 0.84 to 0.80 ($p < 0.05$) and 0.54 ($p < 0.01$), respectively. These effects on loop function probably result from medullary wash-out which thereby contributes to the natriuresis by potentiating the rise in the filtered load of sodium and chloride at high ANP levels. In the absence of changes in GFR and C_{PO_4} the observed rise in C_{Cl} may result from decreased absorption in the medullary collecting tubule. In support of these hemodynamic effects high affinity ANP binding sites were detected in the renal vasculature (3) and in glomeruli (3,4). Whereas no binding sites were found in the loop of Henle, low affinity ANP binding sites were detected in the proximal tubule (4) and in the medullary collecting tubule (3,4).

REFERENCES

1. Kramer, H.J., Lichardus, B. Klin. Wochenschrift (in press) 1986.
2. Kramer, H.J., Kipnowski, J., Stekle, B., Bäcker, A., Predel, H.G., Düsing, R. Klin. Wochenschrift (in press) 1986.
3. Koseki, C., Hayashi, Y., Torikai, S., Furuya, M., Ohnuma, N., Imai, M. Am. J. Physiol. 250: F210-F216, 1986.
4. Healy, D.P., Fanestil, D.D. Am. J. Physiol. 250: F573-F578, 1986.

ATRIAL NATRIURETIC PEPTIDES AND RENIN SECRETION

E. Hackenthal, R.E. LANG, C.P. BÜHRLE

Departments of Pharmacology and Physiology, University of Heidelberg, Heidelberg, Germany

INTRODUCTION

In several studies in vivo, atrial natriuretic peptides(ANP) did either not affect(1,2) or induced a moderate decrease(3,4) of renin secretion from the kidney or plasma renin concentrations. In these studies, ANP produced significant changes of systemic and intrarenal hemodynamics and renal tubular function, all of which are known to participate in the control of renin secretion. It therefore remained unclear, whether ANPs have any direct effect on renin secreting juxtaglomerular cells. We have therefore examined the influence of atrial natriuretic peptide on renin secretion from the isolated rat kidney, in which interference by neuronal, hemodynamic, humoral, and, to some extent, also tubular mechanisms can be excluded. Part of the results have been published in preliminary form(5).

MATERIALS AND METHODS

Kidneys from male Sprague Dawley rats (160-200 g,Ivanovas,Kisslegg, Germany) were perfused in a single-pass system at constant pressure(105 mm Hg) with a modified Krebs-Henseleit medium containing bovine serum albumin(10 g/l,Boehringer,Mannheim) and hydroxyethylstarch(25 g/l,Fresenius, Oberursel) as oncotic substances, as described previously(5). Glomerular filtration rate was measured by the cyanocobalamine method, and renin in perfusates by radioimmunoassay of angiotensin(ANG)I generated during incubation of perfusates with rat angiotensinogen (see 5 for references).

The synthetic rat atrial natriuretic peptide APII(Bachem,Switzerland) has been used in most experiments. Some experiments have also been performed with API, APII and α-ANF(all from Bachem,Switzerland). Indometacin and haloperidol were from Sigma,München, hydralazine from Ciba-Geigy, Basel, and the phosphodiesterase-inhibitor 2-o-propoxyphenyl-8-azapurine-6-one (zaprinast, M&B 22948) from May & Baker, Essex, England.

RESULTS

APII and renin secretion. Infusion of rat atrial natriuretic peptide (APII) into the isolated perfused rat kidney at 0.3, 3, and 30 nM final concentration induced an immediate increase of renin release of 60, 130, and 140 %, respectively, above preinfusion levels(410±80 ng ANGI/h/min). Renal perfusate flow increased from 11.5±0.19 ml/min by 0.11, 0.42, and 0.43 ml/min, respectively, and returned to preinfusion levels during infusion. Glomerular filtration rate was increased at all concentrations.

APII and haloperidol. The natriuretic properties of ANP have been associated with renal dopaminergic D_1-receptors (7). We have therefore examined the response of renin secretion to APII in the presence of haloperidol, a D_1-receptor-antagonist. Infusion of haloperidol produced a slight stimulation of renin secretion, but did not affect the response to APII.

APII and hydralazine. Since stimulation of renin secretion by APII may be an indirect effect, secondary to the induced vasodilatation, the kidney was pre-dilated by infusion of hydralazine(10 µM). Hydralazine stimulated renin secretion by itself (+110 %) and increased perfusate flow from 10.5±0.58 to 12.8±0.32 ml/min. During the additional infusion of APII no further vasodilatation was seen at 0.3 and 3 nM, at 30 nM a small additional vasodilatation of 0.2 ml/min occurred. Despite this lack of significant vasodilatation the response of renin secretion to APII was even more pronounced at all concentrations than in the absence of hydralazine.

APII and indometacin. In order to exclude the possiblity that the effect of APII on renin secretion was mediated by the induction of prostaglandin synthesis and release, APII was infused at the same protocol as above on top of an infusion of indometacin 10 µM. In these experiments the response of renin secretion was higher than in the control experiments(78,118,and 165 % increase).

APII and ß-blockade. By infusion of APII, 30 nM, in the absence or presence of 3 µM propranolol, renin secretion was stimulated by 234±44 % and 251±46 %, respectively, whereas the stimulation of renin secretion by isoproterenol(0.1 µM) was significantly depressed by propranolol(from 613 to 134 % stimulation). This data excludes the possibility that APII stimulates renin secretion by inducing presynaptic release of norepinephrine, which is a well known stimulator of renin secretion by activation of ß-adrenoceptors.

APII and furosemide. In the presence of furosemide(10 µg/ml) the response of renin secretion to the infusion of APII remained unaltered, making it unlikely that APII exerts it's effect on renin secretion indirectly through the socalled macula densa mechanism of renin secretion, which responds to changes of distal tubular sodium load.

APII and inhibition of cGMP-phosphodiesterase. ANPs have been shown to stimulate the particulate guanylate cyclase in vascular smooth muscle cells, and the increase of intracellular cGMP may be responsible for the observed vasorelaxation(see 8). With respect to renin secretion, we have attempted an indirect approach, by infusing the inhibitor of cGMP-phosphodiesterase, zamiprast(M&B 22948). The inhibitor (10 µM) induced a small, but significant increase of renal perfusate flow from 10.65±0.63 to 11.1±0.59 ml/min, as well as a small increase of renin secretion(384±77 to 464±89 ngANGI/h/min). During the additional infusion of APII the response of renin secretion rate was attenuated at all concentrations(40,57,and 89 % increase, respectively). Since the actual effectiveness of M&B 22948 to increase cGMP could not be measured, the role of cGMP in the mediation of the effect of ANP remains unclear.

Other natriuretic peptides. The infusion of API induced a smaller increase of renin release than APII, whereas APIII, α-ANF, or ANF 3-28, on an equimolar basis, were as effective as APII to stimulate renin release.

CONCLUSION

The data suggest that the stimulatory effect of APII on renin secretion is not dependent on prostaglandin synthesis, vasodilatation, dopaminergic receptor activation,presynaptic release of noradrenaline,or macula densa activation.The mechanism by which it stimulates renin secretion remains obscure.

REFERENCES

1. Seymour,A.A., Blaine,E.H., Mazak,E.K., Smith,S.G., Stabilito,I.I., Haley,A.B., Napier,M.A., Whinnery,M.A., and Nutt,R.F., Life Sci. 36: 33-44, 1985.
2. Beasley,D., and Malvin,R.L., Am.J.Physiol. 248: F24-F30, 1985.
3. Burnett,J.C., Granger,Jr.J.P., and Opgenorth,T.J., Am.J.Physiol. 247: F863-F866, 1984.
4. Maack,T., Marion,D.N., Camargo,M.J.F., Kleinert,H.D., Laragh,J.H., Vaugham,Jr.E.D., and Atlas,S.A., Am.J.Med. 77: 1069-1075, 1984.
5. Hackenthal,E., Lang,R.E., and Bührle,C.P., J.Hypertens.3 (suppl.3): S323-S325, 1985.
6. Schwertschlag,U., and Hackenthal,E., Naunyn-Schmiedebergs Arch. Pharmacol. 319: 239-242, 1982.
7. Marin-Grez,M., Briggs,J.P., Schubert,G., and Schnermann,J., Life Sci. 36: 2171-2176, 1985.
8. Winquist,R.J., Faison,E.P., Waldman,S.A., Schwartz,K., Murad,F., and Rapoport,R.M., Proc.Natl.Acad.Sci. 81: 7661-7664, 1984.

SALT LOADING IN SPONTANEOUSLY HYPERTENSIVE RATS FURTHER ELEVATES BLOOD PRESSURE DESPITE ENHANCED RELEASE OF ATRIAL NATRIURETIC PEPTIDES AND EXAGGERATED NATRIURESIS.

M. SAMBHI, M. KOHNO, K. CLEGG

Hypertension Division, Department of Medicine, Sepulveda VA Medical Center, University of California at Los Angeles, CA 91343, U.S.A.

INTRODUCTION

It has been suggested but not established that atrial natriuretic peptides (ANP) may have a role in the mechanisms of hypertension and associated exaggerated natriuresis during volume expansion. The present investigation was undertaken to examine the influence of chronic salt loading on the circulating plasma levels of ANP in spontaneously hypertensive rats (SHR) and to study the concomitant changes in blood pressure as well as urinary excretion of sodium. Normotensive Wistar Kyoto (WKY) rats were studied as controls under the same protocol.

METHODS

Sixteen SHR and sixteen WKY male rats, 18 weeks of age, given standard diet were followed for two weeks. Half of the animals in each group were given 1% sodium chloride in tap water as drinking fluid during this period; the other half received only tap water and served as controls. Twenty-four hours before the end of the study, the animals were placed in single metabolic cages and the urine volume and urinary excretion of sodium were measured. At the end of the metabolic study, systolic blood pressure was measured by the tail cuff method. Animals were decapitated and plasma collected for ANP measurements.

Plasma samples (1-2 ml) were extracted with C-18 Sep-Pak cartridges (Millipore-Waters) prewashed with 5 ml 100% methanol and 5 ml 4% acetic acid. To each plasma sample, 3 volumes of

4% acetic acid was added and immediately loaded onto the cartridge at 1 ml/min. Non-adsorbed material was removed by washing the C-18 with 5 ml distilled water and the bound ANP peptides with 4 ml ethanol: 4% acetic acid (86:14 v/v). The eluate was dried in vacuo (Savant Spin-Vac) and dissolved in 300 ul RIA buffer (0.1 M NaPO4, pH 7.4; 0.05 M NaCl; 0.1% BSA; 0.1% Nonidet P40; 0.01% NaN3). Recovery of ANP from C-18 was determined by adding 100 to 200 pg ANP standard to rat plasma which had previously been treated with dextran coated charcoal to remove endogenous ANP. Extraction and assay for immunoreactive ANP yielded a recovery of 63.9 $\pm$ 3.6% of the added ANP standard.

Radioimmunoassay of ANP was performed using antibody (Peninsula Labs) with the following specificity: 100% cross reactive with human or rat alpha-ANP, rat ANP (8-33), and Atriopeptin III; 60% with ANP (18-28); 10% with Auriculin A; 5% with Atriopeptin II; 1% with ANP (13-28); non-cross reactive with Atriopeptin I. Antibody was reconstituted in RIA buffer as directed by manufacturer. Standard ANP was prepared by dissolving 12.5 ug of Peninsula standard ANP in 12.5 ml 0.1% Acetic Acid and aliquoting 0.2 ml into conical microfuge tubes. The standard was dried in vacuo and stored at -20° C until use. Standard curves (50-5000 pg/ml) were prepared by dissolving the ANP in 200 ul RIA buffer and serial dilution. Assay for ANP was performed by incubating 100 ul Antibody, 100 ul standard or sample and 14000 cpm 125I -ANP (Peninsula) for 48 hrs at 4° C. Bound radioactivity was precipitated by the addition of 50 ul 2% normal rabbit serum and 100 ul goat anti-rabbit IgG serum (Calbiochem-Behring) and incubation for a minimum 2 hrs at 4° C. Precipitated antibody complexes were diluted with 1 ml of RIA buffer and collected by centrifugation at 10000 x g, 30 min, 4° C. Free radioactivity was aspirated from the pellet and the pellet counted in a Micromedic Gamma Counter. Interassay variation was 13.5% (n=10) and the intra-assay variation was 5% (n=20). Standard curves yielded an effective range of sensitivity between 5 and 200 pg ANP, 50% displacement was obtained with 22 pg ANP.

Statistical analysis was done by an unpaired t-test.

RESULTS AND DISCUSSION

Results are listed in Table 1. Urine output and urinary excretion were not significantly different between control WKY and SHR although blood pressure in the SHR was significantly elevated and the plasma level of immunoreactive ANP was two fold higher (p 0.001). It can be concluded that the observed chronic elevation of plasma ANP in the SHR does not in itself result in exaggerated chronic diuresis and natriuresis but may rather be essential for maintaining the hypertensive animal in salt and water balance.

Table 1. Hemodynamic and metabolic changes induced by high salt intake.

	WKY			SHR		
	Control	Salt	P	Control	Salt	P
Plasma ANP pg/ml	125.4 ± 18.7	146.8 ± 26.0	N.S.	254.5 ± 50**	487.0 ± 116.7	p 0.001
B.P. mmHg	114 ± 5	110 ± 7	N.S.	184 ± 7**	199 ± 14	p 0.05
Urine Output ml/24hr/100gBW	3.0 ± 1.0	6.6 ± 2.0	p 0.001	3.9 ± 1.0	11.1 ± 4.1*	p 0.001
Urinary Na excretion mEq/24hr	0.76 ± 0.07	6.20 ± 1.14	p 0.001	1.10 ± 0.20	13.48 ± 3.67**	p 0.001
Weight g	311 ± 14	298 ± 19	N.S.	302 ± 19	311 ± 15	N.S.

Values are expressed as the means ± S.D. * p 0.05, ** p 0.01 WKY vs SHR

It has been reported previously (1,2) that the basal levels of circulating ANP are higher in the SHR than WKY, and this difference is evident during the prehypertensive young age of 4 to 8 weeks. A progressive increase of plasma ANP levels occurs in the SHR concomitant with the rise of B.P. that is proportional to the magnitude of its elevation. These findings suggest that both genetic as well as hemodynamic factors in the SHR may account for the elevated levels of plasma ANP (2). Left atrial pressure in the SHR is known to be higher than that in WKY rats (3). Increased central blood volume and a decreased diastolic compliance of left ventricle in the hypertensive animal are presumably responsible for the elevated left atrial pressure. Higher levels of circulating ANP under these circumstances exist in concert with a higher resetting of pressure natriuresis in the hypertensive kidney. Further work is required to elucidate the cause and effect in this relationship.

The effects of ad lib salt loading were strikingly different in SHR compared with WKY rats as seen in Table 1. The body weight was well matched in all groups of animals, and showed no change after salt loading in either group, thus discounting any significant salt and water retention. Plasma ANP levels did not change significantly in WKY rats but showed an almost two fold rise in the SHR. Urine output and urinary sodium showed marked elevations in the WKY. The urine output approximately doubled and the sodium excretion rose more than six fold. In comparison the responses in the SHR were further exaggerated. Urine volume in the SHR approximately tripled and the urinary sodium excretion rose more than twelve fold. These findings suggest that the in vivo renal response to chronically elevated plasma ANP levels in the SHR is not attenuated and remains active.

Salt loading has been shown to decrease the receptor density but increase the affinity of ANF receptors in normal rat glomeruli (4). Similar studies on the effect of salt loading on the vascular ANP receptors in the SHR have not been reported. In the present studies, salt loading caused no change in the blood pressure of WKY rats. In the SHR, B.P. rose significantly after salt loading despite concomitant marked elevations of plasma ANP levels. Further work is needed to examine the thesis that the observed elevation in ANP levels in the SHR may have prevented more striking elevations of B.P. in response to salt loading than those recorded in this study.

It can also be speculated, however, that the systemic vascular receptors for ANP in the SHR under these conditions demonstrate a relative degree of tachyphylaxis or reduced affinity. It is suggested that the proposed differential response of renal vs vascular receptors for ANP in the hypertensive animal may underlie the phenomenon of exaggerated natriuresis in response to volume expansion. Salt and water balance in the hypertensive is thus achieved and maintained inspite of or perhaps at the expense of elevated blood pressure. Biological primacy of ANP function in the hypertensive animal therefore appears to reside in control of fluid volume and not in regulation of blood pressure.

REFERENCES

1. Imada, T., Takayangi, R., Inagami, T. Bio Chem. Bio. Phys. Res. Commun. 133: 759-765, 1985
2. Gutkowska, J., Horky, K., Lachance, C., Racz, K., Garcia, R., Thibault, G., Kuchel, O., Genest, J. and Cantin, M. Hypertension Suppl. 18(4): I-137-I-140, 1986
3. Noresson, E., Ricksten, S.E., Thoren, P. Acta Physiol. Scand. 107: 9-12
4. Ballermann, B.J., Hoover, R.L., Karnovsky, M.J. and Brenner, B.M. Journal of Clin. Investigation 76(6): 2049, 1985

PLASMA CARDIONATRIN AND VOLUME AND THE RENIN ANGIOTENSIN ALDOSTERONE SYSTEM IN NORMOTENSIVE AND HYPERTENSIVE PREGNANCY.

FIEVET P*, FOURNIER A*, DE BOLD A**, EL ESPER N*, BRUNEL P*, GREGOIRE I*.

* Service de Néphrologie CHU AMIENS
** Queen's University Department of Pathology KINGSTON CANADA

INTRODUCTION

Cardionatrin is the 28 aminoacid atrial natriuretic peptide which is released into the circulation from its storage granules when the atria are stretched, (1,2). This peptide has both remarkable natriuretic and vasodilating properties and suppresses the renin angiotensin aldosterone system. It may therefore be implicated in the pathogenesis of hypertension. So far it has been investigated only in essential hypertension and shown to be increased (3). It has not yet been evaluated in pregnancy induced hypertension (PIH) or preeclampsia. Therefore we measured plasma concentrations of cardionatrin in pregnant women with normal blood pressure as well as in women with PIH and preeclampsia during pregnancy and after delivery, simultaneouly with their plasma volume, blood uric acid, plasma renin activity (PRA) and plasma concentrations of aldosterone(PA).

PATIENTS AND METHODS

Patients : we studied the following groups of patients : (1) normotensive pregnant women ie women with BP < 140 - 90 mmHg before during and after pregnancy : 15 were sutded during pregnancy and 7, 2 months after delivery.(2) women with PIH ie with BP > 140 - 90 during pregnancy on more than 2 ambulatory measurements in sitting position, whereas BP was normal before and after pregnancy : 24 were studied during pregnancy and 14 after delivery.(3)women with preeclampsia ie with PIH complicated by a proteinuria > 1 g/24 H : 11 were studied during pregnancy and 6 after delivery.

Protocol of investigation :The patients were investigated at the out patient clinic between 8 and 10 a.mwhile on a free diet and without any medication. BP reported are those measured after 30 mn of supine position just before the blood samplings through a previously inserted catheter. EDTA tubes were used for cardionatrin, PRA and aldosterone determination. After immediate centrifugation at - 4°C, the plasma were stored at -30° for PRA and aldosterone and at -80° for cardionatrin. Plasma volume was measured by Evan's blue dilution method, the results being expressed in % of normal according to duration of pregnancy established by SMITH et YARBROUGH.

Analytical methods : PRA, aldosterone and cardionatrin were measured by radioimmunoassay. For cardionatrin the RIA was performed after extraction, with an antiserum obtained from rabbits immunized with cardionatrin I (Peninsula Laboratory). The assay sensitivity is 1,5 pg per tube. Its precision is characterized by a coefficient of variation within one assay of 3.8 % and between assays of 9,1 %. Mean ± SD of normal values established in 14 normal women at child bearing age, on a free diet, the blood being sampled after 30 mn of lying position is 54 ± 19 pg/ml.

RESULTS

Table 1. Summarizes the clinical and biological data during pregnancy. It shows that comparatively to the normotensive, the hypertensive women had the same duration of amenorrhea and sodium excretion whereas their PRA, aldosterone, and plasma volume were lower, and their blood uric acid and plasma cardionatrin higher.

mean ± SD	Normotensive n = 15	PIH n = 24	Preeclampsia n = 11
Age yr	26 ± 4	26 ± 4	26 ± 3
Amenorrhea	30 ± 3	33 ± 4	31 ± 3
Mean arterial pressure mmHg	82 ± 8	100 ± 15*	111 ± 30**
Weight before pregnancy kg	65 ± 9	80 ± 14**	65 ± 9
UNa/UCr mmol/mmol	11 ± 3	12 ± 3	9 ± 5
PRA ng/ml/h	7 ± 2	5 ± 2*	3 ± 1**
Aldosterone pg/ml	247 ± 131	276 ± 192	82 ± 109**
Uric acid µmol/l	230 ± 27	313 ± 85	527 ± 102**
PVolume % normal		-17 ± 14	-25 ± 11
Cardionatrine pg/ml	73 ± 45	100 ± 71*	143 ± 93**

Significance of the difference with normotensive * $p < 0.05$, ** $p < 0.01$

In 8 patients with PIH, cardionatrin was measured 2 to 4 times from 22 to 38 week of amenorrhea : there was no significant change with duration of pregnancy.

Table 2. summarizes the changes in the clinical and biological data observed 2 months after delivery and without treatment. It shows that there is a significant drop in cardionatrin levels only in the preeclamptic group where decrease in BP is the most accentuated.

Absolute changes mean ± SD	Normotensive n = 7	PIH n = 14	Preeclampsia n = 6
Mean arterial pressure mmHg	5 ± 11	-7.2 ± 10 S	-19 ± 17*S
PRA ng/ml/h	- 7.6 ± 1.8 S	-2.6 ± 2.4**SS	-1.1 ± 4*
Plasma Aldosterone pg/ml	-258± 122 S	-177 ± 141S	-79 ± 120*S
Plasma Cardionatrin pg/ml	-6 ± 17	-27± 64	-79 ± 56*S

Significance of the changes : S $p < 0.5$; SS $p < 0.1$.
Significance of the difference of the changes with the normotensive : * $p < 0.5$; ** $p < 0.2$.

No linear correlation could be found between absolute values or the changes of plasma cardionatrin with mean arterial pressure, PRA, plasma aldosterone, plasma volume and blood uric acid.

DISCUSSION AND CONCLUSIONS

1/ The sequential study of the normotensive pregnant women does not find a significant decrease of plasma cardionatrin. This contrasts with the data of CUSSON (5) who showed that a group of pregnant women have higher levels of cardionatrin that an other group of non pregnant women. However the number of our patients with paired data is small and when we compared the whole group of 24 normotensive pregnant women with all the data gathered in normotensive non pregnant women (7 after delivery + 14 not previously pregnant women) we find a borderline difference : 73 ± 45 during pregnancy versus 56 ± 15 pg/ml in the absence of pregnancy ($p< 0.10$). These data suggest therefore that pregnancy perse stimulates cardionatrin secretion.

2/ Hypertension develops in PIH and specially in preeclampsia in spite of the fact that both the absolute values of plasma cardionatrin during pregnancy are higher than in controls and that their decreases after delivery (and presumably therefore their increases comparatively to the prepregnant normotensive state) are greater. This excludes both an absolute or relative deficiency of cardionatrin secretion in the pathogenesis of these hypertensions and suggests rather a compensatory role for cardionatrin.

3/ Increased plasma levels of cardionatrin may explain the characteristic contrast between relative hypovolemia and relative hyporeninism and hypoaldosteronism observed during preeclampsia (6) since cardionatrin is known to decrease plasma volume by inducing natriuresis and a shift of plasma into the interstitium as well to suppress possibly renin and certainly aldosterone secretions (7).

REFERENCES

1/ **DE BOLD A.J**. Science.230: 765-770, 1985

2/ **NEEDLEMAN P., ADAMS S.P., COLE B.**Hypertension.7: 469-482,1985

3/ **SAGNELLA G.A.,SHORE A.C.,MARKANDUN N.D.,Mc GREGOR G.A.**Lancet.i:179-181, 1986

4/ **SMITH R.W., YARROUGH C.J.**Am.J. Obst.Gyn.99: 18-20, 1967

5/ **CUSSON J.R.,GUTKOWSKA J., REY E. and Al.** N. Eng.J. Med.313: 1230-1231, 1985

6/ **FIEVET P.,PLESKOV L., DESAILLY I., CARAYON A. and Al.** Nephron.40: 429-432, 1985.

7/ **WEIDMAN P., HJASLER L., GNADINGER MP. et al.** J. Clin. Invest. 1966, 77, 734-742.

ATRIAL NATRIURETIC PEPTIDE AS AN INDICATOR OF CARDIAC AND VOLUME STATE

I. TIKKANEN, C. GRÖNHAGEN-RISKA AND F. FYHRQUIST

The Minerva Institute for Medical Research, P.O. Box 819, SF-00101 Helsinki, Finland, and IVth Department of Medicine, Helsinki University Central Hospital, Helsinki

INTRODUCTION

Peptides with diuretic, natriuretic, and vasodilating properties have been isolated from mammalian atria, and subsequently sequensed and synthetized (1, 2). These peptides are secreted into the circulation during volume expansion and high sodium states, and in disease states such as congestive heart failure (3), renal insufficiency (4), and supraventricular tachycardia (5).

In patients with terminal renal failure requiring dialysis extracellular fluid volume varies between and during each haemodialysis session. Also, these patients frequently suffer from concomitant cardiac failure. The aim of the present study was to correlate plasma atrial natriuretic peptide (ANP) levels in dialysis patients to both volume changes and to cardiac status.

MATERIAL AND METHODS

Twentyfive patients (13 females, 12 males, aged 45 $\pm$ 3,2 years) on maintenance haemodialysis were included in the study. According to clinical examination, chest X-ray, and echocardiography, the patients were subdivided into two groups: 1) Those without signs of cardiac dysfunction (n=14), and 2) those with heart failure with increased cardiac preload (n=11).

Blood samples for determination of ANP (3), plasma renin activity (6), antidiuretic hormone (7), aldosterone (Abbot's kit), and serum sodium and potassium were taken before and after haemodialysis.

Student's t-test for paired or nonpaired observations and linear regression analysis were applied.

RESULTS AND COMMENTS

Before dialysis, plasma ANP levels were elevated in both groups on haemodialysis, but the highest levels were found in patients with concomitant congestive heart failure compared with dialysis patients with normal cardiac function (Table 1). Predialysis plasma ANP levels were in correlation with body weight gain before dialysis (4,9 ± 0,9 %) only in patients with normal cardiac function (r = 0,66, p<0,01), but not in dialysis patients with cardiac failure (r = 0,36, NS).

Table 1. Plasma ANP concentration (mean ± SEM) in patients with terminal renal failure; either with normal cardiac function, or with concomitant congestive heart failure.

Renal insufficiency	ANP (pg/ml) before dialysis	ANP (pg/ml) after dialysis
with cardiac failure	402 ± 60[a]	274 ± 61[c]
without cardiac failure	120 ± 27[b]	59 ± 10[d]

Significance of differences: a vs b, p<0,001; b vs d, p<0,05
b vs c, p<0,05; c vs d, p<0,01

During dialysis, plasma ANP levels decreased both in patients with normal and impaired cardiac function (Table 1). In patients with cardiac failure, however, plasma ANP remained significantly higher than in patients with normal cardiac function. Reduction in plasma ANP during dialysis was in correlation with weight reduction (4,1 ± 0,8%) only in dialysis patients with normal cardiac function (r = 0,70, p<0,01), but not in those with concomitant heart failure (r = 0,09, NS). Changes in body weight, serum sodium and potassium, plasma renin activity, aldosterone, and anti-diuretic hormone did not differ between the two patient groups.

We conclude that hypervolemic overload is an important stimulus to ANP release in terminal renal failure. Additional congestive cardiac failure apparently becomes an overriding determinant of plasma ANP levels, obscuring the effect of fluid retention alone. Thus, ANP may prove a useful indicator both of volume, and particularly, of cardiac state in patients with end-stage renal failure.

REFERENCES

1. Cantin, M. and Genest, J. Endocrine Rev. 6: 101-127, 1985.
2. Needleman, P. and Greenwald, J.E. N. Engl. J. Med. 314: 828-834, 1986.
3. Tikkanen, I., Fyhrquist, F., Metsärinne, K. and Leidenius, R. Lancet ii: 66-69, 1985.
4. Rascher, W., Tulassay, T. and Lang, R.E. Lancet ii: 303-305, 1985.
5. Tikkanen, I., Metsärinne, K. and Fyhrquist, F. Lancet ii: 40-41, 1985.
6. Fyhrquist, F., Soveri, P., Puutula, L. and Stenman U-H. Clin. Chem. 22: 250-256, 1976.
7. Fyhrquist, F., Wallenius, M. and Hollemans, H.J.G. Scand. J. Clin. Lab. Invest. 36: 841-847, 1976.

ATRIAL NATRIURETIC PEPTIDES (ANP) IN RATS WITH CHRONIC RENAL FAILURE.

J. S. PETERSEN, O. M. BECH, E. STEINESS, D. KIRSTEIN* & S. CHRISTENSEN.

Department of Pharmacology, University of Copenhagen, DK-2100 Copenhagen, and *LEO Pharmaceutical Products, DK-2750 Ballerup, Denmark.

INTRODUCTION

In chronic renal failure (CRF) sodium balance is maintained until very low levels of glomerular filtration rate, implying that the sodium excretion per functioning nephron must be increased by some adaptive mechanism (1). The aim of the present study was to investigate the role of ANP in the altered renal sodium handling in rats with CRF. CRF was induced by 5/6 nephrectomy and the rats were maintained on a normal (NSD) as well as on a high sodium diet (HSD) in order to stimulate the adaptive changes in renal sodium excretion. The atrial content of ANP was determined by measurering the natriuretic activity of atrial extracts (AE) and P-ANP was determined by radioimmunoassay.

MATERIALS AND METHODS

16 weeks-old male and female Wistar rats were used. The animals were fed with commercial pellets containing 100 or 800 mmol of sodium per kg dry weight. A homogenous pool of AE was prepared from 45 rats in order to make a dose-response curve. Individual extracts were prepared from 19 control rats and 12 nephrectomized rats (NX-rats). P-ANP was determined from 20 control rats and 20 NX-rats.

For preparation of AE the rats were anaesthetized with halothane and N_2O and soaked by a heparinized syringe placed in the abdominal aorta. The blood was centrifuged at 4000 g, 4^oC for 10 min and stored at -80^oC prior to determination of P-ANP and P-Urea. The hearts were excised and rinsed in cold saline and both atria were dissected out on an ice-cold disc, blotted dry and weighed (55.3 ± 1.5 mg). 9 μl ice-cold medium containing 90 mM glucose, 10 mM NaCl and 40 mM urea were added per mg of tissue. The tissue was then homogenized, boiled for 10 min and centrifuged at 4000 g, 4^oC for 30 min. The supernatant, termed AE, was stored at -80°C prior to bioassay.

For bioassay 200 g female Wistar rats were anaesthetized with Inactin, 120 mg/kg i.p., tracheotomized, catheterized in the bladder and a femoral vein cannula was used for infusion of saline (1.5 ml bolus + 1.5 ml/hr) and injection of test material. After an equilibration period of 2 hr, 4 consecutive 15 min control urine collections were taken. Then a sample of atrial or ventricular extract was injected within 60 sec and urine collections were continued for 2 periods of 15 min each. In all assays the injectionvolume was adjusted to 0.8 ml and only one sample was assayed in each bioassay rat. (2).

The RIA used in this study was Amershams RIA for h-aANP. As standard was used rANP(1-28) which shows cross-reactivity of 90% with h-aANP. The intra-assay variation was 3.9%.

All presented data are mean values $\pm$ SE.

RESULTS

Table 1 shows that P-Urea was significantly increased in all NX-groups corresponding to a higher fractional excretion of sodium (FE_{Na}). When control rats were sodium loaded, FE_{Na} also turned out to increase significantly. The material does not allow an evaluation of the influence of sodium loading for FE_{Na} in the NX-rats as NX-groups were not equally uremic.

Fig. 1 shows the time course of the natriuretic response of AE of 15 mg tissue taken from control rats on NSD. The response is maximal in the first period after injection of test material. This dose produced a natriuretic response of 16-fold increase in sodium excretion, which proved to be approximately half the maximal natriuretic response.

Table 1.

			P-Urea mM	FE_{Na} %
AE :	Normal Na	Contr.	9.8±0.7	-
		NX	52.2±12.9	8.3±2.4
	High Na	Contr.	9.0±0.7	-
		NX	36.8±5.0	35.0±15.8
P-ANP :	Normal Na	Contr.	6.2±0.3	0.5±0.0
		NX	29.3±3.8	5.2±2.1
	High Na	Contr.	7.0±0.7	2.9±0.4
		NX	16.2±1.9	6.4±0.9

① Natriuretic response to atrial Extract ~ 15 mg tissue Control rats, normal Na

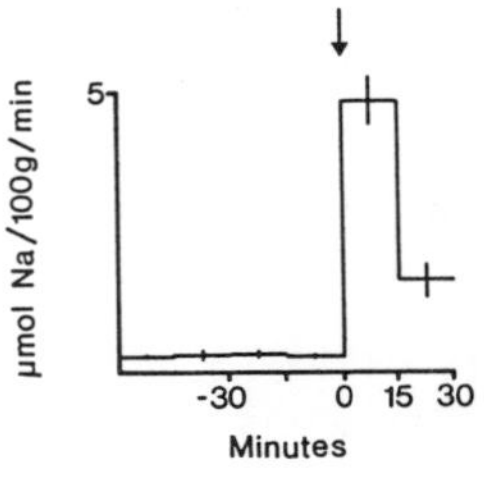

The dose-response curve based upon the AE-pool is shown on Fig. 2. The half maximal effective dose is approximately equal to AE corresponding to 15 mg atrial tissue. There was no effect of extracts corresponding to 15 mg of ventricular tissue taken from the apex of the heart. With the intention of showing any possible relative difference in atrial natriuretic content between control rats and NX-rats, we adjusted all the individual test samples to correspond to 15 mg tissue.

Fig. 3 shows the bioassay responses to AE of 15 mg tissue. The natriuretic activity was unaltered in extracts from NX-rats on NSD compared with control rats on NSD. When the rats were sodium loaded, the natriuretic activity in AE from control rats was significantly increased while it from NX-rats was significantly decreased.

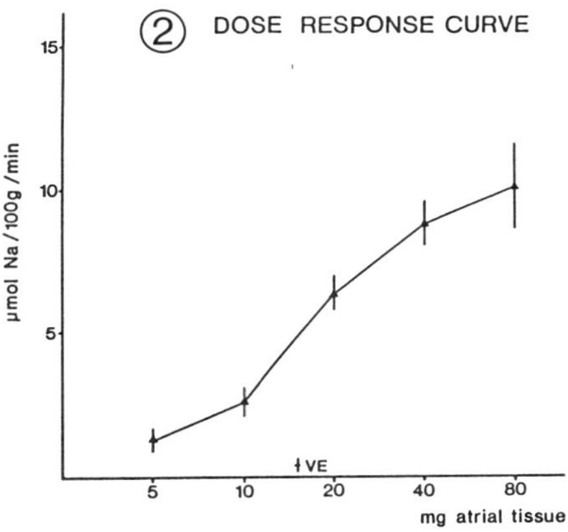

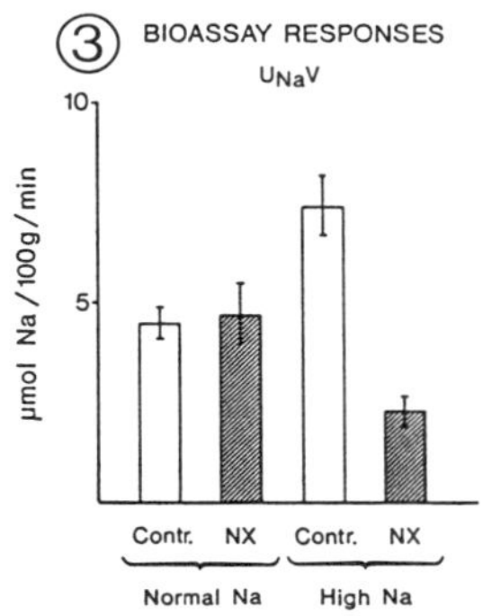

However these data do not reflect the relative differences in ANP-content of extracts. A reflection of the relative content can be obtained by converting the individual natriuretic responses to equivalents of mg atrial tissue in the pooled AE used for preparation of the dose-response curve. These data are shown on Fig. 4.

From this it appears: 1) When control rats gets sodium loaded the atrial content of ANP is increased 2-fold. 2) Uremia in itself does not affect the atrial content of ANP as long as the animal is on a NSD. 3) When NX-rats gets sodium loaded the atrial content of ANP is decreased to half the value of rats on a NSD.

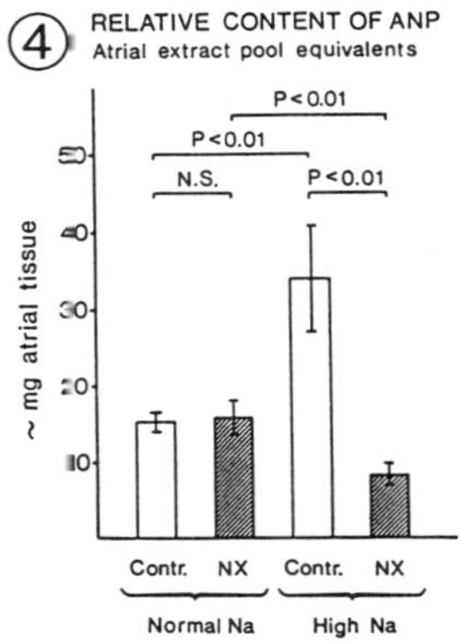

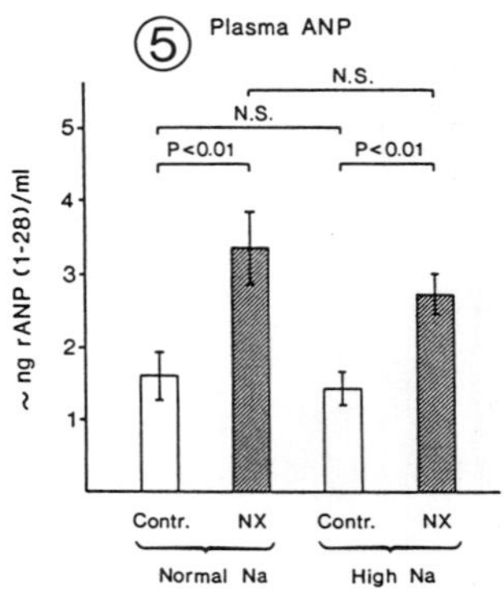

Determination of P-ANP (Fig. 5), showed no significant difference between control rats on NSD and control rats on HSD. However, in the NX-groups P-ANP was increased 2-fold without showing any significant difference between NX-rats on NSD and NX-rats on HSD. There was no correlation between individual P-Urea and P-ANP and neither between individual FE_{Na} and P-ANP.

DISCUSSION

Sodium loading of control rats lead to a 2-fold increase in the atrial stores of ANP, without any simultaneous change in P-ANP. This suggests that sodium loading causes an increase in the atrial stores of ANP, in preparation to a demand of an increase in P-ANP. If the rats had been sodium loaded to a further extent, we might have seen an increase in P-ANP alike the increase reported by others in response to volume loading.

In the NX-rats on NSD we found a 2-fold increase in P-ANP without any simultaneous change in the atrial stores. This can be due partly to a decreased renal clearance and partly to an intracellular adaption in the atrial cells. In CRF sodium retention is expected to stimulate ANP-release, which are in accordance with the increase in P-ANP that we have found. But the atrial stores are not increased which suggests that the atrial cells from uremic rats in contrast to control rats, does not have any reserve capacity which enables them to further increase the ANP-production. This is evident when the intracellular ANP-synthetizing apparatus in uremic rats is further stimulated by sodium loading, since in this situation the stores are depleted to half the value of control rats on NSD. The P-ANP is still 2-fold higher than P-ANP from control rats, which suggests that ANP still acts as a compensatory mechanism, but further sodium loading will probably exceed the maximal load which the ANP-system is able to compensate for.

CONCLUSION

- ANP may be involved in the adaptive increase of fractional sodium excretion during uremia.
- Administration of a high sodium diet to uremic rats may induce depletion of the atrial stores of ANP.
- To which extent a decreased renal clearance of ANP per se is responsible for the increase in P-ANP during CRF, still remains to be solved.

REFERENCES

1. Schultze, R.G., Slatopolsky E., Tall B., Walker W., Levy M., Bricker N.S. Trans Assoc Am Physicians 79: 322-329, 1966.
2. de Bold A.J., Borenstein H.B., Veress A.T., Sonnenberg H. Life Sciences 28: 89-94, 1981.

PLASMA LEVELS OF HUMAN ATRIAL NATRIURETIC PEPTIDE IN CHRONIC UREMIC PATIENTS.

G. CANNELLA, S. GHIELMI*, A. RODELLA*, M. GAGGIOTTI, G. BRUNORI, M. QUINZANINI* and R. MAIORCA.

Departments of Nephrology and *Clinical Chemistry, School of Medicine, Spedali Civili and University of Brescia, Brescia (Italy).

INTRODUCTION

So far, 3 atrial natriuretic polypeptides (ANP) have been isolated from human cardiocytes and, among them, the α-type seems to be preferentially released into the blood stream (1). In normal man, saline infusion or high sodium intake increase plasma α-hANP levels while the opposite is true on low sodium diet (2). These observations seem to suggest that α-hANP is involved in extracellular fluid volume (ECFV) homeostasis. This study was undertaken to obtain some more insight about the involvement of α-hANP in the pathophysiology of body fluid volume in man.

PATIENTS AND METHODS

We studied 7 chronic dialyzed patients (3 m. and 4 f., aged 31 - 46 yrs) and 11 uncomplicated renal patients (4 m., 7 f., aged 29 - 48 yrs) with a glomerular filtration rate (GFR) ranging 7-100 ml/min. All dialyzed patients were anuric and ate unrestricted protein and sodium diets, while patients not in regular dialysis treatment were kept on diets with varying restrictions according to their degree of functional impairment. None of them took hypotensive therapy.

Dialyzed subjects were studied in the morning, 72 hrs after the last hemodialysis, after they had been reclining supine for 30 min. At the end of this period a first blood sample for α-hANP, packed cells volume, serum sodium and osmolarity was drawn through an indwelling catheter inserted in the arterial side of the forearm fistula and a simple ultrafiltration (without diffusion) was started and continued for 3 hrs. Additional blood samples were taken every 60 min from the same sampling site and, in 3 patients, further samples for α-hANP were also taken from the blood outleaving the dialyzing filter. Blood pressure (BP), heart rate (HR) and ECG were continuously monitored. In the 11 non dialyzed patients, resting venous plasma α-hANP samples were taken with the same procedure as above. The assay for plasma α-hANP was done by a direct radioimmunoassay according to the manufacturer's istruction (Peninsula Lab., Belmont, CA). The sensitivity of the method calculated at 95% confidence limit was 7 pg/ml. Data for α-hANP were analyzed by Student's t-test for paired and unpaired samples on log-transformed data. Results are presented as mean ± SE.

RESULTS

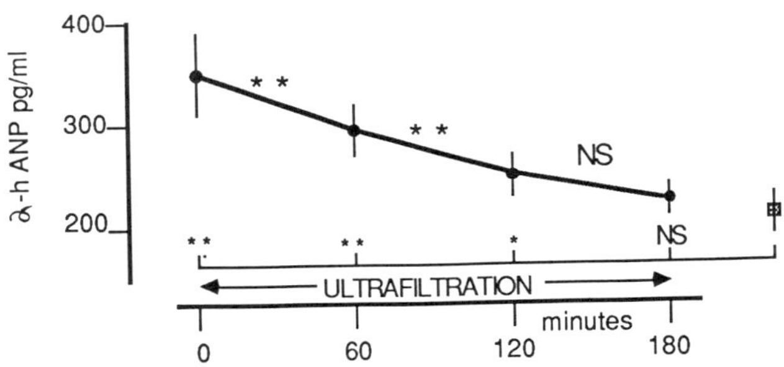

Fig.1 : Effects of reducing the body weight by ultrafiltration on plasma α-h ANP concentration in 7 fluid overloaded dyalized patients (●). Each mean is also compared with that from a group (n=11) of patients with renal disease and variable degree of functional impairement (⊠). Asterisks depict statistical differences .

Resting levels of plasma α-hANP in the 7 dialyzed patients were significantly higher than those of non-dialyzed group (Fig. 1). Body fluid removal by pure ultrafiltration caused an average body weight loss of 2.6 Kg and a nearly 20% decrease in plasma volume, without significant changes in resting levels of mean BP (85 ± 6 mmHg), HR (79 ± 4 b/min), serum sodium (139 ± 1 mmol/ml) and osmolarity (308 ± 3 mosm/l). During ultrafiltration, plasma α-hANP decreased in all patients between 0 and 120 min, then levelled-off until the end

(Fig.1), at which time the final α-hANP levels were no longer significantly higher than those of the non-dialyzed group (Fig. 1). In the 3 patients in whom α-hANP was also measured from dialyzer outlet, no significant arterio-venous gradients for α-hANP concentrations could be seen (n = 9; $P < 0.05$).

DISCUSSION

In our chronically hemodialyzed patients, when they were fluid overloaded, the plasma α-hANP was significantly higher than in non-dialyzed patients with residual excretory function. Since the dialyzed subjects were anuric, one might think that these high α-hANP levels were a mere consequence of the lack of excretory or metabolic clearance of the polypeptide. However, when the patients were dehydrated by ultrafiltration, their plasma α-hANP decreased in all subjects to levels not different from those observed in the non dialyzed group. Therefore, since artefactitious decrease of plasma α-hANP due to polypeptide removal by the filter was excluded, it appears that the fall in plasma α-hANP we observed in dialyzed subjects was dependent mainly on simultaneous decreases in plasma volume and/or ECFV.

These findings seem to suggest that the actual levels of plasma α-hANP are inversely related to those of ECFV. This contention could fit well with an hypothetical scheme proposing α-hANP as a putative natriuretic hormone (3). However, before we are sure of its role, it will be necessary to prove that not only is it influenced by body fluid volumes but also it has effects on renal sodium excretion.

REFERENCES

1. Sugarawa, A., Nakao, K., Morii, N., Sakamoto, M., Suda, M., Shimokura, M., Kiso, Y., Kihara, M., Yamory, Y., Nishimura, K., Soneda, J., Ban, T., Imura, M. Biochem. and Biophys. Res. Comm. 129: 439-446, 1985.
2. Sagnella, G.A., Markandu, N.D., Shore, A.C., Mc Gregor, G.A. Lancet, ii: 1208-1211, 1985.
3. Sagnella, G.A., Mac Greyor, G.A. Nature, 309: 666-667, 1984.

ATRIAL NATRIURETIC PEPTIDE (ANP) AND RENAL FUNCTION: EFFECT OF POSTURE AND DIETARY SODIUM

H. BOBINSKI, J.C. ATHERTON, R. GREEN & L. SOLOMON

Department of Physiology, University of Manchester, and Renal Unit, Royal Infirmary, Manchester, England.

INTRODUCTION

The atria of the heart produce peptides which are released into the systemic circulation in response to an increase in right atrial pressure (1,2). The role of these peptides in the physiological control of renal and cardiovascular function is, however, less well established. We present here studies on the effects of two physiological stimuli - changes in posture and salt intake - on plasma concentrations of ANP and renal function.

METHODS

Posture Study

Nine healthy volunteers (aged 20-44 yr; 42-110 kg; 8 male and 1 female) were studied on their normal salt intake. They were placed head up on a tilt table at 75° for 15 min, then laid supine at 0° for 60 min, then returned to the upright 75° for a further 20 minutes. The evening before the study each consumed 500 mg lithium carbonate. Timed urine samples were obtained immediately before and after tilting and blood samples taken before, during and after the tilt. This enabled us to measure glomerular filtration rate (as the clearance of creatinine - C_{cr}) urine flow rate (v) and the clearance of lithium (C_{Li}) and sodium (C_{Na}). ANP concentrations were measured by radioimmunoassay (3).

Dietary Study

Eleven healthy volunteers (aged 19-36 yr; 54-104 kg; 8 male, 3 female) were studied for 19 days on a low salt diet (10-20 mmole/day). On days 1-5 100 mmole sodium chloride were added and on days 12-19, 300 mmole sodium chloride were added to the diet to give control, low (LNaD) and high (HNaD) in sequence for each subject. On the evening of days 3, 9 and 16 500 mg lithium carbonate was given and on days 4, 10 and 17 urine and plasma samples were obtained and analysed as above.

RESULTS

Tilting subjects for an hour produced an increase in the plasma concentration of ANP from 8.8 ± 0.8 to 12.3 ± 0.9 fmole/ml. On returning to the upright this was reduced again to 9.9 ± 0.9. These changes were accompanied by less dramatic changes in renal function (Table 1). Although there were increases in the clearances of creatinine, lithium and sodium on tilting none of these changes were significant; the only statistically significant effect was an increase in urine flow rate. One reason for the lack of significant change might be that the time over which urine was collected was relatively short. Tilting for longer periods produced significant changes in these variables (4).

Table 1. Effects of change of posture on renal function and plasma concentration of ANP.

	Upright	Recumbent	Significance
C_{Cr} (ml/min)	99.0 ± 10.9	115.2 ± 8.2	NS
V (ml/min)	0.8 ± 0.2	1.3 ± 0.3	<0.05
C_{Li} (ml/min)	32.0 ± 5.7	36.3 ± 3.9	NS
C_{Na} (ml/min)	0.7 ± 0.2	1.1 ± 0.2	NS
P_{ANP} (fmole/ml)	8.8 ± 0.8	12.3 ± 0.9	<0.001

Varying the amount of sodium chloride in the diet produced significant changes in both renal function and plasma concentration of ANP (Table 2). Thus increasing salt in the diet resulted in an increase in glomerular filtration rate, urine flow and clearance of lithium and sodium. Clearance of lithium is a measure of fluid delivered from proximal tubules to loops of Henle (5) and so $C_{cr} - C_{Li}$ gives an indication of reabsorption by proximal tubules. Proximal tubular reabsorption was not significantly different on the two diets (LNaD 72.6 ± 3.9; HNaD 71.1 ± 4.6 ml/min). It can be further shown (4) that $C_{Li} - C_{Na}$ gives a measure of sodium reabsorbed by distal segments of the nephron. Although in absolute terms this was increased on the high salt diet (presumably because of the increased delivery of sodium), when expressed as a fraction of sodium delivered to distal segments it was decreased on the high salt diet (LNaD 99.9 ± 0.1%; HNaD 95.5 ± 0.4; $P<0.001$). Values for proximal and distal reabsorption during control Na diet were intermediate between LNaD and HNaD.

There was also a significant 76% rise in the plasma concentration of ANP on the high salt diet.

Table 2. Effect of salt intake on renal function and plasma concentration of ANP.

	LNaD	HNaD	Significance
C_{cr} (ml/min)	89.2 ± 4.2	110.5 ± 4.3	<0.01
V (ml/min)	0.5 ± 0.1	1.9 ± 0.3	<0.01
C_{Li} (ml/min)	16.7 ± 1.4	39.4 ± 1.4	<0.001
C_{Na} (ml/min)	0.020 ± 0.003	1.8 ± 0.2	<0.001
P_{ANP} (fmole/ml)	7.1 ± 0.8	12.5 ± 2.7	<0.01

DISCUSSION

It can be seen that changing either posture or salt intake has dramatic effects on the circulating concentration of ANP. There are also changes in renal function, particularly with changes in salt diet, when there is an increase in glomerular filtration rate without a concomitant increase in proximal tubular reabsorption; thus the normal mechanisms for glomerulo-tubular balance are disrupted. It is tempting to postulate that the changes in ANP caused the changes in renal function, either by changing renal haemodynamics or by a direct effect on tubular epithelium, but a causal relationship has yet to be established.

REFERENCES

1. Maack, T., Camargo, M.J.F., Kleinert, H.D., Laragh, J.H. and Atlas, S.A. Kidney International 27: 607-615, 1985.
2. Dietz, J.R. Amer. J. Physiol. 247: R1093-R1096, 1984.
3. Sugawara, A., Nakao, K., Morii, N., Sakamoto, M., Suda, A., Shimokura, M., Kihara, M., Yamori, Y., Nishimura, K., Soneda, J., Ban, T. and Imura, H. Biochem. Biophys. Res. Comm. 129: 439-446, 1985.
4. Atherton, J.C., Bobinski, H. & Solomon, L. J. Physiol. 373: 73P, 1986.
5. Thomson, K. Nephron 37: 217-223, 1984.

INVOLVEMENT OF Na^+ TRANSPORT AND NATRIURETIC HORMONES IN THE ANTIHYPERTENSIVE MECHANISM OF CANRENONE.

P. HANNAERT, M. DE MENDONCA, M.L. GRICHOIS, B. THORMANN*, J.P. ABITBOL*, AND R. GARAY.
INSERM U7. Hôpital Necker. Paris 75015. France
* Théraplix Lab. Paris 75013. France.

INTRODUCTION

A key step in the development of some forms of primary hypertension appears to be the disturbance in cell Na^+ homeostasis induced by the interaction of endogenous "ouabain-like" factors (EOLF) with vascular cells having genetic abnormalities in membrane Na^+ transport. Several arguments have suggested to us that Canrenone, an antihypertensive antialdosterone drug, may interfere with this mechanism (1). <u>In vitro</u>, this drug behaves like a partial agonist at the digitalis receptor site of the Na^+,K^+-pump (see for instance ref.1, 2): (i) under basal conditions, canrenone slightly inhibits Na^+,K^+-pump activity. An effect which can explain the previous observation that canrenone administration potentiates the inotropic effect of digitalis in dogs (3), (ii) canrenone is able to restimulate a pump blocked by high doses of ouabain. This effect is likely correlated with its ability to protect against digitalis-induced cardiac toxicity (4) and to reverse the inhibitory effect of digoxin on basal and furosemide-stimulated renin secretion (5).

It is important to note that the above <u>in vitro</u> experiments required canrenone concentrations one order of magnitude higher than those observed in plasma of treated-patients (which are of about 8-10 µM, cited in ref.6). On the other hand, Huot et.al. reported that endogenous "ouabain-like" factors are strongly increased in rats with reduced renal mass under excess Na^+ intake (RRM-salt, ref. 7).

We investigated here : i) if preincubation with canrenone may allow to observe effects <u>in vitro</u> at pharmacological doses and ii) if canrenone may antagonize <u>in vivo</u> the secondary effects of endogenous "ouabain-like" factors on cell Na^+-handling and blood pressure in RRM-salt rats.

MATERIALS AND METHODS.

<u>Animals</u>.

The right kidney and the two poles of the left kidney of Male Wistar rats (225-250g) were removed according to the technique of Huot et.al. (7) and the rats were given a 0.9% NaCl solution (RRM-salt rats). Control rats drank tap water. Canrenone (a gift from Théraplix Laboratories) was administrated intragastrically to RRM-salt rats, at a dose of 60 mg/Kg/day.

<u>Measurement of erythrocyte Na^+ content and Na^+,K^+-pump activity</u>.

Venous blood from healthy human subjects or arterial blood from rats (obtained under pentobarbital anesthesia from a catheter implanted in a carotid) was collected in heparinized tubes. Erythrocyte Na^+ content, Na^+,K^+-pump activity and dose-response curves for pump-inhibition by ouabain, were determined according to previously published methods (1).

RESULTS.

<u>Effect of ouabain on erythrocytes preincubated with canrenone</u>.

Table 1 shows the effect of ouabain on human red cells preincubated for 4 h with pharmacological doses of canrenone. It can be seen that pump-inhibition by ouabain is reduced to about 1/4 and 1/2 at 1 and 10 µM canrenone concentrations respectively.

Table 1. Na^+-pump in human erythrocytes preincubated with Canrenone for 4h.

	Na^+,K^+-pump activity*		
Preincubation	Control	42.5 nM Ouabain	%inhibition
-	2310 ± 15	2075 ± 30	10.2%
1 µM Canrenone	2370 ± 10	2190 ± 10	7.6%
10 µM Canrenone	2365 ± 15	2265 ± 30	4.2%

Values in this Table are given as mean ± range of duplicates. A similar result was obtained in two further experiments.

* Ouabain-sensitive Na efflux, in µmoles $(\text{l.cells} \times \text{h})^{-1}$.

<u>Effect of Canrenone-administration in rats with reduced renal mass</u>.

Table 2 shows systolic blood pressure, erythrocyte Na^+ content and Na^+,K^+-pump activity in the different subgroups of rats studied. It can be seen that the increase in blood pressure in RRM-salt rats is associated with a highly significant decrease in pump activity and increase in erythrocyte Na^+ content. Administration of canrenone to these rats results in a highly significant decrease in blood pressure (Table 2). Erythrocyte Na^+ content tends to decrease and Na^+,K^+-pump activity tends to be restimulated. Both effects are statistically significant.

Table 2. Arterial pressure, volemia, Na^+ pump and erythrocyte Na^+ content in rats with reduced renal mass. Effects of Canrenone administration.

	Control	RRM-salt	RRM-salt +Canr.
S.B.P.[a]	121 ± 5 (10)	183 ± 8 (9)***	156 ± 5 (9)***
Plasm.Prot.[b]	53.2 ± 1.9 (9)	47.2 ± 2.5 (9)	53.4 ± 1.8 (9)
Erythr. Na^+ [c]	4.16 ± 0.11 (14)	4.66 ± 0.06 (20)**	4.40 ± 0.06 (21)*
Na^+pump [d]	10.88 ± 0.41 (11)	7.34 ± 0.29 (21)***	8.64 ± 0.31 (21)**

Mean± SEM. The number of rats is indicated in brackets. *** $p < 0.001$. ** $p < 0.01$. * $p < 0.05$. a. Systolic Blood Pressure, mm Hg. b. Plasma Proteins, g/l. c. Erythrocyte Na^+ content, mmol/l.cells. d. Ouabain sensitive Na^+ efflux, mmoles $(l.cells \times h)^{-1}$.

DISCUSSION.

Preincubation with Canrenone allows to observe antagonistic properties against ouabain at pharmacological doses. This suggests a slow rate of association to the pump, as classically observed for cardiac glycosides.

Canrenone is antihypertensive in RRM-salt rats where: i) aldosterone is strongly decreased and ii) endogenous OLF are increased (7). These results suggest that the interaction of canrenone with digitalis-receptor sites may be more important for its antihypertensive action than the interaction with aldosterone-receptors.

In conclusion, our results suggest that chronic administration of canrenone to subjects with primary hypertension may induce a lowering of blood pressure by antagonism with endogenous "ouabain-like" factors at the vascular wall.

REFERENCES

1. GARAY, R.P., J. DIEZ, C. NAZARET, G. DAGHER and J.P. ABITBOL. 1985. . Naunyn-Schmiedeberg's Arch. Pharmacol. 329: 311-315.
2. FINOTTI, P. and P. PALATINI. 1981. J.Pharmacol.Exp.Ther. 217: 784-790.
3. MARCHETTI, G., E. VITOLO, G.F. DiFRANCESCO, B. CAVALLARO and C. SPONZILLI. 1983. Arch. Int. Pharmacodyn. ther. 266: 250-263.
4. YEH, B.K., B.N. CHIANG and P.K. SUNG. 1976. Am. Heart J. 92: 308-314.
5. FINOTTI, P. and A. ANTONELLO. 1982. Clin. Pharmacol. Ther. 32: 1-6.
6. MUGGE, A., W. SCHMITZ and H. SCHOLZZ. 1984. Klin. Wschr. 62: 717-723.
7. HUOT, S.J., M.B. PAMNANI, D.L. CLOUGH and F.J. HADDY. 1983. Am. J. Nephrol. 3: 92-99 .

INHIBITION OF THE ERYTHROCYTE Na+, K+-PUMP BY MAMMALIAN LIGNANS : A POSSIBLE LINK WITH ENDOGENOUS DIGITALIS

P. Braquet, N. Senn*, A. Esanu, and R. Garay*

Institut Henri Beaufour, 17, av. Descartes, F-92350 Le Plessis Robinson (France)

* INSERM U7, Hôpital Necker, 161, rue de Sèvres, F-75015 Paris (France)

Introduction

Natural products formed by oxidative dimerization of phenols, most lignans belong to the vegetal world. However, related structures have been found recently in human and animal urines (1,2). These mammalian lignans are characterized by the presence of the meta hydroxyl group on each aryl cycle of a dibenzyl-gamma-butyrolactone framework (Fig. 1, ref 3).

The main lignan identified in mammalian urine is enterolactone (Fig. 1). The corresponding methylated derivatives (Fig. 1) as well as enterodiol (deriving from the opening of the lactone cycle) have also been characterized, but in lower quantities.

The biological role of mammalian lignans has been never clearly evaluated : (i) their renal excretion increases during the luteal phase of the menstrual cycle and pregnancy in humans and the vervet monkey (1,2) (ii) in contrast, it decreases in postmenopausal women and during breast cancer (4); (iii) lignans could exert a protective effect against intestinal cancer (5); (iv) significant differences have been noted between the blood and seminal concentrations in man and the monkey (6).

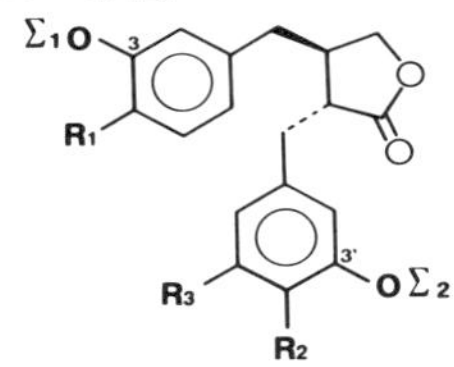

trans-2,3-bis benzyl- -butyrolactone

Σ1	Σ2	R1	R2	R3	PRODUCT	ORIGIN
H	H	H	H	H	1 - Enterolactone	Mammalian urines
Me	H	H	H	H	2 - 3-O-methylenterolactone	Mammalian urines
Me	Me	H	H	H	3 - Di-O-methylenterolactone	Mammalian urines
H	H	OMe	OMe	H	4 - Prestegane A	Mammalian urines and steganotaenia araliacea
Me	H	OMe	OMe	H	5 - Prestegane B	
Me	Me	OMe	OMe	H	6 - Di-O-methylmatairesinol	
Me	Me	OMe	OMe	OMe	7 - 5'-methoxymatairesinol	Synthetic

Fig. 1 :Chemical structure of mammalian lignans and related compounds

There is a certain structural analogy between lignans present in mammals and digitalis since these two compounds have in common a lactone cycle : butanolide and butenolide respectively. These chemical similarities suggested to us that mammalian lignans could interact at the digitalis receptor site of the Na^+, K^+-pump. Indeed, identification of endegenous digitalis is still an unsolved problem even though various hypotheses have been advanced (7-9). Thus, the existence of such regulators is still a controversial subject.

We therefore investigated here the effect of enterolactone, methyl and oxymethyl derivatives on the Na^+, K^+-pump in human red blood cells.

Methods

Preparation of red cells

Venous blood from healthy donors was collected in heparinized tubes and centrifuged at 1750 g for 10 min at 4°C. The plasma and buffy coat were aspirated and the red cell pellet was used immediately.

Na^+-loading procedure

In order to study the effect of internal Na^+ content on Na^+, K^+-pump activity, five aliquotes of cells containing different Na^+ contents were prepared by using a previously described PCMBS method (10). Briefly, red cells washed twice with isotonic NaCl, were resuspended to a hematocrit of about 4 % in the different cold loading media. Five different loading-media were prepared by mixing varying amounts of Na^+ and K^+ media. The Na^+-medium contained (mM) : 150 NaCl, 2.5 Na phosphate buffer (pH 7.2 at 4°C), 1 $MgCl_2$ and 1 EGTA (neutralized with Tris up to pH 7.2 at 4°C). The K^+-medium contained (mM) : 150 KCL, 2.5 K phosphate buffer (pH 7.2 at 4°C), 1 $MgCl_2$ and 1 EGTA (neutralized with Tris up to pH 7.2 at 4°C). PCMBS was added to both media up to a final concentration of 20 μM. The osmolarity of the loading-media was adjusted to 295 $\pm$ 5 mOsm.

The red cell suspensions were incubated in the loading-solutions for 20 h at 4°C. The suspension media were renewed once 6 h incubation. At the end of the treatment with PCMBS, the cells were spun down at 1750 g for 5 min at 4°C and the supernatants were discarded.

The red cells were resuspended at a hematocrit of 10 % in a "recovering medium" containing (mM) : 145 NaCl, 5 KCl, 2.5 Na^+ phosphate buffer (pH 7.4 at 37°C), 1 $MgCl_2$, 4 cysteine, 10 glucose, 3 inosine and 2 adenine. The final pH was adjusted to 7.4 at 37°C with Trizma base. The Na^+-depleted cells were resuspended in a recovery solution in which Na^+ was replaced by K^+. The cell suspensions were incubated at 37°C for 1 h. At the end of this recovery step, the cells were spun down at 1750 g for 5 min at 4°C and the supernatants were discarded.

Measurement of Na^+, K^+-pump activity

Ouabain-sensitive Na^+ efflux was taken as a measure of Na^+, K^+-pump activity (10).

Fresh or Na^+ loaded erythrocytes were washed five times with cold 110 mM $MgCl_2$ and resuspended in Mg-sucrose medium efflux medium at a hematocrit of 20-25 %. The Mg-sucrose medium contained (mM) : 75 $MgCl_2$, 85 sucrose, 10 MOPS-TRIS buffer (pH 7.4 at 37°C) and 10 glucose. The osmolality was adjusted to 295 $\pm$ 5 mOsm. A pormeasure hematocrit, intracellular Na^+ and K^+ by flame photometry and hemoglobin absorbance at 541 nm by spectrophotometry (10).

0.5 ml of the cell suspensions in Mg-sucrose medium were added to two tubes containing 2 ml of Mg-sucrose-K media and to two tubes containing 2 ml of Mg-sucrose-K media with 100 μM ouabain. The Mg-sucrose-K medium was prepared by adding KCl up to a final concentration of 2 mM to a Mg-sucrose medium. The tubes were incubated for 30 min at 37°C (in control experiments we observed that fluxes were linear for more than 30-40 min). At the end of the incubation period the tubes were chilled at 4°C for 1 min and the centrifugated at 1750 g for 4 min at 4°C. The supernatants were transfered into tubes for Na^+ analysis in an Eppendorf flame photometer. Na^+ standards (checked with commercial standards, Merck, Darmstadt) were prepared in water and compared with those prepared in the different efflux media.

In control experiments no evidence of red cell lysis during the incubation in the efflux media could be detected.

Ouabain-sensitive Na^+ efflux (V) was calculated from the difference in external Na^+ concentration between tubes with and without ouabain (DNa) in accordance with the following formula :

$$V = \frac{DNA \times (100\text{-}Ht)}{f \times Ht \times t} \quad \textit{(Eq.1)}$$

where : Ht is the final hematocrit, t : incubation time (30 min) and f : 0.85 is the correction factor for the interference of the Mg-sucrose-K media on the Na^+-reading of the Eppendorf flame photometer.

Determination of the IC_{50} of pump-inhibition by ouabain

Ouabain-sensitive Na^+ efflux was measured in fresh erythrocytes as a function of ouabain concentration according to a previously published protocol (10). The IC_{50} for pump-inhibition by ouabain was determined for each subject studies.

Calculation of apparent affinity for internal Na^+ and maximal rate of Na^+ efflux

For each studied subject, ouabain-sensitive Na^+ efflux (V) was plotted as a function of internal Na^+ content. As previously described (11), the stimulation of ouabain-sensitive Na^+ efflux (V) by internal Na^+ is clearly sigmoidal (S-shaped) and can be expressed by the equation :

$$V = \frac{V_{max}}{[(1 + K_{Na} / (Na)_i]^3} \quad \textit{(Eq.2)}$$

where V_{max} is the maximal rate of ouabain-sensitive Na^+ efflux, K_{Na} represents the apparent dissociation constant for internal Na^+ $(Na)_i$ and 3 is number of inner pump sites for internal Na^+.

Equation (2) can be rearranged as follows : $(Na)_i / (V)^{1/3} = [K_{Na} / (V_{max})^{1/3}] + [(Na)_i / (V_{max})^{1/3}]$ *(Eq.3)*

The left member of equation (3) was plotted against $(Na)_i$ K_{Na} and V_{max} were obtained from the intercept with the abscissa and slope respectively (see ref 11 for further details).

Radioimmunoassay

Displacement by means of lignans of digoxin marked by ^{125}I linked with an antidigoxin antibody was perfomed using the Becton Dickinson equipment in accordance with a previously described technique (8).

Drugs used in this study

Ouabain and digoxin were supplied by SIGMA (St Louis, Mo, USA). The lignans were obtained mainly by total synthesis (12). However, a sampling of various natural compounds was obtained using the urine of pregnant women in accordance with the following protocol : urines were chromatographied in the presence of a neutral resin Amberlite XAD-2. After elution by ethanol, the solvent was evaporated in a vacuum and the conjugates were hydrolyzed by a Helix pomatia juice; the lignans were then purified by successive chromatographies in accordance with the protocol of Setchell et al (3). Their characterization was performed using the linked gas-chromatography / mass spectrometry method.

Results

Effect of lignans on ouabain-sensitive Na^+ efflux

Figure 2 presents the results obtained with all the lignans on the sodium pump of the human erythrocyte. A significant inhibition was obtained with 3-oxy-methylenterolactone, prestegane B and enterolactone (IC_{50} = 6.8 x 10^{-4} M; 7.4 x 10^{-4} M and 9.1 x 10^{-4} m). These results represent a difference with ouabain of about 3 orders of magnitude *(Fig. 2).* The inhibitory activity is inversely proportional to the number of oxy-methylated groups borne by the aromatic ring, no significant inhibition being observed with matairesinol, prestegane A or the synthetic compound methoxy-5' matairesinol *(Fig. 2).*

Effect of lignans on the for IC_{50}ouabain

None of these lignans was able to modify significantly the IC_{50} for ouabain.

Apparent affinity for internal Na^+ and maximal rate of Na^+ efflux

3-oxy-methyl enterolactone increased K_{Na} and decrease V_{max}. Similar results were obtained with prestegane B (Table 1).

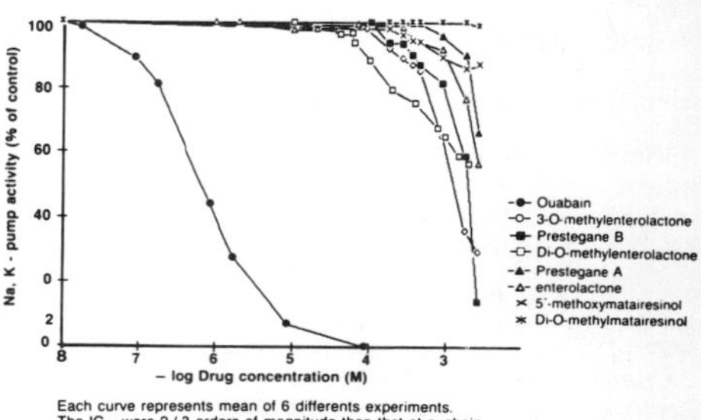

Each curve represents mean of 6 differents experiments.
The IC_{50} were 2 / 3 orders of magnitude than that of ouabain.

Fig. 2 : Inhibitions of the Na^+, K -pump in human red cells by mammalian lignans and related compounds.

(Table 1) : Effect of lignans on the apparent affinity for internal Na^+ and maximal rate of Na^+ efflux.

Compound	K_{Na} (mmol / l.cells)	V_{max}[mmol (l.cells x h)$^{-1}$]
Control	2.9 ± 0.4 (6)	7.4 ± 1.0 (6)
3-oxy-methyl-enterolactone	5.6 ± 0.3 (5)	5.0 ± 1.3 (5)
Prestegane B	4.0 ± 0.6 (5)	4.6 ± 0.6 (5)

Values in this table are given as mean ± SD. The number of experiments is given in brackets.

Interference of lignans with the radioimmunoassay of digoxin

Prestegane B and enterolactone interfere only slightly with the radioimmunoassay of digoxin : thus at 10^{-3} M, enterolactone and prestegane B shift respectively only 16.2 % and 24.3 % of the tracer (digoxin) (see table 2). Thus the crossed reactivity is lower than 2 x 10^{-4} %.

(Table 2) : interference of lignans with the radioimmunoassay of digoxin. Mammalian lignans (10^{-3} M) interfere *slightly* with the RIA of digoxin (%) :

HPM (enterolactone)	:	16.2
Prestegane A	:	4.1
Prestegane B	:	24.3
Di-O-methylenterolactone		11.1
3-O-methylenterolactone		20.7

Discussion

Experimental and clinical evidences strongly suggest the existence of one or several endogenous regulators of the sodium pump (for a recent review see ref 7). However the chemical structure(s) and the production sites are still unknown despite the fact several approaches have been made (7-9).

The physiological role played by mammalian lignans is still poorly known. The presence of a lactone ring (butanolide), a structure also present in the digitalic series (butenolide) suggested to us that lignans were potential canditates for an inhibitory activity on the sodium pump. The results we have obtained on Na^+, K^+-pump of human erythrocytes this assumption : 3-oxy-methylenterolactone, prestegane B and enterolactone inhibit the sodium pump with a decreasing potentiality. Nevertheless the inhibition capacity is still very much lower than that exerted by ouabain. The inhibitory potency seems to be associated with the presence of an hydroxyl or oxymethyl group in meta position, the para substitution generally leading to a loss of activity.

A further substitution on the other meta position abolishes the activity.

The Na^+, K^+-pump inhibition by lignans does not appear to be competitive with that of ouabain suggesting that they do not act at the digitalis receptor site.

Lignans decrease both, the apparent affinity for internal Na and the maximal rate of cation translocation (another difference withouabain see ref 10).

The fundamental question raised here is to know if these lignans are the endogenous digitalic factors or if they are only potentially related compounds.

According to De Wardener and al. (7), endogenous digitalic factors have the following properties : (i) low molecular weight, lower than 500 Dalton, (ii) resistance to heat and proteolytic enzymes, (iii) relative stability in the presence of acid solutions, (iv) absence of amino acids. Furthermore they are polar substances which appear to possess a sugar (9). In chromatographic systems, endogenous digitalic factors have a retention time close to that of steroids. Lignans possess some of these characteristics [molecular weight $<$500 Dalton, stable to heat and acids, destruction in an alkaline medium, absence of amino acids, polar molecules eluted between oestradiol and oestriol in chromatographic systems (2)].

However it is important to note that the urinary concentrations of enterolactone and its methylated derivatives (= 1 μM, ref 4) are at least 2 to 3 orders of magnitude lower than those required to inhibit the sodium pump. It is thus difficult to believe that lignans in the form of aglycones are endogenous. However, natural lignans present in urine possess an osidic group and it is a well known fact that the aglycones of digitalic drugs (and/or the corresponding butanolides) are far less active than the corresponding heterosides (and/or butenolides; ref 13). We cannot therefore exclude the possibility that glycosyl derivatives (and/or butenolide) of mammalian lignans may be endogenous digitalic compounds.

References

1. Stich, S.R., Toumba, J.K., Groen, M.B., Funke, C.W., Leemhuis, J. and Woods, G.F. Nature 287 : 738-740, 1980.
2. Setchel, K.D.R., Lawson, A.M., Mitchel, F.L., Adlercreutz, H., Kirk, D.N. and Axelson, M. Nature 287 : 740-742, 1980.
3. Setchel, K.D.R., Lawson, A.M., Conway, E., Taylor, N.F., Kirk, D.N., Cooley, G., Farrant, R.D., Wynn, S. and Axelson, M. Biochem. J. 197 : 447-458, 1981a.
4. Adlercreutz, H., Fotsis, T., Heikkinen, R., Dwyger, J.T., Woods, M., Goldin, B.R. and Gorbach, S.L. The Lancet ii : 1295-1299, 1982.
5. Setchel, K.D.R., Lawson, A.M., Borriello, S.P., Harkness, R., Gordon, H. and Morgan, D.M.L. The Lancet ii : 4-7, 1981b.
6. Dehenin, L., Reiffsteck, A., Jondet, M. and Thibier, M. Reprod. Fert. 66 : 305-309, 1982.
7. De Wardener, H.E. and Clarkson, E.M. Physiol. Rev., 65 : 658-759, 1985.
8. Godfraind, T. and Fagoo, M. (1985) Symposium "Cardiac Glycosides 1785-1985" (Ed. Erdmann) pp 34 (in press).
9. Cloix, J.F., Crabois, M., Wainer, I.W., Ruegg, V., Seller, M. and Meyer, P. Biochem. Res. Commun., 131 : 1234-1240, 1985.
10. Garay, R.P., Diez, J., Nazaret, C., Dagher, G. and Abitbol, J.P. Naunyn-Schmiedeberg's Arch. Pharmacol. 329 : 311-315, 1985.
11. Garay, R.P. and Garrahan, P.J. J.Physiol. 231 : 297-325, 1973.
12. Robin, J.P. and Braquet, P. (1986) J. Med. Chem. (in preparation).
13. De Pover, A. and Godfraind, T. Naunyn-Schmiedeberg's Arch. Pharmacol. 321 : 135-139, 1982.

EFFECTS OF HUMAN ALFA NATRIURETIC ATRIAL PEPTIDE ON ALDOSTERONE SECRETION IN VITRO.

N.FRISINA, M. BUEMI, F. SQUADRITO, I. MACRI'
ISTITUTO MEDICINA INTERNA UNIVERSITA' DI MESSINA.

There are several evidences on the effects of atrial natriuretic peptide on aldosterone output in intact animals (1) in human (2) and in vitro (3),but the results are variable. To study this discrepancy, the behaviour of aldosterone output was evaluated in isolated and superfused bovine adrenal glands during superfusion with human alfa atrial natriuretic alfa peptide (h-alfa-ANP) alone, with angiotensin II (AII) or dopaminergic drug antagonist metaclopramide (MCP).

MATERIALS & METHODS

Bovine adrenal glands were used. The glands were removed and tissue immediatly placed in a cold Kreebs-Ringers bicarbonate (KRBC) buffer (ph 7,4) conteining 200 mg% glucose and gassed with a mixture O_2-CO_2 (95:5); the adrenal medulle was rapidly separated and the cortex cutted into slices of 2x2 mm. Therefore 500 mg. of tissue was used in each experiment obtained from at least six adrenal glands. One ml chambers termostically controllated at 37° C were used for superfusion. Superfusion was carried with KRBC alone (controls) or with A II (10^{10} M) or MCP (10^{10}M) or h alfa ANP (10^{10}M,10^{8}M, 10^{6}M) or A II (10^{10}M)and h alfa ANP (10^{6}M). Aldosterone assay was carried out on aliquots of perfusion fluid removed at 0,5,10,20,30 and60 min. after the start of superfusion. Aldosterone was assayed by RIA - Analysis of variance was performed and when significant it was fallowed by multiple impaired test.

RESULTS AND DISCUSSION

Data of our present observation, reported on Table I, suggest that ANP markedly blunts the aldosterone response to AII but it does not decrease the aldosterone response to MCP or basal aldosterone production in isolated and superfused bovine adrenal glands.

These findings do not support previous data obtained with atrial extract or other syntetic natriuretic factor which inhibited both basal and stimulated aldosterone secretion in intact animals (3) and in isolated rat adrenal cells (4) . This our result on basal aldosterone secretion agrees with other results in rats (1-5) and in humans (2) . We think that this difference between h-alfa-ANP and atrial peptide of rat on basal aldosterone secretion is due to differences in species.

The mechanism by which h-alfa-ANP blocks the aldosterone response to angiotensin II cannot be clarify by the present experiments. This effect is indipendent of dopaminergic modulation (6) because h-alfa-ANP does not inhibit the aldosterone secretion stimulated by dopaminergic antagonist metoclopramide.

Future studies of the mechanism by which atrial peptide inhibits aldosterone response to A II should provide additional information concerning the role of the h-alfa-ANP on the control of aldosterone secretion and natriuresis.

TIME - min.	0	5	20	60
CONTROLS	6.4±0.08	6.4±0.13	6.6±0.12	6.4±0.08
h ANP 10^{6}M	6.6±0.12	6.8±0.10°	6.7±0.01^{x}	6.5±0.10
A II 10^{10}M	6.4±0.09	18.1±0.27^{x}	12.7±0.19^{x}	6.3±0.26
A II+hANP	6.3±0.07	11.3±0.28^{x}	8.71±0.07^{x}	6.5±0.11
MCP 10^{10}M	6.4±0.18	11.5±0.2^{x}	11.6±0.25^{x}	10.2±0.26^{x}
MCP+hANP	3.3±0.06	12.1±0.11^{x}	11.1±1.08^{x}	10.3±0.06^{x}

TAB. I: Aldosterone output in isolated, superfused, bovine adrenals during superfusion with KRBC alone or with KRBC containing h-alfa ANP (10^{6}M) or A II (10^{10}M) MCP (10^{10}M) alone or in association - 0=P 0,2

X= P 0.001

REFERENCES

1) Chartier L.E., Schiffrin G., Thibaut and R. Garcia, Endocrinology 115:2026-29,1984.

2) Richards A.M., Nicholls M.G., Ikram M., Webster M.W., Sandle T.G. and Espiner E.A.: Lancet I., 545-56,1985.

3) Atarascki K., Mubrow P.J., Franco Saenz R., Suyder R. and Raap J. Science 224+992-994,1984.

4) Goodfriend T.L., Elliot M.E., Atlas SA., Life Science 35, 1675,82,1984.

5) Nakamura M.,Adaguchi K., Shimizu T., Nakamura Y., and Okaurato M., European Journal of Pharmacology 117,285-86,1985.

6) Frisina N., Costa G. and Buemi M.: Clinical Endocrinology, 19,741-745,1983.

INTERACTION OF PLATELET-ACTIVATING FACTOR WITH NATRIURESIS AND DIURESIS INDUCED BY THE SYNTHETIC ATRIAL NATRIURETIC FACTOR [Ser 99 - Tyr 126] IN ANAESTHETIZED DOG

Pierre Thievant, Joelle Baranes, Pierre Etienne Chabrier, Christine Guilmard, Sylvie Regnier and Pierre Braquet

Institut Henri Beaufour, 17 Avenue Descartes, F-92350 Le Plessis Robinson (France)

Introduction

The intravenous infusion of platelet-activating factor (1-O-alkyl-2(R)-acetyl-glycerophosphocholine : PAF, PAF-acether, AGEPC), a potent mediator of anaphylaxis is associated with peripheral vasodilatation, plasma leakage and arterial hypotension (for rev see ref 1). Perfusion of most vital organs is therefore impaired : renal blood flow (RBF) and glomerular filtration rate (GFR) are both decreased markedly, as a consequence of increased renal vascular resistance (RVR, ref 2). Recent studies indicate that the effects of PAF-acether on peripheral circulation are mediated by vasodilatory prostaglandins (PGs), since indomethacin prevents both plasma leakage and hypotension (3). However it was found that the renal effects of PAF are mediated by additional substances, since PGs synthesis inhibition did not prevent RBF, GFR and urinary sodium to fall despite adequate peripheral arterial perfusion (3). Furthermore it has been recently shown that PAF-acether induces *in vivo*, the appearance in the plasma of a tryptic-like activity (Etienne et al., in preparation).

In contrast, it has been shown that mammalian atria contain potent natriuretic and vasoactive peptides which have been termed atrial natriuretic factor (ANF), atrial natriuretic peptides, cardionatrin, atriopeptin and auriculin (for rev see ref 4). Several laboratories have purified, sequenced and synthesized atrial peptides including the [Ser 99 - Tyr 126] fragment which displays natriuretic and vasoactive properties of crude atrial extract (for rev see ref 4). The most striking effects of ANF are to increase GFR, RBF and urinary flow, *in vivo* in various species (5). *In vitro*, in isolated perfused rat kidneys, ANF increased GFR and either enhanced or decreased RVR depending upon pre-existing vascular tone (6). In addition to natriuresis, ANF relaxed rat aortic strips (7) and reduced blood pressure of anaesthetized rats (8). These effects of ANF are independent of PG release.

Since PAF-acether and ANF display : (i) reverse effects on natriuresis, GFR and RBF (ii) similar hypotensive effect although different in duration, we investigated a possible interaction between these two mediators, using specific tools like the specific PAF-acether antagonists BN 52021 (9) and the antiproteasic agent aprotinin.

Materials and methods

- C_{16}-PAF-acether (1-O-hexadecyl-2(R)-acetyl-glycerophosphocholine) and the synthetic ANF [Ser 99 - Tyr 126] were purchased from Novabiochem (Switzerland).
- Sodium pentobarbital was obtained from Clin-Midy Labs. (Paris, France) and aprotinin from SPECIA Labs. (Paris, France).
- BN 52021 (3-[1,1-dimethylethyl]hexahydro-1,4,7b-trihydroxy-8-methyl-9H-1,7α-[epoxy-methano]-1H,6αH-cyclopenta[c]furo[3',2' : 3,4]cyclopenta[1,2-d]furan-5,9,12[4H]-trione) was produced by IHB-Research Labs. (Le Plessis, France).
- All the drugs were dissolved in a saline medium (NaCl 9 ‰) except BN 52021 in dimethyl sulfoxide (DMSO) in a volume of 0.1 ml/kg and PAF-acether in a saline-bovine serum albumin (0.5 ‰).

Methods

Mongrel dogs of either sex (12-18 kg) purchased from Lessieux (95 Bray Lû, France) were anaesthetized with pentobarbital (35 mg/kg, iv), intubated and ventilated with compressed air via a logic O_2 respirator (Minerve, France). Anaesthesia was maintained by a constant pentobarbital perfusion (5 mg/kg per hour) during all the experimentation. After laparotomy, each ureter was separately canulated at the base of the bladder for continous urine collection. The experimental protocol consisted in two 15 min collection periods (control periods) followed by a further three 15 min periods after drug or solvent administration (iv). Urinary volume was measured and Na^+ and K^+ excretions were determined by flame photometry (Delhomme, France).

Five series of experiments were performed (6 animals per group) :

Group 1 : Specific effect of ANF	: - ANF (5 μg/kg, iv) in saline - saline (control solvent) 5 min before ANF
Group 2 : Specific effect of PAF-acether	: - PAF-acether (0.06, 0.150, 0.300 and 0.600 μg/kg, iv) in saline/BSA medium - saline/BSA medium (control solvent) 5 min before ANF
Group 3 : Specific effect of BN 52021	: - BN 52021 (5 mg/kg, iv) in DMSO 5 min before saline - DMSO (control solvent) 5 min before saline
Group 4 : PAF-acether / ANF interactions	: - PAF-acether (0.1 μg/kg, iv) 5 min before ANF (5 μg/kg, iv) - saline 5 min before ANF (5 μg/kg, iv)
Group 5 : BN 52021 / ANF interactions	: - BN 52021 (5 mg/kg, iv) 5 min before ANF (5 μg/kg, iv) - DMSO 5 min before ANF (5 μg/kg, iv)
Group 6 : Aprotinin / ANF interactions	: - aprotinin (Zymofren® 10.000 KIU/kg, iv) 5 min before ANF (5 μg/kg,iv) - saline 5 min before ANF (5 μg/kg, iv)

In all experiments, drugs were given in a bolus. Results were given as mean ± SEM. Each dog was its own control. Differences between control, experimental and recovery periods were analyzed by the two ways analysis of variance. Simultaneous comparisons at the different periods between pairs of groups were also made by analysis of variance.

Results

- Effect of [Ser 99 - Tyr 126] ANF on diuresis and electrolyte excretion in the anaesthetized dog.

Administration of ANF (5 μg/kg, iv) induced a significant increase (i) in diuresis (6 to 8 fold) (ii) in natriuresis (5 to 8 times) (iii) and in kaliuresis to a lesser extent (2 to 3 times). This action was relatively short since it did not exceed 15 minutes and the second and third collection periods were not significantly different from the control period.

- Effect of PAF-acether on sodium excretion in the anaesthetized dog.

PAF-acether injection reduced sodium excretion by 210, 330, 600 and 960 μEq/15 min from baseline values at 0.060, 0.150, 0.300 and 0.600 μ/kg respectively. After each bolus sodium excretion returned to control values within 30 min.

- Effect of the PAF-acether antagonist BN 52021 in diuresis and electrolyte excretion in the anaesthetized dog.

Used alone, BN 52021 was totally devoid of effect on both diuresis and electrolyte excretion (data not shown). The solvent (DMSO) was also devoid of effect (data not shown).

- Effect of PAF-acether on [Ser 99 - Tyr 126] ANF-induced diuresis and electrolyte excretion in the anaesthetized dog

Administered preventively 5 min before ANF, PAF-acether (0.1 μg/kg, iv) pratically abolished the effect of the peptide. These effects were equally pronounced in diuresis, natriuresis and kaliuresis (see Fig. 1 for details). For example ANF alone induced an increase from 2.60 ± 0.65 ml/15 min to 22.00 ± 5.05 ml/15 min ($p<0.001$) and this effect of ANF was reduced to 4.4 ± 1.80 ml/15 min when PAF-acether was injected preventively 5 min beforehand ($p<0.001$ compared with ANF alone).

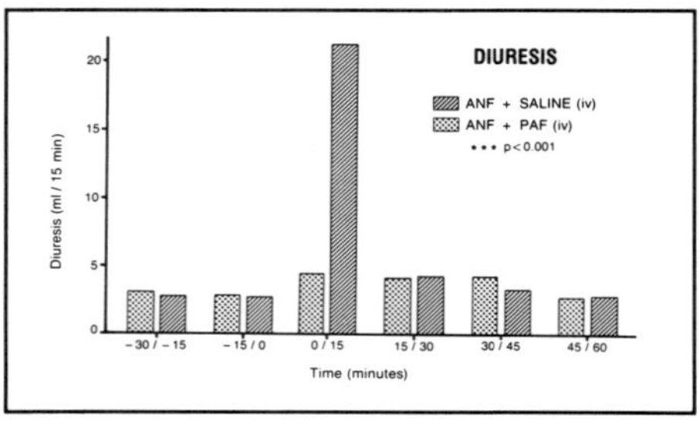

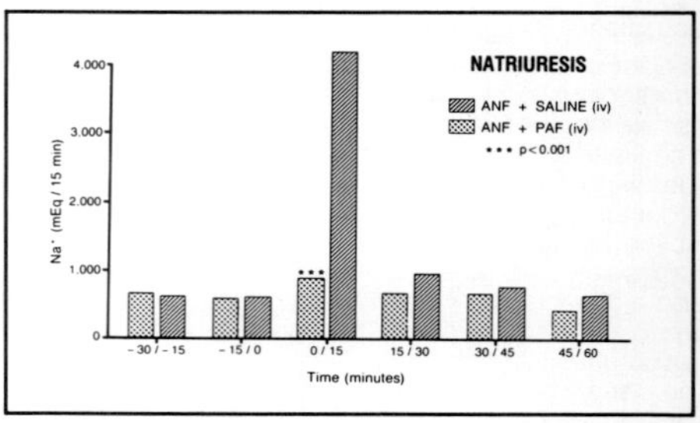

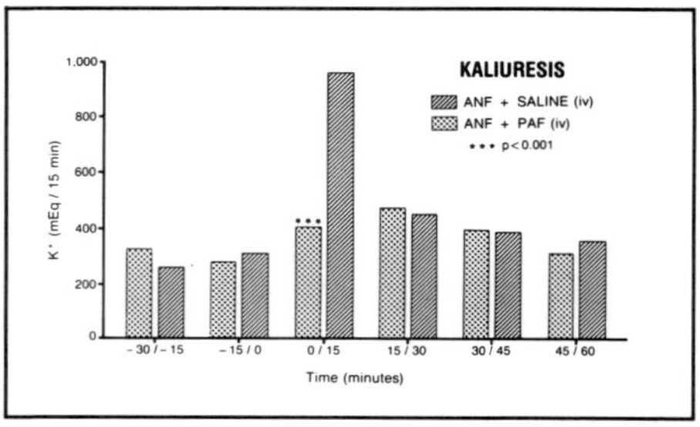

Fig. 1 : Effect of C_{16}-PAF-acether on ANF [Ser 99 - Tyr 126]-induced diuresis and electrolyte excretion in the anaesthetized dog.

- Effect of BN 52021 on [Ser 99 - Tyr 126] ANF-induced diuresis and electrolyte excretion in the anaesthetized dog.

In contrast to PAF-acether, administered preventively, BN 52021 (5 ml/kg, iv) potentiates the effect of ANF on diuresis, natriuresis and kaliuresis (see Fig. 2 for details). For example concerning natriuresis, ANF alone increases approximately 6 fold Na^+ excretion (control period 236 ± 123 μEq/15 min, ANF period 1320 ± 880 μEq/15 min, $p<0.001$). When BN 52021 was administered before ANF, natriuresis increased approximately 10 fold (control period 320 ± 115 μEq/15 min, ANF period 3140 ± 800 μEq/15 min, $p<0.001$).

Effect of aprotinin on [Ser 99 - Tyr 126] ANF-induced diuresis and electrolyte excretion in the anaesthetized dog.

Aprotinin (10.000 KIU/kg, iv) given 5 min before ANF does not affect the duration nor the amplitude of the effect of the peptide on diuresis, natriuresis and kaliuresis (data not shown).

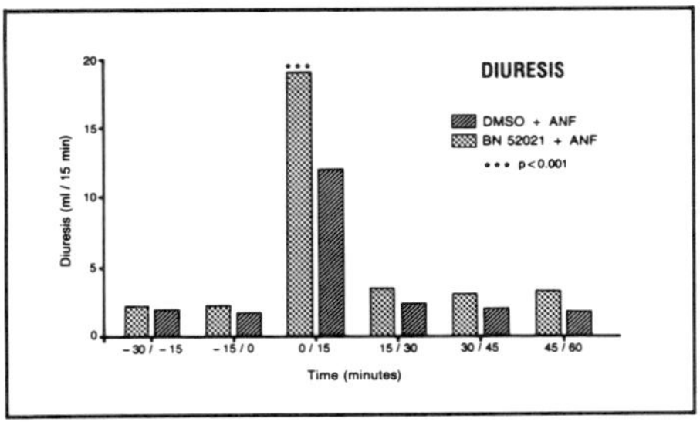

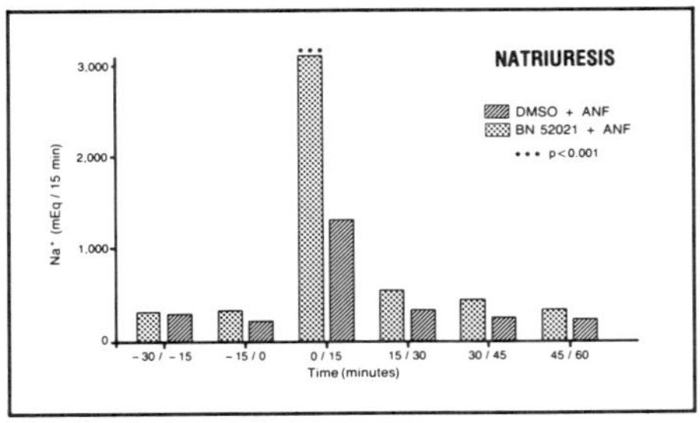

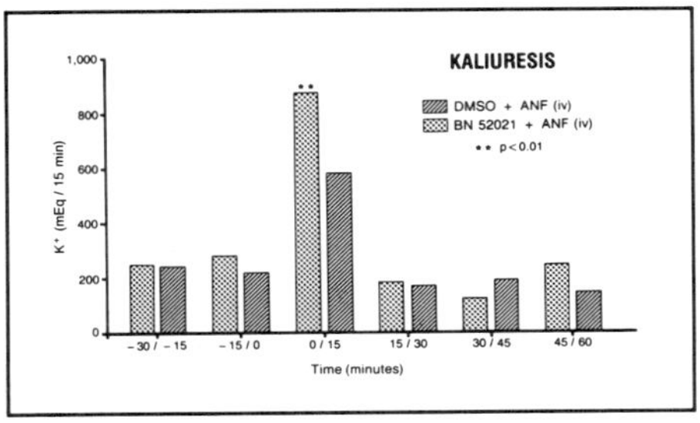

Fig. 2 : Effect of the PAF-acether antagonist BN 52021 on ANF [Ser 99 - Tyr 126]-induced diuresis and electrolyte excretion in the anaesthetized dog.

Discussion

As classically observed the synthetic [Ser 99 - Tyr 126] ANF induces increases in diuresis, natriuresis, and also kaliuresis to a lower extent, in the anaesthetized dog. These effects are immediate and have a short duration (approximately 15 min).

In contrast, PAF-acether induces a dose-dependent decrease in sodium excretion, this parameter returns to control values within 30 min. On the basis of this result, we used a 0.1 μg/kg dose for PAF-acether/ANF dual experiments in order to avoid too massive an effect of the ether lipid. These effects of PAF-acether on renal function are significantly inhibited by the specific antagonist BN 52021 (3).

Surprisingly (i) pretreatment with PAF-acether 5 min before ANF practically abolishes the effect of the peptide on both diuresis and electrolyte excretion. (ii) The PAF-antagonist BN 52021 which is devoid of effects per se on diuresis and electrolyte excretion, potentiate the effect of the synthetic ANF. This effect is observed only with respect to amplitude but not duration. Since we have recently shown that PAF-acether induces *in vivo*, the appearance in the plasma of a tryptic-like activity (Etienne et al., in preparation) we performed a similar experiment with aprotinin, an anti-proteasic agent. At the dose used (10.000 KIU/kg, iv) pretreatment with aprotinin does not affect the duration nor the amplitude of the effects of ANF. Different findings were observed in anaesthetized rats by Thibault et al. (10) who recorded a prolongation of the effect of the peptide with only a slight increase in amplitude.

Our results give rise to several questions. Firstly how does PAF-acether antagonize the effect of ANF in this model : among the possible hypotheses, it can be assumed that PAF-acether increases the catabolism of ANF since it induces a very rapid increase in plasma protease activity. This effect lasts from 15 to 20 min and practically disappears around 30 min. Secondly, how can PAF-antagonist alone potentiate the effects of ANF. It can be assumed that PAF-antagonist may act by its indirect anti-proteasic effect since we demonstrated that although BN 52021 does not inhibit tryptic activity *in vitro*, it counteracts PAF-induced proteolytic activity *in vivo* (Etienne et al., in preparation). This could strengthen the assumption that an endogenous PAF or PAF-like compound may be involved in the regulation of homeostasis. A second explanation for our results is that ANF could raise the level or release of PAF-acether which itself inhibits the action of ANF by a feedback mechanism, as has already been demonstrated for angiotensin/prostaglandins system (13).

In another respect it was recently demonstrated that PAF-acether increases GTPase activity in platelets and consequently may affect the level of cyclic GMP (14). This contrasts with the action of ANF which has been proved to increase the level of cyclic GMP in many systems. These two antagonistic effects may provide a possible explanation, at molecular level, for the results observed.

Further studies will be necessary to obtain better comprehension of these interrelations.

References

1. Braquet, P., Touqui, L., Vargaftig, B.B. and Shen, T.Y. J. Med. Chem. (in press). - 2. Vemulapalli, S., Chiu, P.J.S. and Barnet, A. Hypertension 6 : 489-493, 1984. - 3. Plante, G., Hebert, R.L., Lamoureux, C., Braquet, P. and Sirois, P. Pharmacol. Res. Com. (in press). - 4. Needleman, P., Currie, M.G., Geller, D.M., Cole, B.R. and Adams, S.P. TIPS 506-509, Dec. 1984. - 5. Maack, T., Camargo, M.J.F., Kleinert, H.D., Laragh, J.H. and Atlas, S.A. Kidney int. 27 : 607-615, 1985. - 6. Camargo, M.J.F., Kleinert, H.D., Atlas, S.A., Sealey, J.E., Laragh, J.H. and Maack, T. Am. J. Physiol. 246 : 447-456, 1984. - 7. Auguet, M., Delaflotte, S., Garay, R., Cantin, M., Clostre, F. and Braquet, P. Regul. peptides supp. 4 : 104-109, 1985. - 8. Sasaki, A., Kida, O., Kangawa, K., Matsuo, H. and Tanaka, K. Eur. J. Pharmacol. 109 : 405-407, 1985. - 9. Braquet, P., Drieu, K. and Etienne, A. Actual. Chim. Ther. 13 : 237-254, 1986. - 10. Thibault, G., Garcia, R., Cantin, M. and Genest, J. Can. J. Physiol. Pharmacol. 62 : 645-649, 1984.

CIRCULATING NATRIURETIC FACTOR IN THE PATHOGENESIS OF GENETIC HYPERTENSION OF RENAL ORIGIN.

P.Ferrari[*], HE.de Wardener[o], JA.Millet[o], L.Torielli[*], M.Ferrandi[*], G.Bianchi[**]
[*]Farmitalia Carlo Erba Centro Ricerche, Nerviano - [o]Research Laboratories Charing Cross, London - [**]Istituto Scienze Mediche Università di Milano

INTRODUCTION

A circulating natriuretic factor, able to inhibit the cellular Na^+-K^+ pump, has been described in human essential and animal sperimental hypertension (1,2). Increases of this circulating factor seem to be linked to a kidney defect in sodium and water excretion. The Milan hypertensive strain of rats (MHS) spontaneously develops hypertension due to a genetically determined, renal abnormality which produces a transient Na^+ retention during the prehypertensive phase (3). To verify whether a circulating natriuretic factor could be involved in the pathogenesis of MHS hypertension, we have measured in MHS and their normotensive controls (MNS) at different ages the Na^+ transport through the Na^+-K^+ pump in red blood cells (RBC), and the ability of rat plasma to stimulate "in vitro" the glucose 6-phosphate-dehydrogenase (G6PD) as index of the plasma capacity to inhibit the Na^+-K^+ ATPase activity(4).

METHODS

Male MHS and MNS rats were used at different ages: 25-30 day-old (prehypertensive), 50-70 day-old (hypertensive), 150-160 day-old (established hypertensives). Blood pressure was measured both as systolic blood pressure (SBP) at the tail and as mean blood pressure (MBP) on the carotid artery through a chronic catheter. Na^+ fluxes were measured in fresh washed RBC cells, as described elsewhere (5). The Na^+-K^+ pump was calculated as ouabain-sensitive Na^+ efflux, Na^+-K^+ cotransport as ouabain-insensitive, bumetanide-sensitive Na^+ efflux and Na^+ permeability as ouabain and bumetanide-insensitive Na^+ efflux. The G6PD stimulating activity of the rat plasma was measured by a cytochemical technique, as described elsewhere (4).

RESULTS

Fig. 1 shows the Na^+ fluxes through the RBC membrane of MHS and MNS, as function of age and blood pressure levels. At the prehypertensive age (25 day-old) the Na^+-K^+ pump is equal in MHS and MNS RBC, while the Na^+-K^+ cotransport is faster in MHS, up to 70 days of age. When hypertension has fully developed in MHS (70 and 150 days of age) their RBC Na^+-K^+ pump is significantly inhibited than in MNS. The Na^+-K^+ cotransport is still faster in 70 day but becomes equal in the two strains at older age.

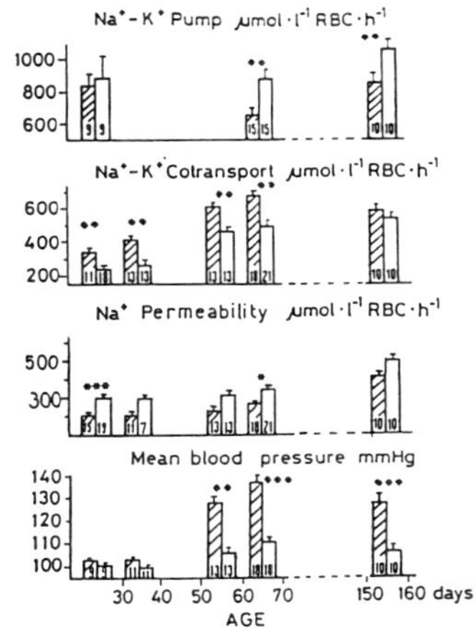

FIG. 1

Mean blood pressure, Na-K pump, Na-K cotransport and Na passive permeability of fresh RBC from MHS and MNS at different ages. Values are±mean ± SEM. Number of animals in the bars.

The plasma ability of MHS and MNS to stimulate the G6PD is reported in Table 1. At 21 days the MHS already show a significantly raised plasma capacity to stimulate G6PD than MNS, but this activity becomes more evident in adult 55 day-old MHS than MNS.

TABLE 1- Blood pressure and G6PD plasma stimulating activity of MHS and MNS rats at different ages.

Age (days)	21		55	
Strain	MNS	MHS	MNS	MHS
SBP (mmHg)	117.5±1.3*	124.3±1.8	133.6±1.0***	172.0±1.1
G6PD Stim.activity (unit .ml^{-1})	7.8±1.8***	100.0±27.4	23.4±8.3***	586.0±88
N°animals	7	7	7	7

Values are mean±SEM. *$p < 0.05$ ***$p < 0.001$ by t Student analysis.

DISCUSSION

This work demonstrates that the RBC Na^+-K^+ pump activity is inhibited in adult hypertensive MHS than MNS and the plasma of MHS is able to stimulate G6PD (i.e. to inhibit Na^+-K^+ ATPase), during the development of hypertension. Much experimental evidence supports the existance of a renal abnormality which produces at tubular level an increased Na^+reabsorption during the prehypertensive phase (3,5). Moreover, experiments on the activation of the tubuloglomerular feedback (TGF) mechanism (6) showed that in young MHS this mechanism is essentially absent while it is activated in adult hypertensive MHS, indicating that prehypertensive MHS behave like volume expanded animals. The rise with age of the plasma G6PD stimulating activity and the parallel inhibition of RBC Na^+-K^+pump in MHS support the hypothesis that the levels of a circulating Na^+-K^+pump inhibitor are increased in MHS as consequence of the renal defect that produces Na^+retention and in turn hypertension in this rat strain.

REFERENCES

1. MacGregor G.A. et al.: Clin. Sci. 61: 17, 1981
2. Millett J.A. et al. : J. Endocrin. 108: 69, 1986
3. Bianchi G. et al.: Circ. Res. 36&37: 153, 1975
4. Fenton S. et al.: J. Endocrin. 94: 99, 1982
5. Ferrari P.et al.: Clin. Sci. 63: 61, 1982
6. Persson E. et al.: Acta Physiol. Scand. 122: 217, 1984

LACK OF CORRELATION BETWEEN PLASMA OUABAIN-LIKE FACTOR AND URINARY SODIUM EXCRETION IN ESSENTIAL HYPERTENSIVE PATIENTS.

P. DELVA, M. DEGAN, C. CAPRA, M. DE GASPERI, M. MENEGAZZI AND A. LECHI.

Clinica Medica, University of Verona Medical School, Policlinico, 37134 Verona, Italy.

INTRODUCTION

It has been proposed that a circulating ouabain-like factor may act as a modulator of sodium excretion and that primary renal impairment in patients with essential hypertension might be compensated for by high plasma levels of this putative natriuretic hormone (1). Natriuretic peptides have recently been isolated from atria, but their biological effect is not mediated by Na^{+}-K^{+} pump inhibition (2). On the contrary, the natriuretic hormone described by De Wardener (1) is thought to cause both natriuresis and depolarization of arteriolar muscle cells by means of the same effect on the cell membrane, i.e. inhibition of the Na^{+}-K^{+} pump.

In an attempt to investigate the role of this putative Na^{+}-K^{+} pump inhibitor on sodium homeostasis, we have measured plasma ouabain-like activity and urinary Na^{+} excretion in a group of normotensive and hypertensive subjects in order to correlate these parameters.

MATERIALS AND METHODS

We studied 23 normotensive (NT) and 37 essential hypertensive (EH) subjects on an unrestricted sodium diet (60-190 mmol/day). All patients were hospitalized, and the diagnosis was made after a complete clinical and laboratory investigation. None of the EH patients exhibited metabolic disorders, ischaemic heart disease, cerebrovascular or kidney disease and none of them was obese. The normotensive subjects were healthy donors with a proven familial history of normotension for at least two generations. Plasma ouabain-like activity was assessed, following Devynck et al. (3), by measuring the plasma-induced kinetic modifications of tritiated ouabain binding to human erythrocytes. The red cells were incubated in the presence of six different ouabain concentrations ranging from 1.5 to 30 nmol/l. The addition of plasma exclusively affects the affinity of ouabain binding, so plasma ouabain-like activity was arbitrarily expressed by (K'd-Kd)/Kd where K'd and Kd represent the apparent dissociation constants of ouabain in the presence and in the absence of plasma respectively. Daily 24-h urine collections were analyzed for sodium, potassium and creatinine excretion.

RESULTS

Despite a wide scattering of values and a substantial overlap between the two groups, the mean value of plasma ouabain-like activity was significantly higher in EH as compared to NT (Table 1).

We did not find any significant correlation between plasma ouabain-like activity and either urinary sodium or potassium excretion.

Table 1. Clinical and laboratory data (values expressed as means ± SD).

Group	Age (yrs)	Blood pressure (mm Hg) diastolic	Blood pressure (mm Hg) systolic	$\frac{K'd-Kd}{Kd}$
Normotensive	37 ± 8	75 ± 5	116 ± 7	0.216 ± 0.430
Hypertensive	40 ± 11	109 ± 13	166 ± 20	0.947 ± 1.328*

* Wilchoxon's test, $p < 0.01$

DISCUSSION

As the ability of plasma to compete with ouabain for a specific membrane receptor may be considered as reflecting its potential Na^+-K^+ pump inhibitor activity (3), our results confirm previous reports (3-4) on the existence of a plasma regulator of this membrane cation transport system and its elevation in essential hypertension.

The main question raised by the present study concerns the pathophysiological relevance in renal excretion of this potential Na^+-K^+ pump inhibitor. In fact, we were unable to confirm the positive correlation, postulated by De Wardener and recently confirmed by Devynck (3), between the plasma levels of this factor and sodium excretion. Nevertheless, given the complexity of the factors that normally influence sodium excretion, our results are not sufficient to exclude a role for this factor in renal sodium handing.

In conclusion, the recently proposed identity of ouabain-like factor and the putative natriuretic hormone remains uncertain, as does its possible role in essential hypertension.

REFERENCES

1. De Wardener, H.E. and Mac Gregor, G.A. Lancet i: 1450-1454, 1982.
2. Maack, T., Camargo, M.J.F., Kleinert, H.D., Laragh, J.H. and Atlas, S.A. Kidney Int. 27: 607-615, 1985.
3. Devynck, M.A., Pernollet, M.G., Rosenfeld, J.B. and Meyer, P. Brit. Med. J. 287: 631-634, 1983.
4. Hamlyn, J.M., Ringel, R., Schaeffer, J., Levinson, P.D., Hamilton, B.P., Kowarsky, A.A. and Blaunstein, M.P. Nature 300: 650-652, 1982.

ATRIAL NATRIURETIC PEPTIDE DURING WATER IMMERSION IN HEALTHY VOLUNTEERS

T. TIKKANEN, I. TIKKANEN, F. FYHRQUIST, K. METSÄRINNE, K.J. TÖTTERMAN

Unit of Clinical Physiology, the Minerva Foundation Institute for Medical Research, P.O. Box 819, 00101 Helsinki, Finland

INTRODUCTION

Atrial natriuretic peptide (ANP) is a diuretic and natriuretic hormone secreted from atrial myocytes in response to increased cardiac filling pressure (1, 2). ANP also suppresses release of renin and aldosterone (1, 2). Water immersion to the neck causes diuresis and natriuresis, which has been related to increased central blood volume (3). Decreased activity of renin-angiotensin-aldosterone axis and suppression of antidiuretic hormone (ADH) release have been observed during immersion (3). However, additional factors have been suggested to be involved in immersion-induced natriuresis. It was therefore of interest to study plasma ANP levels during water immersion.

METHODS

Eight healthy male volunteers, aged 25-38 years, were studied. They were on their normal diet but during the experimental day, only tap water, 200 ml/hr, was given. Starting at 15.00 hr, subjects were seated for 1 hr, and then immersed (34°C) to the neck for 2 hr, and finally sat outside the bath for 1 hr.

Voided urine volumes, sodium excretion, pulse rate, and blood pressure were measured. Plasma ANP (4), renin activity (5), aldosterone (Abbot's kit), and ADH (6) were measured by radioimmunoassay.

Student's t-test for paired data was applied. The results are expressed as mean $\pm$ S.E.M.

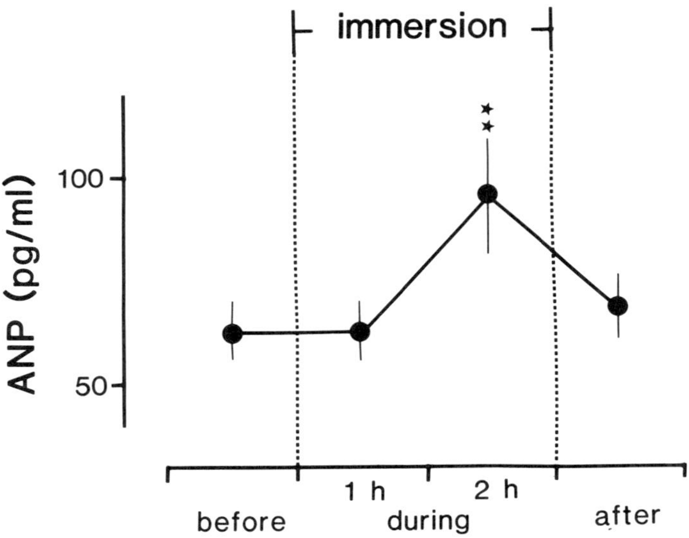

Fig. 1. Plasma ANP concentration before, during, and after head-out water immersion in healthy volunteers. **p<0,01 compared with control period before immersion.

RESULTS AND CONCLUSIONS

During immersion, urine output and sodium excretion increased (Fig. 2). Both systolic and diastolic blood pressure decreased slightly. During the first hour of immersion, plasma ANP concentration did not change (64 $\pm$ 6,5 vs 63 $\pm$ 6,8 pg/ml before immersion, NS) but rose to 95 $\pm$ 9,6 pg/ml (p<0,01) during the second immersion hour. After immersion, plasma ANP declined to control levels (Fig. 1). Plasma renin activity and aldosterone decreased during immersion, while ADH, which was low even before immersion, did not change (Fig. 3).

Thus head-out water immersion causes both suppression of renin aldosterone axis and stimulation of ANP release. We conclude that ANP may be involved in immersion-induced natriuresis.

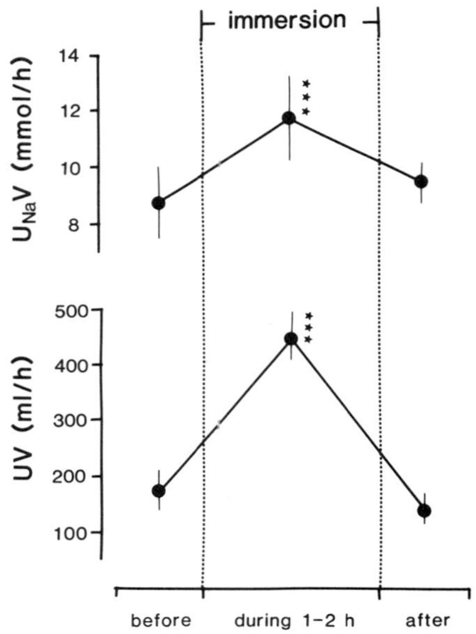

②

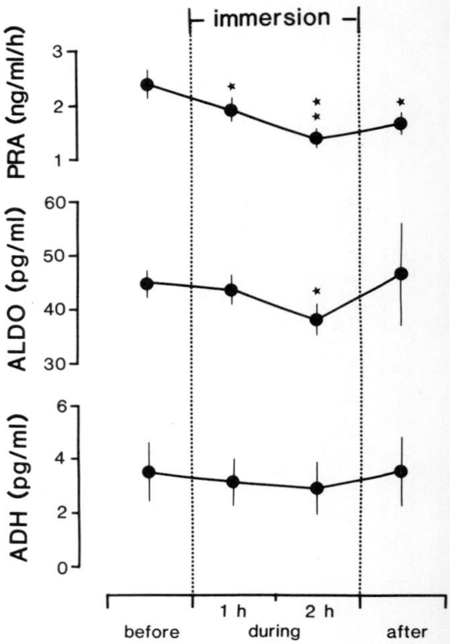

③

Fig. 2. Urinary sodium excretion ($U_{Na}V$) and urine output (UV) before, during and after water immersion. ***p<0,001 compared with control period before immersion.

Fig. 3. Plasma renin activity (PRA), aldosterone (ALDO), and antidiuretic hormone (ADH) before, during and after water immersion. *p<0,05, **p<0,01 compared with control period before immersion.

REFERENCES

1. Cantin, M. and Genest, J. Endocrine Rev. 6: 107-127, 1985.
2. Needleman, P. and Greenwald, J.E. N. Engl. J. Med. 314: 828-834, 1986.
3. Epstein, M. Contr. Nephrol. 41: 174-178, 1984.
4. Tikkanen, I., Fyhrquist, F., Metsärinne, K. and Leidenius, R. Lancet ii: 66-69, 1985.
5. Fyhrquist, F., Soveri, P., Puutula, L. and Stenman U-H. Clin. Chem. 22: 250-256, 1976.
6. Fyhrquist, F., Wallenius, M. and Hollemans, H.J.G. Scand. J. Clin. Lab. Invest. 36: 841-847, 1976.

VI. AQUARETICS

SYMPOSIUM ON AQUARETICS: INTRODUCTION

L.B. KINTER

Department of Pharmacology, Smith Kline and French Laboratories, Swedeland, PA 19479, USA

INTRODUCTION

Diuretics form a large and successful class of therapeutic agents useful in the treatment of volume-expanded states resulting from cardiovascular and renal pathologies and disease processes (1). Conventional diuretic agents interfere with renal salt reabsorption, resulting in greatly increased renal salt loss (1). Water lost as a consequence of the imposed "saliuresis" is that required to excrete the additional solute load. Loss of salt in excess of water, however, can result in potentially life-threatening hyponatremia.

Several groups have sought to describe new diuretic agents which would allow excretion of water in excess of solute as a treatment for hyponatremic states. Wiebelhaus first described the concept and identified a series of potentially water-diuretic compounds in 1974 (2). Demeclocycline and lithium carbonate were the first agents used clinically to produce positive free water clearances ("aquaresis") in patients (3,4). Both agents, however, have slow onsets of action, serious toxic liabilities and poorly understood mechanisms of action (5,6). Leskal and colleagues have described aquaretic activity associated with administration of the prostaglandin E_2 analog, 9-desoxy,16,16-dimethyl PGE_2 in experimental animals (7). This analog has been reported to be aquaretic in humans and effective to treat hyponatremia in a patient (8). The mechanism of action of 9-desoxy,16,16-dimethyl PGE_2 is not understood (8). Drs. Manning and Sawyer first described diuretic vasopressin antagonists in 1980 (see ref. 9). The aquaretic activity of these vasopressin receptor antagonists is now well documented in experimental animals, and the mechanism of action thought to be well understood; aquaretic activity in humans, however, has yet to be demonstrated.

The proposed therapeutic utilities for aquaretic agents include diseases and pathological conditions associated with excessive body water (e.g. hyponatremia, congestive heart failure, Syndrome of Inappropriate Antidiuretic Hormone, cirrhosis, and edema states; see 6-10). It is notable that, in contrast to saliuretics, aquaretics are not considered likely to be of general use in the management of hypertension.

It has previously been proposed that with the advent of selective water-diuretic agents, it is appropriate to consider an extended nomenclature for diuretic agents to distinguish mechanisms of action (11). Thus:

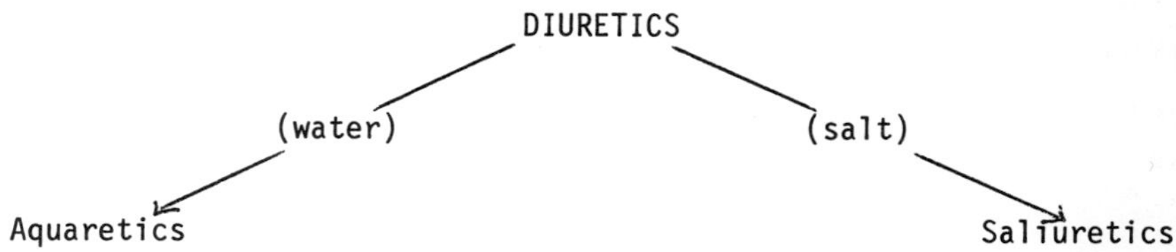

Beyond their demonstrated and proposed therapeutic utilities, the significance of clinically successful aquaretics is that with these agents, it will be possible for the first time to selectively and conveniently manipulate body water content, independent of body salt content. Thus, with aquaretic and saliuretic agents, it will be possible to pharmacologically control, in a predictable fashion, both the quantity and composition of extracellular fluid.

REFERENCES

1. Mudge, G. In: The Pharmacological Basis of Therapeutics (Ed. A.G. Gilman, L. Goodman and A. Gilman), Macmillan, New York, 1980, pp. 885-915.
2. Wiebelhaus, V., Sosnowski, G., Maas, A., and Brennan, F. In: Recent Advances in Renal Pharmacology and Physiology (ed. L.G. Wesson and G.M. Fanelli), Univ. Park Press, Baltimore, 1974, pp. 331-347.
3. Forrest, J., Cox, M., Hong, C., Morrison, G., Bia, M., and Signer, I. N. Engl. J. Med. 298:173-177, 1978.
4. Oster, J., Epstein, M. and Ulamo, H. Curr. Ther. Res. 20:797-801, 1976.
5. Hays, R. In: The Pharmacological Basis of Therapeutics (Ed. A.G. Gilman, L. Goodman and A. Gilman), Macmillan, New York, 1980, pp. 916-928.

6. Earley, L.E. (This volume).
7. Christensen, N.J., Bygdeman, M., Green, K., et al. Pflugers Arch. 402:360-363, 1984.
8. Leksall, L. (This volume).
9. Kinter, L., Huffman, W., Stassen, F., et al. (This volume).
10. Schrier, R. (This volume).
11. Kinter, L., Huffman, W., Wiebelhaus, V., et al. In: Diuretics (ed. J. Puschett and A. Greenberg), Elsevier Science Publishing Co., New York, 1984, pp. 72-81.

SOME AQUARECTIC AGENTS OTHER THAN VASOPRESSIN ANALOGS

L.E. EARLEY

Department of Medicine, University of Pennsylvania School of Medicine, Philadelphia, Pennsylvania

The ability to excrete dilute urine may be impaired in at least three different ways that are of clinical importance. In some patients with heart or liver failure and avid sodium retention, the isotonic reabsorption of filtrate in proximal portions of the nephron may be so great that the limited delivery of fluid to diluting sites in distal nephron segments may be inadequate to permit the excretion of an amount of water sufficient to balance intake. Over relatively long periods of time, the continued intake of water would lead to hyponatremia. Aquaresis in this situation would be achievable by reducing isotonic reabsorption in proximal portions of the nephron so long as the distal diluting functions were not impaired.

In very rare situations patients with excessive intake of water due to primary polydipsia may become hyponatremic with only modest impairment in the ability to excrete dilute urine. Thiazide diuretics impair urinary dilution by interfering with electrolyte reabsorption in the distal neprhon where reabsorption normally generates dilute urine. This limit of diluting ability is quantitatively so modest that water retention is not a usual complication of therapy with thiazides. However, if the intake of water is extraordinarily large, as has been the case in some patients, then the interference with urinary dilution by thiazides may result in clinically important retention of water.

The most common intrarenal mechanism of water retention is the continued reabsorption of dilute tubular fluid in the vasopressin sensitive distal segments of the nephron due to the inappropriate presence of vasopressin, or to the presence of drugs that mimic the action of vasopressin or amplify the effects of small amounts of the hormone. The effect of vasopressin to promote inappropriate retention of water and hyponatremia can be approached pharmacologically in several ways. Aquaretics could be designed that interfere with the synthesis or release of vasopressin, that compete with the binding of vasopressin to its receptors, or that interfere with some biochemical step in the cellular action of vasopressin. The serendipitous observation of polyuria associated with agents employed therapeutically for reasons unrelated to the kidney led to the discovery of their aquaretic property. Shortly after lithium carbonate achieved widespread use in the treatment of the manic phase of manic-depressive disorders, polyuria and polydipsia were recognized as common side effects of the treatment. This observation led to the use of lithium to successfully increase the excretion of water in patients with the syndrome of inappropriate secretion of antidiuretic hormone and to investigations of the mechanism of its polyuric effect.

In laboratory studies, it was shown that the polyuria induced by lithium in rats was unresponsive to vasopressin and only partially responsive to cyclic-AMP, when compared to normal rats and to the Brattleboro rat with inherited complete central diabetes insipidus (Fig. 1). This observation suggested that lithium interferes with the action of vasopressin, and since the polyuria is responsive to cyclic-AMP, the interference by lithium appears to be at the step of generation of clyclic-AMP. These conclusions are strengthened by in vivo observations on the urinary bladder of the toad as shown in Fig. 2. In these experiments, lithium in clinically therapeutic

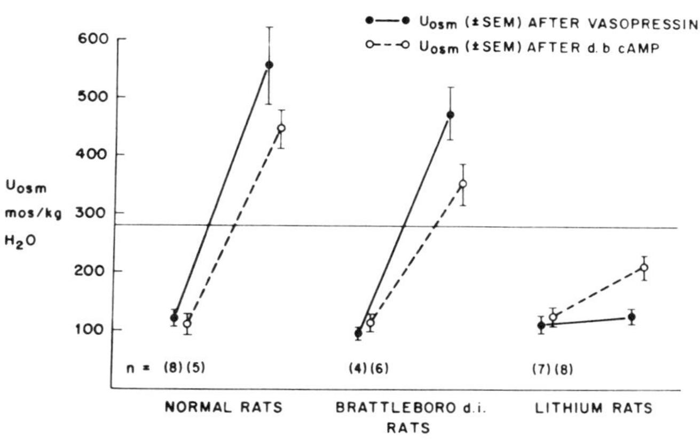

Fig. 1. Effect of vasopressin or cyclic-AMP on urine osmolality during water diuresis in normal or diabetes insipidus rats and normal rats receiving lithium. (Reprinted with permission from ref. 2).

concentrations is substituted for sodium in the hypotonic mucosal medium in the experimental bladders, and an equimolar substitution for sodium with choline is used in the medium of the control bladders. Vasopressin-induced osmotic water flow was reduced approximately 50 percent in the bladders exposed to lithium, but lithium had no effect to decrease the osmotic flow of water induced by cyclic-AMP. It is interesting to note that this effect of lithium to interfere with the hydro-osmotic effect of vasopressin requires that the ion be applied to the mucosal surface of the epithelium. Furthermore, the inhibitory effect of lithium on vasopressin is blocked by amiloride. These observations indicate that lithium gains access to its biochemical target by transport across the epithelial apical membrane.

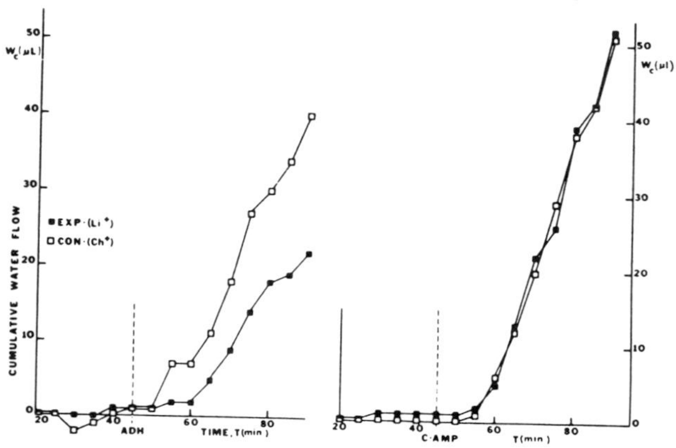

Fig. 2. Effect of lithium (EXP) on vasopressin-induced (ADH) or cyclic-AMP induced (c-AMP) osmotic water flow across toad urinary bladder. Open symbols (CON) are control hemibladders. (Reprinted with permission from ref. 3)

The aquaretic effect of lithium may not be limited to its effect to inhibit the biochemical pathway of vasopressin action. When administered chronically to rats, lithium has been shown to reduce proximal tubular absorption of water and electrolytes. Lithium also reduces both basal and vasopressin induced sodium transport by the urinary bladder of the toad as shown in Fig. 3. In the Brattleboro rat with a genetic absence of vasopressin, lithium increases urine flow and free water clearance (Fig. 4). These observations support the view that lithium interferes with the reabsorption of sodium (and passively, water absorption) in proximal portions of the nephron, resulting in the delivery of an increased volume of tubular fluid to distal sites where larger volumes of dilute urine are generated.

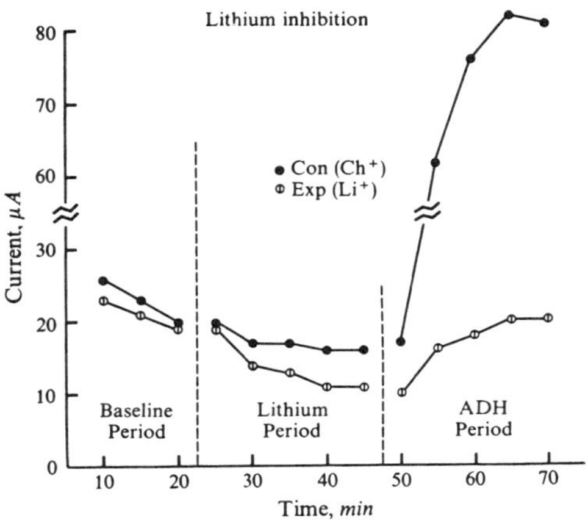

Fig. 3. Effect of lithium to reduce basal and vasopressin-induced (ADH) short-circuit current in totad urinary bladder. Open symbols (EXP) are hemibladders exposed to lithium from 20 minutes through the remainder of the experiment. (Reprinted with permission from ref. 4).

Other effects of lithium on water balance have been suggested. There is some evidence that lithium may produce primary polydypsia in the rat and that the ion may interfere with the production and/or secretion of vasopressin,

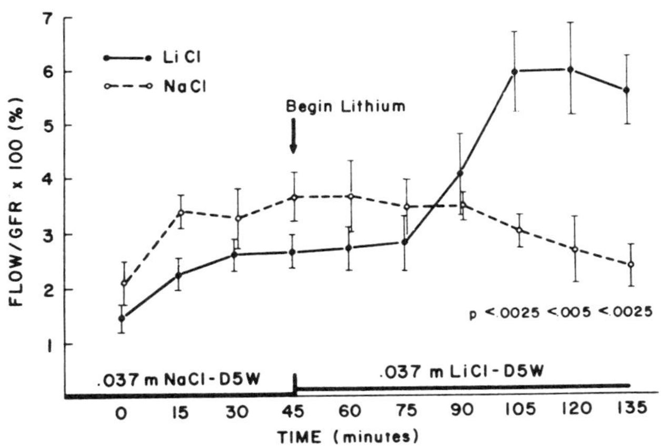

Fig 4. Effect of lithium chloride infusion to further increase fractional water excretion in diabetes insipidus Brattleboro rats. (Reprinted with permission from ref. 5).

resulting in central diabetes insipidus. It is likely that these are uncommon and minor consequences of lithium therapy.

The next aquaretic to emerge from clinical observation was demethylchlortetracycline, or demeclocycline. This antibiotic has been used in relatively high doses in the treatment of acne. Patients undergoing such treatment were noted to have polydipsia and polyuria, and these symptoms led to studies that substantiated the antibiotic as an aquaretic. Fig. 5 shows the maximum urine osmolality after water deprevation and vasopressin in groups of patients receiving three different doses of demeclocycline. At the higher dose of the antibiotic, patients were barely able to raise urine osmolality to isotonic levels. Two of these patients were unable to achieve negative free water clearance during osmotic diuresis. These same investigators examined the effect of demeclocycline on osmotic water flow across the toad bladder. As shown in Fig. 6, increasing concentration of demeclocycline in the serosal bath inhibited vasopressin induced water flow up to 75 percent. The antibiotic had some effect to inhibit cyclic-AMP induced water flow, but at higher concentrations of the antibiotic, the inhibitory effect on cyclic-AMP

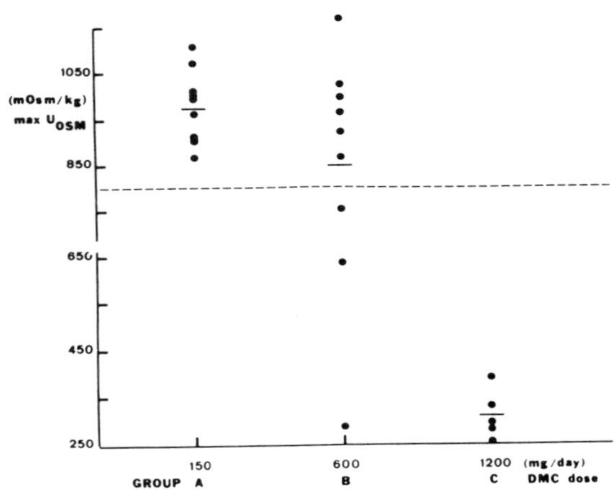

Fig. 5. Dose related effect of demeclocycline to decrease maximal urine osmolality in humans after water deprivation and injection of vaspressin. (Reprinted with permission from ref. 6).

was less than half the inhibitory effect on vasopressin. These observations suggest that demeclocycline interferes with vasopressin induced water absorption both by impairing the generation of cyclic-AMP and at some step beyond cyclic-AMP. This conclusion is further supported by studies in renal medullary tissue showing that increasing concentrations of demeclocycline result in progressive declines in vasopressin stimulated adenylate cyclase activity as well as declines in cyclic-AMP stimulated protein kinase activity (Fig. 7).

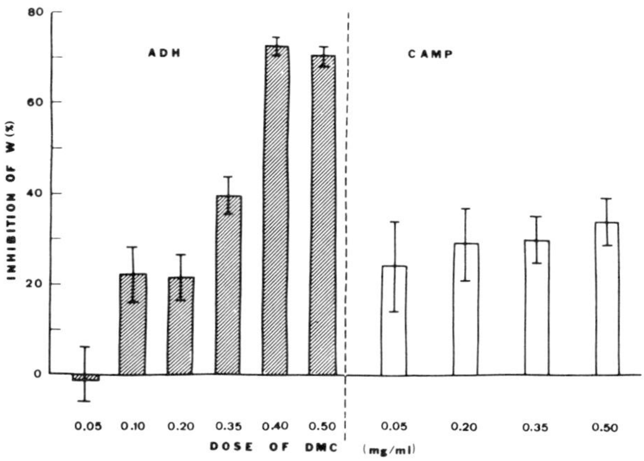

Fig. 6. Effect of demeclocycline (DMC) to inhibit osmotic water flow across toad urinary bladder after addition of vasopressin (ADH) or cyclic-AMP (c-AMP). Values are compared to hemibladders not receiving demeclocycline. (Reprinted with permission from ref. 7).

Demeclocycline appears to be superior to lithium as a clinically useful aquaretic, both in terms of its effectiveness in promoting the excretion of water and in terms of its lack of potential side effects and toxicity. Forrest, et al reported the use of demeclocycline to treat a relatively large group of patients with the syndrome of inappropriate antidiuretic hormone secretion secondary to neoplasia or intracranial disease. A summary of their results is shown in Fig. 8. These investigators also compared the therapeutic efficacy of lithium and demeclocycline in three patients and found demeclocycline to be superior in its effect to promote the excretion of water and correct the hyponatremia (Fig. 9).

Because of the multiple effects of lithium involving secretion of thyroid hormone, cardiac excitability, the central nervous system, the adrenal, and other systems, and because of the superior clinical aquaretic effectiveness of demeclocycline, the latter agent became the drug of choice in the management

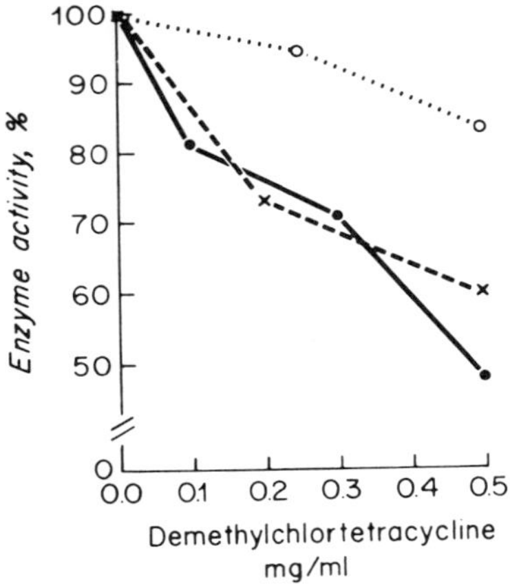

Fig. 7. Effect of increasing media concentration of hemeclocycline on enzyme activity in human renal medulla in vitro. Solid circles = vasopressing stimulated cAMP; open circles = cAMP phosphadiasterase; x = cAMP stimulated protein kinase. (Reprinted with permission from ref. 8.).

(Fig. 8)

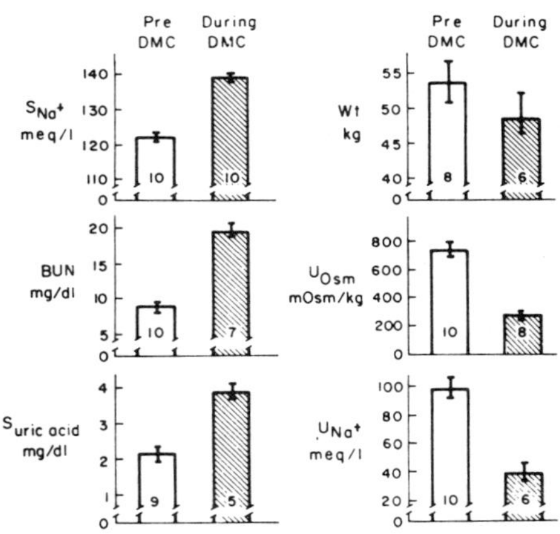

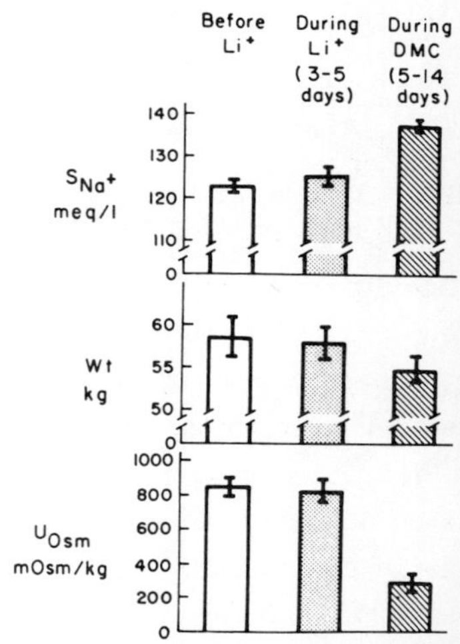

Fig. 8. Effects of demeclocycline (DMC) in patients with the syndrome of inappropriate secretion of antidiuretic hormone. (Reprinted with permission of ref. 9).

Fig. 9. Comparison of effects of lithium (Li^+) and demeclocycline (DMC) in patients with the syndrome of inappropriate secretion of antidiuretic hormone (Reprinted with permission from ref. 9).

of chronic water retention due to inappropriate secretion of vasopressin. In many clinical settings the retention of water is a transient abnormality that is best managed by manipulation of intake and/or urine output. Even when the syndrome is chronic, the steady state retention of water may be modest and treatment with drugs is unnecessary. The ultimate in specificity for aquaretics will be the advent of non-antidiuretic analogs of vasopressin that can be conveniently administered and that block the antidiuretic effect of endogenous vasopressin without producing unwanted effects of their own.

REFERENCES

1. Forrest, J.N., Jr., Cohen, A.D., Torretti, J., Hemmelhock, J.M. and Epstein, F.H. J. Clin. Invest. 53: 1115-1123, 1974.
2. Singer, I., Rotenberg, D. and Puschett, J.B. J. Clin. Invest. 51: 1081-1091, 1972.
3. Singer, I. and Franko, E.A. Kidney Int. 3: 151-159, 1973.
4. Forrest, J.N. and Singer, I. In: Disturbances in Body Fluid Osmolality, Am. Physiol. Soc., USA, 1977, pp. 309-340.
5. Singer, I. and Rotenberg. D. Ann. Internal Med. 79: 679-683, 1973.
6. Feldman, H.A. and Singer, I. J. Pharmacol. Exptl. Therap. 190: 358-364, 1974.
7. Dousa, T.P. Mayo Clinc. Proc. 49: 188-199, 1974.
8. Forrest, J.N., Cox, M., Hong, C., Morrison, G., Bia, M. and Singer, I. N. Engl. J. Med. 298: 173-177, 1978.

VASOPRESSIN ANTAGONISTS: MODEL AQUARETIC AGENTS

L.B. KINTER[1], W. HUFFMAN[2], F. STASSEN[3], and S. CHURCHILL[4]

Departments of Pharmacology[1], Molecular Pharmacology[2] and Peptide Chemistry[3], Smith Kline and French Laboratories, Swedeland, PA 19479, USA, and Department of Physiology[4], Harvard Medical School, Boston, MA 02115, USA

INTRODUCTION

Drs. Manning and Sawyer and their colleagues were the first to report vasopressin analogs having intrinsic vasopressin-antagonist activities in anesthetized rats (1-5). We have previously shown that these and other diuretic vasopressin analogs have high affinity for renal vasopressin binding sites, and specifically antagonize renomedullary vasopressin-stimulated adenylate cyclase (6). The structures of some represented antagonists are shown in Figure 1.

PEPTIDE VASOPRESSIN ANTAGONISTS

Pmp-X-Phe-Val-Asn-Cys-Pro-Y-Z

Pmp =

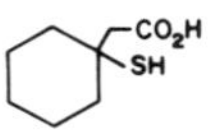

SK&F #	X	Y	Z
101926	D-Tyr(Et)	Arg	NH_2
101498	D-Tyr(Et)	Arg	Gly-NH_2
101071	D-Phe	Arg	Gly-NH_2
100885	D-Tyr	Arg	Gly-NH_2

Fig. 1. Structures of representative aquaretic vasopressin antagonists.

We have demonstrated a relationship between antagonist potency to inhibit renal adenylate cyclase *in vitro* and aquaretic potency *in vivo* in experimental animals (6-8). We have explored unexpected differences in species sensitivity to specific antagonists, and have identified the structure [des Gly^{9}d$(CH_2)_5$ ^{1}D-Tyr(Et),^{2}Val^{4}] arginine vasopressin (SK&F 101926) as a potent vasopressin antagonist and aquaretic agent in all species tested to date (8-11). In this paper we will review the current key literature, and demonstrate some of the biological activities and potential therapeutic utilities of vasopressin receptor antagonists.

Human Renal Tissue In Vitro

The effects of vasopressin analogs to inhibit vasopressin-stimulation of adenylate cyclase in renal medullary membranes has been reported (8). The most potent antagonists are those with the D-Tyr(Et) substitution at position 2 (inhibition constants, Ki, on the order of 10^{-9}M, ref. 8). In contrast to experience with agonists, removal of the terminal glycine residue resulted in no loss, and an actual increase in antagonist potency (8,12). The rank order potency of a series of antagonists was different in human than in rat or pig renomedullary tissue (8). It was concluded from these studies that caution must be exercised in applying structure-activity data from one species to another. Findings were extended with the report that the antagonists $d(CH_2)_5$-Tyr(Et)VAVP and SK&F 101926 inhibited vasopressin-stimulated adenylate cyclase in isolated medullary and papillary collecting ducts and medullary ascending limbs of human nephrons *in vitro* (13). Taken together these studies suggest that potent antagonists exist with which to inhibit human V_2 receptors.

Squirrel Monkeys

Vasopressin analogs have been reported to inhibit vasopressin-stimulated adenylate cyclase in squirrel monkey kidney *in vitro*, and to stimulate aquaresis *in vivo* (8,14). A strong correlation was reported for rank order potency of different analogs to inhibit vasopressin adenylate cyclase *in vitro*, and to increase renal water excretion *in vivo* (8). The most potent structures were those having D-Tyr (alkyl) substitutions at position 2 (8). An example of the aquaretic activity of the vasopressin antagonist SK&F 101926 is shown in Fig. 2.

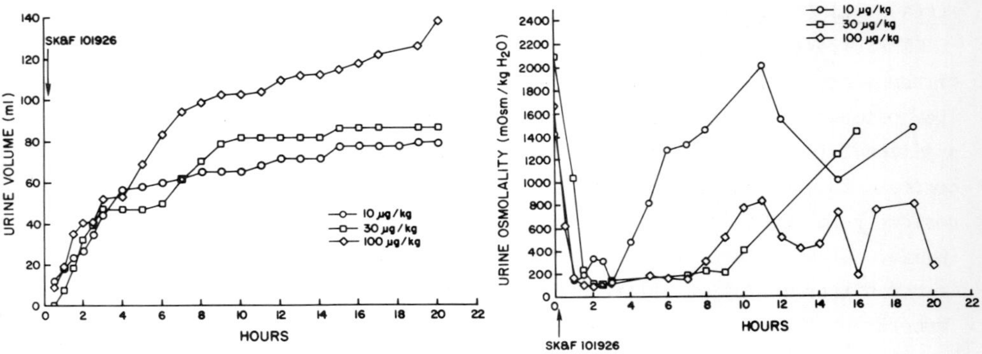

Fig. 2. Effect of increasing doses (10-100 μg/kg, i.v.) of SK&F 101926 on urine volume (left panel) and urine osmolality (right panel) in conscious trained squirrel monkeys.

The studies were conducted in individual squirrel monkeys previously prepared with indwelling arterial and venous catheters (22), and trained and studied using metabolic chairs and individual isolation chambers. SK&F 101926 was administered intravenously with an indwelling catheter from outside of the chamber; all monkeys had free access to food and water throughout the study. Baseline urine osmolality was >1400 mOsm/kg H_2O. A dose-dependent increase in cumulative urine volume to levels exceeding 50 ml (or 5% of body weight) in 4 hr was observed. Urine osmolality was diluted rapidly to hypotonic levels (<100 mOsm/kg/H_2O) with the effect of increasing doses being principally upon duration of the maximal hypotonic response. No increase in urinary solute excretion was detected in spite of the maximal rates of urine flow (see 14). Taken together, these studies show that potent vasopressin antagonists, such as SK&F 101926, are effective aquaretic agents with prolonged durations of action in conscious squirrel monkeys.

Dogs

Diuretic vasopressin analogs were initially reported to be remarkably ineffective in conscious dogs (9,10). Stassen et al. reported that the most potent antagonists of vasopressin-stimulated renal adenylate cyclase in both cortical and medullary renal membranes of dog kidney were those with D-Tyr(Et) substitution at position 2 (16). The potency (Ki) of SK&F 101926 in dog kidney is ~1 x 10^{-9}M. Activity of two vasopressin antagonists in several conscious dog models has been reported (11,17). The results show that vasopressin antagonists with D-Tyr (O-et) substitutions at position 2 are potent aquaretic agents capable of antagonizing exogenously administered AVP in conscious dogs. The lack of activity in dogs of antagonists having Tyr (alkyl) (17) or D-Phe (9) substitutions at position 2 may be due to reduced potency and/or partial agonist activity, at cortical or medullary AVP receptors (16).

Rats

Diuretic vasopressin analogs have been most extensively studied in rats. Pioneering studies of Manning and Sawyer first identified diuretic vasopressin analogs in this species (1-7). These findings were confirmed and extended in conscious rats (18,19). The structure-activity relationships for antagonist inhibition of rat renal adenylate cyclase *in vitro* and aquaresis *in vivo* have been described, and a high correlation between *in vitro*/*in vivo* rank order potencies established (7,8). The most potent antagonists identified are those with D-Tyr (alkyl), D-Phe, and B-Leu and D-Ile substitution at position 2. The aquaretic and vasopressin antagonist activities of SK&F 101926 in rats have been extensively described (7,8,12,14,19).

The effects of vasopressin antagonists on renal hemodynamics in conscious rats (Long Evans strain) have been carefully described (20). These studies showed that infusion of selective antipressor (V_1) or antidiuretic (V_2) antagonists had no effects on effective renal blood flow or glomerular filtration rate. Unexpectedly, the combination of V_1 plus V_2 antagonists was associated with a selective decrease (-40%) in GFR. The aquaretic activity of the V_2 antagonist was uneffected by presence of the V_1 antagonist. The mechanism was unexplained, but the result suggests that certain vasopressin antagonists may effect renal hemodynamics in rats.

Animal Models of Clinical States

Vasopressin antagonists have been studied for effectiveness to prevent dilutional hyponatremia in rats (21,22). These groups described the effects of two antagonists, $d(CH_2)_5$Tyr(Et)VAVP and SK&F 101926, respectively, to block the development of dilutional hyponatremia in rat models of Syndrome of Inappropriate Antidiuretic Hormone (SIADH). We have recently shown that SK&F 101926 will also reverse established hyponatremia in a conscious rat SIADH model (19).

Ishikawa and colleagues have used vasopressin antagonists to investigate the long suspected role of non-osmotically released vasopressin in glucocorticoid- and mineralocortoid-deficient rats (23). It was shown that vasopressin was responsible for water retention in the mineralocorticoid-deficient state, and impaired water excretion in the glucocorticoid-deficient state.

Dr. Hofbauer and colleagues have used vasopressin antagonists to investigate the role of vasopressin in the development of desoxy-corticosterone-salt (DOCA) hypertension in rats (24-27). These studies showed that not only do both pressor and antidiuretic vasopressin activities contribute to the development of DOCA-salt hypertension, but that V_2 agonist activity is required to prevent potentially lethal hypernatremia.

A notable finding from Dr. Hofbauer's studies is the apparent tachyphalaxis to both vasopressin and diuretic vasopressin antagonists following chronic administration of the $d(CH_2)_5$ D-Tyr(Et)VAVP in rats (24). Infusion (24-72 μg/d for 7 days by osmotic minipump) resulted in a large increase in water intake on day 1, which attenuated to baseline levels over the following 3 to 5 days. Subsequent challenge on day 6 or 7 with either additional antagonist (200 μg, s.c.) or vasopressin (50 ng, i.v.) failed to elicit responses in either water intake or urine osmolality in antagonist-infused rats (24).

We probed this phenomena using vasopressin-deficient Brattleboro strain rats homozygous (DI) or heterozygous (Het, control) for diabetes insipidus. All rats were housed individually in metabolism cages, and associated to a daily metabolic protocol. Following collection of baseline parameters, osmotic minipumps (Alzet model 2001), loaded to deliver the potent V_1/V_2 antagonist ($d(CH_2)_5$ D-PheVAVP, ref. 18, 2.5 μg/hr), were implanted intraperitoneally under ether anesthesia. The rats were studied for an additional 14 days (Fig. 3).

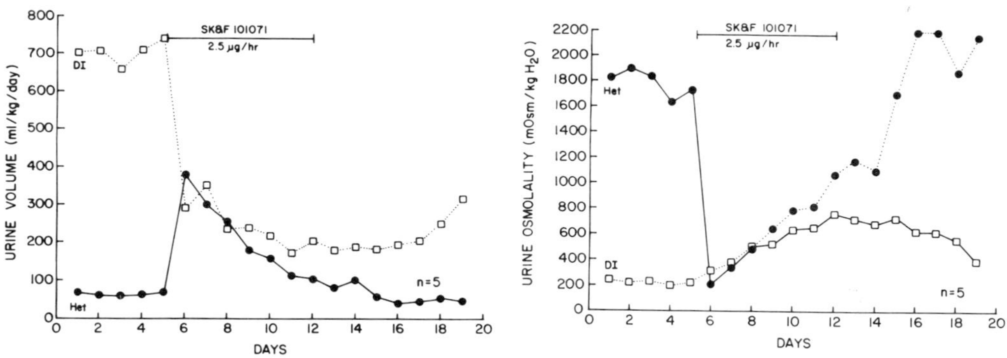

Fig. 3. Effect of SK&F 101071 (2.5 μg/hr) on daily urine volume (left panel) and average daily urine osmolality (right panel) in conscious Brattleboro strain rats homozygous (■) and heterozygous (●) for diabetes insipidus. Horizontal bar denotes the minimum duration of SK&F 101071 infusion.

Intraperitoneal infusion of SK&F 101071 in vasopressin-replete (Het) rats was associated with a rapid aquaretic response which was maximal within the first 24 hr and attenuated over the following 6-8 days. Upon apparent exhaustion of the pumps, Uosm rapidly returned to control levels. In vasopressin-deplete (DI) rats, an opposite antidiuretic response was associated with infusion of SK&F 101071. The daily levels of Uosm achieved in DI rats were similar to the levels measured in Hct rats over the duration of the infusion period. Taken with the results of Dr. Hofbauer's group, these results suggest that following chronic exposure in rats, vasopressin antagonist-associated partial agonist activity may result in changes in epithelial vasopressin receptor regulation and subsequently dominate the responsiveness of vasopressin-sensitive terminal nephron segments.

ACKNOWLEDGEMENTS

We would like to acknowledge D. Ashton, J. McDonald, G. Heckman, and G. Dytko for expert technical assistance; F. Ali, W. Bryan, J. Callahan, M. Moore, J. Silvestri, H. Green, and N. Yim for synthesis of vasopressin analogs; Drs. B. Berkowitz, M. Wasserman, R. Beeuwkes, and S. Crooke for continued support and useful discussions; and S. Tirri for assistance in manuscript preparation.

REFERENCES

1. Bruszynski, M., Lammek, D., Manning, M., et al. J. Med. Chem. 23:364-368, 1980.
2. Manning, M., Klis, W., Olma, A., et al. J. Med. Chem. 25:414-419, 1981.
3. Manning, M., Lammek, B., Kolodziejczyk, A., et al. J. Med. Chem. 24:701-706, 1981.
4. Manning, M., Lammek, B., Kolodziejczyk, A., et al. J. Med. Chem. 24:408-414, 1981.
5. Manning, M., Olma, A., Klis, W., et al. J. Med. Chem. 25:45-50, 1982.
6. Stassen, F., Erickson, R., Huffman, W., et al. J. Pharmacol. Exp. Ther. 223, 50-54, 1982.
7. Stassen, F.L., Huffman, W.F., Wiebelhaus, V.D., et al. In: Diretics: Chemistry, Pharmacology and Clinical Applications (Ed. J. Puschett and A. Greenberg), Elsevier Science Publishing Co., New York, 1984, pp. 64-71.
8. Stassen, F.L., Heckman, G., Schmidt, D., et al. In: Vasopressin (Ed. R. Schrier), Raven Press, New York, 1985, pp. 145-154.
9. Stassen, F.L., Bryan, W., Gross, M., et al. In: The Neurohypophysis: Structure, Function and Control, Progress in Brain Research, vol. 60, Ed. B.A. Cross and G. Leng, Elsevier Science Publishing Co., New York, 1983.
10. Kinter, L., Stassen, F., Horner, E., et al. Kidney Int. 23, 259, 1983.
11. Kinter, L., Mann, W., Heckman, G., et al. Kidney Int. 25, 304, 1984.
12. Manning, M., Olma, A., Klis, W., et al. Nature 308(12):652-653, 1984.
13. Kim, J. and Schrier, R. In: Vasopressin (Ed. R. Schrier), Raven Press, New York, 1985, pp. 155-158.
14. Kinter, L.B., Dubb, J., Huffman, W., et al. In: Vasopressin (Ed. R. Schrier), Raven Press, New York, 1985, pp. 553-561.
15. Kass, D., Salzman, F., Fuller, C., et al. Am. J. Physiol. 242:F649-F656, 1982.
16. Stassen, F., Heckman, G. and Huffman, W. J. Pharm. Expl. Ther. 232:100-105, 1985.
17. Kinter, L.B., Mann, W., Brennan, F. et al (this volume).
18. Kinter, L.B., Huffman, W., Wiebelhaus, V.D., et al. In: Diuretics: Chemistry, Pharmacology and Clinical Applications, Ed. J. Puschett and A. Greenberg, Elsevier Science Publishing Co., New York, 1984, pp. 72-81.
19. Kinter, L.B. and Dytko, G. (this volume).
20. Gellai, M. In: Vasopressin (Ed. R. Schrier), Raven Press, New York, 1985, pp. 167-170.
21. Laszlo, F., Csati, S. and Balaspiri, L. Acta Endocrinologica 106:56-60, 1984.
22. Kinter, L.B. and Dytko, G. Kidney Int. 1986 (in press).
23. Ishikawa, S., Kim, J. and Schrier, R. In: Vasopressin (Ed. R. Schrier), Raven Press, New York, 1985, pp. 171-180.
24. Hofbauer, K.G., Mah, S.C., Baum, H.P., et al. J. Cardiovasc. Pharmacol. 6:S184-S191, 1984.
25. Hofbauer, K.G., Mah, S.C., Wood, J.M., et al. J. Hypertension 2 (Suppl. 3):333-335, 1984.
26. Hofbauer, K.G., Studer, W., Mah, S.C., et al. J. Cardiovasc. Pharmacol. 6:S429-S438, 1984.
27. Hofbauer, K., Opperman, J., Mah, S.C., et al. In: Vasopressin (Ed. R. Schrier), Raven Press, New York, 1985, pp. 159-165.

THE ANTI-ANTIDIURETIC EFFECT OF A STABLE PROSTAGLANDIN-E_2 ANALOG IN CONSCIOUS SHEEP AND MAN

L. G. LEKSELL AND C-J. WALLIN

Department of Anesthesiology and department of Physiology I, Karolinska Institutet, 104 01 Stockholm, Sweden

The syndrome of inappropriate antidiuretic hormone release (SIADH), also referred to as the Schwartz-Bartters syndrome is characterized by too high levels of circulating antidiuretic hormone (ADH) in relation to the actual fluidbalance of the organism. The inadequately high plasmalevel of ADH (p-ADH)produces the triad water retention, dilutional hyponatremia and increased renal Na^+-excretion which is typical for the syndrome (1-2). This is of clinical importance as various causes, among others nausea, arterial hypotension and artificial ventilation may induce 10 to 1000-fold increases in the normal (1-5 pg/ml) plasmalevels of ADH (2). The hazards of a reduced plasma sodium (p-Na^+) were beautifully illustrated in a recent large study by Anderson et col (3). These investigators found that a p-Na^+ below 130 mmol/l caused a severalfold increase in the mortallity rate of a large population of hospitalized patients.

The SIADH-syndrome with areduced excretion of free water is of particular interest in anesthesiology and intensive care were patients often suffer from insufficient production of urine. In patients that had undergone hysterectomy at the Karolinska hospital with a normal pre-, peri- and postoperative period (insignificant bloodloss, positive fluidbalance and soforth) mean p-ADH was 41 $\pm$ 15 and 29 $\pm$ 12 pg/ml 1 and 3 hours respectively after the end of the operation. High levels of p-ADH (16 $\pm$ 1 pg/ml) were also found in an unsampled group of patients treated at the intensive care unit (ICU) of the Karolinska hospital. The latter group offers particular problems. These patients are often artificially ventilated which i) by itself, through its effects on central hemodynamics, augments the secretion of ADH ii) puts their intake, and to a ceratin extent output, of fluids and electrolytes under the control of the physician. Furthermore as the ICU patients often suffer from severe infections and septicemia they are catabolic and produce large volumes of endogenous water. Put together this makes it hazardous to evaluate the fluid and electrolyte balance of the severly ill patient. The diagnosis of SIADH is difficult to make in the common clinical setting as the classical signs of the syndrome often are veiled by the intravenous (iv) administration of large volumes of solutions rich in electrolytes together with the injection of loop-diuretics in large dosages.

Prostaglandins (PG) antagonize ADH-induced permeabillity changes in the toadbladder (4) and the isolated renal collecting duct (5). The intrarenal infusion of PGE_1 augments both free water clearance (C_{H2O}) and renal Na^+-excretion (6). The natural occurring PGs also cause an increase in body temperature and affect gastrointestinal function eliciting nausea, factors which by themselves stimulate ADH-secretion. However, these "side-effects" can be negliable to moderate when a synthetic PG-analog is given.

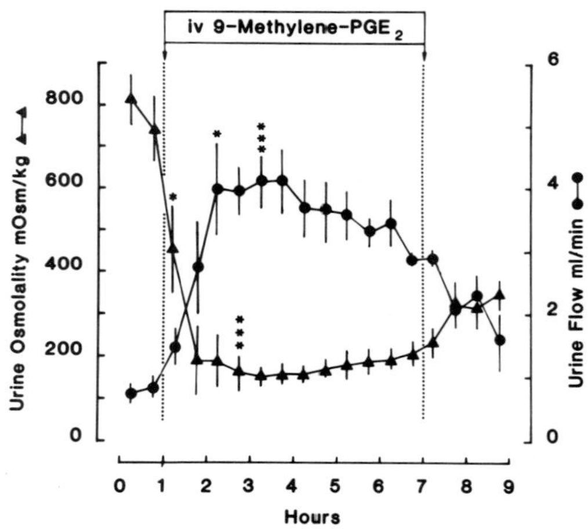

Fig. 1. The effects on urine osmolality and urine flow caused by the iv infusion of 9-methylene-PGE_2 24 µg/min for six hours in the euhydrated sheep. Mean ± SE, *$P < 0.05$, ***$P < 0.001$.

In our search for some substance of possible use in the clinical treatment of SIADH and similar conditions we decided to study the effect on the fluid balance of the stable PG-analog 9-deoxo-16,16-dimethyl-9-methylene-PGE_2 (9-methylene-PGE_2).

Studies in the conscious sheep

In the euhydrated concious sheep the six hour iv infusion of 9-methylene-

PGE_2 (24 ug/min) decreased urine osmolality (U_{osm}) and increased urine flow (UF) causing a conspicous water diuresis (Fig. 1). Free water clearance increased from a preinfusion value of approximately -1.2 to a maximum around +1.8 ml/min 150 min after the infusion was started. The C_{H2O}-curve remained altough slightly depressed towards the end, positive throughout the 6 hour infusion. The net water loss increased p-osm from approximately 290 to 300 mOsm/kg. Parlell to this, in accordance with classical PG-studies, the infusion produced a marked increase (fivefold) in renal Na^+-excretion.

In the hyperhydrated sheep the iv infusion of the analog (24 ug/min) abolished the antidiuretic effect of exogenous ADH (0.5 mU/min iv) (7).

Studies in the male volunteer

In the male volunteer the two hour iv infusion of 9-methylene-PGE_2 induced similar changes in U_{osm} and UF to those in the previous section (Fig. 2). This occurred without causing any changes in the clearance for

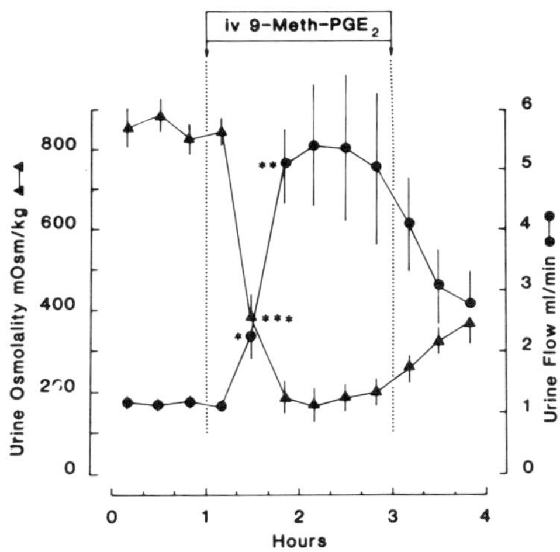

Fig. 2. Changes of urineosmolality and urine flow induced by the iv infusion (o.5 ml/min) of 9-methylene-PGE_2 (40 µg/ml) for 2 hours in the euhydrated male volunteer. Mean ± SE, ***$P < 0.001$ to preinfusion baseline. Reprinted with permission from ref.8 .

paraaminohippuric acid or inulin (C_{In}). However as can be seen in Fig. 3 (shown as the clearance for each ion divided by C_{In}) the renal tubular reabsorbtion for Na^+, Ca^{++} and Mg^{++} increased while that for K^+ decreased(8).

Hormonal effects caused by the PG-analog could partly explain the renal Na^+-retention and the excretion of K^+. Aldosterone in plasma increased from around 170 to 270 pmol/l ($P < 0.05$) in response to the infusion. The concentration of parathyroid hormone in plasma did not change. There are indications that p-ADH and renal excretion of ADH rose in response to the infusion, however these results are not conclusive.

Studies in the patient

Six patients, 3 admitted to the ICU and 3 to the neurosurgical department of the karolinska hospital, that had suffered major trauma or severe postoperative complications, were treated with the iv infusion of 9-methylene-PGE_2 (20 ug/min) for two hours. All patients were artificially ventilated, 5 with a positive endexpiratory pressure of 5 to 10 cm of H_2O. Their mean p-Na^+ was 133.2 ± 2.9 mmol/l and their p-osm was 277.8 ± 6.7 mOsm/kg. As a result of the infusion C_{H2O} went from negative (-1.5 ml/min) to positive (+1.1 ml/min), and remained positive throughout the 9-methylene-PGE_2 administration.

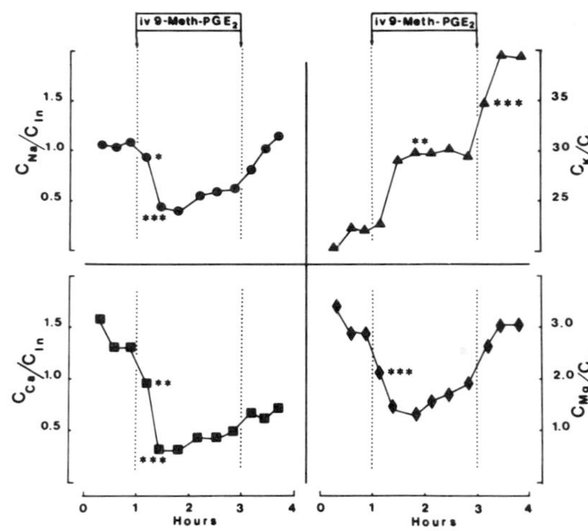

Fig. 3. The Na^+, Ca^{++} and Mg^{++}retaining and K^+ excretory effects induced by the iv infusion (0.5 ml/min) of 9-methylene-PGE_2 (40 µg/ml) for two hours in euhydrated male volunteers (n=6). Values are expressed as the clearance (C_X) for respective ion divided by clearance of inulin (C_{In}). Mean ± SE, $^{***}P < 0.001$ compared to preinfusion baseline. Reprinted with permission from ref.8 .

On 6 patients that had undergone hysterectomy 9-methylene-PGE_2 was given in the same way as in the previous section. This produced a slight increase in C_{H_2O} however C_{H_2O} never turned from negative to positive.

Conclusions

There exists an obvious need to obtain some water diuretic agent for the clinical treatment of SIADH and SIADH-like conditions. The hospitalized patients suffering from water retention and dilutional hyponatremia are today treated with a combination of Na^+-administration and diuretic drugs that are mainly natriuretic. The administration of Na^+ to these patients that already suffer from increased extracellular volume endangers their cardiovascular function and may induce acute cardiac failure. The loss of Na^+ caused by the administration of loop-diuretics appears unlogical as these patients already suffer from a low p-Na^+.

The results reported here illustrate the desirable characteristics of a diuretic agent suitable in the treatment of SIADH, ie an anti-anti-diuretic quality in combination with renal retention of Na^+. However the PG-analog 9-methylene-PGE_2, discussed here does not appear to be effective enough in the clinical treatment of SIADH. There are indications that the infusion of the actual PG-analog causes an increased secretion of ADH, furthermore its anti-antidiuretic quality is not potent enough to produce a water diuresis in the patients with levels of p-ADH around 30 pg/ml such as in those that had undergone hysterectomy. The use of 9-methylene-PGE_2 is also limited to males and nonfertile females as the compound is an effective abortive agent (9). Eventually other PG-analogs may be more efficient than 9-methylene-PGE_2 for the eventual treatment of SIADH. However the development of strong ADH-analogs that are antagonists and compete with ADH at its renal receptor appear to be the most promising lead in the search for an agent suitable for the treatment of SIADH.

The investigations reported here were approved by the Ethical Committee of Karolinska hospital and the National Board of Health and Welfare, department of Drugs, Uppsala, Sweden.
The investigations were supported by the swedish Medical Research Council, Stockholms Läns Landsting and by grants from the Karolinska Institute, Jeanssons Stiftelse and Hiertas Stiftelse.

1. Bartter, F.C. and Schwartz W.B. Am. J. Med. 42:790-806, 1967.
2. Robertson, G.L. J. Lab. Clin. Med. 101:351-371, 1983.
3. Anderson, R.J.,Chung, H-M.,Kluge, R. and Schrier, R. Ann. Intern.Med. 102:164-168, 1985.
4. Lipson, L.C. and Sharp, G.W.G. Am. J. Physiol. 220:1046-1052, 1971.

5. Grantham, J. and Orloff, J. J. Clin. Invest. 47:1154-1161, 1968.
6. Johnston, H.H., Herzog, J.P. and Lauler, D.P. Am. J. Physiol. 213: 939-946, 1967.
7. Christensen, N.J., Bygdeman, M., Greén, K., Jonasson, H., Rundgren, M., Wallin, C-J., Vesterqvist, O. and Leksell, L.G. Pflüg. Arch. 402:360-363, 1984.
8. Leksell, L.G., Christensen, N., Vesterqvist, O. and Wallin, C-J. Clin. Physiol. 4:449-459., 1984.
9. Bygdeman, M., Bremme, K., Christensen, N., Lundström, V. and Green, K. Contraception. 22(5):471-483, 1980.

VASOPRESSIN IN PATIENTS WITH LIVER AND CARDIAC DISEASE

Berne Yee, Robert L. Cosby and Robert W. Schrier

Division of Renal Diseases, University of Colorado Health Sciences Center, 4200 East Ninth Avenue, Box C-281, Denver, Colorado 80262

Hyponatremia is a marker of abnormal water metabolism and frequently complicates the clinical course of patients with cirrhosis and chronic congestive heart failure (CHF) (1,2,3,4,5). Both of these hyponatremic disorders are associated with an increased total body sodium and a larger excess of total body water.

Recent studies support a role for a decrease in effective arterial blood volume (EABV) in this sodium and water retention (1,2,7,8,9,10,11,12,13,14). This decrease in EABV may be due to peripheral vasodilation and thus an increase in arterial vascular holding capacity, the development of portosystemic fistulae, decreased cardiac output, and/or a decreased plasma oncotic pressure. The sympathetic tone is increased in response to the decrease in EABV, and non-osmotic release of vasopressin ensues and may contribute to this impairment in water metabolism (9).

Role of Vasopressin in Cirrhosis

The pathogenesis of the impairment in water metabolism has been intensively studied. It appears to be related to intrarenal factors such as decreased delivery of filtrate to the diluting segments of the nephron and increased vasopressin (AVP) activity (14,15).

Studies to increase distal delivery and to evaluate intrarenal factors have included infusion of isotonic mannitol (16), head out water immersion (HWI) (7,10), infusion of ascitic fluid (17), saline (18), saline plus albumin (16), and peritoneovenous shunting (12,19). The difficulty in these maneuvers is separating the intrarenal mechanism from AVP suppression since these maneuvers all expand extracellular fluid volume. Furosemide can improve free water clearance in cirrhosis without expanding extracellular volume which supports a role for decreased distal delivery (20). However, the free water clearance induced by furosemide was unaffected by infusions of AVP which further supports an intrarenal mechanism. In this regard, furosemide may not only increase distal fluid delivery but may also block the renal effect of AVP (21).

Before a sensitive assay for AVP became available the role of vasopressin in cirrhosis was conflicting. However, suggestive evidence for increased AVP activity was demonstrated by Strauss et al (22). These authors showed that ethanol ingestion increased urine flow and decreased urine osmolality in patients with decompensated cirrhosis and normal glomerular filtration rate, suggesting that ethanol inhibited the release of AVP.

Reznick et al (15) have used peritoneovenous shunting in decompensated cirrhotic patients and measured plasma concentrations of AVP. They observed that despite improvement in sodium and water excretion in the perioperative period AVP levels remained elevated. Continued follow-up of these patients showed that AVP levels decreased with a further rise in serum sodium and serum osmolality but AVP levels continued to be elevated as compared to normals. Unfortunately, these investigators did not use water loading to assess the suppresibility of plasma AVP. Nevertheless, these results implicated a role for both an intrarenal mechanism and AVP in the water retention of cirrhosis.

Using a sensitive radioimmunoassay for AVP, most investigators report elevated levels of cirrhosis (1,2,7,9,15,23). We have shown a significant negative correlation between the ability to excrete a water load and plasma concentrations of AVP (2,9). We studied twenty-six patients with cirrhosis and various degrees of ascites or peripheral edema (9). They were studied using standard water loading (20 ml/kg), hormonal profiling, and evaluation of renal function with inulin and PAH clearances. These patients segregated into 2 groups: excretor (>80% water load excretion in 5 hr) and non-excretor patients (<80% water load excretion in 5 hr). The non-excretor group demonstrated higher urine osmolalities, lower basal serum sodium concentration, lower serum osmolality, lower serum albumin, higher plasma renin activity, aldosterone, norepinephrine, and AVP as compared with excretor patients. Furthermore, we were able to demonstrate a significant correlation between plasma norepinephrine and AVP concentrations. The physiologic importance of this finding was supported by the negative correlation between plasma norepinephrine and the percentage of water load excreted. Using plasma norepinephrine levels as a measure of baroreceptor activity (24), the AVP response appears to be due to a non-osmotic release in response to a decrease in EABV.

We tested this hypothesis using HWI, a maneuver known to augment EABV as assessed by increased intracardiac pressures and cardiac index, in a group of non-excretor cirrhotic patients. HWI was shown to increase renal sodium and water excretion in association with suppression of plasma renin, aldosterone, NE and AVP (7). However, a decrease in systemic vascular resistance was observed during HWI and implicated in the attenuation of the central blood volume expansion and thus of EABV (7).

On this background, we attempted to correct the abnormal water handling by using a combination of HWI and a NE infusion to prevent the fall in systemic vascular resistence (14). Systemic hemodynamics were assessed by Swan-ganz catheter and correction was attempted using HWI alone, NE infusion alone, and the combined maneuver using HWI and NE infusion. HWI alone caused only a modest increase in percent water load excreted 28.3 ± 6.3 to 60.0 ± 11.1 ($p<0.05$). There was a similar increase using NE infusion alone with an increase in water load excretion to 61.0 ± 9.5 ($p < 0.05$). Most importantly, we were able to completely reverse the abnormal sodium and water handling with the combined maneuver (HWI and NE), as water load excretion increased to 94.6 ± 9.4 ($p<0.001$). AVP suppression was similar in the HWI versus HWI plus NE studies. These results, therefore, support both AVP and an intrarenal mechanism in the abnormal water metabolism in cirrhotic patients.

In contrast to our results, in a recent report using HWI (23) the investigators were unable to demonstrate consistent suppression of AVP in cirrhosis and this may have been due to the heterogeneity of the population examined. In a previous study by the same group (10), an increase in free water excretion was demonstrated during HWI but unfortunately plasma AVP levels were not measured. Our studies show that AVP is important in the pathogenesis of the abnormal water metabolism in cirrhosis.

Furthermore, cirrhosis develops over a period of time and the hemodynamic consequences and renal sodium and water retention varies between earlier and later stages (9,11,14,25). We have been able to classify these patients based upon their response to a 5 hr water load test (25): Class I -Excretor (>80% water load excretion in 5 hr), Class II - Non-excretor (40-80% water load excretion in 5 hr), Class - III Non-excretor (< 40% water load excretion in 5 hr), and Class IV - Hepatorenal Syndrome. Morbidity and mortality parallel this classification scheme.

Role of AVP in CHF

The cardiovascular system maintains tissue perfusion to meet the body's metabolic needs. In heart failure, a host of homeostatic mechanisms are activated to maintain this balance (6). One of the compensatory responses is an increased sodium and water retention by the kidney.

The abnormal sodium and water handling in chronic congestive heart failure appears also to be related to a decrease in the EABV. This afferent mechanism is in response to either a decreased cardiac output or decreased vascular resistance. Models of low output (26,27,28) and high output (29,30) heart failure have advanced this concept of a decreased EABV. When compensatory mechanisms like mycardial dilation, increased contractility and hypertrophy are not able to maintain cardiac output, peripheral vascular constriction occurs as a circulatory response to maintain perfusion pressure. The neurohumoral vasoconstrictor systems in the heart failure are activated and include activation of sympathetic nervous system, renin-angiotensin system, and vasopressin (31). The non-osmotic release of vasopressin may be due to activation of baroreceptor mechanisms with subsequent impairment in water excretion (32). Pressure changes are sensed by aortic and carotid sinus baroreceptors and stimulte AVP secretion. Left atrial distention may inhibit AVP secretion (33); however, chronic distension blunts this effect and the high pressure baroreceptors therefore predominate. Moreover, a defect in the central control of AVP release is suggested by its nonsuppressibility with ethanol challenge (3) and inappropriate responses to osmotic (34) and nonosmotic (4,35) manipulations. Furthermore, water load excretion correlates inversely with plasma levels of AVP. The water retention may also be due to intrarenal factors that cause decreased fluid delivery to the distal diluting segments of the nephron. Studies in our laboratory suggest that both intrarenal mechanisms and elevations in AVP are involved. Intrarenal mechanisms were evaluated with mannitol and furosemide. There have been a host of studies demonstrating high plasma AVP levels in hyponatremic patient with chronic congestive heart failure (1,4,8,21). We were able to demonstrate inappropriately elevated plasma AVP levels in 30 of 37 hyponatremic patients with CHF (21). These findings were dissociated from diuretic use since 14 of the patients were not receiving diuretics.

We have recently examined renal water excretion and plasma AVP levels in response to an acute water load before and after improvement in cardiac performance using afterload reduction with vasodilator therapy (8). Twenty-five patients with severe CHF (New York Heart Association Class III - IV) were studied. Patients received 2 water loads of 15 ml/kg. One before and the second after vasodilator therapy with captopril or prazosin. Hemodynamics were monitored before and hourly for 5 hours using Swan-ganz catheter. They were classified according to their basal AVP levels (Group I - elevated basal AVP levels and Group II - suppressed basal AVP levels). Group I patients had more severe cardiac function as defined by higher pulmonary capillary wedge pressures and a lower cardiac index. In addition, they had significantly higher plasma renin and aldosterone levels and a further impairment in water load excretion as compared to Group II.

Moreover, water excretion improved with an improvement in cardiac function. Also an inverse correlation was found between plasma AVP and the percentage of the water load excreted. This study supports the notion that patients with more severe impairment in cardiac function have greater impairment in water load excretion and higher plasma AVP concentrations.

Finally, as with cirrhotic patients, there is information to suggest an intrarenal mechanism contributing to the impairment in water excretion. Group II patients demonstrated suppressed levels of AVP yet they continued to have a significant impairment in their ability to excrete a water load. This implies non-AVP factors, most likely an intrarenal mechanism producing a decrease in distal delivery of filtrate.

In summary, the impairment in water excretion in both cirrhosis and CHF exhibit many similarities. Both are a continuim of disease with impairment of water excretion correlating with severity of disease. The afferent stimulus for this impairment is believed to be a decrease in EABV. Finally, the mechanism for impairment in water excretion involved both intrarenal factors and increased plasma AVP levels. In addition, morbidity and mortality may parallel the severity of disease as measured by hormonal profiles and degree of impairment of water excretion.

REFERENCES

1. Bichet DG and Schrier RW, IN: Vasopressin, (Ed. RW Schrier), Raven Press, New York, 1985, pp 525-534.
2. Bichet DG, Szatalowicz VL, Chaimovitz C and Schrier RW, Ann Intern Med, 96:413-417, 1982.
3. Goldsmith SR and Dodge D, Am J Cardiol 55:1354-1357, 1985.
4. Godsmith SR, Francis GS, Cowley AW, Levine TB and Cohn JN, J Am Coll Cardiol 6:1385-1390, 1983.
5. Szatalowicz VL, Arnold PE, Chaimovitz C, Bichet DG, Berl T and Schrier RW, N Engl J Med 305:263-266, 1981.
6. Skorecki KL and Brenner BM, Am J Med, 72:323-338, 1982.
7. Bichet DG, Groves BM and Schrier RW, Kidney Int, 24:788-804, 1983.
8. Bichet DG, Kortas C, Mettauer B, Manzini C, Marc-Aurele J, Rouleau JL and Schrier RW, Kidney Int, In Press.
9. Bichet DG, Van Putten VJ and Schrier RW, N Engl J Med, 307:1552-157, 1982.
10. Epstein M, Pins DS, Schneider N, Levinson R, J Lab Clin Med, 87:822-839,1976.
11. Nicholls KM, Shapiro MD, Groves BM and Schrier RW, Kidney Int, In Press.
12. Nicholls KM, Shapiro MD, Kluge R, Chung HM, Bichet DG and Schrier RW, Hepatology, 6:235-238, 1986.
13. Schrier RW, Gastroenterology 84:870-872, 1983.
14. Shapiro MD, Nicholls KM, Groves BM, Kluge R, Chung HM, Bichet DG and Schrier RW, Kidney Int, 28:206-211, 1985.
15. Reznick RK, Langer B, Taylor Br, Seif S and Blendis LM, Gastroenterology, 84:713-718, 1983.
16. Vlahcevic ZR, Adham NF, Jick H, Moore EW and Chambers TC, N Engl J Med, 272:387-391, 1965.
17. Zipser RD, Hoefs JC, Speckart PF, Zia PK and Horton R, J Clin Endocrinol Metab 48:895-900, 1979.
18. Watkins L Jr, Burton JA, Haber E, Cant JR, Smith FW and Barger AC, J Clin Invest, 57:1606-1617, 1976.
19. Blendis LM, Greig PD, Langer B, et al, Gastroenterology, 77:119-125, 1979.
20. Schrier RW, Lehman D, Zacherle B and Early LE, Kidney Int, 3:30-34, 1973.
21. Szatalowicz VL, Miller PD, Lacher JW, Gordon JA and Schrier RW, Clin Sci, 62:235-238, 1982.
22. Strauss MB, Birchard WH and Saxon L, Trans Assoc Am Physicians, 69:222-228, 1956.
23. Epstein M, Weitzman RE, Preston S, Denunzio AG, Mineral Electrolyte Metab, 10:155-165, 1984.
24. Grossman SH, Davis D, Gunnells JC and Shand DG, 4:566-571, 1982.
25. Cosby RL, Yee B, Shapiro MD, Nicholls KM and Schrier RW, Kidney Int, 29:184, 1986.
26. Lifschitz MD and Schrier RW, Am J Physiol 225:1364-1370, 1973.
27. Schrier RW and Humphreys MH, Circ Res, 29:479-489, 1971.
28. Schrier RW, Humphreys MH and Ufferman RC, Circ Res, 29:490-498, 1971.
29. Epstein FH, Post RS and Mc Donald M, J Clin Invest, 32:233-241, 1953.
30. Epstein FH, Shadle OW and Ferguson TB, J Clin Invest, 32:543-547, 1953.
31. Riegger AJG, Eur Heart J, 6:479-489, 1985.
32. Schrier RW, Berl T, and Anderson RJ, Am J Physiol, 236:F321-F322, 1979.
33. De Torrente A, Robertson GL, McDonald KM and Schrier RW, Kidney Int, 8:355-361, 1975.
34. Uretsky BF, Verbalis JG, Generalovich T, Valdes A and Reddy PS, Am J Physiol, 248:H396-H402, 1985.
35. Goldsmith SR, Francis GS, Levine TB, Cowley AW and Cohn JN, J Am Coll Cardiol, 2:1080-1083, 1983.

REVERSAL OF HYPONATREMIA IN EXPERIMENTAL SCHWARTZ-BARTTER SYNDROME WITH A VASOPRESSIN ANTAGONIST (SK&F 101926).

L.B. KINTER[1], G. DYTKO[1], W. HUFFMAN[3], and F. STASSEN[2].

Departments of Pharmacology[1], Molecular Pharmacology[2] and Peptide Chemistry[3], Smith Kline and French Laboratories, Swedeland, PA 19479, USA

INTRODUCTION

Hyponatremia is now increasingly recognized as a relatively common clinical disorder (1,2,3). Multifactorial in origin, hyponatremia is often associated with inappropriate plasma vasopressin levels, and has potentially life-threatening neurological sequalae (1). The vasopressin antagonist desGlyd^9(CH_2)$_5$^{1}D-Tyr(Et)2Val^{9}AVP (SK&F 101926) is a potent water diuretic (aquaretic) agent potentially useful in the treatment of hyponatremia (4,5 - see Fig. 1). We and others have previously shown that vasopressin antagonists including SK&F 101926 are effective in preventing development of hyponatremia in rat models of experimental Schwartz Bartter Syndrome (or Syndrome of Inappropriate Antidiuretic Hormone, SIADH) (6,7). In this paper we report the use of SK&F 101926 to effectively reverse established hyponatremia in SIADH.

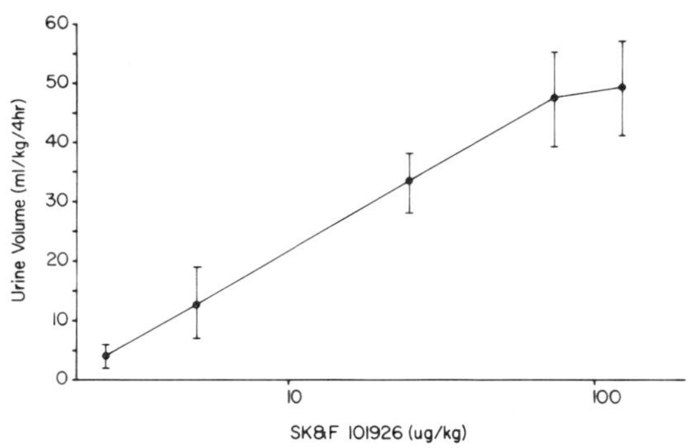

Fig. 1. SK&F 101926-associated dose-dependent water diuresis in hydropenic rats. The increases in urine volume are largely independent of changes in solute excretion (see 5,6).

METHODS AND MATERIALS

Male Sprague-Dawley rats (210-350 g, Charles River Laboratories) were prepared with gastric and caudal artery catheters using previously described surgical techniques (6). The arterial catheter, used for blood sampling, was continuously infused with 5% dextrose (0.6 ml/hr). Arginine vasopressin (AVP, Bachem, Belmont, CA) was continuously infused intraperitoneally using an implantable osmotic minipump (Alzet model 2001, Alza Corporation, Pal Alto, CA) at a total dose of 1 IU/day. Plasma AVP levels >10 pg/ml would be anticipated using this procedure (8). After 1 day of equilibration, tap water (5% body weight) was infused via the gastric catheter. Following development of hyponatremia, vehicle (0.9% NaCl) or SK&F 101926 (1-[β-mercapto,β,β-cyclopentamethylenepropionic acid, 2(O-ethyl) D-tyrosine, 4-valine, 8-arginine, 9-desglycine] vasopressin; prepared by SK&F Peptide chemists; 10 μg/kg) was administered intra-arterially. Plasma osmolality (Precision Systems Model 5004, Sudbury, MA) was monitored as an index of hyponatremia (6). All values are expressed as means ± SEM. Statistically significant differences were determined by application of Student's "t" test; significance is defined as $p<.05$.

RESULTS AND DISCUSSION

Plasma osmolality (Posm) levels associated with each step of the protocol are shown in Figure 2. Initial (pre-surgery) Posm was 292 ± 2 mOsm/kg H_2O. Twenty-four hr following placement of catheters and initiation of the AVP infusion, Posm was not significantly decreased. Following gastric administration of water, Posm significantly decreased to 260 ± 4 mOsm/kg ($p<.001$). Administration of placebo had no effect on established hyponatremia over the 4 hr observation period. Administration of SK&F 101926 reversed the hyponatremia, and returned Posm to control levels within 2 hr (Fig. 3). No overshoot was observed.
SK&F 101926 is a potent aquaretic which selectively increases renal excretion of water in rats (see 6,9 and Fig. 1). SK&F 101926 displaces AVP from renal vasopressin receptors, and blocks AVP stimulation of renal epithelial adenylate cyclase *in vitro* in renomedullary membranes and in isolated collecting tubule segments (4,10). In SIADH, SK&F 101926 blocks the antidiuretic action of AVP, selectively enhances renal water

excretion, and thus permits rapid excretion of the water load. Since most patients with hyponatremia have detectable plasma AVP levels (1), it is likely that aquaretic vasopressin antagonists, like SK&F 101926, will be useful in the treatment of clinical hyponatremia.

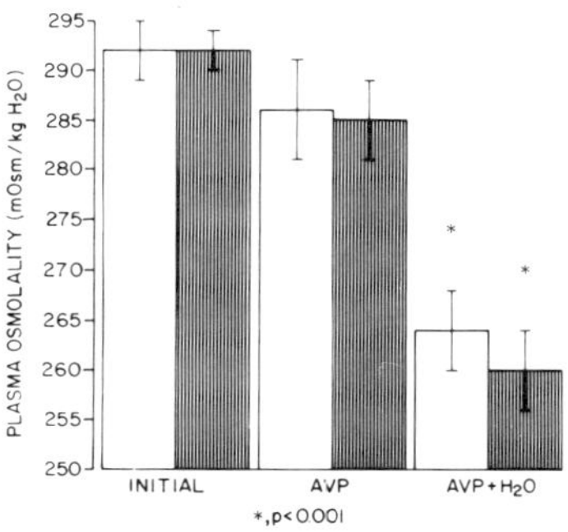

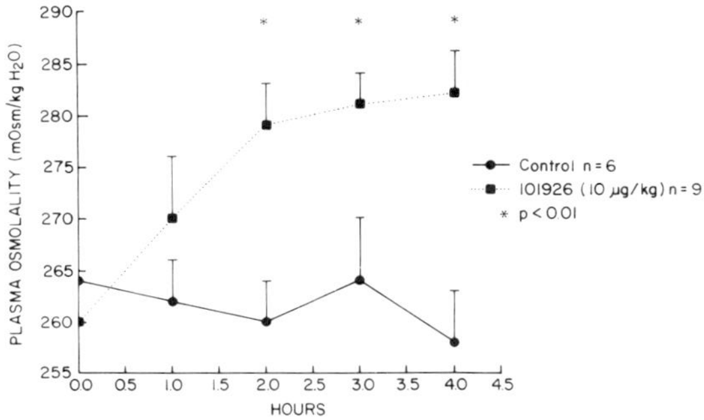

Fig. 2. Baseline plasma osmolality in rats before surgery (initial), 24 hr after initiation of AVP infusion (AVP) and 2 hr following administration of the gastric water load. Open bars are rats (n=6) to receive vehicle; closed bars are rats (n=9) to receive SK&F 101926 (see Fig. 3).

Fig. 3. Plasma osmolality as a function of time following establishment of hyponatremia (Fig. 2) and administration of vehicle (●) or SK&F 101926 (10 μg/kg, ■).

REFERENCES

1. Anderson, R.J., Chung, H.M., Kluge, R., and Schrier, R.W. Ann. Intern. Med. 102:164-168, 1985.
2. Ayus, J.C., Krothapalli, R.K., Armstrong, D.L. Am. J. Physiol. 248:F711-F719, 1985.
3. Ayus, J.C. Krothapalli, R.K. and Arieff, A. Am. J. Med. 78:897-902, 1985.
4. Stassen, F., Heckman, G., Schmidt, D. In: Vasopressin (Ed. R. Schrier), Raven Press, New York, 1985, pp. 145-154.
5. Kinter, L.B., Dubb, J., Huffman, W., Brennan, F., and Stassen, F.L. In: Vasopressin (Ed. R. Schrier), Raven Press, New York, 1985, pp. 553-561.
6. Kinter, L.B., Dytko, G., Ashton, D., McDonald, J., Huffman, W., and Stassen, F. J. Cardiovasc. Pharmacol. (in press), 1986.
7. Lazlo, F., Csati, S. and Balaspiri, L. Acta. Endocrinol. 106:56-60, 1984.
8. Cheng, S.W.T., North, W.A. and Gellai, M. Ann. N.Y. Acad. Sci. 394:473-480, 1982.
9. Kinter, L.B., Huffman, W., Stassen, F., and Churchill, S. (This volume).
10. Kim, J.K. and Schrier, R.W. In: Vasopressin (Ed. R. Schrier), Raven Press, New York, 1985, pp. 155-158.

THE VASOPRESSIN ANTAGONIST SK&F 101926 IS A SELECTIVE AQUARETIC AGENT IN DOGS

L.B. KINTER[1], W. MANN[1], F. BRENNAN[1], W. HUFFMAN[3], and F. STASSEN[2]

Departments of Pharmacology[1], Molecular Pharmacology[2] and Peptide Chemistry[3], Smith Kline and French Laboratories, Swedeland, PA 19479, USA

INTRODUCTION

The vasopressin analog desGly^{9}d$(CH_2)_5{}^1$D-Tyr(Et)^{2}Val^{4}AVP (SK&F 101926) has previously been reported to be a potent vasopressin antagonist and aquaretic agent in anesthetized and conscious rats and in squirrel monkeys (1,2,3). In these studies we report the effects of SK&F 101926 on cardiovascular and renal hemodynamics and renal solute and water excretion in conscious dogs. The results show that SK&F 101926 selectively increases water excretion in dogs. The mechanism of action is antagonism of vasopressin at renal V-2 receptors. At diuretic doses, SK&F 101926 has no significant effects on blood pressure, heart rate, renal plasma flow, or glomerular filtration rate in conscious dogs. However, at these doses, SK&F 101926 blocks the pressor and bradycardic responses to exogenous vasopressin.

METHODS AND MATERIALS

Cardiovascular Hemodynamics and Renal Solute Excretion:

Trained beagle dogs were prepared with intra-arterial Vascular-Access-Ports (VAP) using standard aseptic surgical techniques (4). Following a 2-week recovery period, 18 hr fasted dogs were prepared for continuous collection of urine (bladder catheter), monitoring of heart rate and blood pressure (VAP), and intravenous drug administration (vascular catheter). Following collection of baseline parameters, SK&F 101926 was administered intravenously (30 to 1000 μg/kg) at 30 minute intervals. Blood pressure and heart rate were monitored continuously. Urine was collected at 10 min intervals. Vasopressin challenges were administered at the beginning and end of the protocol to test SK&F 101926-associated pressor blockade.

Vasopressin Antagonism In Vivo:

Trained female mongrel dogs (fasted 18 hr) were orally water-loaded (to suppress endogenous vasopressin) and infused (5 ml/min) with 5% dextrose. Following establishment of water diuresis, an infusion of exogenous vasopressin (10 ng/kg plus 0.25 ng/kg/min) was initiated, and the dextrose infusion carefully monitored to match urinary loss for the duration of the study. Once the antidiuretic response to vasopressin had plateaued, SK&F 101926 (6.3 μg/kg) was administered, and the response followed for 60 min or more.

Arginine vasopressin (AVP) was obtained from Bachem; SK&F 101926 (1-[β-mercapto-β,β-cyclopentamethylenepropionic acid, 2-(O-ethyl) D-tyrosine, 4-valine, 8-arginine, 9-desglycine] vasopressin) was prepared by SK&F Peptide chemists. Vascular-Access-Ports (see ref. 4) were obtained from Norfolk Medical Products, Inc., Skokie, IL.

RESULTS AND DISCUSSION

In conscious dogs increasing doses of SK&F 101926 increased urine flow rate (V) and diluted urine osmolality (Uosm) in a dose-dependent fashion (Fig. 1). Threshold was between 30 and 100 μg/kg; peak V approached 2.0 ml/min; Uosm was diluted to ~150 mOsm/kg H_2O. There were no significant increases in sodium, potassium, creatinine (and hence glomerular filtration rate) or urea excretion associated with SK&F 101926

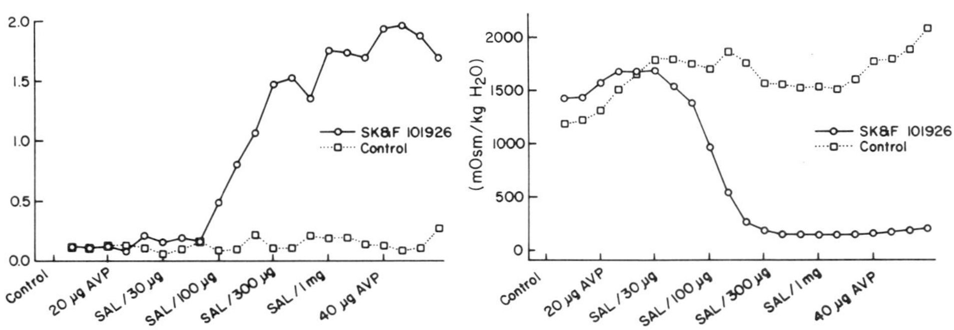

Fig. 1. Effect of increasing doses of SK&F 101926 (30 μg/kg to 1 mg/kg) on urine flow rate (left panel) and urine osmolality (right panel) in 4 conscious dogs. SAL, 0.9% NaCl vehicle.

administration in this model. SK&F 101926 administration had no effect on mean blood pressure or heart rate at any dose tested (Figure 2); the presence of SK&F 101926 blocked the pressor and bradycardiac responses to 40 ng of AVP.

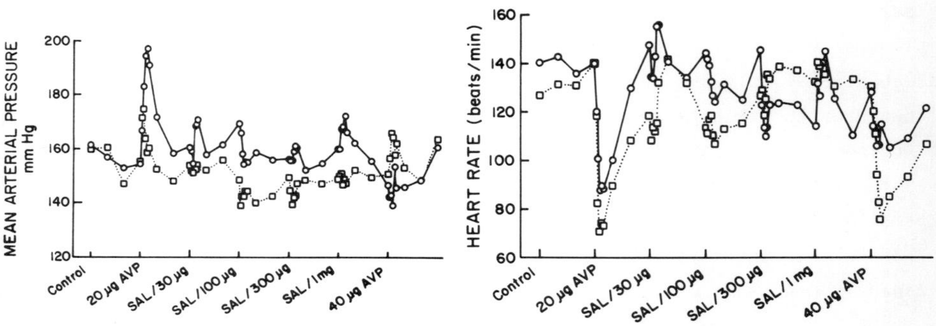

Fig. 2. Effect of increase of SK&F 101926 on mean arterial pressure (left panel) and heart rate (right panel) in 4 conscious dogs (see Fig. 1 for legend).

SK&F 101926 (6.3 μg/kg) reversed the antidiuretic action of exogenously administered AVP in conscious water-loaded dogs in which endogenous AVP secretion is suppressed (Fig. 3). The onset of AVP antagonist-like activity was within 30 min; peak V approached 2 ml/min (not shown); Uosm was diluted from levels greater than 1200 to ~150 mOsm/kg H_2O. It is notable that SK&F 101926 is a potent antagonist of AVP stimulation of adenylate cyclase in dog renomedullary membranes (see 5); the Ki for SK&F 101926 is ~1×10^{-9}M in that preparation.

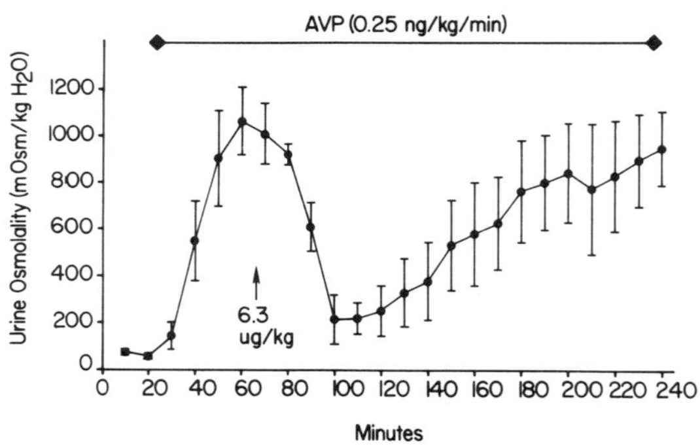

Fig. 3. Effect of SK&F 101926 (6.3 μg/kg) to antagonize vasopressin (AVP) antidiuresis in 3 conscious dogs undergoing water diuresis.

We conclude from these studies that SK&F 101926 is a selective water diuretic (aquaretic) agent in conscious dogs. SK&F 101926 is effective in both hydropenic and water-loaded AVP-infused dogs, tending to be more potent in the latter. The mechanism of action of SK&F 101926 is consistent with antagonism of renal epithelial vasopressin receptors *in vivo*.

ACKNOWLEDGEMENTS

We would like to acknowledge P. Woodward, M. Gross, D. Schmidt, and G. Heckman for experimental assistance; Dr. M. Landi and staff for expert care of our dog colony; and S. Tirri for assistance in manuscript preparation.

REFERENCES

1. Stassen, F., Heckman, G., Schmidt, D. *In*: Vasopressin (Ed. R. Schrier), Raven Press, New York, 1985, pp. 145-154.
2. Kinter, L.B., Dubb, J., Huffman, W., Brennan, F., and Stassen, F.L. *In*: Vasopressin (Ed. R. Schrier), Raven Press, New York, 1985, pp. 553-561.
3. Manning, M., Olma, A., Klis, W. Nature *308*(12):652-653, 1984.
4. Mann, W.A., Landi, M.S., Horner, E., Woodward, P., Campbell, S., and Kinter, L.B. Lab Animal Sci. (in press), 1986.
5. Stassen, F., Heckman, G., Huffman, W. J. Pharm. Expl. Ther. *232*:100-105, 1985.

VII. DIURETICS AND HYPERTENSION

THE ANTIHYPERTENSIVE MECHANISM OF DIURETICS

E.Ambrosioni, C.Borghi, S.Boschi, F.V.Costa, A.Mussi, Cattedra e Servizio di Farmacologia Clinica,Policlinico S.Orsola,Università di Bologna,Italy.

INTRODUCTION

Diuretics are still the most widely used drugs for the treatment of arterial hypertension but the mechanism by which they lower blood pressure is still a controversial question. Two main mechanisms have been considered:

1) Depletion of extracellular fluid volume (ECF) with reduction of plasma volume (PV)
2) Decreased peripheral vascular resistance (PVR) due to a "vasodilator" action of these drugs.

It is now widely accepted that while ECF and PV depletion account for the initial antihypertensive effect of diuretics, their long-term effect is due to a decrease in PVR. In the present paper we will briefly review some of the hemodynamic and cellular ionic changes induced by diuretics in order to attempt an explanation of their effects on PVR.

Plasma Volume and Extracellular Fluid Changes

Even if the data from the literature are somehow conflicting, the majority of the studies have shown that during the first days of therapy, diuretics produce a decrease in PV of about 300-400 ml and a fall in ECF of about 2 L (1,2). After the initial decrease, there is no further reduction in ECF or PV, on the contrary, in the long-term, PV ,ECF and cardiac output return to pre-treatment values while blood pressure remains low (3,4). These data support the hypothesis that PV fall is probably not the main mechanism by which diuretics reduce blood pressure in the long term. Also severely salt-restricted diets can produce the same effects on PV,ECF and blood pressure (5) while oral salt loading (20-30 Gm daily) is able to re-expand ECF despite concomitant

thiazide diuretics administration and it also restores hypertension in the long-term (6). These data suggest that modifications in sodium balance (and not only volume changes) are responsible for blood pressure reduction induced by thiazide diuretics. Finnerty (7) showed that, after acute furosemide i.v. administration , PV and and blood pressure have a significant fall, but re-expansion of PV with dextran does not cause any increase in blood pressure. However, if volume is re-expanded with a saline solution, blood pressure and sodium balance have parallel changes (8). These data further reinforce the hypothesis that sodium balance is a determinant factor in the antihypertensive action of diuretics and that a re-expansion of ECF is needed, rather than of PV alone, to counterbalance the antihypertensive effects of diuretics.
To explain how the reduction in ECF can lower blood pressure, one should consider several hypothesis. Firstly, environmental pressor stimuli seem to be blunted by ECF reduction. Secondly, the volume depletion and the reduction in cardiac output could activate baroreceptor reflexes. Thirdly, it has been supposed that feedback mechanisms are activated in response to the decrease in cardiac output observed during the early phases of diuretic therapy.
Tobian (9) postulated the hypothesis that thiazides and related compounds, induce a "reverse autoregulation" leading to a fall in PVR. Diuretics, reducing ECF, would produce a decrease in central venous pressure, in venous return and in cardiac output. The chronic cardiac output reduction could be the cause of a progressive fall in PVR and blood pressure. This hypothesis however, has never been experimentally demonstrated.

Decreased Peripheral Vascular Resistance

Even if there is a general agreement that PVR are reduced during chronic diuretic therapy, the intimate mechanism leading to this reduction has never been fully explained. One of the early hypothesis took into account the dehydratation of arteriolar wall with a decrease in intracellular Na^+ resulting in an increase in the arteriolar diameter with consequent fall in PVR. The reduction of arteriolar Na^+ content could also explain why diuretic administration is associated with a decrease in vascular reactivity to norepinephrine and angiotensin II and with a reduction in sympathetic nerve responsiveness (10). Studies in animals have failed to demonstrate a reduction in water and sodium arteriolar content after diuretic therapy but studies in man, performed using blood cells, have shown that diuretic treatment causes a decrease in intracellular Na^+ and K^+ (11,12,13). These changes in cellular electrolyte balance could give an useful support for understanding the mechanisms by which diuretics reduce PVR.

Electrolyte Balance and Thiazide Diuretics

There is a general agreement in the literature, that sodium content of blood cells is abnormally high in essential hypertension and it has been hypothesized that the increase in Na^+ (and probably in Ca^{++}) could be involved in the pathogenesis of essential hypertension. However, even if intracellular Na^+ (Na_i) plays an important role in blood pressure regulation, it is K^+ which plays the most important role. In particualr, the membrane potential , and thus the arterial tone, is directly dependent on the intra/ extracellular K^+ ratio (K_i/K_e) as shown by the Nernst equation (Resting Membrane Potential $=-61.5 \log K_i/K_e$). In previous studies we have shown that diastolic blood pressure is related directly to Na_i and inversely to K_i , but that the best correlation was found when we considered, instead of K_i alone, the K_i/K_e ratio (14,15). This suggests that the cellualr model we used (lymphocyte) is a good model for indirectly studying what happens in arterial smooth muscle cells. Treatment with hydrochlorothiazide (8 weeks) is able to cause significant changes in electrolyte balance as shown in Table 1.

	Na_e	K_e	Na_i	K_i	Na_i/Na_e	K_i/K_e
Placebo	141 ± 2	$4.2\pm.2$	110 ± 10	438 ± 27	$0.78\pm.07$	105 ± 8
Diuretic	$138\pm2^{**}$	$3.7\pm.2^{**}$	$95\pm9^{**}$	$405\pm23^{**}$	$0.68\pm.07^{**}$	$111\pm10^{**}$

Table 1 : Changes in intra and extracellular Na^+ and K^+ in 18 hypertensive patients treated for 8 weeks with hydrochlorothiazide, 25 mg/daily.
** = $p<0.001$.

Treatment with hydrochlorothiazide induced a reduction in both extra and intracellular Na^+ and K^+ however, the reduction in K_i was lesser than the reduction in K_e , therefore the K_i/K_e ratio rose signficantly in about 50% of patients. When we considered separately responders (decrease of at least 10% in diastolic blood pressure) and nonresponders to diuretic therapy, we observed that the two groups had different changes in electrolyte balance as shown in Table 2

	Na_e	K_e	Na_i	K_i	Na_i/Na_e	K_i/K_e	P.R.A.	Aldosterone
Responders	-2%	-15%	-21%	- 4%	-22%	+15%	+100%	+37%
Non Responders	-2%	- 9%*	- 6%***	-10%*	- 5%***	+ 1%***	+120%	+91%***

Table 2 : Percent changes induced by hydrochlorothiazide in responders (n.9) and nonresponders (n.9) after 8 weeks of therapy. * =p<0.05; ***=p<0.001.

Responders were characterized by a greater decrease in Na_i and Na_i/Na_e but by a lesser decrease in K_i with a much greater increase in K_i/K_e than nonresponders. This different response could be due to the greater increase in aldostrerone observed in nonresponders. In fact, even if P.R.A. had a similar increase in responders and nonresponders, nonresponders had a much greater rise in aldosterone. These data are in accordance with those from Laragh (16) and suggest that aldosterone, causing intracellular Na^+ increase and K^+ decrease, could be responsible for the lack of the favourable electrolyte changes of non responders. In fact, diastolic blood pressure reduction was directly related to the Na_i/Na_e decrease (r=0.88) and to the K_i/K_e decrease (r=0.90) while diastolic blood pressure decreased least in those subjects in whom aldosterone had the greatest rise (r=-0.65). Therefore, the reduction in PVR induced in responders by diuretic treatment, could be explained , on the basis of these data, as the consequence of changes in membrane potential due to the hyperpolarization of cell membrane (linked to the increase in K_i/K_e) and to the reduced vascular sensitivity to pressor agents.

CONCLUSIONS

The antihypertensive mechanism of action of diuretics has been attributed to various volume and hemodynamic changes but it has been clearly demonstrated that the ultimate mechanism by which they lower blood pressure in the long term is a reduction in PVR. The intra and extracellular changes in Na^+ and K^+ we observed could be the basic mechanism leading to PVR decrease. It should be also considered that membrane potential regulates not only vascular tone but it is also related to baroreceptors activity, to cardiac contractility and to renal ionic reabsorption. Thus, the "reverse auto - regulation " hypothesized by Tobian, is not excluded by our studies but should be explained on a ionic basis . If hypertension is caused by a renal defect in sodium and water excretion with consequent increase in PV and cardiac output followed by autoregolatory increase in PVR, the reverse autoregulation could be explained as a consequence of the reduction in Na_i and of the increase in K_i/K_e induced by diuretics. A direct demonstration of the effects of diuretics and K^+ sparing drugs on memebrane potential has been recently given in a study (16) showing that diuretic-treated patients developing hypokalaemia have a decrease in myocardial memebrane potential and that amiloride is able to re-increase membrane potential. Aldosterone production seems to be an important factor for the antihypertensive effect of diuretics since blood pressure has an insatisfactory decrease in those subjects in whom aldosterone rise is greater.

REFERENCES

1. Shah, S., Khatri, I., Freis, E.D. Am. Heart J. 95: 611-618, 1978.
2. Freis, E.D. Am. Heart J. 106: 185-187, 1983.
3. Conway, J., Lauwers, P. Circulation XXI: 21-27, 1960.
4. Tarazi, R.C., Dustan, H.P., Frohlich, E.D. Circulation, 41: 709-717, 1970.
5. Murphy, J.F. J. Clin. Invest. 29: 912-916, 1950.
6. Winer, B.M. Circulation, 23: 211-216, 1961.
7. Davidov, M., Gavrilovich, L., Mroczek, W., Finnerty, F.A. Jr., Circulation XL: 349-355, 1969.
8. Finnerty, F.A. Jr., Davidov, M., Kakaviatos, N. Circulation, XXXVII: 175-183, 1968.

9. Tobian, L. Fed. Proc. 33: 138-145, 1974.
10. Zsotér, T.T., Hart, F., Radde, I.C. Circ. Res. XXVII: 717-725, 1970.
11. Araoye, M.A., Khatri, I.M., Yao, L.L., Freis, E.D. Am. Heart J. 96: 731-737, 1978.
12. Ambrosioni, E., Costa, F.V., Montebugnoli, L., Cavallini, C., Magnani, B. Drugs Exptl. Clin. Res. VII: 757-762, 1981.
13. Poston, L., Jones, R.B., Richardson, P.J., Hilton, P.J. Clin. Exp. Hypertens. 3: 693-701, 1981.
14. Ambrosioni, E., Costa, F.V., Borghi, C., Mussi, A., Boschi, S. J Hypertension 3: S69-S71, 1985.
15. Ambrosioni, E., Costa, F.V., Borghi, C., Mussi, A. Postgrad. Med. J. (in press) 1986.
16. Stewart, D.E., Ikram, H., Espiner, E.A., Nicholls, G.A. Br. Heart J. 54: 290-297, 1985.

METABOLIC EFFECTS OF LONG-TERM DIURETIC TREATMENT.

J.L.Rodicio, J.M. Alcazar, J.Nieto, B.Miranda, L.M. Ruilope.
Service of Nephrology. 1º Octubre Hospital. Madrid, Spain.

INTRODUCTION.

In the last two decades diuretics have been amply considered as the first choice drug for the treatment of essential arterial hypertension. In 1978, the Expert Committee of the World Health Organization(1) recommended the use of stepped-care treatment starting with a diuretic or a beta-blocker alone or in combination. A third drug mainly a vasodilator should be added when necessary.

The usefulness of diuretics has been clearly shown and 50 per cent of the patients can be controlled when they are used as monotherapy(2).This percentage raises to 85 per cent when a second drug is added(3). The treatment of arterial hypertension has been proved to be adequate for the prevention of mortality, cerebral strokes and renal damage(4, 5). Nevertheless, its efficacy to diminish the incidence of coronary heart disease seems to be low or evenmore negative(6). The absence of a preventive effect for the heart has been considered as secondary to the modifications of plasma lipids (7, 8) and carbohydrates metabolism(9) induced by the diuretics mainly the thiazides.

Other side-effects attributable to diuretics are hypokalemia, hypomagnesemia and hyperuricemia. The decrease of serum potassium can induce cardiac arrithmias (10) and probably worsens the control of blood pressure(11). Hyperuricemia has been considered as a risk factor for ischemic heart disease (12)besides contributing to renal damage and to the appearance of acute gouty arthritis.

The aim of this study has been to investigate the metabolic effects of long-term treatment of essential hypertension when a diuretic has been used as the first step drug. Whenever needed, a betablocker alone or in combination with a vasodilatador was added following the stepped care protocol of the WHO.

MATERIAL AND METHODS.

A total of 1093 patients diagnosed as having essential hypertension have been followed for five years; 428 out of the total(47% males, 53% females; aged between 16 and 80 years) have received the same treatment during the follow-up period and were included in the study. The initial visceral damage of the patients was low, proteinuria was present in 13% of the cases, grade 3 or 4 retinopathy in 6.5% and electrocardiographic signs of ischemia and/or myocardial infarction in 13%.

The stepped-care therapeutic permited us to include the patient in one of the following groups:

		(n)	%
Group 1-	Non pharmacological treatment	55	13
Group 2-	Group 1+ hydrochlorothiazide (50-100 mg/d) and amiloride (5-10 mg/d)	141	33
Group 3-	Group 2 + Propranolol (80-200 mg/d)	92	21
Group 4-	Group 3 + hydralazine(50-200 mg/d)	59	14
Group 5-	Propranolol(80-400 mg/d)	81	19

Those patients presenting initially with high levels of serum glucose and uric acid were initially included in the Group 5.

In every patient clinical and analytical controls have been performed after 1, 6, 12, 18, 24, 36, 48 months of treatment. This paper contains the results of the evolution of serum cholesterol, triglycerides , potassium, glucose, creatinine and uric acid during the follow-up. Biochemical parameters were measured by means of an SMAC-Technicon.

The statistical analysis of the results was performed by means of an IBM Personal computer using the Student`s t test for paired and unpaired data and the analysis of variance.

RESULTS.

Blood pressure control.

As can be seen in Table 1 the blood pressure(BP)control was adequated and similar in the 5 groups studied. The Table II represents the mean ,standard deviation and P signification at initial and 60 months of treatment of the biochemical paramaters

Cholesterol.

The levels of serum cholesterol increased significantly($p<0.01$)in groups 2 and 3 in which the diuretic was used alone or in combination with propranolol after 36 and 48 months of therapy and remained elevated after 60 months. Nevertheless, no significant change was observed when a vasodilator was added to both drugs (Group 4). in Group 1 and 5 there was no significant variation of this parameter.

TABLE I.

EVOLUTION OF THE LEVELS OF BP:

		INITIAL	36 months	60 months
G-1	SBP mmHg	166±23	144±16*	141±15*
	DBP "	103±11	86±8*	85±9*
G-2		174±29	143±15*	143±16*
		110±13	90±10*	87±9*
G-3		190+13	150±18*	152+17*
		119±18	95±13*	93±13*
G-4		195±30	153±17*	152±21*
		124+16	98±11*	95±15*
G-5		170±26	155±21*	152±19*
		112±10	98±11*	93±7*

*$p<0.01$ vs Initial

Triglycerides.

A significant increase of serum triglycerides was observed after 1 month of treatment in group 2 and 3, returning to basal values after one year and declining progressively and significantly there after. A significant decrease during the follow-up was also observed in the groups 1 and 5 but not in group 4.

Potassium.

The initial values of group 1 were significantly higher when compared to any of the others groups. When analyzed separately we did not find differences between the initial and the following values of potassium in any of the group studied. However, the levels of potassium in group 2 were significantly lower when compared to groups 1 and 5 in any point during the evolution. Furthermore the percentage of hypokalemia presentation at the end of follow-up was higher in group 2 (3.3%) than in group 1 (1.1%).

Glucose.

Patients in groups 2, 3 and 4 exhibited a significant increase of this parameter after 36 to 48 months of therapy ($p<0.05$). On the contrary in group 1 and 5 that did not receive diuretic treatment blood glucose did not vary along the study.

TABLE II.

BIOCHEMICAL ALTERATIONS IN LONG-TERM DIURETIC TREATMENT IN ESSENTIAL HYPERTENSION.

GROUP	N	PARAMETER	INITIAL	60 MONTHS	P
G-1	55	Glucose (mg/dl)	93±13	96±13	N.S.
		Cholesterol(mg/dl)	205±37	220±66	N.S.
		Triglycerides(mg/	151±72	118±77	p<0.01
		Potassium(mEq/L)	4.2±0.4	4.3±0.36	N.S.
		Creatinine(mg/dl)	1.0±0.35	0.95±0.2	N.S.
G-2	141	Glucose(mg/dl)	97±18	100±17	p<0.05
		Cholesterol(mg/dl)	205±41	226±46	p<0.01
		Triglycerides(mg/dl)	147±63	123±58	p<0.01
		Potassium(mEq/L)	4.1±0.46	4.0±0.41	N.S.
		Creatinine(mg/dl)	1.03±0.5	1.1±0.30	N.S.
G-3	92	Glucose(mg/dl)	103±23	113±35	p<0.01
		Cholesterol(mg/dl)	210±40	228±41	p<0.01
		Triglycerides(mg/dl)	161±80	134±53	p<0.01
		Potassium(mEq/L)	4.0±0.5	4.05±0.5	N.S.
		Creatinine(mg/dl)	1.1±0.34	1.08±0.34	N.S.
G-4	59	Glucose(mg/dl)	95±17	119±51	p<0.01
		Cholesterol(mg/dl)	209±32	220±37	N.S.
		Triglycerides(mg/dl)	161±42	150±50	N.S.
		Potassium (mEq/L)	3.95±0.46	4.0±0.6	N.S.
		Creatinine(mg/dl)	1.2±0.4	1.2±0.3	N.S.
G-5	81	Glucose(mg/dl)	106±37	110±50	N.S.
		Cholesterol(mg/dl)	211±39	221±33	N.S.
		Triglycerides(mg/dl)	173±70	150±76	p<0.05
		Potassium(mEq/L)	4.0±0.4	4.4±0.5	p<0.05
		Creatinine(mg/dl)	1.1±0.3	1.3±0.4	N.S.

Creatinine.

There was a tendency for higher values of in the initial serum creatinine of group 4 (this group included, as expected, the most elevated blood pressure levels and degree of visceral damage). During the evolution there was no significant change was observed in this parameters in any of the groups studied.

In a group of 131 patients the evolution of the electrocardiographic signs of left ventricular hypertrophy have been evaluated during the study. A regression of those signs has been observed independently of the type(s) of drug(s) used to control blood pressure.

DISCUSSION.

The biochemical consequences of long-term diuretic treatment differ considerably in the literature(8, 13). Certain groups have described an increase of total cholesterol and of its lipoprotein fractions, mainly LDL (6), while for others no change of serum cholesterol level has been observed (14). In opposition to our results the addition of propranolol to the diuretic prevented the diuretic-induced increase of cholesterol in some series (8). When a non selective beta-blocker such as propranolol is used alone an elevation of total cholesterol together with a decrease of HDL has been described (4). In our series, the elevation of serum cholesterol related to diuretic use appears later than expected according to the literature and seems to be prevented by the addition of a vasodilator such as hydralazine.

Most of the authors have found an stabilization or an increase in serum triglycerides levels during the treatment of essential hypertensives with diuretics (15). On the contrary, we have observed a progressive fall of serum triglycerides in all our groups but in 4 in which a vasodilator was used. These differences could be due to the type of diuretic employed in our study the association a thiazide and a distal diuretic amiloride, was used . In fact the Oslo Study (7) finds that during a shorter follow-up period and using the same diuretic no variation was observed in serum triglycerides. Other possible explanations for these differences could be a genetic influence in different groups of population and also change in dietary habits.

The consequence of the lipid pattern alteration could give raise to the failure in preventing myocardial ischemia (2) or evenmore could promote is worsening(6) in patients treated with diuretics for periods above 10 years.

The percentage of hypokalemia was in our series clearly lower than previously reported when a thiazide is used alone. In this case low serum potassium can appear in as much as 48% on the patients(16). Blood glucose exhibited a raise after 3 or 4 years of diuretic treatment. This increase has been ascribed to the depletion of potassium. In our series the presence of hypokalemia was low and it probably indicates that other factors are influencing carbohydrate metabolism.

Renal function as measured by serum creatinine does not seem to change during the follow-up period. Meanwhile electrocardiographic changes of left ventricular hypertrophy showed a progressive regression that seems to be mainly dependent on the adequate control of blood pressure more than in the type of drug used to get it (17).

REFERENCES.

1.- Who Expert Committee Arterial Hypertension. Tech.Rep.Ser.1978: 628.Geneve. WHO.
2.- Veterans Administration Cooperative Study Group on antihypertension Agents. J.A.M.A. 248: 1966-2003, 1982.
3.- FREIS. Circulation 53: 589.595, 1976.
4.- The Australian Therapeutic Trial in mild hypertension. Lancet I: 1261-1267, 1982.
5.- Multiple Risk Factor Intervention Trial Research Group. J.A.M.A. 248: 1465-1477, 1982.
6.- LEREN P, HELGELAND A.- Am.J.Med. 80:(suppl 2A): 3-6, 1986.
7.- HELGELAND A.- Am.J.Med. 69: 725-732, 1980.
8.- WEIDMANN P, VEHLINGER D, GERBER A.- J.Hypertension 3: 297-306, 1985.
9.- SARRETT R.J., McCARTNEY P., KEEN H.- Diabetologia 22: 79-84, 1982.
10.- ATWOOD J., GARDIN J.- Arch.Intern.Med. 145: 1185-1187, 1985.
11.- KAPLAN N., CARNEGIE A., RASKIN P., HELLER J., SIMMONS S.- N.Engl. J.Med. 312: 746-749, 1985.
12.- FESSEL J., SIGELAMB A., JOHNSON E.- Arch.Intern.Med.132:44-54,1973.
13.- AMES R., HILL P.- Circulation 65: 899-904, 1982.
14.- BERGLUND G., ANDERSSON O.- Lancet I: 744-747, 1981.
15.- GRIMM R., LEON A., HUNNINGHALKE D., LENZ K., HANNAN P., BLACKBURN H.- Ann. of Int.Med. 94: 7-11, 1981.
16.- MORGAN D.B., DAVIDSON C.- Br. Med. J. 280: 905-908, 1980.
17.- ARRIBAS F., MIRANDA B., RUILOPE L.M., ALCAZAR J.M., NIETO J., RODICIO J.L.- Kidney Int. 28(3), 584 (1985).

ANTIHYPERTENSIVE DIURETICS-OLD AND NEW

M.P. SAMBHI

Hypertension Division, Department of Medicine, Sepulveda VA Medical Center, University of California at Los Angeles, Sepulveda, CA 91343, U.S.A.

Antihypertensive diuretics were one of the first synthetic compounds introduced in medicine. These medicinal agents are used widely and their use is on the increase. Diuretics have been the cornerstone of antihypertensive therapy and with the development of new compounds with fewer long term metabolic side effects, diuretics may continue to hold this primacy.

Studies on localization of the site of action of diuretics in different segments of the nephron, have made enormous contribution to advances in renal physiology. The studies on the cellular mode of action of diuretics are an invaluable aid in the identification and characterization of ionic transport processes in renal as well as extrarenal cells.

This paper will briefly review some of the new and prototype members of the various types of antihypertensive diuretics. A historical reference only is made to the older members.

PRE THIAZIDE DIURETICS

Organomercurials

These compounds exhibit "High Ceiling" type of diuresis and saluresis. Since the major mode of action of mercurials is to block the active chloride transport in Henle's Loop, greater loss of chloride than sodium occurs. On prolonged use hypochloremic alkalosis can result leading to loss of activity that can be restored by induction of intracellular and urinary acidosis.

Mercurials have been shown to exert antihypertensive effect, however, therapeutic use in long term treatment is limited by toxicity, renal and hemopoietic and by the need for parenteral administration.

Carbonic Anhydrase Inhibitors

Acetozolamide was the first sulfonamide diuretic and paved the way for the subsequent synthesis of Thiazides. Acetozolamide is a weak diuretic, causing greater loss of sodium than chloride. Bicarbonate loss can result in hyperchloremic acidosis and limit further diuretic response. These agents thus were not suitable for prolonged use and not very effective for the treatment of hypertension.

THIAZIDE DIURETICS (BENZOTHIADIAZINES)

Thiazides (1) represented the first true saluretic, promoting excretion of sodium and chloride in approximately equal proportions. The acid base disturbances associated with prethiazide diuretics are eliminated with the use of thiazides, however, other well known metabolic deviations are common such as hypokalemia, hypomagnesemia, hyperuricemia, hyperglycemia and less frequently hyperlipidemia.

Enhanced Na excretion is not accompanied by equal amount of free water excretion. More Na and K than H_2O excretion may result in hypertonic urine and dilution hyponatremia which is corrected by suppression of vasopressin release and by intact ability to excrete dilute urine. In the absence of above functional mechanisms, vasopressin antagonists or Acquaretics will prove useful (in presence of excessive vasopressin release such as heart failure). Thiazides appear to increase water permeability of distal tubule and collecting duct independent of vasopressin mechanisms and thus induce antidiuresis in diabetics insipidus. Reduction in G.F.R. adds to this effect. Na reabsorption is inhibited in early distal segment mainly by inhibiting the Mg and K dependant ATPase, with no effect on Na-K ATPase. On prolonged use, natriuretic effect is limited by declining G.F.R. and by increasing aldosterone secretion and by enhanced distal exchange for potassium. K loss is accelerated by increased delivery of Na ions to the distal tubule. Initial natriuresis leads to volume contraction and antihypertensive effect. On prolonged use partial restoration of fluid volumes and escape from diuretic effect is observed but antihypertensive action continues.

Clinical Use. Diuretic dose response curve of hydrochlorothiazide is relatively flat beyond a daily dose of 100 mg. Antihypertensive dose response curve has never been studied in its entirety but is believed to level off similarly. In recent years the standard dose of 50 mg B.I.D., has been considered higher than optimal, and progressively lower doses are being recommended. The therapeutic floor and ceiling of a thiazide dose in different patients can vary with state of hydration, salt balance, racial origin and the status of renin-angiotensin aldosterone system.

The introduction of thiazides for treatment of hypertension in 1957-1958, was a landmark, as the long term administration of then available fluid retaining sympathetic blockers and vasodilators became possible for the first time with the addition of thiazides. Prevailing opinion at the time recommended treatment of moderate and severe hypertension and thiazides as components of polytherapy proved unequalled.

In recent years, the era of large clinical trials designed to assess the benefit risk ratio of drug treatment of asymptomatic mild hypertension, thiazide diuretics and their long term metabolic effects, have been the focus of attention and unresolved controversy. For the treatment of vast numbers of subjects with mild hypertension, thiazides compared to most other antihypertensive drugs are less expensive and reputed to cause less symptomatic side effects. In the recently completed M.R.C. Trial, however, 18 to 20% of the male subjects receiving thiazide diuretics, withdrew from treatment because of symptomatic side effects. As monotherapy of hypertension in unselected populations, thiazides are effective in 35 to 45% of the cases in achieving goal blood pressure.

THE SEARCH FOR BETTER DIURETICS

Table I, II and III, list the site and mode of action of diuretics. Table IV gives a partial list of functional improvements sought or achieved in synthetic molecules since the synthesis of the first thiazide compounds.

Table 1. Principal Site of Action of Diuretics

Proximal tubule	Carbonic Anhydrase Inhibitors
Ascending Loop of Henle	High Ceiling Diuretics
Early Distal Tubule	Thiazides and Sulfonamides
Late Distal & Collecting Duct	Antikaluretics

Table 2. Cellular Mode of Action of Diuretics

Diuretics are not inhibitors of Na+-K+-ATPase-But Alter:

a. Permeability of tubular membrane
b. Ion transport systems
c. Potential differences in the nephron

Table 3. Cellular Mode of Action of Diuretics

Carbonic Anhydrase Inhibitors:

Inhibition of the enzyme in the cytosol, brushborders and peritubular membranes of the proximal tubule

Thiazides and Sulfonamides

Inhibition of active sodium transport in early distal tubule

Loop Diuretics

Inhibit the stereospecific receptors in the ascending loop thus inhibit the passive sodium transport

Antikaluretics (Non Aldosterone)

Block sodium channels in distal nephron and thus diminish passive potassium secretion

Table 4. Improvements sought and partially achieved over Hydrochlorothiazide by devising new molecules

Prolonged action

Efficacy in the present of renal insufficiency

To balance the saluretic and diuretic effects to promote free water clearance in proportion to sodium loss

To counteract K and Mg loss

To attenuate the diabetogenic effect

To attenuate or abolish Hyperuricemia

To increase the saluretic and diuretic potency with diminishing effect on electrolytes and on blood sugar and uric acid

To increase the antihypertensive effect with diminishing diuretic and saluretic actions

To dissociate the antihypertensive effect from the diuretic and saluretic action

NON THIAZIDE SULFONAMIDE DIURETICS

Many compounds in this class have features common with thiazides. Chlorthalidone is a much longer acting agent. Metolazone, also long acting, shares the site of action with thiazides but extends it to the proximal tubule, and hence is effective in the presence of renal insufficiency. Loop diuretics such as Furosemide and Bumetanide are high ceiling diuretics for use in renal failure and edema states.

Indapamide

Indapamide (2) is a non thiazide sufonamide, methyl indoline derivative of Sulfamoyl benzamide. Its empirical formula is: 4 chloro N (2 methyl-1-indolinyl) 3-Sulfamoyl-benzamide.

Mode and site of action. The molecule exhibits a two pronged action: The Methylindoline moiety is highly lipid soluble and binds strongly to elastin in vascular smooth muscle; and decreases vascular reactivity and peripheral resistance in experimental animals and hypertensive patients.

The sulfamoyl benzamide moiety is shared with chlorthalidone and hydrochlorothiazide and has similar diuretic actions on distal convoluted tubule and a similar profile of side effects.

However, at maximally effective antihypertensive dose of 2.5 mg daily (equivalent to 50 mg HCT) chemical side effects are relatively less common and may be negligible except hypokalemia.

Pharmacokinetics. The drug is rapidly and completely absorbed from oral route and undergoes extensive hepatic metabolism: only 5% appears unchanged in urine. Elimination ½ life is 14-18 hours and the drug does not accumulate in body and thus has a potential advantage over thiazides in renal insufficiency. With the use of the recommended dose of 2.5 mg/day, B P begins to fall in one week but may take 12 weeks to reach maximum. Higher doses do not significantly increase the antihypertensive effect, but increase the side effects.

Adverse Effects. Symptomatic side effects are similar to those with thiazides but are less common. Chemical side effects are also claimed to be less common as compared with thiazides. Hypokalemia does occur and in about 3% of patients may be clinically significant. Elevations of blood glucose, uric acid and changes in lipid profile are reported to be uncommon with 2.5 mg daily of indapamide. However, in certain patients and at higher doses, all these effects that are common with thiazides can potentially occur with indapamide.

Clinical use in Hypertension. Long acting, once a day-effective antihypertensive diuretic with a profile of side effects that is potentially safer than that of thiazides. In a controlled trial on mild to moderate hypertension 50% of 644 patients achieved goal B P in 3 months with 2.5 mg a day (3). In a randomized, double blind trial in 83 patients with mild to moderate hypertension, 1 mg, 2.5, 5 mg of indapamide daily was equally effective in lowering B P (4). Indapamide 2.5 mg has been shown to be as effective as 50 mg of hydrochlorothiazide or 5 mg of bendroflumethiazide (5, 6).

Xipamide

Xipamide (4-chloro-5 sulfamoyl 2', 6' salicyloxylidide) a non thiazide sulfonamide, is a salicylic acid derivative with structural resemblance to chlorthalidone and to furosemide (7).

Mode and site of action. Mode and site of action of this long acting diuretic are ill defined and disputed. Existing studies are contradictory. The diuresis produced by Xipamide has similarities to that evoked by furosemide on one hand and by hydrochlorothiazide on the other, yet Xipamide does not behave either as a typical thiazide or a loop diuretic (8). Currently its major site of action is considered to be the distal tubule, perhaps different from that of thiazides.

Characteristics of Xipamide Diuresis. Similarities to loop diuretics: Diuresis is high ceiling and over a 24 hour period the maximal diuresis approaches that with furosemide. Xipamide is an effective diuretic in renal failure. The slight loss of calcium in urine resembles the action of furosemide and is opposite to that of hydrochlorothiazide. This observation however has been disputed and requires confirmation (9). It has been suggested that Xipamide may act as a loop diuretic but micro-puncture studies have not supported the thesis (9, 10).

Similarities to Thiazides: Xipamide decreases free water clearance and increases osmolar clearance during maximal water diuresis (10). During hydropenia (vasopressin induced) Xipamide and hydrochlorothiazide increase osmolar clearance with no significant effect on free water reabsorption. Xipamide perhaps acts in distal convoluted tubule however the action may be different or more extensive as compared to hydrochlorothiazide since the actions of the two in animal experiments are additives (11).

Pharmacokinetics. Xipamide is completely absorbed after oral administration, reaching peak concentration (3 mg/L-with a dose of 20 mg) within 1 or 2 hours. It has a high bioavailability (73%). The calculated volume of distribution is 2 liters (8). Approximately half of the administered drug is excreted unchanged about one quarter as a glucuronide conjugate in the urine and only a trace (3%) is excreted in the feces. The half life in plasma is about 7 hours and is not significantly prolonged in renal failure since extrarenal clearance (1.5 L/hour) remains adequate.

Adverse effects. Symptomatic side effects are reported to be mild and infrequent not requiring drug withdrawal. The reported incidence in various studies has varied between 1 to 10%. Symptoms appear to be related to diuresis and blood pressure reduction such as dizziness, fatigue, anorexia, nausea, headache, leg cramps, dry mouth, polyuria and nocturia.

The general profile of chemical side effects with Xipamide treatment is similar to other sulfonamide diuretics (12), and can all occur in a proportion of subjects receiving the drug.

Hypokalemia, hypomagnesemia, hyperuricemia, hyperglycemia have been observed. Some studies have suggested that potassium loss with Xipamide is similar to that with Furosemide and is less than that observed with hydrochlorothiazide or chlorthalidone (13, 14).

Clinical use in Hypertension. Xipamide is a long acting, once daily diuretic effective as monotherapy of mild to moderate hypertension as well as combined therapy with other agents. Its efficacy in this regard is comparable to that of thiazide and other sulfonamide diuretics. Larger doses tend to enhance efficacy somewhat, however, at the expense of side effects such as hypokalemia. Its efficacy in the presence of compromised renal function and its diuretic potency render it as useful agent in hypertension associated with renal failure. Early studies employed the dose of 40 mg daily, however, the average optimal monotherapy dose in hypertension has been shown to be 10 to 20 mg daily. In some patients (white) 5 mg a day can suffice (12).

NEW SALURETICS

Muzolimine

Muzolimine is a new non sulfonamide, highly ceiling, loop diuretic, undergoing clinical evaluation. In a crossover study against hydrochlorothiazide plus amiloride, muzolimine compared favorably regarding blood pressure reduction. In the 4 weeks study in patients with hypertension no decrease in serum potassium or increase in cholesterol, triglycerides, uric acid or blood glucose was observed. Symptomatic side effects were rare. Muzolimine monotherapy appeared to be effective in treatment of hypertension without untoward side effects (15, 16).

URICOSURIC DIURETICS

Tienilic Acid

A major advance was made with the development of this first uricosuric diuretic. Tienilic acid is a phenoxy acetic acid derivative, related to ethacrynic acid. Except its uricosuric property, it closely resembled thiazide diuretics in action and efficacy (17). Because of occasional but serious hepatotoxicity, it was taken off the market soon after its release.

Indacrinic Acid

Indacrinone, a new indanone derivative, with structural resemblance to ethacrynic acid, can acutely increase uric acid excretion and prevent the chronic elevation in serum uric acid caused by thiazides. Indacrinone administered alone increases urine flow rate and urinary sodium, potassium and hydrogen ion excretion for 8 hours. Uricosuria occurs in first 4 hours, followed by urate retention during the subsequent 24 hours, with no net change in serum uric acid (18). Addition of amiloride 2.5 mg to indacrinone 10 mg once a day, lowered the urinary excretion of potassium, hydrogen ion and calcium, and potentiated the natriuresis. Serum electrolytes and uric acid remained normal (18).

A promising new approach is being taken in mixing the two enantiomers of racemic indacrinone in optimal proportions to produce an isouricemic diuretic (19). The (-) enantiomer is more potent as a natriuretic agent and the uricosuric property predominantly resides with the (+) enantiomer.

NEW ANTIKALURETICS

Amiloride

Amiloride is a pyrazine-carbonyl-guanidine, that is unrelated in structure to other antikaluretic or diuretic agents. Its empirical formula is: 3, 5-diamino-N (aminoiminomethyl) 6-chloropyrazine carboxamide monohydrochloride dihydrate.

Mode and site of action. Amiloride acts by blocking sodium channels in the distal tubule independant of aldosterone. It is the most potent inhibitor of sodium entry through sodium channels operated by electric potential. At higher doses the drug also inhibits electroneutral Na^+/H^+ exchange. This inhibition of active sodium transport is coupled with a reduction of passive potassium secretion. Amiloride thus acts as a sparing agent for K^+ and Mg^{++} and reduces the urinary excretion of calcium (20).

Pharmacokinetics. Amiloride is excreted unchanged; almost 50% in the urine and 40% in the feces over 72 hours, half life is 6 to 9 hours. Amiloride is weakly bound to plasma proteins and is filtered and secreted into renal tubules. Renal clearance is unaffected by urine flow or PH or by probenecid.

Adverse effects. Hyperkalemia and metabolic acidosis can develop in susceptible people or in renal insufficiency. On addition of amiloride to previous therapy with hydrochlorothiazide, certain patients, particularly the elderly may develop "Amiloride Hyponatremia" (21). Lithium toxicity induced by amiloride combined with HCT in a phychiatric patient has been reported. Amiloride reduces the taste intensity of Na+ and Li+ salts and of sweeteners, probably through inhibition of sodium channels operative in the perception of taste (22).

Clinical Use. In patients with mild to moderate hypertension, amiloride 5 mg added to HCT 50 mg daily appears to be no more effective than HCT alone with K supplements in reducing blood pressure or in preventing hypokalemia (23). The addition of amiloride does however exert an additional sparing effect on Mg++, and may be more effective than K supplements in preventing hypokalemia especially if higher doses of added HCT are used (23, 24). Amiloride addition leads to the normalization, not only of plasma K but also of total body K. Plasma renin angiotensin and aldosterone, however, are further elevated with the addition of amiloride to HCT (25). Amiloride added to a beta blocker can prove to be nearly as effective in lowering blood pressure as when it is added to HCT, without causing biochemical deviations.

The addition of amiloride to HCT provides superior management of patients with nephrogenic diabetes insipidus as compared with HCT alone (26). The combination of HCT and amiloride either alone or with allopurinol is reported to be clinically effective in reducing the rate of calcium nephrolithiasis (27). Amiloride reduces urinary calcium slightly itself, however, more strongly potentiates the HCT induced reduction of urinary calcium.

Thirty three patients with primary calcium nephrolithiasis exhibiting inherited increase in red cell oxalate transport, all had the abnormality corrected with the use of HCT 50 mg and amiloride 5 mg daily (28). Unlike triamterene, amiloride does not increase urinary prostaglandins. Accordingly the documented potentiation of triamterene nephrotoxicity by non steroidal anti-inflammatory agents is not observed if amiloride is used instead of triamterene (29, 30).

Amiloride at higher doses (10-40 mg daily) (31), is useful in the management of several hypokalemic disorders such as primary and secondary aldosteronism, Bartter's Syndrome and K losing nephropathy.

In primary aldosteronism, plasma K rises and blood pressure falls with amiloride treatment. Additional antihypertensive drugs are usually required to achieve normotension. In these patients amiloride causes elevations in plasma renin activity as well as in plasma aldosterone. In Bartter's Syndrome on the other hand, plasma aldosterone is elevated but plasma renin activity falls with amiloride treatment (32). Thus the use of a converting enzyme inhibitor alone or in combination with amiloride is recommended for the treatment of hypokalemia associated with secondary aldosteronism because a suppression of plasma aldosterone levels is achieved rather than the elevation observed with amiloride alone (33).

For similar reasons, the use of aldosterone antagonists and furosemide in the management of patients with liver cirrohsis is generally preferred to the use of HCT in combination with amiloride.

REFERENCES

1. Peters, G., In: Antihypertensive Therapy. Ed Gross, F., Springer-Verlag, N.Y., 1966, pp 31-58
2. Carretta, R. et al, Eur. Journal Clin. Pharmacol. 24: 579, 1983
3. Passeron, J. et al, Postgrad Med. Journal, 57(2): 57, 1981
4. Capone, P. et al, Clin. Therapy, 5: 305, 1983
5. Morledge, J.H., American Heart Journal, 106: 229, 1983
6. Bing, R.F. et al, British Journal Clinical Pharmacol. 12: 883, 1981
7. Prichard, B.N.C. and Brogden, R.N., Drugs 30: 313-332, 1985
8. Knauf, H. and Mutschler, E., Europ. J. Clin. Pharmacol. 26: 513-520, 1984
9. Gold, C.H. and Viljoen, M., Clinical Pharmacol. and Therapeutics, 25: Part 1: 522-527

10. Hempelmann, F.W., Arzeneimittel-Forschung 25: 259-260, 1975b
11. Hempelmann, F.W., Leuschner, F. and Liebenow, W., Arzeimittel-Forschung 25(2): 252-255, 1975
12. Leary, W.P. and Reyes, A.J., Current Therap. Research 34: 888-899, 1983
13. Leary, W.P. and Asmal, A.C., Current Therap. Research 24: 656-661, 1978b
14. MacGregor, G.A., Banks, R.A., Markandu, N.D. and Roulston, J., British Journal of Clincal Pharmacology, 13: 859-863, 1982
15. Ferrara, L.A., Strazzullo, P., Scillitani, A., Mancini, M., Gagliardi, R., European Journal Clin. Pharmacol., 28(3): 241-244, 1985
16. Wicker, Pierre and Clementy, J., Clinical Pharmacol. and Therapeutics, 39(5): 537, 1986
17. Freis, E., and Sambhi, M.P. et al, New England Journal of Medicine, 301(6): 293-297, 1979
18. Ravenscroft, P.J., Hall, G.R., Ahokas, J.T., Emmerson, B.T., Tobert, J.A., Clinical Pharmacol. Therapeutics 28(1): 45-51, 1980
19. Blaine, E.H., Fanelli, G.M., Irvin, J.D., Davies, R.D., Clinical Exp. Hypertension, 4(1-2): 161-176, 1982
20. Ryan, M.P., Magnesium, 3(4-6) 274-288, 1984
21. Tarssanen, L., Huikko, M., Rossi, M., Acta Med. Scand., 208(6): 491-494, 1980
22. Schiffman, S., Lockhead, E., Maes, F.W., Proc. Natl. Acad. Science, 80(19): 6136-6140, 1983
23. Dorevitch, A., Baruch, E., American J. Psychiatry, 143(2): 257-258, 1986
24. Larochelle, P., Logan, A.G., Can. Medical Assoc. Journal, 132(7): 801-805, 1985
25. Svendsen, U.G., Ibsen, H., Rasmussen, S., Leth, A., Nielsen, M.D., Dige-Petersen, H., Giese, J., Clinical Pharmacol. Ther., 34(4): 448-453, 1983
26. Alon, U., Chan, J.C., American J. Nephrol., 5(1): 9-13, 1985
27. Maschio, G., Tessitore, N., D'Angelo, A., Fabris, A., Pagano, F., Tasco, A., Graziani, G., Aroldi, A., Surian, M., Colussi, G., Mandressi, A., Trinchieri, A., Rocco, F., Ponticelli, C., Minetti, L, American J. Medicine, 71(4): 623-626, 1981
28. Baggio, B., Gambaro, G., Marchini, F., Cicerello, E., Tenconi, R., Clementi, M., Borsatti, A., New England J. Med., 314(10): 599-604, 1986
29. Favre, L., Vallotton, M.B., Prostaglandins Leukotrienes Med., 14(3): 313-319, 1984
30. Spence, J.D., Wong, D.G., Lindsay, R.M., Lancet, 2(8446): 73-75, 1985
31. Jackson, P.R., Ramsay, L.E., Wakefield, V., British J. Clin. Pharmacol., 14(2): 257-263, 1982
32. Griffing, G.T., Aurecchia, S.A., Sindler, B.H., Melby, J.C., Journal Clin, Pharmacol., 22(11-12): 505-512, 1982
33. Griffing, G.T., Melby, J.D., Clinical Exp. Hypertension, 5(6): 779-801, 1983

THE PHYSIOLOGY OF NATRIURETIC MECHANISMS IN THE KIDNEY.

KLAUS THURAU

Department of Physiology, University of Munich, Munich, West Germany.

Since it was firmly estabilished in the 60ies by De Wardener, Levinsky and several groups that urinary NaCl excretion in the high salt state remains elevated even when glomerular filtration rate is experimentally prevented from increasing, or even kept below control, it became clear that a) an increase in GFR is not essential for an increased NaCl and volume excretion and b) that the tubular cells somehow recognize the high salt state and respond to it by reducing their NaCl and volume reabsorption rate. Also excluded, besides the increase in GFR, were known regulating systems such as aldosterone, ADH and others. The mistery of a third factor was born and kept a large number of laboratories in the whole world busy, trying to uncover the secret. It was De Wardener, who continously kept the idea alive that a specific humoral natriuretic mechanism must exist. For a surprising number of years no real breakthrough could be made and it is only recently that this field in renal research has obtained new momentum and produced results which justifies a lecture today on endogenous natriuretic principles. The subject of natriuretic principles is of particular interest in the context of the discussion on pathophysiological mechanisms associated with development of arterial hypertension as retention of NaCl or a shift in its compartimental distribution are observed phenomena during hypertension. Excluded from this presentation is the action of pharmacological, natriuretic substances and the description is limited to mechanisms, inherent in the organism, which allow the kidney to excrete an excess intake of salt in order to maintain a normal, i.e. physiological milieu interior. Because the work of unmasking the physiologic natriuretic principles is currently in progress in several laboratories, the presentation can be nothing but a description of the actual status quo, a now fast moving field.

The data currently available strongly indicate that not one but several natriuretic mechanisms exist which act upon the kidney, which can be separated at the present time with respect to their site and mode of action as well as to their physical and biochemical properties.

Three major sites within the nephron have been identified at which functional changes occur during volume expansion to allow for the excretion of an increased amount of NaCl and volume.
A) At the juxtaglomerular apparatus where the control of the glomerular filtration rate ty the tubuloglomerular feedback is being reset.
B) In the proximal convolution, where filtered, i.e. glomerular born material in the tubular fluid has been found to inhibit NaCl and volume reabsorption and
c) in the distal part of the nephron, i.e. the late distal and collecting duct system, where NaCl and volume reabsorption is reduced by a low identified substance.

<u>As to the adjustment of GFR by tubulo-glomerular feedback during volume expansion or high salt inatke.</u>

Fig. 1 shows at left a schema of the nephron with the proximal convolution, the loop of Henle, wich returns to the vascular pole of its own glomerular, then the distal tubule and finally the collecting duct. The point of contact between the end of ascending loop of Henle and the vascular pole, the JGA, is shown in more detail in the middle where the encircled region marks

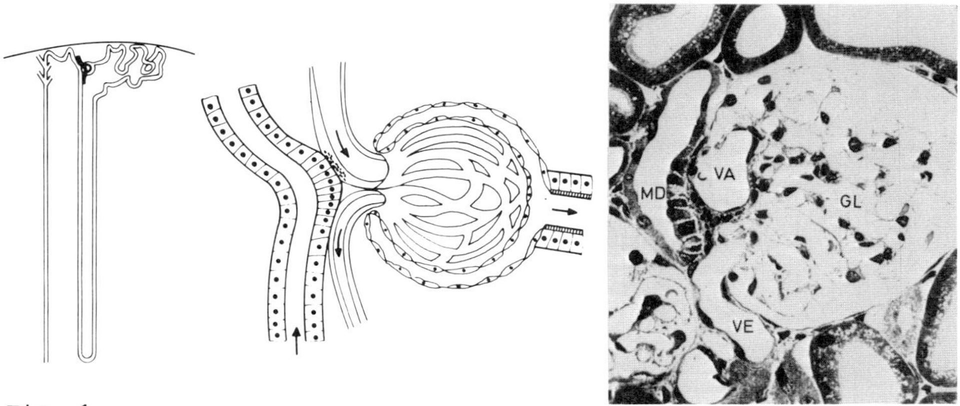

Fig. 1.

the JGA. Here are the afferent and efferent arterioles. Attached to the vascular pole is the ascending limb of Henle's loop, contacting the vessels through the macula densa cells. Because of the reabsorptive activity of the ascending limb, a flow depend signal is generated at this site of the nephron, which is received by the macula densa cells and triggers the local renin activity.

It is through the activation or the inhibition of the angiotensin system in the JGA that the SNGFR is adjusted to the nephron's capacity to reabsorb it and thereby controlled by the tubuloglomerular feedback. On the right, a histological slice shows the region of the JGA.

Fig. 2 demonstrates the special structural appearance of the macula densa receptor cells, which sense the NaCl concentration in the tubular fluid.

An important intrarenal mechanism to facilitate the excretion of NaCl is the increase in GFR. This increase is in large part due to the fact that the sensitivity of the feedback, controlling filtration rate, is reduced.

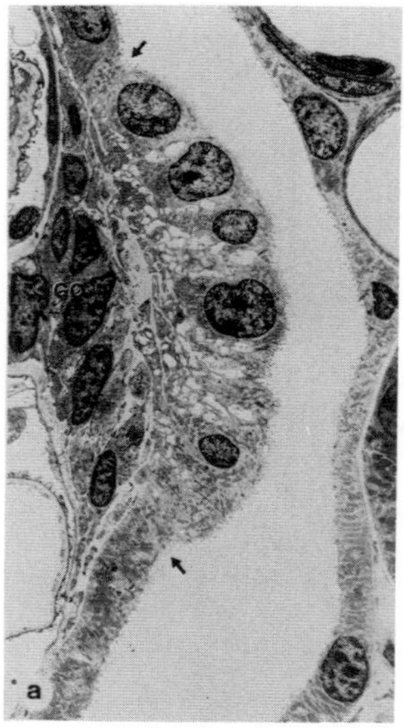

Fig. 2.

The idea of a humoral control of natriuresis implies that the humoral principle should be detectable in the plasma and transferable to a non-diuretic animal inducing natriuresis.

For a number of postualted natriuretic substances, this criterion is not fulfilled. Plasma exchange alone from an expanded to a non-expanded animal hardly produces natriuresis in the antidiuretic animal. Two groups, that of Sonnenberg in Toronto and that of De Warderner in London found it needs also the infusion of the urine into the assay animal to make it natriuretic. Wheter a natriuretic hormone, which is excreted by the kidney and present in the urine, is responsible for this effect or whether it is the reinfused urinary volume and NaCl which facilitate the onset of natriuresis, is still a matter of debate.

Taking the various results from different groups togheter, it is fair to state that at present time the evidence for a transferable natriuretic substance present in the plasma is still weak.

Two groups of investigators, that of Dr. Györy from Sidney

and that of Dr. Häberle in our Department have produced evidence at the single nephron level that the tubular fluid harvested from the proximal tubule of a volume expanded animal when transferred in the proximal tubule of a nonexpanded animal, leads to a reduction in proximal reabsorption activity. Therefore, the proximal convolution appears to be a second site along the nephron where the function is changed in the high salt state.

Fig. 3 shows a graph from Dr. Györy's recent paper. He measured the steady state concentration difference for sodium across the proximal tubular epithelium in stationary droplets, plotted on the abscissa in non-expanded and volume expanded animals, after instillation of harvested tubular fluid marked as "urine" or artificial solution. The important finding is that tubular fluid

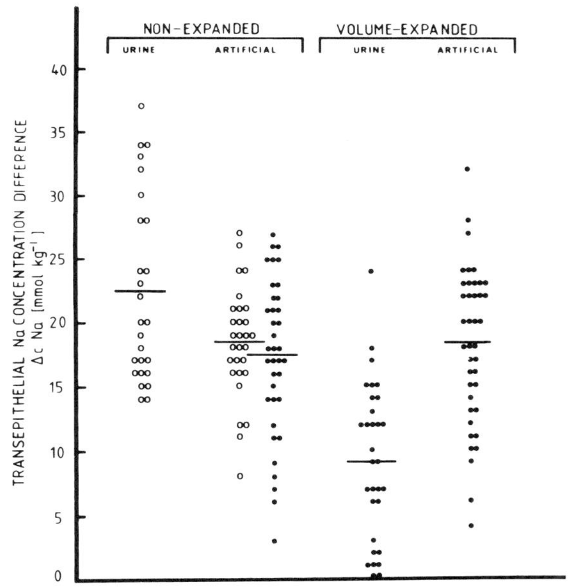

Fig. 3

Transepithelial concentration differences of Na measured with an artificial solution in the non-expanded state and again in the volume expanded state in the same animals (●) and with harvested proximal tubular fluid also in the same animals (●). There is marked overall reduction in ΔcNA with harvested tubular fluid. The (○) show similar experiments in another group of rats but only in the non-expanded state, and show, this time, a general increase in ΔcNa with harvested proximal tubular fluid of non-expanded animals harvested during volume expansion shows a much reduced Na concentration gradient, reduced to about 50% of normal.

A normal concentration gradient is estabilished in the proximal convolution even during volume expansion when the artificial tubular fluid is instilled. This led Györy to postulate that a natriuretic agent exists in the glomerular born tubular fluid during volume expansion which inhiibts proximal -ubular NaCl reabsorption.

Similar conclusions, namely that proximal volume reabsorption during volume expansion is inhibited by a luminal agent were drawn by Häberle from microperfusion experiments.

First, proximal tubular fluid was harvested from salt deprived and from salt loaded rats and used as perfusate in the proximal tubule. This allows the control values for the flow dependent reabsorption rate to be estabilished. Thereafter, harvested fluid was transferred from a low sodium tubule into a high sodium tubule and vice versa.

The tubule of the low Na animal is now being perfused with tubular fluid harvested during the high salt state. A comparison of the reabsorption rates ujder these two conditions will answer the question whether or not an inhibitory agent for volume reabsorption has been tranferred from the high salt animal.

Thereafter, the control experiment has been repeated to assure steady state over the time of the experiment.

Fig. 4: On the right panel, the decrease of reabsorption rate is shown when the tubule of a low-salt rat is perfused with tubular fluid from a high-salt animal. The inhibition of reabsorption in the expanded animals becomes also visible when their tubules are being perfused with fluid harvested from low-salt animals. This is shown on the left.

Fig. 5 shows the characteristics of flow-dependent reabsorption rates. The solid symbols are control and low salt values,

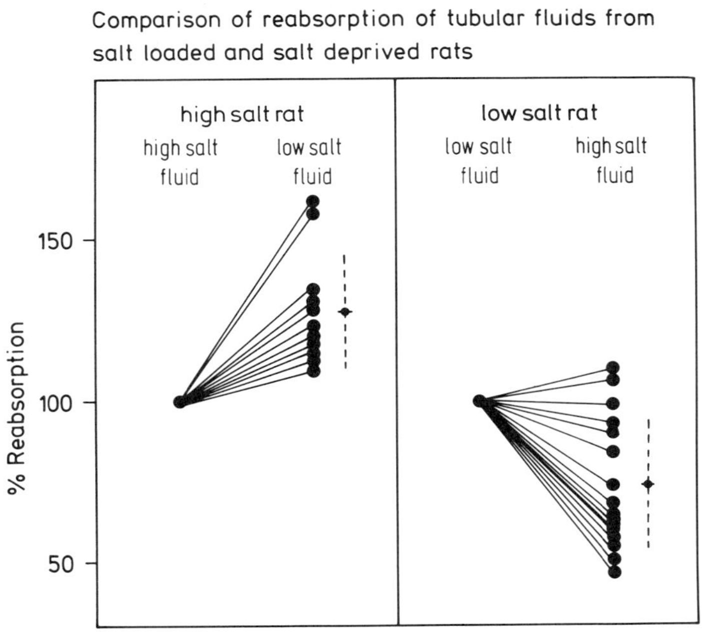

Fig. 4.

the open symbols salt loaded values. The slope of the values obtained with tubular fluid from salt loaded animals is significantly reduced indicating inhibition of proximal fluid reabsorption by a glomerular born agent or agents acting from the luminal site.

Two years ago, while Dr. Gÿory was working with us as visiting professor in Münich, we applied the electron microprobe technique to analize the intracellular Na concentration of proximal tubular cells under the same condition of volume expansion during which he found the prox. NaCl reabsorption inhibited by 50%. If the entrance step for Na across the luminal membrane into the cell is reduced while the pump remains uninhibited, one would expect a decrease in intracellular Na concentration.

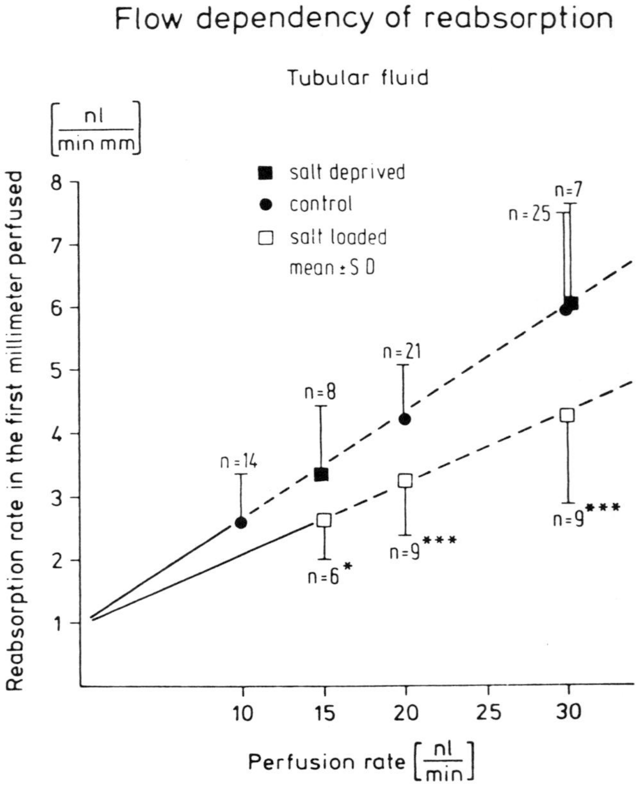

Fig. 5.

The intracellular Na concentration would increase if the pump activity is primarily inhibited during volume expansion. The intracellular Na concentration is 19.3 mmol per kg wet weight in the control and increases to 23.4 mmol during volume expansion. Cl also increases from 15.8 to 21.3.

These data point to an inhibition of the pump activity at the basolateral membrane during volume expansion. Together with the finding of Häberle and Györy that an inhibitory agent is present in the tubular fluid during volume expansion which acts from the luminal site, the present data led one to assume that the inhibitory agent must cross the tubular cell to interfere with the active transport step at the basolateral side. Such a mode of action of a regulatory agent for volume reabsorption is not exceptional. ADH, for example, acts from the basolateral side to affect the H_2O permeability of the luminal membrane.

Altough the data of Häberle and Gÿory are consistent in themselves, it must be noted that the evidence for existence of a luminal agent is still purely phenomenological and that no information is yet available as to the nature of this agent. It appears unlikely that it is a peptide, since the peptidase activities located at the brush border of the prox. tubule make it unlikely for a peptide to cross the luminal membrane intact and to act at the basolateral site. One candidate could be the substance of De Wardener extracted from the urine which he claims to be a non peptide. But this is highly speculative.

This brings me to a natriuretic principle, which, at the present time, appears to be the most documented and defined mechanism operating at a very distal site of the nephron.

In 1964 Jamieson and Palade reported on the existence of granules containing cells in the atria of the heart, which could not or only to a much lesser extent be found in the ventricular myocardium. The original idea of catecholamine-stores was soon discarded, and it was only three years ago that these granules received again great attention: de Bold and coworkers from Kingston in Canada injected an extract from the atrium of the heart into a rat and observed a pronounced natriuresis and diuresis. They concluded from their data that a naturally occurring natriuretic substance exists in the granules of the atrial tissue.

Already about 30 years ago the atria of the heart were discovered to be an important site for the regulation of body volume. It was at that time that Gauer and Henry performed their fundamental work demonstrating the physiological role of atrial volume receptors for the regulation of ADH secretion.

De Bold together with Flynn were the first to publish data in Life Sciences, which clearly mark an important step towards the identification of this natriuretic substance, using extracts from over 1200 rat atria. They found, using reverse phase high pressure liquid cromatography, natiuretic activities in four distinct chromatographic regions. From region 1 they purified a peptide with potent natriuretic properties and named it cardionatrin I.

Dr. Schnermann and Briggs in our Department have further investigated the physiological action of this atrial natriuretic substance. Urine flow increases approx. ten fold immediately after the injection of the extract from one atrium in rats and returns also fast to almost control values within 10-20 min. Concomitant to the incresed urine volume there is an increase in Na excretion. In extracts from ventricles natriuretic activities are practically absent. This is consistent with the observed intracardial distribution of the Palade-granules, which are practically absent from the ventricular tissue.

Potassium excretion is enhanced to some extent by the atrial extract.

The auriculi of the atria appear to be the major site of the natriuretic activity. Per unit tissue, both left and right auriculi contain the highest natriuretic and diuretic activity in the atria. Other vascular tissues except the atria such as vessels, aorta, or muscle are practically void of natriuretic activities. It appears that the atrial natriuretic peptide does not inhibit NaCl and volume reabsorption in the proximal tubule and therefore is not identical with the luminal agent postulated by Gÿory and Häberle. Neither atrial extracts, whether obtained from animals kept on a low or from those kept on a high diet inhibited proximal volume reabsorption.

Neither were any effects found by Schnermann and Briggs along Henle's loop, and cardionatrin appears not to be a kind of endogenous furosemide.

Experimental evidence has been produced by Sonnenberg from Toronto and Briggs and Schnermann showing consistently that cardionatrin inhibits NaCl reabsorption beyond the loop, especially in the late distal and collecting duct segments. Whether this is caused by transport inhibitory or changes in permeability as suggested by Trefor Morgan remains to be estabilished. An inhibition of collecting duct NaCl reabsorption is consistent with results produced 7 years ago by Bengele and Alexander in Boston, who, in micropuncture experiments, found collecting duct sodium reabsorption to be inversely related to the degree of NaCl and volume expansion.

Hence, the evidence today strongly suggests the existence of a natriuretic peptide in the atria of the heart, which inhibits NaCl reabsorption in a rather distal part of the nephron. The localization is interesting: if it were to act upon ascending limb of Henle's loop, it would automatically affect the CCS, thereby affecting H_20 reabsorption as well. The more distal locality makes it possible to uncouple to a large extent NaCl from H_20 excretion and to make the regulation of NaCl independent of H_20. A similar aspect certainly applies to the action of aldosterone.

The atrial peptide has an additional effect, which facilitates NaCl excretion. It resets the tubuloglomerular feedback and allows the formation of a larger filtrate, as demonstrated by Schnermann and Briggs.

One way to test the efficacy of the feedback is to determine the single nephron filtration rate in either at a proximal or at a distal puncture site. The proximal collection technique necessitates the installation of an oil block into the late proximal tubule, blocking the flow through the loop and thereby omitting a signal at the macula densa. The SNGFR formed under these conditions is maximal for the given BP. Measuring the filtrate beyond the macula densa in the distal tubule maintains flow through the loop and the feedback signal at the macula densa, thus adjusting SNGFR to a lower value to achieve tubulo-glomerular balance.

The difference is diminished during the infusion of natrial extract. The diminished sensitivity of the feedback control is further documented by the results of experiments in which a given strenght of signal is applied to the macula densa by micropuncture techniques before and after atrial extracts. In control, the given signal reduces SNGFR by 37%, whereas the same signal leads to a reduction of SNGFR of only 8% after the infusion of the atrial extract.

The exact nature of the interrelationship between volume expansion and the activity of tha atrial mechanism is far from being understood. The extractable natriuretic activity appears not to vary with the state of salt intake. Such a relationship may not to be relevant at all, since it might well be the activity in the plasma, which could determine the renal response. Data obtained by radioimmunoassay for the atrial natriuretic factor favour such a mechanism.

One other observation is of interest: vagotomy abolishes the natriuresis following atrial distension. This may indicate a trophic role of the vagal innervation of the atria. Again, these are open questions, which need further analysis.

INTRACELLULAR ELECTROLYTES IN ESSENTIAL HYPERTENSION DURING TREATMENT WITH TORASEMIDE

C. Spieker, W. Zidek, W. Häcker, W. Schmidt, W. Tenschert and H. Vetter
Med. Univ.-Poliklinik, Albert-Schweitzer-Str. 33, 4400 Münster, FRG

INTRODUCTION

Diuretics do play an important role in the treatment of hypertension. But still the mechanism of the blood pressure lowering effect of diuretics in hypertension is not entirely clarified. Whereas the reduction in blood volume and consequently in stroke volume can be demonstrated initially, this is not found during long term treatment. On the other hand a decrease in total peripheral resistance has been described, which may be responsible for the long term reduction in blood pressure (1). The mechanism, by which diuretics influence vascular tone, is still unknown. In this context the direct action of diuretics on the pathogenetic factors in essential hypertension may be suspected. Among those interest has focussed on intracellular free calcium in arterial smooth muscle cells and other tissues in the last years. Such an increase in intracellular free calcium which has been demonstrated in red blood cells from essential hypertensives and from spontaneously hypertensive rats as well as in arterial smooth muscle cells from spontaneously hypertensive rats (2) can be expected to cause vasoconstriction by the well known effect of calcium on electromechanical coupling in contractile tissues. Therefore the effect of a loop diuretic on intracellular free calcium was examined. Furthermore intracellular natrium in red blood cells was measured, as the diuretic induced natriuresis can be expected to alter intracellular natrium stores.

METHODS

The study was performed on 87 essential hypertensives aged between 28 to 65 years old, who had previous been untreated or the hypertensive therapy was withdrawn for 4 weeks. In a randomized trial 42 patients received 2,5 mg Torasemide and 45 patients 5 mg Torasemide once daily. In all patients diastolic blood pressure was more than 100 mm Hg before treatment. The trial was performed over a period of 6 months. In both groups doubling of the dosage was performed in those patients who had an insufficient blood pressure after 4 weeks (diastolic blood pressure more than 90 mm Hg). Blood pressure and intracellular natrium and calcium activities in red blood cells were performed with ionselective electrodes after washing the red blood cells in an isotonic solution containing choline hydrogen tartrate with 5 mmol/l NaCl. Then the cells were centrifuged, frozen to -18° C and thawed in order to disrupt the cell membranes. The measurements were thus performed in the hemolysate, containing not only the cytoplasm but also parts of the cell membrane. The results are given as ion activities in the following, referring to liter of free cell water.

RESULTS

Blood pressure measurements and the evaluation of the intracellular sodium and calcium were performed at the beginning of the trial and after 4, 12 and 24 weeks. Blood pressure normalisation (90 mm Hg) was observed after 4 weeks treatment in 21 of 42 patients receiving 2,5 mg Torasemide daily and in 26 of 45 patients with 5 mg Torasemide daily. Fig. 1 shows the results of the intracellular sodium (A) and calcium (B) measurements. There was a marked decrease of intracellular free calcium after 4 weeks treatment and a slight increase after 12 weeks which was nearly similar after 24 weeks. Intracellular sodium activity showed a tendence to increase after 4 weeks, which was significant only after 12 weeks and showed after 24 weeks a slow decrease.

DISCUSSION

The results show that treatment with 2,5 mg Torasemide daily and 5 mg Torasemide daily were equal effective. There was a decrease in intracellular free calcium together with a slight increase in intracellular free sodium. Blood pressure continued to decrease during the whole period of therapy. As to the mechanism by which intracellular calcium is essentially lowered, the possibilities should be considered. First there may be a direct effect on the membrane transport mechanism or the cellular calcium binding properties. Secondly, with regard to a possible humoral pathogenesis of hypertension, a suppressor of humoral factors may be the cause. In animal experiments it could be demonstrated that in the SHR hypovolemia suppresses humoral factors causing hypertension in a normotensive rat. This suggests that diuretics may also act by inducing a slight hypovolemia which in turn causes a suppression of a humoral factor. However, at present it is not certain whether this experimental analogy corresponds to the pathophysiological mechanisms in human hypertension. Possibly a suppression of humoral factors by hypovolemia is only one component in the blood pressure lowering effect of diuretics. The results further show a discrepancy between the changes in intracellular natrium and calcium activity during treatment with Torasemide. Increase in intracellular free natrium may be explained by an inhibition of natrium-kalium-cotransport which has mainly been described as an effect of Furosemide. Similar results on the diuretic induced changes of intracellular sodium have been described by Walter and Distler (3).

In summary the study demonstrates that the decrease in blood pressure during antihypertensive treatment with the diuretic Torasemide is associated with a decrease in intracellular free calcium in red blood cells. Intracellular free natrium however does not seem to be directly linked to the changes in vascular tone. The study further supports the hypothesis that intracellular free calcium is an important regulator of vascular tone in essential hypertension.

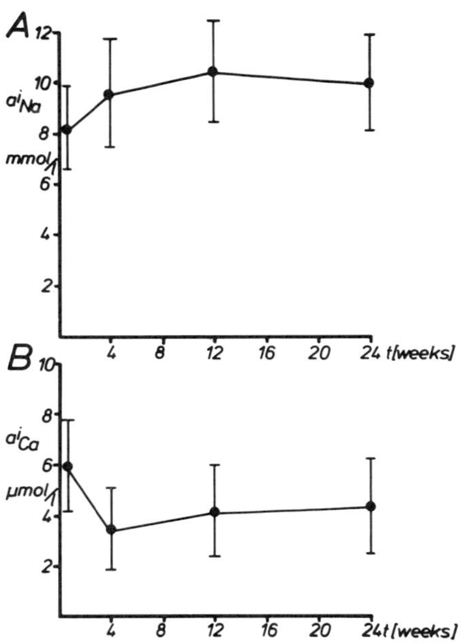

Fig. 1

REFERENCES

1. Reis, E.D. How diuretic lower blood pressure. Am. Heart J. 1983, 106 : 185
2. Zidek, W., Kerenyi, T., Losse, H. and Vetter, H. Intracellular Na^+ and Ca^{++} in aortic smooth muscle cells after enzymatic isolation in spontaneously hypertensive rats. Res. Exp. Med. 1983, 183: 129-132
3. Walter, U., Distler, A. Effects of ouabain and furosemide on ATP-ase activity and sodium transport in erythrocytes of normotensives and of patients with essential hypertension. In: Intracellular Electrolytes and Arterial Hypertension. Zumkley, H, Losse, H., Stuttgart, Thieme, 1980

THE ISOLATED PERFUSED RAT KIDNEY AS A MODEL FOR THE STUDY OF DIURETICS IN HYPERTENSION

P. Salvati, R.G. Ferrario and G. Bianchi

Farmitalia Carlo Erba Centro Ricerche, Nerviano (Milano) and Istituto di Scienze Mediche dell'Università degli Studi di Milano, Milano (Italy)

INTRODUCTION

Many abnormalities in cell membrane ion transport mechanisms had been found in hypertension. Amongst them the ouabain-resistant, bumetanide-sensitive Na^+-K^+cotransport reported to be either slower or faster in different subgroups of essential hypertensives (1). In genetically hypertensive rats also, Na^+-K^+ cotransport had been found to be either decreased, -SHR rats-, or increased, -MHS rats- (2,3). Possibly loop diuretics, which selectively inhibit Na^+-K^+ cotransport, could have a more pronounced effect in both hypertensive rats and humans with elevated Na^+-K^+ cotransport. To test this hypothesis in rats, the activity of bumetanide (B) was studied in comparison to amiloride (A) and hydrochlorothiazide (H) in MHS isolated perfused kidneys.

METHODS

The study was carried out in 26 MHS rats, 75-85 g body weight, before the development of hypertension and in 25 matched normotensive controls (MNS). The isolated kidney was perfused according to the technique of Epstein F.H. (4) slightly modified by us (5), using 6.7% bovine albumin (fraction V) in Krebs Henseleit saline as recirculating medium. After 30 min of equilibration, 3 five min control samples of urine and perfusate were taken, followed by 3 five min clearance periods for each cumulative concentration of respectively B, A and H (tenfold increases from 10^{-8} to 10^{-4}M). Cr^{3+}EDTA clearance was used to estimate GFR; urine volume (UV), urinary Na^+ (UNa^+) and urinary K^+ (UK^+) excretions were evaluated as previously described (5).

RESULTS

% Tubular Na^+ reabsorption (% TNa^+reabs) of control kidneys exceeded 99% of the filtered load and remained stable over a period of 90 min, as well as UV and UNa^+. Only a moderate decline of GFR was observed after 1 hour of perfusion. On the other hand kidneys perfused under our conditions did not fail to acidify urine unlike reported by others (6) (FIG.1). In table 1 in vitro kidney function is compared with in vivo values of age matched conscious rats.

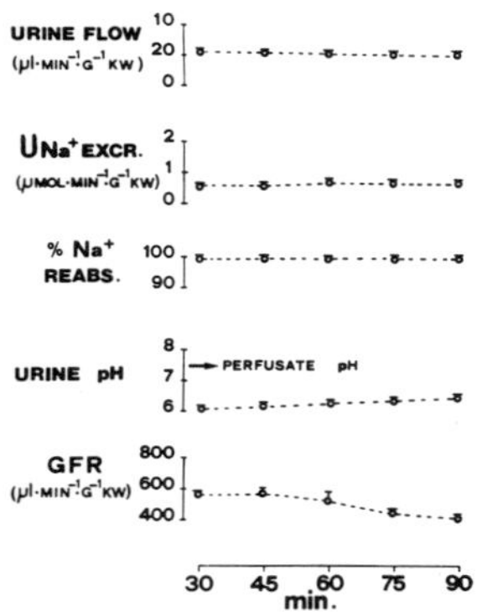

FIG. 1- Functional stability of isolated control kidneys (MNS rats) perfused with Krebs-Henseleit saline containing 6.7 g/dl fraction V bovine albumin. Values are means ± SEM of 8 experiments.

TABLE 1-MNS kidney function in vitro (n= 8) and in vivo (n= 12).

	Isolated kidney[a)]	Intact rats
UV[(b)]	11.1±0.9	6.6±0.5
% TNa^+reabs.	99.3±0.1	99.8±0.01
GFR[(b)]	571.6±61.9	1337±60
U/P ratio	50.2±2.9	200-250
Urine pH	5.9±0.1	5-6

a) 1st hour of perfusion

b) $\mu l.min^{-1}.g^{-1}$ kidney wt

TABLE 2 shows results on the highest concentration (10^{-4}M) for each diuretic. % TNa^+ reabs. significantly decreased for all agents in both strains: statistically significant differences were not found amongst A, B and H in MNS, whereas B had a stronger effect in MHS as compared to both A and H. The K^+-sparing diuretic A increased the Na^+/K^+ ratio in both strains, its effects being stronger in MHS. In MHS also B increased the Na^+/K^+ ratio, due to its selectively more pronounced activity on UNa^+. Urine pH was increased only by A and H to the same degree in both strains, as expected from their mechanism of action.

TABLE 2- Effects of diuretics (10^{-4}M) on kidney function. Means$\pm$SEM of the last two clearance periods are reported (6 rats each group).

	% TNa^+Reabs.		Na^+/K^+		Urine pH	
	MNS	MHS	MNS	MHS	MNS	MHS
Controls[a)]	99$\pm$0.1	97$\pm$0.2	2.2$\pm$0.4	3.2$\pm$0.3	6.4$\pm$0.1	6.7$\pm$0.1
B	94$\pm$0.8**	75$\pm$1.9**	3.0$\pm$0.4	6.6$\pm$0.3**	6.6$\pm$0.1	6.9$\pm$0.1
A	97$\pm$0.7*	91$\pm$0.4*	27$\pm$1.9*	64$\pm$4.7**	7.2$\pm$0.1**	7.7$\pm$0.1**
H	97$\pm$0.4*	94$\pm$0.6*	1.6$\pm$0.1	2.4$\pm$2.3	7.4$\pm$0.2**	7.8$\pm$0.1**

*$p<0.05$ **$p<0.01$ from the corresponding controls by Dunnett's test.
a) at the same perfusion time (75 min).

CONCLUSIONS

The major limitation of using cell-free isolated perfused kidney preparations are time dependent changes. However under our experimental conditions the ion transport characteristics remained stable over the experimental time, closely approaching the *in vivo* values. Our preparation also proved to be a suitable model for studying the mechanism of action of diuretics, as renal function changes induced by B, A and H were consistent with their known tubular activity in humans. MHS rats, characterized by a faster Na^+-K^+ cotransport (3), showed a selectively higher natriuretic response to the loop diuretic bumetanide. Our results suggest that also the subgroup of hypertensive patients with a faster erythrocyte Na^+-K^+cotransport might show an enhanced sensitivity to bumetanide.

REFERENCES

1. D.C. Tosteson et al. : Clin. Sci. 62:5s, 1981
2. M. De Mendoca et al. : Kidney Intern. 21 suppl.11: S-69, 1982
3. G. Bianchi et al.: Hypertension 7: 319, 1985
4. F.H. Epstein et al.: Am. J. Physiol. 243:F284, 1982
5. P. Salvati et al.: J. of Hypertension 2 suppl. 3: 351, 1984
6. B.D. Ross : Clin. Sci. Mol. Med. 55: 513, 1978

ANTIHYPERTENSIVE MECHANISMS OF MUZOLIMINE

D. RUSSO, E. COFELICE, G. CONTE, A. GIUNTA°, S. MAIONE°, G. ROMANO, M. SABBATINI, A. TESTA, P. VENIERO, A. DAL CANTON, V.E. ANDREUCCI.
Departement of Nephrology and Internal Medicine°, 2nd Faculty, Naples.

INTRODUCTION

This study was performed to investigate both the antihypertensive mechanism(s) and the efficacy of Muzolimine, a loop diuretic with no structural similarity to other loop diuretics.

METHODS

The study was carried out in 13 outpatients with mild to moderate hypertension and normal renal function. After a 2-week washout period, baseline Blood Pressure (BP), Body Weight (BW), Plasma Volume (PV), Plasma Renin Activity (PRA) and Serum Aldosterone (A) both in the supine and standing position, Total Peripheral Resistances (TPR), 24-hr urinary volume (V), Na^+ and K^+ excretion ($U_{Na}V$, U_KV) were recorded. Muzolimine was then administered at the daily dose of 30 mg, given at 8.00 a.m.. Measurements were repeated after 2, 4, 8, 12, 16 weeks of treatment. Salt intake was free throughout the study. PV was measured by Evans' blue method, PRA and A by radioimmunoassay, Sodium and Potassium by flame photometry, TPR were calculated from systemic Blood Pressure and Cardiac Output indirectly measured by echocardiography.
Results were expressed as Mean $\pm$ SE. Student's "t" test was used for statistical analysis.

RESULTS

The effects of Muzolimine on BP, BW, PV, TPR are reported in Table 1. Both Systolic and Diastolic Blood Pressure (SBP and DBP) was reduced significantly after 2 weeks of treatment. The antihypertensive efficacy of

Muzolimine was persistent throughout the study. BW and PV were significantly reduced after 2 weeks of treatment, but returned to basaline values. TPR were steadly and significantly reduced after week 2. The effects of Muzolimine on PRA, A, $U_{Na}V$, U_KV, and V are summarized in Table 2. PRA, A, V, $U_{Na}V$, and U_KV rose significantly at week 2 and 4 of treatment.

Table 1. Effects of Muzolimine in 13 patients. Numbers are Means and (SE).

Weeks	0	2	4	8	12	16
SBP	160.2	136.3°°	138.2°°	137.1°°	134.3°°	139.2°°
(mmHg)	(3.2)	(3.0)	(2.3)	(2.3)	(2.0)	(2.4)
DBP	105.5	89.2°°	89.2°°	89.6°°	89.6°°	88.4°°
(mmHg)	(1.6)	(2.9)	(5.0)	(2.0)	(1.8)	(1.9)
BW	66.9	66.5°	66.6	66.8	67.2	67.0
(Kg)	(2.8)	(2.8)	(2.8)	(2.7)	(2.8)	(2.9)
PV	2499	2226°	2400	2590	2582	2450
(ml)	(148)	(131)	(122)	(103)	(116)	(119)
TPR	2107	2140	1768°	1694°°	1690°°	1639°°
(Dyne/sec/cm^{-5})	(41.6)	(38.8)	(47.1)	(45.1)	(47.9)	(39.7)

Table 2. Effects of Muzolimine in 13 patients. Numbers are Means and (SE).

Weeks	0	2	4	8	12	16
PRA Standing	2.4	5.4°°	4.5°°	2.0	1.3	1.6
(ng/ml/hr)	(0.5)	(1.7)	(1.7)	(0.3)	(0.4)	(0.3)
PRA Supine	1.1	3.7°°	1.9°°	0.9	1.0	0.9
	(0.2)	(1.2)	(0.3)	(0.2)	(0.1)	(0.2)
A Standing	139	201°°	173°°	141	146	153
(pg/ml)	(11)	(18)	(14)	(13)	(11)	(13)
A Supine	126	156°°	145°°	124	130	130
	(17)	(16)	(12)	(16)	(15)	(18)
$U_{Na}V$	193	240°°	232°°	178	200	198
	(12)	(13)	(17)	(11)	(15)	(12)
U_KV	64	78°°	74°°	64	70	65
	(6)	(5)	(3)	(5)	(6)	(6)
V	1400	1703°°	1625°°	1542	1576	1580
(ml/24hr)	(110)	(67)	(143)	(123)	(119)	(109)

° $p < 0.05$ °° $p < 0.025$

DISCUSSION

This study shows that Muzolimine is a well effective treatment of mild to moderate essential hypertension. The antihypertensive effect of Muzolimine can be secondary to ECF volume depletion for a transient time (2 to 4 weeks), as suggested by both the reduction in PV, BW, and the rise in TPR, PRA, A, V, and $U_{Na}V$. After 4 weeks, however, ECF volume reverts to basaline, as shown by normalisation of PV, BW, and hormones. Thus, other mechanism should account for the steady antihypertensive effect of Muzolimine. Our results suggest that a reduction in TPR is the long term antihypertensive mechanism of Muzolimine. This is in keeping with studies showing a vasodilating action of Muzolimine (1 - 2). The reduction in TPR can be secondary to depletion of sodium and water in the vessel wall, with improved lumen/wall ratio (3), and a reduced reactivity to vasopressor substances. Recent reports of the ability of the loop diuretics to increase urinary excretion of Prostaglandin E (4) suggest a PGE-mediated vasodilating effect of Muzolimine.

REFERENCES

1. Rovelli, E.G., Carnovali, M. In: Recent Advances in diuretic therapy (Ed. Andreucci V.E.), Excerpta Medica, 1983, pp. 112-115.
2. Rossi, F., Lampa, E. In: Proceedings of the International Congress of Pharmacology. (Ed. International Society of Pharmacology), Paris 1978, pp. 631.
3. Reinech, J.H., Stein, J.H. In: The Kidney (Ed. Brenner BM, Rector FC), Saunders Company, 1981, pp. 1097-1131.
4. Katayama, S., Atallah, A.A. and Lee, J.B. Am. J. Physiol. 247:555-561, 1984.

INDAPAMIDE: ANTIHYPERTENSIVE ACTIVITY AND RENAL EFFECTS

G. TRAMONTI, C. DONADIO, M. BONADIO, P. LORUSSO, C. BIANCHI

Cattedra di Nefrologia Medica, Centro Nefrologico, Clinica Medica 2,

University of Pisa, Pisa, Italy

INTRODUCTION

Indapamide is a sulphonamide derivative with definite antihypertensive activity. The aim of this study is the evaluation of the antihypertensive efficacy and the effect on renal function of Indapamide in hypertensive patients with different degrees of renal function.

MATERIAL AND METHODS

Twenty four adult patients, 2 male and 22 female, were studied. Their main clinical data were as follows:

- age 29-64 years, mean 46.2
- systolic BP 144-208 mmHg, mean 169
- diastolic BP 87-125 mmHg, mean 104
- plasma creatinine 0.4-1.7 mg/dl, mean 0.82

Indapamide* was administered in the morning at a daily dose of 2.5 mg. In 10 patients this dosage was doubled to 5 mg starting at the 8th day of treatment. The length of treatment was 2 weeks. Supine and standing BP were measured 6 times on different days of the pre-treatment period (one week). Urine output, creatinine cl and potassium cl were determined twice and glomerular filtration rate (GFR) and effective renal plasma flow (ERPF) once in the pre-treatment period. Blood pressure, urine output and potassium cl were also checked on the 3rd, 7th and 13th days of therapy, while creatinine cl was checked on the 7th and 13th and GFR and ERPF on the 13th only. The

---

*Ipamix, Gentili S.p.A., Pisa, Italy

measurement of GFR and ERPF was carried out by the noninvasive bladder cumulative method (1).

RESULTS

The results are reported in the following table.

	number of cases	days of treatment 0	3	7	13
SUPINE BP	24				
SYSTOLIC		169±3.3	157±4.5*	153±3.6*	151±3.6*
DIASTOLIC		104±1.7	101±2.3	98±2.2*	96±2.3*
mmHg					
STANDING BP	24				
SYSTOLIC		166±3.9	151±3.6*	147±3.3*	148±3.6*
DIASTOLIC		111±1.8	109±2.1	106±2.1*	104±2.1*
URINE OUTPUT l/day	15	1.12±0.07	1.29±0.10	1.18±0.07	1.24±0.08
CREATININE Cl ml/min	18	96.6±9.3		100.4±9.6	92.6±10.0
G F R ml/min	7	72.4±10.1			70.4±7.2
E R P F ml/min	6	286.6±28.8			276.4±27.6
POTASSIUM Cl ml/min	15	7.6±0.8	14.5±1.3*	11.3±1.1*	10.5±1.1*
PLASMA POTASSIUM mEq/l	17	4.2±0.1	3.6±0.1*	3.7±0.1*	3.5±0.2*

mean ± SEM * $p < 0.005$

DISCUSSION

In this group of patients with mild to moderate hypertension Indapamide was effective in lowering systolic and diastolic BP. This effect was evident in both supine and standing positions, without causing orthostatic hypotension.

In approximately half of the patients studied diastolic BP in the supine position decreased during treatment to less than 95 mmHg (responders). In the remaining patients the antihypertensive efficacy of Indapamide was poor (non responders).

Systolic and diastolic pressures were significantly reduced starting from the 3rd and from the 7th days of treatment respectively and showed a continuous decrease in the short period of our study (two weeks). This behaviour suggests that a more prolonged period could normalize BP in a higher number of patients.

The antihypertensive efficacy of Indapamide did not seem to be influenced by the renal function of the patients. In fact creatinine cl was lower than 80 ml/min in 4 out of 12 responders and in 3 out of 12 non responders. On the other hand Indapamide did not influence renal function since creatinine cl, GFR and ERPF were remarkably stable during treatment.

The diuretic effect of Indapamide was generally moderate. It was higher in the responders (mean increase of urine output 53% of the basal value) than in the non responders (43%).

Finally, an important decrease of plasma potassium during therapy with Indapamide was observed. This was due to a marked increase of renal cl of potassium. In 6 patients a supplement of potassium was necessary. No difference between responders and non responders was observed with regard to this hypokalaemic effect.

In conclusion, our results, which are in agreement with those previously reported in a comprehensive review (2), indicate that Indapamide is an antihypertensive drug which does not influence renal function. Hypokalaemia represents a clinically important side effect of Indapamide. For this, periodic determination of serum electrolytes should be performed at appropriate intervals.

REFERENCES

1. Bianchi, C., Donadio, C. and Tramonti, G. Nephron 28 : 53-57, 1981.
2. Chaffman, M., Heel, R.C., Brogden, R.N., Speight, T.M. and Avery, G.S. Drugs 28 : 189-235, 1984.

IN VITRO EFFECTS OF FUROSEMIDE ON RABBIT BLOOD VESSELS

F. ANDREASEN & J.H. CHRISTENSEN

Institute of Pharmacology, University of Aarhus
DK-8000 Aarhus C - Denmark

INTRODUCTION

A search in the litterature does not allow any firm conclusions concerning a possible furosemide effect on vascular smooth muscle in arteries and veins and in different regions. On the one hand there is clinical evidence indicating a relaxing effect on the large central veins (1), and a concentration dependent effect on the rat portal vein has been demonstrated in vitro (2). On the other hand the immediate measurable effect on the arterial side has been an increase in peripheral vascular resistance (3), and an increase in the mean blood pressure (4). A relaxing in vitro effect on arteries has only been demonstrated in concentrations above 300 µg/ml (5).

There are two purposes with the present paper: 1) To quantitate the effect of furosemide on vascular muscle at a therapeutic level. We chose a comparison between furosemide 20 µg /ml and nitroglycerin 0.5 µg/ml. 2) To study the effect of the two drugs also in Krebs-Henseleit-solutions with 45 g serum albumin per liter and in heparinized blood plasma.

MATERIALS AND METHODS

We have tested several vessels from the rabbit including the caval veins, the femoral vein, and the lateral ear vein. In these preliminary experiments none of them gave a contractile response sufficient for the study of drugs which may or may not have the ability to relax smooth muscle. In the present paper we report results obtained from experiments with the central ear artery and the portal vein of the rabbit.

We have constructed an apparatus (6) which allows the study of smooth muscle reactivity in a 5-6 ml volume tissue bath where pH and pO_2 can be kept at the desired level also if the organ bath is a protein solution or blood plasma.

Nerve specific electrical field stimulation was obtained from a Grass stimulator in connection with a constant current unit. The frequency was 10 HZ, the pulse duration 0.5 msec, the train duration 10 sec, and the interval between the trains was 10 min.

Table 1.

Furosemide effect on rings of rabbit ear artery
n=16, Mean ± SD. Initial tension adjusted to 1 g.

RESTING TENSION (reduction in g)		EL-CONTRACTIONS	
Furosemide 20 µg/ml	Nitroglycerin 0.5 µg/ml	Furosemide 20 µg/ml	Nitroglycerin 0.5 µg/ml
- 0.03 ± 0.03 *	- 0.08 ± 0.05* *	1.31→1.05 ± 0.61 ± 0.63 *	1.23→0.73 ± 0.62 ± 0.43* *

(* $p<0.01$)

The results of experiments with rings of the rabbit ear artery are shown in Table 1. Significant drug responses on el-stimulation as well on resting tension were achieved by furosemide as well as by nitroglycerin at the concentration levels studied. The percentage responses ranged from a few percent to 40 % and the responses were always more pronounced for nitroglycerin. Rather similar and statistically significant responses were found for rings of the rabbit portal vein.

The effect of furosemide and nitroglycerin on the response to adrenaline and noradrenaline was carried out on rings from the rabbit ear artery and portal vein. No effect on maximal answer was seen and no significant effect on the EC_{50} ranges was observed.

Table 2 shows the effect of substituting the tissue bath fluid with Alb K-H or heparinized human donor plasma. It is obvious that the addition of albumin accentuates the differences in response between furosemide and nitroglycerin and the same tendency is found in plasma. The relatively high plasma binding of furosemide (98,6 % (7)) may offer the whole or a partial explanation for that finding.

Table 2.

Influence of albumin (45 g HSA/l) and plasma. Rabbit ear artery - Average percentage reductions. (n=11-16).

	Initial resting tension/g	Furosemide 20 µg/ml	Nitroglycerin 0.5 µg/ml	F/N
	RESTING TENSION			
K-H	1.0	3	8	0.38
Alb K-H	1.0	0	9	0
Plasma	2.6	2	18	0.11
	EL-CONTRACTIONS			$p<0.01$
K-H	1.0	20	40	0.50
Alb K-H	1.0	7	45	0.18
Plasma	2.6	10 (NS)	27	-
				$p<0.01$

REFERENCES

1. Dikshit, K, Vyden, J.K, Forrester, J.S, Chatterjee, K, Prakash, R, Swan, H.J.C. N Engl J Med. 289: 1087-1090, 1974.
2. Biamino, G, Wessel, H.J, Nöring, J, Schröder, R. Int J Clin Pharmacol. 12: 356-368, 1975.
3. Franchi, F, Malfanti, P.L, Scardi, A, Pedenovi, P, Bisci, G, Barletta, G.A, Fabbri, G. Cardiology 71: 331-340, 1984.
4. Andreasen, F, Hansen, U, Husted, S.E, Mogensen, C.E, Pedersen, E.B. Br J Clin Pharmac. 18: 65-74, 1984.
5. Kreye, V.A.W, Bauer, P.K, Villhauer, I. Eur J Pharmacol. 73: 91-95, 1981.
6. Andreasen, F, Christensen, J.H, Poulsen, B. J Pharm Methods. In press.
7. Andreasen, F, Hansen, U, Husted, S.E, Jansen, J.A. Br J clin Pharmacol. 16: 391-397, 1983.

COMPARISON OF TORASEMIDE AND INDAPAMIDE IN THE TREATMENT OF ESSENTIAL HYPERTENSION

N. SPANNBRUCKER, I. ACHHAMMER, W. HÄCKER
Med. Univ. Klinik, Bonn and Boeringer Mannheim GmbH, FRG

INTRODUCTION

In view of increasing evidence, that in treatment of essential hypertension even a small dosage of diuretics is effective and successful the present trial was designed to compare the efficacy of a low dose regimen of torasemide (TO) with Indapamide (IN).

METHODS

In a controlled, double-blind multicentre trial over 12 weeks either 2.5 mg TO or 2.5 mg IN were given to 66 patients with essential hypertension. Inclusion criteria were diastolic blood pressure (DBP) between 100 mm Hg and 115 mm Hg, no antihypertensive treatment within 4 weeks before start of the trial and a supposed response to diuretic therapy. Exclusion criteria were DBP below 100 mm Hg and above 115 mm Hg as well as systolic blood pressure (SBP) above 220 mm Hg.

At start of the study (A 1) the patients were randomly assigned to take either 2.5 mg TO or 2.5 mg IN, and the basal clinical investigations and labaratory tests were performed. Patients came back to the investigators office after 1 week (A 2), 2 weeks (A 3) and 4 weeks (A 4) for control investigations. In addition, at A 4 in all patients with DBP higher than 100 mm Hg the dosage of TO or IN could be doubled. Further control investigations were performed after 5 weeks (A 5), 8 weeks (A 6) and at the end of the trial after 12 weeks (A 7).

Blood pressure (BP), body weight (BW) and pulse rate (PR) were controlled during each appointment (A 1 - A 7). At A 1, A 4, A 6 and A 7 blood was withdrawn for determination of serum sodium, potassium, calcium, cloride, magnesium, creatinine, uric acid and glucose. In addition, at A 1 and A 7 control of SGOT, SGPT, yGT as well as haemoglobin, leukocytes and platelets was performed. Urine was collected for 24 hours at A 1, A 4 and A 7 for the determination of excreted volume, sodium, potassium, creatinine and proteine.

RESULTS

66 patients compleated the entire 12 week trial: 39 male and 17 female. 32 patients received TO (group 1) and 34 patients received IN (group 2) as antihypertensive agent. Both groups showed no signifcant differences in BW, age and sex distribution. Because of the possibility of dose adjustment 4 weeks after start of the trial 4 subgroups were formed, retrospectively. In group 1 23 patients received 2.5 mg TO during the entire study (subgroup 1.1), whereas in 9 patients the dose of TO was doubled to 5 mg after 4 weeks (subgroup 1.2). At the end of the study in 7 of these patients the mean DBP was equal or below 90 mm Hg. 2 patients in this subgroup 1.2 did not respond to therapy. In group 2 24 patients received 2.5 mg IN during the entire trial (subgroup 2.1). 10 patients were switched to 5 mg IN at A 4 (subgroup 2.2). In this subgroup 6 patients were responder to the therapy. In the other 4 patients mean DBP was equal or above 95 mm Hg at the end of the study.

In the main groups 1.1 and 2.1 mean DBP at entry was 106.5 mm Hg and 105.6 mm Hg, respectively. From A 1 to A 7 mean DBP dropped significantly to 84.1 mm Hg in subgroup 1.1 and to 81.9 mm Hg in subgroup 2.1 without significant differences between these groups. In patients receiving 2.5 mg TO ther was still a significant reduction in mean DBP from 91.1 mm Hg at A 4 to 84.1 mm Hg at A 7. In contrast, in subgroup 2.1 change of mean DBP from 86.7 at A 4 to 81.9 mm Hg at A 7 was not significant.Between the 2 subgroups 1.1 and 2.1 ther was a pronounced but not significant difference in mean DBP at A 1, A 3 and A 4.

Mean SBP fell significantly from 167.2 mm Hg at A 1 to 146.0 at A 4 and 137.6 mm Hg at A 7 in subgroup 1.1. In subgroup 2.1 mean SBP dropped from 158.4 mm Hg at A 1 to 141.0 at A 4 and to 136.0 mm Hg at A 7. Between both groups there was a significant difference at A 1, whereas there were no significant differences from A 2 to A 7.

Mean BW in the patients receiving 2.5 mg TO (subgroup 1.1) decreased significantly from 78.3 kg at A 1 to 76.4 kg at A 4. The further change to 76.4 kg reached no significance to A 4, whereas it was significant different to the BW at A 1. In subgroup 2.1 mean BW decreased significantly from 72.8 kg at A 1 to 70.8 kg at A 4. At the end of the study a further but not significant decrease in mean BW to 68.1 kg was observed. Between the 2 groups 1.1 and 2.1 there was a marked but not significant difference in mean BW from A 1 to A 7.

In the time course of serum concentrations for sodium, potassium, calcium, cloride, uric acid and creatinine significant changes were obtained only for potassium. In subgroup 1.1 mean serum concentration of potassium decreased significantly from 4.5 mmol/l at A 1 to 4.1 mmol/l at A 4. The further change to 4.3 mmol/l reached no significance to A 1. In subgroup 2.1 serum potassium decreased significantly from 4.5 mmol/l at A 1 to 4.1 mmol/l at A 4. In contrast to subgroup 1.1 the further change of potassium to 4.0 mmol/l at A 7 was statistical significant.

None of the patients had notable changes in the clinical status oe symptoms during the 12 week trial.

CONCLUSIONS

The results demonstrate a comparable efficacy of 2.5 mg TO and 2.5 mg IN in the treatment of essential hypertension. The responder-rates as well as average decrease and time course of lowering systolic and diastolic blood pressure were similar for both drugs. No adverse reations were reported in both groups. In contrast to indapamide, torasemide did not relevantly influence laboratory parameters during the entire trial.

MODIFICATIONS IN CARDIOVASCULAR NOREPINEPHRINE RESPONSIVENESS BY DIURETIC TREATMENT IN MILD RENAL PARENCHYMAL DISEASE

H. SCHIFFL

Medizinische Klinik Innenstadt der Universität München, 8000 München 2, West Germany

Introduction.

The mechanisms by which diuretics cause vasodilation in hypertension associated with early renal disease are still not completely understood. Reduction of the expanded extracellular fluid volume and removal of accumulated sodium are undoubtedly vital elements in their therapeutic profile (1,2). Nevertheless, the dissociation between the natriuretic and hypotensive efficacy of a thiazide diuretic in patients with severe renal failure points to additional extrarenal factors (3). Moreover, the diuretic-aggravated release of renin can be expected to oppose the blood pressure lowering effects of these agents.

In patients with early stage parenchymal kidney disease and mild renal failure, pressor responsiveness to norepinephrine (NE) tends to be enhanced despite the presence of normal or slightly increased plasma NE levels. This disturbance could possible predispose or contribute to the development of renal hypertension, because it is even noted in patients with normal blood pressure (4,5). To gain information on the mechanisms of the interaction between diuretics and the sympathetic axis, we assessed the body sodium-blood volume state, the renin-aldosterone system, the catecholamines and the responsiveness to NE and angiotensin II before and after 6 weeks muzolimine monotherapy or combination treatment with muzolimine and nifedipine in normals and renal patient.

Subjects and Methods.

27 patients with hypertension of chronic renal disease and 27 sex- and age-matched normal subjects were studied. The patients included 8 females and 19 males (mean = 41 $\pm$ 7 (SD) years. The diagnosis was chronic glomerulonephritis in 20 patients, nephroangiosclerosis in 4 patients, and chronic pyelonephritis in 3 patients. Blood pressure was in all patients consistently over 140/90 mm Hg under outpatient condition, they were clinically stable and did not show evidence of congestive heart failure, of cardiac arrhythmia or of edema. The patients were instructed to adhere to their usual diet, but not to add salt to their food.

Patients were treated with placebo for 4 weeks. Thereafter, they received either muzolimine (mean dose 25 $\pm$ 8 ($\pm$ SD) mg/day) or muzolimine (mean dose 24 $\pm$ 8 ($\pm$ SD) mg/day) and nifedipine, 20 mg t.i.d., for 6 weeks. Studies were performed at the end of the placebo phases and the treatment periods. Body weight, blood pressure (using a standard cuff and syphygmomanometer or an automatic blood pressure recorder), plasma sodium, potassium (flame photometry), creatinine, calcium (autoanalyzer), and haematocrit, plasma volume (isotope dilution technique using 125 I-human serum albumin), plasma renin activity, aldosterone (radioimmunoassay), and plasma catecholamines (radioenzymatic method) were measured after the completion of a 24 hour urine collection for sodium, potassium, calcium and norepinephrine excretion rates and exchangeable sodium (by isotope dilution technique using 24 Na). The pressor responsiveness to intravenously infused NE or angiotensin II was tested in supine position. From the dose-response curve, two parameters were derived, namely, a) the threshold dose of NE or angiotensin II, i.e. the extrapolated dose causing a zero change in blood pressure, and b) the pressor dose, i.e. the dose of pressor agents necessary to elevate the mean (NE) or diastolic (angiotensin II) blood pressure by 20 mm Hg (2,5).

Statistical methods included the paired and unpaired, two-tailed non parametric Wilcoxon signed-rank tests.

RESULTS

FINDINGS BEFORE DIURETIC-BASED TREATMENT

Under basal conditions, carefully matched normal subjects and patients with hypertension (166/110 $\pm$ 12/7 mm Hg) and mild renal failure (GFR 48.6 $\pm$ 6.1 ml/min 1.73 m^2) had no differences in mean heart rate, body weight, haematocrit, blood volume, plasma sodium, potassium, calcium, NE, PRA and angiotensin II pressor dose, urinary sodium, potassium, calcium and NE excretion rates. Exchangeable body sodium and plasma aldosterone tended to be higher ($P < 0.001$), and NE threshold and pressor dose were significantly ($P < 0.001$) lower in the patients than in the normal subjects.

FINDINGS AFTER 6 WEEKS OF MUZOLIMINE MONOTHERAPY OR COMBINATION TREATMENT WITH MUZOLIMINE AND NIFEDIPINE

Compared to placebo conditions, muzolimine significantly lowered the supine and upright blood pressure ($P < 0.001$). Muzolimine also reduced body sodium ($P < 0.001$), body weight ($P < 0.001$) and plasma potassium ($P < 0.001$), and tended to increase plasma creatinine, renin and aldosterone levels, as well as urinary calcium excretion ($P < 0.001$). The cardiovascular responsiveness to NE, as indicated by significant increases in the NE threshold and pressor dose ($P < 0.001$), was reduced by the diuretic. Muzolimine treatment was associated with a slight increase in the AII pressor dose. The other parameters were not consistently altered by the diuretic.

Combination therapy with muzolimine and nifedipine caused a more pronounced decrease in blood pressure than muzolimine monotherapy. NE threshold and pressor doses under treatment no longer differed from the corresponding values in untreated normal subjects. Body weight, heart rate, blood volume, exchangeable sodium, plasma creatinine and electrolytes, urinary electrolyte excretion rates, plasma and urinary NE levels were not consistently altered, but PRA and plasma aldosterone were significantly increase by combination treatment ($P < 0.001$).

DISCUSSION

Compared with 27 age- and sex-matched normal subjects, the major alterations, in our 27 patients with early renal disease and hypertension were an expansion of extracellular fluid volume and body sodium and an inappropriate NE pressor responsiveness despite the presence of normal plasma NE levels. The latter abnormality was characterised by lower NE threshold and pressor doses, but the slope of the NE dose-blood pressure response curve was comparable in all study subjects. The cardiovascular hyperresponsiveness to NE was unrelated to the age or sex of the patients, the status of renal function or to the etiology of the renal lesion, and could not be explained by altered kinetics of infused NE, by disturbed cardiac invervation or by diminished baroreceptor sensitivity.

The distinct hyperresponsiveness of the cardiovascular system to this vasoconstricting stimulus may be a primary, pressure-independent event, as this abnomality may be present in the prehypertensive phase of chronic renal disease, too. However, during the course of renal hypertension development, structural alterations may cause the arteries to hyperreact to NE. Whether and to what extent defects in sodium and/or calcium handling by the human vascular smooth muscle cell membranes may play a pathogenic role in chronic renal disease is presently unknown. Nevertheless, this hypothesis has received strong experimental support (6,7). The possibility, that a lack of depressor substances (8,9) could contribute to enhanced pressor reactivity is speculative, but deserves consideration. Correction of a true abnormality in noradrenergic blood pressure control mechanisms by addition of a calcium channel blocker led to normotension in our patients.

Six weeks of treatment with the loop diuretic muzolimine caused a 8 % decrease in blood pressure in our patients. Whatever the underlying cellular/and hormonal mechanisms are diuretics may decrease blood pressure in renoparenchymal disease by lowering an abnormally high cardiovasular NE pressor reactivity without causing an equivalent increase in noradrenergic nervous activity and by removal of excess body sodium. The marked renin stimulation with only limited decreases in A II pressor reactivity may contribute to an increased angiotensin II dependence of diuretic-treated hypertension, thus partly counteracting the antihypertensive potency of the diuretic agent.

REFERENCES

1) Wollam, G.K., Tarazi, R.C., Bravo, E.L., Dustan, H.P.: Am J Med 79, 929-938, 1982

2) Schiffl, H., Weidmann, P., Beretta-Piccoli, C., Cottier, C., Seiler, A.J., Ziegler W.H.: Eur J Clin Pharmacol 23, 215-220, 1982

3) Jones, B., Nanra, R.S.: Lancet 2, 1258-1260, 1979

4) Beretta-Piccoli, C., Weidmann, P., Schiffl, H., Cottier, C., Reubi, F.C.: Kidney Int 22, 297-303, 1982

5) Schiffl, H., Weidmann, P., Beretta-Piccoli, C., Cottier, C., Mordasini, R., Riesen, W., Ziegler, W.H.: Clin Nephrol 19 (Suppl 1), 101-108, 1983

6) Zimlichman, R.R., Chamovitz, C., Chaichenco, Y., Goligorsky, M., Rapaport, J., Kaplanski, J.: Clin Sci 67, 161-166, 1984

7) Huot, S.J., Pamnani, M.B., Clough, D.L., Buggy, J., Bryant, H.J., Harder, D.R., Haddy, F.J.: Hypertension 5 (Supp I) I-94 - I-100, 1983

8) Wilson, T.W.: Clin Pharmacol Ther 39, 94-101, 1986

9) O'Connor, D.T., Preston, R.A., Mitas, J.A., Frigon, R.P., Stone, R.A.: Hypertension 3, 139-147, 1981

MUZOLIMINE VERSUS CAPTOPRIL IN LOW AND MILD HYPERTENSION

V. CANONICO, G. MORGANO, M. PETRETTA, R. BREGLIO, G. CONFORTI, C. TEDESCHI, D. BONADUCE, M. CONDORELLI.
Institute of Internal Medicine, 2nd School of Medicine, Naples, Italy.

INTRODUCTION

Diuretics are widely used alone or in combination with other antihypertensive drugs in the treatment of hypertension. However, their value is somewhat reduced by side effects as hypokaliemia, hyperuricemia, increasing in cholesterol, triglycerides and glucose (1). Muzolimine (M) is a new loop diuretic with some peculiar structural and physiochemical properties compared with other diuretics (2). Preliminary reports have assessed that M possess a power diuretic action similar to that of furosemide togheter with antihypertensive activity (3). Recently some Authors have assessed in cross-over studies that the hypotensive effect of M is comparable to that of other thyazides (4). The aim of this study was to compare the hypotensive effect of M at low dosage with Captopril (C), a well known antihypertensive drug (5).

MATERIALS AND METHODS

Thirty patients (pts) with mean age of 52 years suffering from primary hypertension at 1st and 2nd degree by W.H.O. classification were enrolled. The pts after 30 days (15 for wash-out and 15 for placebo run-in) were randomized to M (20 mg/day) or C (100 mg/day) administration and followed the study design as shown in Fig. 1.

Fig. 1.

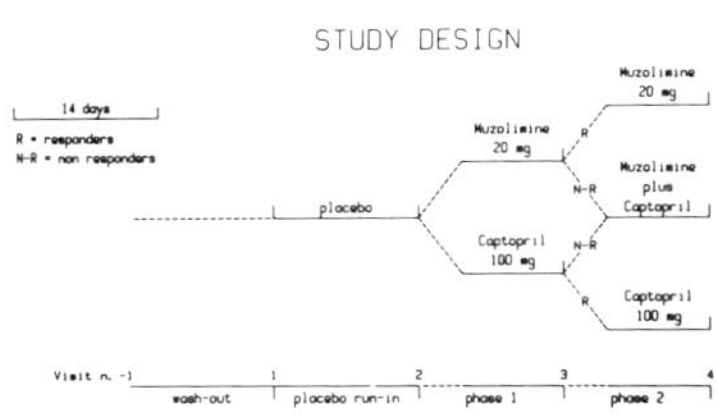

At 14th day the pts having diastolic blood pressure under 90 mmHg were considered like "responders" (R) and followed the same therapy for other 14 days; at the same time if antihypertensive therapy had failed to lower blood pressure adequately, the pts were considered like "non-responders" (NR) and continued for other 14 days with association of both drugs. At the end of wash-out and active treatment the following biochemical parameters were evaluated: glucose, urea, creatinine, uric-acid, sodium, potassium, total cholesterol, triglycerides, AST, ALT and blood cells count; furthermore, body weight and diuresis at every step of study design were controlled.

RESULTS

Results are reported in Fig. 2.

Fig. 2.

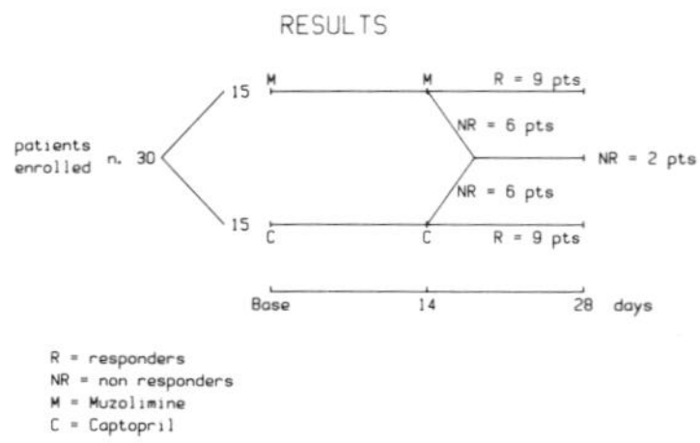

After the 1st phase there were 9 pts R in M and 9 pts R in C group, all of them continued the treatment, while there were 6 pts NR for M and 6 pts NR for C treatment that continued with association of both drugs. In Fig. 3

Fig. 3.

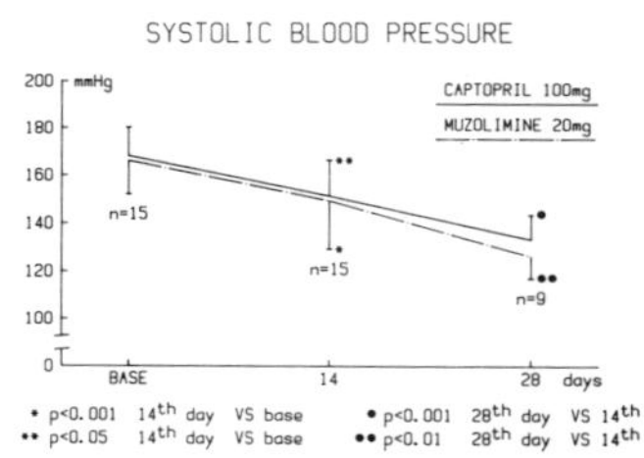

is shown systolic blood pressure prophile in dashed line for M and continuous line for C: a statistical significant reduction was observed. In Fig. 4

Fig. 4.

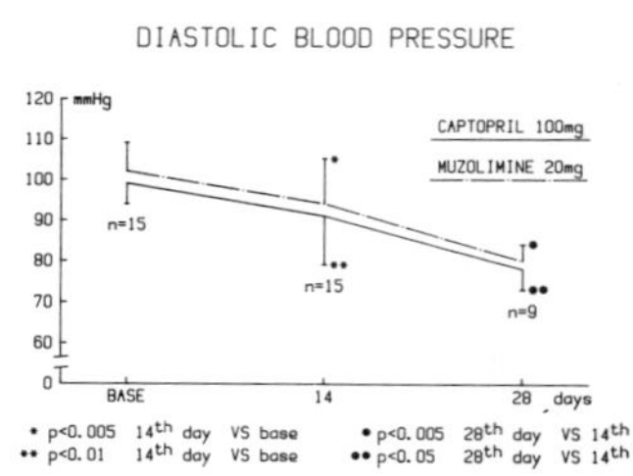

is shown the diastolic blood pressure prophile, in dashed line for M and continuous line for C: a significant reduction was observed at 14th and 28th day. In Fig. 5

Fig. 5.

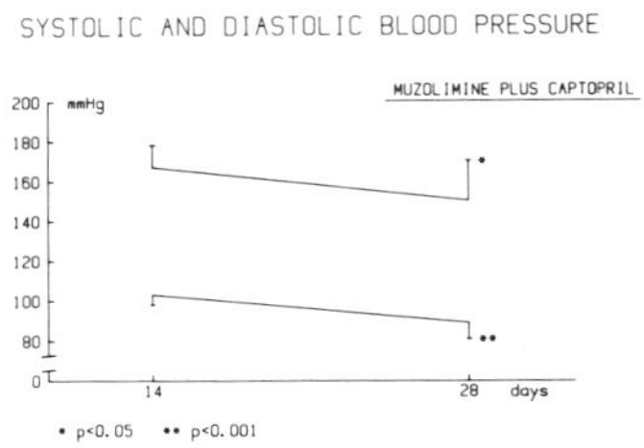

are reported the results of 12 pts NR that continued the trial with association C + M: the results at 28th day were compared with those at 14th day and resulted a significant reduction for diastolic and systolic blood pressure.
In M group the body weight was Kg 73 ± 10 at baseline, Kg 73 ± 10 after placebo run-in and Kg 72 ± 10 at 14th day of therapy ($p < 0.001$ vs baseline); in the 9 R pts the body weight at 28th day was Kg 71 ± 10 ($p < 0.001$ vs baseline). In the C group the body weight was Kg 70 ± 12 and Kg 70 ± 10 at beseline and at the end of placebo run-in respectively, while was Kg 69 ± 12 after 14 days of therapy ($p < 0.001$ vs baseline). In 12 NR pts the body weight at 28th day was Kg 67 ± 10 ($p < 0.001$ vs baseline). In 9 R pts of M group the diuresis at 28th day was 1766 ± 200 ml, while it was 1188 ± 196 ml at the end of run-in period ($p < 0.001$). In 9 R pts of C group the diuresis at 28th day was 1177 ± 204 ml, while it was 1100 ± 100 ml at the end of run-in period (p= ns). In 12 NR pts the diuresis at 28th day was 1508 ±144 ml, while it was 1116 ± 133 ml at the end of run-in period ($p < 0.001$).

DISCUSSION

Loop diuretics such as Furosemide are not currently used in the therapy of hypertension because of their short acting action which implies at least 2 or 3 daily doses (4). In our study M, 20 mg once day, showed antihypertensive efficacy like C, an ACE inhibitor, whose efficacy is well established. In particular our data show that M has a powerful antihypertensive effect on both systolic and diastolic blood pressure without side effects. Thus M can be widely used in first line therapy of mild and moderate hypertension.

REFERENCES

1. Pagano, G., Dal Molino, V. and Carta, Q. Z. Kardiol. 74 Suppl.2: 80-83, 1985.
2. Meng, K., Loew, D., Stoepel, K. and Hoffmeister, F. Curr. Med. Res. Opin. 4: 555-563, 1977.
3. Loew, D., Ritter, W. and Dycka, J. Eur. J. Clin. Pharm. 12: 341-344, 1977.
4. Ferrara, L.A., Strazzullo, P., Siciliani, A., Mančini, M. and Gagliardi R. Eur. J. Clin. Pharm. 28: 241-244, 1985.
5. Gavras, H., Brunner, H.R. and Turini, G.H. N. Engl. J. Med. 298: 991-998, 1978.

THE HYPOTENSIVE ACTION OF INDAPAMIDE

L.I.JUNCOS, J.C.CORNEJO, C.FERRER.
National University and Instituto Privado de Especialidades Médicas
Córdoba - Argentina.

Three main theories have been advanced to explain the antihypertensive action of diuretics. The first two are related to their sodium depleting effects; that is, blood pressure lowering results from a reduction in extracellular fluid volumen or in the water, sodium and calcium content of the arterioles. The third theory states that some diuretics maintain their chronic hypotensive action through a direct vasodilator effect. As far as thiazides are concerned, numerous studies have shown such action is dependant on a significant diuresis (1-2). It has been stated that Indapamide excerts its hypotensive action by means of a calcium blocking effect. (3) However, it has not been shown that a vasodilator effect "in vivo" is not dependant on sodium depletion.

PATIENTS AND METHODS

16 hypertensive patients were studied in two groups. The first of them included 8 patients with normal renal function (NRF)(serum creatinine of 1.4 mg/dl or less). All of them received no medication for 2 weeks prior to the study. Then, body weight (BW) sitting systolic (SBP) and diastolic blood pressure (DBP), serum sodium (S_{Na}), and serum potasium (S_K) were measured before and after receiving 5 mg of Indapamide twice a day for 3 days.

The second group included 8 chronic hemodialysis (CHD) patients (glomerular filtration rate less than 7 cc/min). During a 3 day control period (C), no dialysis was performed and placebo was given twice a day. The experimental (E) period took place seven days later but now Indapamide was given for 3 days in doses of 10 mg twice a day. BW, SBP, DBP, S_{Na}, and S_K were checked prior to and after each period. Urinary output (UO) was measured during the C and E periods. Medications other than vitamins and aluminum hidroxide were discontinued 14 days prior to the study.

In both NRF and CHD groups, BW, SBP, DBP, S_{Na} and S_K were analized by the one way analysis of variance. In the CHD group, the least significant difference was utilized to compare the data obtained at the begining and at the end of both the C and E periods, and also the differences between periods. UO was analized assuming a log-normal distribution.

RESULTS

The mean values obtained are shown in the table. Mean BW decreased 1.360 ± 0.55 Kg in the NRF group. This difference though was not statistically significant. The mean SBP decreased by 13.75 ± 8.40 mmHg ($p=<0.01$) and the mean DBP by 12.50 ± 7.07 mmHg ($p=<0.01$). There was statistically significant positive correllation between the falls in BW and in mean SBP on the one hand (r= 0.85) and BW and mean DBP on the other hand (r=0.94)

TABLE

Group	Weight (kg) B*. A#.	SBP (mmHg) B. A.	DBP (mmHg) B. A.	S_{Na} (mEq/L) B. A.	S_k (mEq/L) B. A.	UO (cc)
NRF	58.750-57.390	160.0º146.0	108.7º 96.2	140.0-140.0	4.5-4.3	----
CHD-C	56.130º57.870	157.2º170.0	86.2º100.0	142.8-141.8	4.1º5.5	1160.0
CHD-E	56.580º58.080	148.7º172.5	85.0º 99.3	139.1-140.5	3.9º5.6	1208.0

*Before #After °p=<0.01

UO in the CHD group showed no significant differences between periods. Mean BW increased 1.74 ± 0.31 Kg during the C period ($p=<0.01$) and 1.5 ± 0.23 Kg during the E period ($p=<0.01$). Mean SBP also increased during both the C (+12.50 ± 4.91 mmHg) and the E (=23.75 ± 7.89 mmHg) periods; both changes were statistically significant ($p=<0.05$). Mean DBP increased 13.75 ± 3.03 mmHg and 14.37 ± 2.41 mmHg during the C and E periods respectively. Both changes were statistically significant ($p=<0.01$). S_{Na} did not change in either group or period. S_K increased significantly during both, the C and E periods ($p=<0.01$).

Although mean BW, mean SBP and mean DBP increased in C and E there was a significant correlation only between the changes in BW and DBP in the E period (r=0.72). The changes in meanSBP and mean DBP were not different when comparing the C and E periods in the CHD group.

COMMENTS

Indapamide has a well proven effect upon the cortical diluting segment of the nephron. In addition, some studies seem to show a direct action on peripheral vascular resistance (4) perhaps related to a calcium channel blocking effect. Thus the drug would have two discrete actions: diuresis and vasodilation. For the latter however, as with other diuretics, volumen depletion could be an "in vivo" requirement.

In this study, the 8 NRF patients responded to Indapamide lowering their SBP and DBP. This response correllated with a parallel fall in BW. The blood pressure lowering effect could be related in these patients to either diuresis or vasodilation or both.

The 8 CHD patients did not show an increment in UO when given Indapamide in doses twice as large as those given to the NRF group. Furthermore, these patients BW increased similarly both during the C and E periods. SBP and DBP increased significantly in this group in both periods although these changes did not correllate with changes in BW, except for SBP during the E period.

That Indapamide failed to induce an increment in diuresis in the CHD group is not surprising, since it is well known that at these levels of renal function none or minimal effect is achieved. But, in the absence of diuresis, Indapamide not only failed to decrease blood pressure, but also was unable to prevent the mild elevation seen during the C period. In this respect it should be underlined there were two control groups: one with NRF and the other the same CHD patients during the C period.

Of course we realize that in patients with renal failure there may be other variables wich could be responsable for the lack of response. However, we believe our findings suggest that the hypotensive effect of Indapamide is dependant upon its diuretic action as has been shown for other diuretics (5). Our results do not negate a direct vasodilator effect on resistance vessels. They do indicate though, that such action is either very mild or dependant upon an effective diuretic action.

REFERENCES:

1. Freis, E.D.:Hypertension, Proceedings Council High Blood Pressure Research, November 1958. New York:American Heart Association, 1959.
2. Freis, E.D. et al: Ann. N.Y.Acad. Sci 71:450, 1958
3. Mironneau,J.,Gargouil,Y.M. La Revue de Medicine 32:26, 1977.
4. Finch,L.,Hicks,P.E. J.Pharmacol. 58:282, 1976
5. Leth, A.: Circulation 42:479. 1970.

ETOZOLIN INDUCED URINE EXCRETION OF WATER AND SOLUTES IN PATIENTS WITH HYPERTENSION

C.ROMANO, B.COPERCINI, P.GHIRINGHELLI, E.GNOCCHI[+], F.PECCHINI

Division of Nephrology and Nuclear Medicine Service[+]
Hospital of Cremona - Italy

INTRODUCTION

Etozolin is a new diuretic, thiazolidone derivate, not related to sulphonamide: it differs from the other loop diuretics for a longer action profile, similar to the benzothiodiazides' one. The drug is metabolized in the active form ozolinone, that prolongs single-dose efficacy longer than 24 hours.

Aim of the present study is to evaluate its effects on arterial blood pressure(BP) and its action as regarding water and solutes excretion and urine acidification processes.

MATERIALS AND METHODS

Study involved ten patients with essential hypertension(six female and four male), 16 to 65 years old, mean age 47, with normal renal function. Every other drug withdrawn for at least 7 days balance, 3 days control and 7 days treatment periods. Sodium and potassium content of the diet was stable, while water intake free. Etozolin dose varied from 200 to 400 mg/day, given in the morning. After control period, basal plasma levels of renin activity(ARP), aldosterone, parathyroid hormone(PTH), electrolytes, uric acid, pH, osmolarity and creatinine were studied; the same data controlled the last day of treatment. Osmolar and free-water clearances and fractional electrolytes excretion were also simultaneously seen. ARP and aldosterone were determined after two hours of supine and standing position. Urine data daily measured during control and treatment periods.

RESULTS

Etozolin induced important($p<0,005$)reduction in both systolic(170±19 to 138±13)and diastolic(105±7 to 88±9,9)BP with a significant($p<0,05$)ARP release both in rest(1,41±1,1 to 2,07±1,6 ng/ml)and standing(1,93±1 to 4,74±3,4). Not varied plasma aldosterone and PTH. The drug increased urine output($p<0,001$) and chloride excretion($p<0,05$)(Fig. 1),but not clearly calcium, sodium and potassium;slightly lowered phosphate and uric acid. Urine osmolarity showed a significant fall($p<0,05$)with an increase of free-water clearance

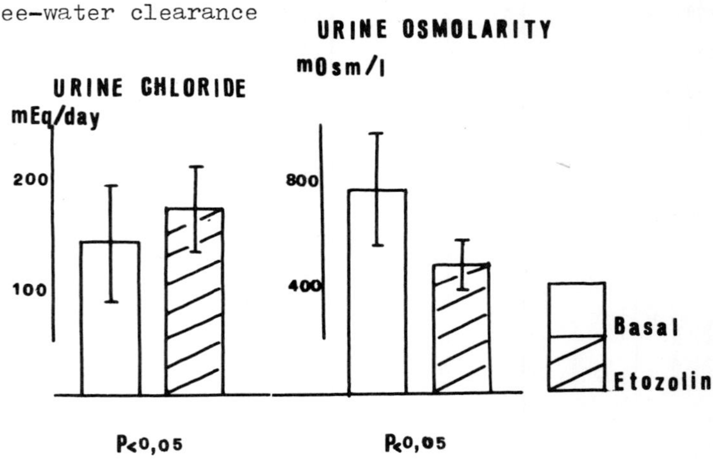

Fig. 1. Increase of chloride excretion and reduction of urine osmolarity due to Etozolin.

Urine pH decreased with a greater(but not significant)output of titratable acid and ammonium. No changes in serum electrolytes; only some patients had a slight reduction in potassium. Moderate increase of plasma creatinine and uric acid. Blood pH not varied, while bicarbonate resulted slightly higher.

DISCUSSION

Etozolin given once a day induced fall in both systolic and diastolic BP during a week treatment. Drug increased urine volume and free-water clearance for all the period and decreased urine osmolarity in reason of reduced distal fluid absorption due to depressed medulla osmolarity. Electrolytes excretion increased mostly in first days,returning below or to basal levels by the end of treatment for enhanced proximal tubular absorption and compensatory increase in distal tubular absorption(1). Urine chloride was higher than sodium presumably for a greater inhibition of chloride transport in ascending limb of Henle(2). Only a slight increase in calcium excretion not confirmed known effect of furosemide(3)due to inhibition of calcium absorption in the thick ascending limb(4). Potassium excretion increased to lesser extent.

Tendency to urine pH fall and ammonium-titratable acid increase may be result of decreased H^+ and NH_4 diffusion out of lumen via intercellular pathway and of increased ammonium excretion secondary to fall in tubular pH and to greater flow rate(5). ARP grew for juxtaglomerular stimulation due to renal underperfusion(2);stimulation of sympathetic nervous system also plays a role. Glomerular filtrate showed a slight decline due to increased intratubular hydrostatic pressure(2)(5)and decreased glomerular capillary pressure. Uric acid excretion reduced for enhanced proximal reabsorption of urate or inhibition of excretion.

REFERENCES

1. Greven J.,Kolling B. In: Recent advances in diuretic therapy. Excerpta Medica(Nov.4-6,1982)Ed.V.E.Andreucci,pp.37-45.
2. Greven J.,Klein H.,Heidenreich O. Naunyn-Schmiedeber's Archives of Pharmacology. 304: 289-296,1978.
3. Pecchini F.,Andreucci V.E.,Savi M. Giorn.Clin.Med. 47: 191-200,1966.
4. Bourdeau J.E. In: Divalent ion homeostasis(Eds.B.M.Brenner and J.H.Stein),Churchill Livingstone,1983,p.23.
5. Hropot M.,Fowler N.,Karlmark B.,Giebisch G. Kidney International. 28: 477-489,1985.

CALCIUM METABOLISM IN ESSENTIAL HYPERTENSIVE PATIENTS TREATED WITH ETOZOLIN.

P. MORACHIELLO, U. COLI, S. LANDINI, A. FRACASSO, F. RIGHETTO, F. SCANFERLA, R. GENCHI, G. BAZZATO.

Department of Nephrology and Dialysis, Umberto I Hospital, Venice-Mestre, Italy.

INTRODUCTION

Calcium and Phosphate metabolism abnormalities have been shown to be present either in experimental (1) or in clinical studies (2) in essential hypertension (E.H.). Among these, the most frequent relief is an overactivity of the parathyroid glands (3). Furthermore diuretics as thiazides commonly employed in such pathological condition, as first step therapy, exert some well known actions on mineral metabolism: a reduction of Ca excretion in hypercalciuric states (4), a modification of Ca intestinal absorption (5) and an increased bone mineralization (6). From these considerations, we have investigated, in E.H. patients (pts), the effects on mineral metabolism induced by Etozolin (E) a diuretic compound acting on Henle's loop (7) with a considerable antihypertensive property (8).

PATIENTS AND METHODS

15 pts (10 M - 5 F) aged 38-46 ys with E.H. underwent the following protocol: a) 1 week (wk) of baseline study with placebo; b) a 12 wks study period with E (400 mg/day). During periods a-b, daily and weekly controls were performed: among the first, we included blood pressure (BP), heart rate (HR), body weight (wt), urine volume (U.Vol.) blood and urine Na-K-Ca-P-Mg, uric acid and creatinine; among the latter, serum ionized Ca (S.I.Ca^{++}), PRA, aldosterone, PTH (COOH), calcitonin, bone GLA protein, alkaline (alk.) phosphatase, urine cAMP were controlled. The statistical evaluation was performed with the Student's t test.

RESULTS

A significant reduction of BP was obtained (from mean values of 185/102 to 145/83 mmHg $P < 0.003$) after 2 wks maintaining on normal range during the study period. In the meantime HR increased from 68±8 to 75±8 $P < 0.05$. Serum creatinine remained unchanged (mean value 1.08±0.12 mg/dl); contrariwise, uric acid rose from 4.85±0.8 to 7.5±1.6 mg/dl $P < 0.005$ at the end of study. The variations of PRA, aldosterone, U. Vol., Na and K excretion and the parameters of mineral metabolism during E treatment are reported in Table 1 and 2.

Table 1

Patients	S.I.Ca^{++} mg/dl	S.$PO_4^{=}$ mg/dl	S.PTH ng/ml	Calcit. pg/ml	Alk. phosph. U/l	PRA ng/ ml/hr	Aldost. ng/ml
basal values	3.79± 0.1	3.2± 0.7	0.55± 0.2	69± 22	137± 40	3.78± 2.2	200± 90
12 wk after	4.1± 0.6	4.3± 0.7	0.4± 0.3	92± 28	117± 33	1.4± 0.7	118± 38
P	< 0.007	< 0.001	< 0.02	< 0.02	< 0.01	< 0.003	< 0.005

Table 2

Patients	U.Vol ml/ 24 hr	U.Na mEq/ 24 hr	U.Ca mg/ 24 hr	U.PO_4 mg/ 24 hr	U.Mg mg/ 24 hr	U.cAMP n mol dl/VFG	U.K mEq/ 24 hr
basal values	1287± 198	116± 20	126± 25	614± 98	66+ 11	4.8± 0.4	39± 7
12 wk after	2250± 494	214± 50	200± 57	470± 72	70± 15	2.3± 0.7	52± 10
P	< 0.001	< 0.001	< 0.001	< 0.007	NS	< 0.0001	NS

DISCUSSION

E. has shown an important diuretic and natriuretic effect as reported by Others (9). It has to be stressed that this action has not been followed by an activation of the renin-angiotensin system. Regarding calcium metabolism, we have found some results that may be explained by a reduction of parathyroid activity. In fact after E treatment, resulted decreased PTH, alk. phosphatase, $PO_4=$ and cAMP urine excretion, while increased appeared S.I. Ca^{++}, s. $PO_4=$, calcitonin and calciuria. Similar data have been obtained in E.H. pts treated with Ca-channel blockers by our group (10): besides the well established diuretic action, it may be assumed that E acts like a Ca-channel blocker. It has still to be explained whether parathyroid inhibition is directly related to E or the effect is consequent to the increased S.I. Ca^{++}. Moreover E action on divalent jons tubular transport may play a primary role on these metabolic changes. However further studies on intestinal Ca absorption and bone metabolism will be necessary for a complete evaluation of the role of E on mineral metabolism.

REFERENCES

1. Holloway, E.T., Bohr, D.F. Circul. Res. 33: 678-685, 1973.
2. Mc Carron, D.A. N. Engl. J. Med. 307: 226-228, 1982.
3. Mc Carron, D.A., Pingree, P., Rubin, R.J., Gaucher, S.M., Molitch, M., Kurtzik, S. Hypertension 2: 162-168, 1980.
4. Yendt, E.R., Cohanim, M. Kidney Int. 13: 397-402, 1978.
5. Barilla, D.E., Tolentino, R., Kaplan, R.A., Pak, C.Y.C. Metabolism 27: 125-131, 1978.
6. Wasnich, R.D., Benfante, R.J., Yano, K., Heilbrun, L., Vogel, J.M. New Engl. J. Med. 309: 344-346, 1983.
7. Greven, J. Heidenreich, O. Arzneimittel-Forschung-Drug Res. 27: 1755-1757, 1977.
8. Kopp, H. Fortschritte der Medizin 96: 1194-1198, 1978.
9. Scheitza, E. Arzneimittel-Forschung 27: 1807-1814, 1977.
10. Morachiello, P., Coli, U., Landini, S., Fracasso, A., Righetto, F., Scanferla, F., Bazzato, G. In: Mineral Metabolism Res. in Italy (Wichtig Ed. Milan) 1985, in press.

IMPROVEMENT IN EXERCISE-INDUCED DIASTOLIC BLOOD PRESSURE CHANGES BY DIURETIC TREATMENT

C. MONTANARI and A. VERGANI

Department of Cardiology, Istituti Clinici di Perfezionamento, Milan, Italy

INTRODUCTION

Antihypertensive drugs would not seem to be very useful in controlling BP variations caused by phisical activity. Not many studies have been carried out in this regard, with the exception of those relative to beta blocking agents; these, however, show that at submaximal levels of effort there are not any significant reduction in SBP and DBP, and, if there are, BP decreases are of a value almost identical to the differences between the resting BP before and after treatment. In other words, the slope of SBP and DBP in relationship to the changes in workload, tends to be substantially the same, or even becoming sharper after antihypertensive therapy. It is quite probable that there may be drugs capable of minimizing this tendency (1,2).

MATERIALS AND METHODS

A group of 163 untreated patients suffering from mild essential hypertension was chosen. After a control period of at least 3 wk, during which both unstable BP and secondary hypertension were excluded, the subjects underwent an exercise test characterized by increases in external workload of 25 W every 3 min. The test was suspended upon reaching the target HR according to Sheffield (3), or due to muscular exhaustion. HR, SBP and DBP were recorded at the end of every step of effort. Subsequently the patients were assigned at random with one of 7 foreseen treatments. After 2 mo, the ergometric procedures were repeated, only in responders who showed a DBP _ 90 mmHg, at the end of treatment. Only 118 patients (72.4%), 84 m and 34 f (mean age: 50.1 $\pm$ 8.8 yrs; range 29 - 68 yrs) were admitted to the trial; they were treated with Acebutolol, 400 mg (n=31), Penbutolol, 40 mg (n=9), Metoprolol,

200 mg (n=13), Clonidine, 0.300 mg (n=9), Spironolactone, 100 mg (n=9), Indapamide, 2.5 mg (n=19) and Muzolimine, 15 mg (n=26). The SBP and DBP data, obtained at every exercise step before an after treatment, was plotted against the relative W value, in order to obtain BP/W slopes, which were analyzed by the usual inferential techniques.

RESULTS

As far as modifications of SBP and DBP at rest are concerned, all therapies significatively ($p < 0.05$, or more) reduced BP to around 135/85 mmHg, with a mean change of approximately -10/-15 mmHg.

The results obtained in exercise tests are shown in Fig. 1.

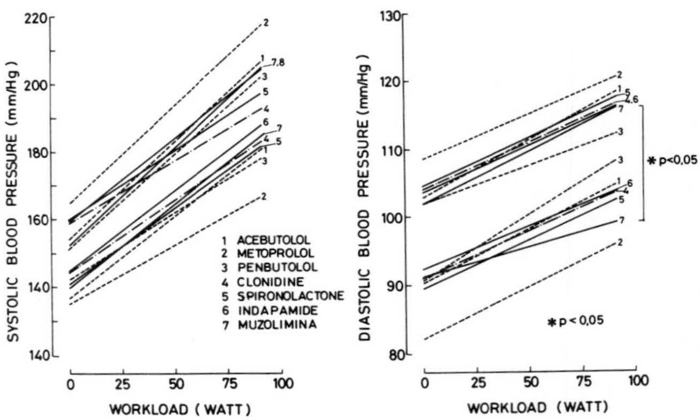

Fig. 1. Changes in SBP and DBP during graded exercise. Correlations between BP and W values are highly statistically significant ($p < 0.01$).

The SBP/W ratio was substantially the same in controls and in treated subjects. Beta blocking agents seemed to decrease SBP/W slopes more noticeably.

Statistical analysis did not reveal any difference between DBP/W ratios, before and after treatment, with the sole exception of muzolimine (from 0.153 mmHg/W to 0.090 mmHg/W, $p < 0.05$). It is noticeable that, whilst not reaching a significant statistical level, there is a tendency in slope increase in patients treated with beta blockers with ISA (penbutolol: +0.060; metoprolol: +0.022); moreover, in the case of latter drug, DBP values in relationship to external workload are always lower than those found with other drugs, notwithstanding slope increase. It must be remarked that patients treated with beta blockers did not reach the target HR at the end of exercise test: muscular exhaustion occurs at a HR of 113-117 bpm, against an expected HR of 145-150 bpm ($p < 0.01$).

CONCLUSIONS

Notwithstanding that all therapies proved to be effective in normalizing hypertension, they are unable to control the SBP changes induced by effort. The slight slope reduction after beta blockers treatment may be ascribed to changes in CO. DBP increases are only affected by a loop diuretic such as muzolimine. This phenomenon would not seem to find an explanation in the volume depletion induced by the drug, since 15 mg daily would not seem to have a marked diuretic effect, and because neither spironolactone or indapamide induces a similar slope reduction. The possibility that muzolimine directly counteracts the effects of adrenergic system at vascular level is denied by the evidence that alpha or beta receptors blockade does not cause changes in DBP/W ratio. It is quite probable that the favourable action of muzolimine is due to activation of PG system, which, besides producing direct dilatation of vascular bed, modulates the renin-angiotensin activity.

In clinical terms, muzolimine would seem to be the drug most indicated in treatment of exercise induced BP raises, also because, differently from beta blocking agents, it does not exclude a physiological HR adjustment during exertion.

REFERENCES

1. Lund-Johansen, P. and Bakke, O.M. Br. J. clin. Pharmac. 7: 169-174, 1979
2. Roja, M., Cumetti, C., Vergani, A., Montanari, C. and De Cristofaro, A. Drugs Exptl. Clin. Res. 11 (12): 851-860, 1985

ANTIHYPERTENSIVE ACTIVITY AND TOLERABILITY OF THIOBUTIZIDE ALONE OR IN FIXED COMBINATION WITH POTASSIUM CANRENOATE IN ESSENTIAL HYPERTENSION.

P.DESSI'-FULGHERI, F.BANDIERA, M.OPPES, P.MADEDDU, F.COCCO, S.RUBATTU, N.GLORIOSO, C.M.TROFFA, A.RAPPELLI.

Cattedra di Patologia Medica II, University of Sassari, SASSARI (Italy).

INTRODUCTION

Diuretics have a number of well known adverse effects such as hyperglycaemia (or reduced carbohydrate tolerance), hyperlipidemia, hyperuricemia and hypokaliemia (1,2,3). The latter seems to mediate, at least in part, the negative effects on carbohydrate methabolism through a reduction of insulin release (4). The aim of our study has been to compare the antihypertensive and metabolic effects of a thiazide diuretic alone, thiobutizide, versus a combination of thiobutizide plus a potassium sparing agent, potassium canrenoate.

PATIENTS AND METHODS

The study has been planned as a randomized between-patient, single-blind comparison between the fixed combination of thiobutizide 5 mg+ potassium canrenoate 50 mg (Group A) and thiobutizide alone 5 mg (Group B). After at least a 2-week wash-out period all patients assumed a placebo tablet once daily for one week. At the end of the placebo period 30 patients (16 male and 14 female; mean age 50.5±8.1 yrs) whose diastolic blood pressure was between 95 and 115 mmHg were randomly allocated to Group A or B for the duration of 12 weeks. Lying and standing blood pressure, heart rate, body weight, plasma sodium and potassium were evaluated every 2 weeks. In addition fasting glucose, plasma Mg, uric acid, total and HDL cholesterol, tryglicerides, oral glucose tolerance test (OGTT:40 g/m²), HbAlc, plasma renin activity (PRA) and urinary aldosterone (UA) were measured before and at the end of the study period with active treatment.

Statistical analysis was performed by Student's t test for paired or unpaired data. The values are expressed as mean±SEM. OGTT results were analyzed as the sum of blood glucose values obtained at time 0, 30, 60, 90, 120 and 180 min of each OGTT (5).

RESULTS

The Table summarizes the principal results obtained in our study.

Table

	GROUP A before	GROUP A after	GROUP B before	GROUP B after
Syst.BP mmHg	166.6±3.2	135.3±2.5**	167.3±3.2	146.5±4.1**#
Diast.BP mmHg	106.6±1.7	84.2±1.1**	106.0±1.7	97.8±6.1#
Uric acid mg/dl	5.5±0.4	6.0±0.3	5.8±0.4	6.1±0.3
Blood Gluc. mg/dl	89.7±2.2	91.8±2.1	91.0±1.8	93.8±1.4
Total chol.mg/dl	230±13	224±11	237±14	232±9
HDL chol.mg/dl	44±2.2	42±1.7	40±1.0	41±1.3
Tryglic. mg/dl	139±9	130±6	141±6	139±6
HbA1c(% Hb)	5.4±0.2	5.0±0.2	5.8±0.1	6.2±0.3
Plasma Na^+ mEq/l	141.8±1.4	141.1±1.3	142.1±1.2	140.3±0.5
Plasma K^+ mEq/l	4.2±0.1	4.1±0.1	4.4±0.2	3.8±0.2*
Plasma Mg mg/dl	2.2±0.1	2.1±0.1	2.3±0.1	2.1±0.1
OGTT mg/dl	738±27	730±26	705±28	757±31
PRA ng/ml/h	2.3±0.3	3.4±0.5	2.1±0.3	5.7±0.5*##
UA μg/24h	7.6±1.1	10.6±0.7	8.1±1.3	14.6±0.4*##
Body Weight, Kg	69±2	68±2	69±3	67±2

*=p<0.05, ** = p<0.01 before versus after

#=p<0.05, ## = p<0.01 Group B versus Group A

At the end of the study 73% of the patients of Group A were normotensive (diastolic blood pressure ≤ 90 mmHg) whereas 47% of patients of Group B achieved normalization of their blood pressure. None of the patients in Group A showed impairment of the OGTT whereas 2 out of 15 patients of

Group B developed an impaired OGTT at the end of the study. Hypokaliemia (less than 3.0 mEq/l) occurred in two patients of Group B.

DISCUSSION

Our results showing a better antihypertensive response in patients treated with the combination of thiobutizide plus K canrenoate with respect to those treated with the thiazide diuretic alone, might be explained by the lesser stimulation of the renin angiotensin system. The latter finding might be in turn the result of a less pronunced hypokaliemia obtained through the potassium sparing action of K canrenoate. The preservation of a normal serum potassium level, in addition, may contribute to the better carbohydrate tolerance observed in patients treated with the association as compared to the occurrence of some deterioration of glucose metabolism in patients treated with thiobutizide alone.

REFERENCES

1. Kaplan, N.M. Am.J.Cardiol. 51: 621-627, 1983.
2. Amery, A., Bulpitt, C., de Schaepdryver, A., Fagard, R., Hellemans, J., Mutsers, A., Berthaux, P., Deruytteere, M., Dollery, C., Forette, F., Lund-Johansen, P., Tuomileheto, J. Lancet I: 681-683, 1978.
3. Murphy, M.B., Kohner, E., Lewis, P.J., Schumer, B., Dollery, C.T.: Lancet II 1293-1295, 1982.
4. Conn, J.W. N.Engl.J.Med. 273: 1135-1138, 1965.
5. Lindgarde, F., Malmquist, J., Balke, B. Acta Diabet.Lat. 20: 33-37 1983.

K-RICH/Na-POOR SALT REDUCES BLOOD PRESSURE IN HOSPITALIZED PATIENTS

F. Arzilli, S. Taddei, L. Graziadei, E. Bichisao, R. Giovannetti, A. Salvetti
Clinica Medica I, University of Pisa (Italy)

INTRODUCTION

It is still controversial whether the reduction of Na as well as the increase of K intake in hypertensive patients can reduce blood pressure [1,2,3,4], and the mechanisms which account for blood pressure decrease following a low Na intake are still debated. Aim of the study was to assess the efficacy of a K-rich/Na-poor salt (NaCl 50%, KCl 25%, $K_3C_6H_5O_6$ 15%) in lowering blood pressure levels.

PATIENTS AND METHODS

Ten in-patients (pts) with mild (7 pts) to moderate uncomplicated essential hypertension diagnosed on average 3.4 years previously, 6 males, aged 39.5 years (range 28-53), entered the study. After a previous withdrawal of any antihypertensive treatment followed by 5 days of hospitalization, pts with DBP $\geq$95 mmHg, on a standard diet containing about 20-40 mEq/Na + 4 g of common salt (CS) were randomly given in double-blind condition 2 g b.i.d. either of CS (5 pts) or K-rich/Na-poor salt (K-Na, 5 pts) to add to the food for further 8 days. The following parameters were measured:

every day: blood pressure (BP), heart rate (HR), body weight (BW) and 24 hours (hr) urinary sodium and potassium (UNa, UK);

every 4 days (days: 0, 5, 9, 13): plasma renin activity (PRA), plasma nor-adrenaline (PNA), plasma sodium (PNa) and potassium (PK) measured in sitting position; provocative tests: cold pressure test (CPT), mental stress (MS) and a hand-grip (HG) recording BP and HR. PRA was measured by RIA, PNA by HPLC-EC, sodium and potassium by flame photometry, BP and HR by mercury sphygmomanometer and by pulsatory method.

Statistical analysis was performed by using parametric test (two-way ANOVA according to a split-plot design with multiple comparisons) for quantitative data, and non-parametric tests for qualitative data.

RESULTS

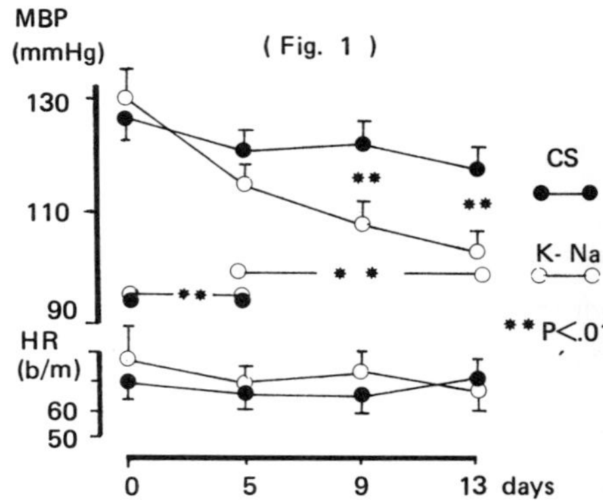

At the 5th day of hospitalization the homogeneity check of patients distribution was satisfactory as far as BP, provocative tests response and humoral data are concerned. Mean blood pressure (MBP) significantly (P<0.01) decreased in both groups at the 5th day of hospitalization and, in the following 8 days, it significantly (P<0.01) decreased only in the K-Na salt treated group. HR did not significantly change showing a similar trend in both groups (Fig. 1, mean values ± S.E.M.).

Humoral data are reported in the following table (mean values±S.E.M.):

	K-Na				CS			
	0	**5**	**9**	**13**	**0**	**5**	**9**	**13 days**
UNa	**204.6**	**78.2**	**55.4**	**54.8**	**151.8**	**113.6**	**105.4**	**101.0**
(mEq/24hr)	(34.7)	(9.1)	(13.5)	(5.2)	(28.3)	(23.6)	(12.1)	(6.8)
cumulative balance	**100.2**		**62.9**		**100.8**		**109.9**	
(mean of 4 days)	(11.0)		(3.6)		(7.9)		(4.3)	
UK	**64.6**	**43.2**	**62.0**	**57.6**	**45.0**	**55.8**	**49.8**	**51.6**
(mEq/24hr)	(15.9)	(5.9)	(6.0)	(2.6)	(10.4)	(4.9)	(4.9)	(4.4)
cumulative balance	**43.6**		**54.3**		**53.0**		**50.6**	
(mean of 4 days)	(3.5)		(2.1)		(2.8)		(1.4)	
PNa	**138.0**	**137.8**	**137.0**	**138.4**	**140.2**	**141.0**	**139.2**	**140.4**
(mEq/l)	(4.6)	(2.6)	(1.6)	(2.2)	(3.9)	(2.6)	(1.6)	(1.2)
PK	**3.8**	**3.7**	**3.9**	**4.2**	**3.6**	**3.7**	**3.8**	**3.7**
(mEq/l)	(0.2)	(0.2)	(0.2)	(0.2)	(0.1)	(0.1)	(0.2)	(0.1)
BW	**74.4**	**72.8**	**72.2**	**71.6**	**77.6**	**76.4**	**75.8**	**75.4**
(kg)	(5.9)	(5.5)	(5.4)	(5.3)	(5.4)	(5.1)	(5.3)	(5.2)
PRA	**1.13**	**0.89**	**1.46**	**1.42**	**1.29**	**1.70**	**1.44**	**1.44**
(mg/ml/h^{-1})	(0.4)	(0.4)	(0.7)	(0.7)	(0.7)	(0.7)	(0.7)	(0.8)
PNA	**383.4**	**312.6**	**374.6**	**245.0**	**351.0**	**257.8**	**291.6**	**342.4**
(ρ/ml)	(67.5)	(57.9)	(83.4)	(32.9)	(40.1)	(30.5)	(34.4)	(30.8)

Both groups showed in the first 4 days the same UNa excretion which was practically unchanged until the 13th day in the CS group. On the contrary in the K-Na group, UNa significantly (P<0.05) dropped by about 50% com-

pared to the CS group. UK excretion similar in both groups at the 5th day, tended to increase only in K-Na group. PNa did not consistently change in each group, whereas PK tended to increase only in the K-Na group. BW showed the same decrease in both groups (on average 1 kg). PNA did not differ significantly between the two groups and among the days of treatment. However in both groups, PNA tended to decline at the 5th day of hospitalization and thereafter in the CS group it tended to increase but in the K-Na group it tended to decrease at the 13th day. PRA values of the two groups did not differ between themselves during the various trial periods. However in the CS group they showed a trend towards increasing at the 5th day without any further significant changes in the subsequent days, whereas in the K-Na group PRA, which was slightly decreased at the 5th day, tended to increase at the 9th and 13th day. No differences between the two dietetic regimens were detectable as regards MBP during HG and CP. On the contrary the K-Na group showed a significant ($P<0.04$) MBP decrease to MS as compared to the CS group:
In the following table the response of MBP (Δ% between baseline value of MBP and at the maximal response) after provocative tests is reported:

	K-Na				**CS**			
	0	**5**	**9**	**13**	**0**	**5**	**9**	**13 days**
	%	%	%	%	%	%	%	%
CPT	13.9	13.7	17.6	17.0	11.9	15.5	11.8	12.3
HG	12.7	12.7	12.3	11.4	17.8	15.4	14.1	12.4
MS	10.7	7.9	9.7	6.0	18.6	17.3	15.3	17.2

CONCLUSIONS

In this study, performed in a metabolic unit, the compliance of the pts to the dietetic regimens was satisfactory as shown by the fact that UNa excretion equalled the intake. During the first 4 days when Na intake was similarly reduced to about 100 mEq/24hr, BP declined similarly in both groups. However, owing to the well known effect of hospitalization, one can not assess if this mild reduction of Na intake is responsible for the BP decrease. When the Na intake was further reduced by about 50% in the K-Na group, BP further dropped as compared to the CS group whose BP values remained practically unchanged. These findings suggest that a reduction of Na intake below 100 mEq/24hr linked to a small increment of K intake (about 20 mEq/24hr) is able to decrease BP. The lowering BP effect of a K-Na diet might be explained either by its action on the volume and/or on the vasoconstrictor components. The first hypothesis seems unlikely since the loss in BW was similar in both groups. For the second hypothesis one might observe that PNA behaviour was similar in both groups, but it tended to decline only in the K-Na group, whose vascular reactivity to MS but not to stronger stimuli (CP, HG) was reduced. These findings suggest that a reduced sympathetic nervous activity by itself and/or a reduced vascular response to it, might be involved [5]. Our data evidencing that a reduced Na intake by about 200 to about 100 mEq/24hr did not significantly stimulate PRA, might be explained by the fact that the inverse relationship between Na excretion and PRA (the so called nomogram) is probably due to the stiffness of this relationship below 100 mEq/24hr [6]. However it can not be excluded that, owing to the hospitalization, a decline in renin stimulation due to a reduced sympathetic nervous system activity occurred. Altogether these data are in agreement with the fact that a moderate Na reduction did not exert any evident stimulus on the renin angiotensin system. However in the K-Na group a further reduction of UNa excretion was achieved (up to 50 mEq/24hr), and since the PRA/UNa relationship is now in the stiff part of the curve, one might expect a clear stimulation of the renin angiotensin system. The reasons why a further reduction of Na intake did not stimulate PRA or SNS, are not readily understandable but the blunting action of these two hypertensive systems might concur to the antihypertensive effect of low Na in these patients. Two only possible explanations are likely: the small (indeed!) increments of K intake, and the intrinsic characteristics of patients (salt-sensitive).

REFERENCES

1 - Mac Gregor G.,Hypertension,7,628-637,1985

2 - Watt G.C.M.,Edwards C.,Hart J.T.,Hart M.,Walton P.,Foy C.J.W.,Br. Med.J.,286,432-436,1983

3 - Fujita T.,Ando K.,Hypertension,6,184-192,1984

4 - Richards M.A.,Espiner E.A.,Maslowski A.H.,Nicholls A.G.,Ikram H.,-Hamilton E.J.,Wells J.E.,Lancet 1,757-761,1984

5 - Holly J.M.P.,Evans S.J.W.,Goodwin f.J.,VandenBurg M.J.,Ledingham J.M. Lancet,1,1384-1387,1981

6 - Salvetti A.,Pedrinelli R.,Magagna A.,Poli L.,Sassano P.,Arzilli F., Nephron 26,189-194,1980

COMBINATION OF NIFEDIPINE AND CHLORTHALIDONE IN THE TREATMENT OF HYPERTENSION

L.A.FERRARA, T.MAROTTA, F.PASANISI, P.MASTRANZO, M.MANCINI
Institute of Internal Medicine and Metabolic Diseases- Clinica Medica, 2nd Medical School- University of Naples, Italy

INTRODUCTION

In the Seventies the World Health Organization suggested the use of diuretics or beta blockers as first-line drugs for the treatment of arterial hypertension (1), confining the use of vasodilators (hydralazine, prazosin) to the combined treatment. Recently calcium entry blockers, particularly nifedipine and verapamil, frequently replaced thiazide as first-line drug in old or low-renin hypertensives. The use of new combinations including this class of drugs is therefore under extensive investigation. Whilst previous studies showed the rationale of the combination of beta blockers and calcium antagonists, in particular nifedipine (2), the usefulness of its combination with diuretics is still controversial. In fact, a possible reflex increase in plasma renin activity (PRA) has been suggested to reduce the antihypertensive effect of the two drugs.

Aim of this study was to evaluate the antihypertensive effect of the addition of chlorthalidone to slow-release nifedipine.

PATIENTS AND METHODS

Seven patient (4M, 3F), age range 39-64 yrs, with primary uncomplicated arterial hypertension entered the study. Their informed consent was previously requested and obtained. An isocaloric well balanced diet (2000 kcal) without salt restriction was prescribed for two weeks whilst all antihypertensive drugs were withdrawn. Afterwards patients were given slow-release nifedipine 20 mg b.i.d. for a period of 6 weeks; at the end of the monotherapy chlorthalidone 25 mg o.d. was added for the following 6 weeks.

Supine and standing blood pressure (BP) and heart rate (HR) were measured twice in a quiet room by an automatic recorder (Sentron) at baseline, after 6 weeks of nifedipine monotherapy and after 6 weeks of the combined treatment. On the same occasions the following parameters were also measured:

plasma renin activity (PRA) after 1 hr of standardized walking;

24 hr urinary excretion of sodium and potassium.

Statistical analysis: the results are expressed as mean± standard deviation. Statistical analysis of the results was performed by one-way analysis of variance. Multiple comparisons were assessed according to Duncan's test (3).

RESULTS

Body weight of the patients did not change over the treatment period (76±5; 76±5; 75±5; at baseline, at 6 and at 12 weeks of treatment respectively). Supine and standing BP were reduced by the sole nifedipine but a further, significant fall was observed when chlorthalidone was added. No significant change in heart rate was observed throughout the study (Table 1).

	supine			standing		
	SBP	DBP	HR	SBP	DBP	HR
	(mm Hg)		(beats/min)	(mm Hg)		(beats/min)
baseline	158±17	91±8	72±7	166±18	100±7	80±6
monotherapy	151±11	89±6	80±8	149± 9*	92±7*	92±7
combination	138± 7*°	83±5*°	77±7	140± 8*	87±5*	93±7

Table 1: Blood pressure and heart rate at baseline, after the monotherapy and after the combination.
Significance vs. baseline: *$p<.01$.
Significance vs. monotherapy: °$p<.05$.

Nifedipine alone slightly and not significantly increased PRA (from 3.6±2.2 ng/ml/hr to 5.1±2.6), but a three-fold increase in PRA was observed (10.7±9; $p<.05$ vs baseline) when chlorthalidone was added.

No significant change, on the other hand, was observed in daily urinary excretion of sodium (236±69 mEq/24hr at baseline, 212±74 after nifedipine and 214±75 after nifedipine+chlorthalidone) and potassium (68±21, 69±16 and 63±27 mEq/24hr at baseline,at the end of monotherapy and at the end of the combination, respectively).

DISCUSSION

Studies on the effectiveness of a combined treatment with calcium antagonists and diuretics are still few and particularly concerning the use of verapamil (4). In this study we have looked at the antihypertensive efficacy of the combination of slow-release nifedipine with chlorthalidone, given to the patients after a 6-week period of nifedipine alone. The monotherapy reduced BP and the addition of the diuretic induced a further marked fall in both SBP and DBP. Regarding the possible increase in the activity of the renin-angiotensin-aldosterone axis, which would be expected using such an association, we observed a three-fold increase in PRA which, however, did not reduce the effectiveness of the combination and did not change significantly the urinary excretion of sodium and potassium. It is possible that the increase in PRA might not be followed by a corresponding increase in plasma aldosterone, since its secretion has been suggested to be calcium-mediated and might be reduced by nifedipine. This explanation might account for the lack of changes in urinary electrolytes excretion.

Our data support the usefulness of the combination of nifedipine + chlorthalidone, since the observed increase in PRA does not lead to sodium retention, which could theoretically reduce the effects of the treatment.

RFERENCES

1. Arterial Hypertension - Report of WHO Expert Committee. Technical Report Series No 628, 1978.
2. Bühler, F.R., Hultèn, H.L., Kiowski, W. and Bolli, P. Drugs 25 (Suppl. 2): 50-57, 1983.
3. Winer, B.J. In: Statistical principles in experimental design. Mc Graw-Hill Scientific Publication, London, 1971.
4. Corea, L., Bentivoglio, M., Verdecchia, P., Provvidenza, M. In: Calcium antagonists and the treatment of hypertension (Eds. J.L. Reid and A.J. Pickup), published by Royal Society of Medicine No. 62, London,1984, pp. 23-30.

CARDIOVASCULAR REFLEX AND SYSTEMIC HEMODYNAMICS RELATIONSHIP IN PATIENTS WITH ESSENTIAL HYPERTENSION UNDER CHRONIC TREATMENT WITH INDAPAMIDE

R. CARRETTA, B. FABRIS, S. MUIESAN, M. BARDELLI, F. FISCHETTI, R. LEPRINI, G. BELLINI, *A. BIANCHETTI, L. CAMPANACCI

Institute of Medical Pathology of University; *Dept. of Anaesthesia, Ospedale Maggiore; Trieste, Italy

INTRODUCTION

In a previous study we have shown that chronic treatment with indapamide increases baroreceptor sensitivity and reduces vascular reactivity, to pressor doses of noradrenaline (1). These observations suggest an action of the drug on blood vessels. To further investigate this point, we performed this study with the aim of establish whether the changes in baroreceptor sensitivity induced by chronic treatment with indapamide could be related to changes in vascular peripheral resistances.

MATERIALS AND METHODS

The study was performed in 10 patients - 6 males and 4 females, aged 22-45 - with uncomplicated essential hypertension. Each patient was randomly assignated either to therapy with indapamide 2.5 mg/day or placebo. After three months of therapy with placebo or indapamide the drug administration was reversed following a cross-over criterion. At the end of each three months period of treatment, an hemodynamic study was performed. In the morning, after an overnight fasting, under local anaesthesia, an agocannula was inserted in the brachial artery and then right atrial catetherization was performed. Intraarterial blood pressure was continuously recorded through a Statham P23 transducer. Cardiac output was determined by the dye dilution technique. Baroreceptor sensitivity was assessed by the phenylephrine method. The results were expressed as mean $\pm$ standard deviations. Statistical significativity of the differences was evaluated by T Student's test for paired data.

RESULTS

Three months of therapy with indapamide resulted in a significant reduction of the blood pressure (from 116 $\pm$ 18 to 105 $\pm$ 15 mmHg, $p < 0.01$) while heart rate did not change. At the same time, cardiac index increased, from 3.70 $\pm$ 0.6 to 3.96 $\pm$ 0.7 $l/min/m^2$ ($p < 0.01$) while total peripheral resistances decreased from 2750 $\pm$ 405 to 2040 $\pm$ 715 $dynes/sec/cm^{-5}/m^2$ ($p < 0.01$). Baroreceptor sensitivity was increased after indapamide treatment (Fig. 1). An inverse correlation was found between changes in total peripheral vascular resistances and changes in baroreceptor sensitivity (Fig. 2).

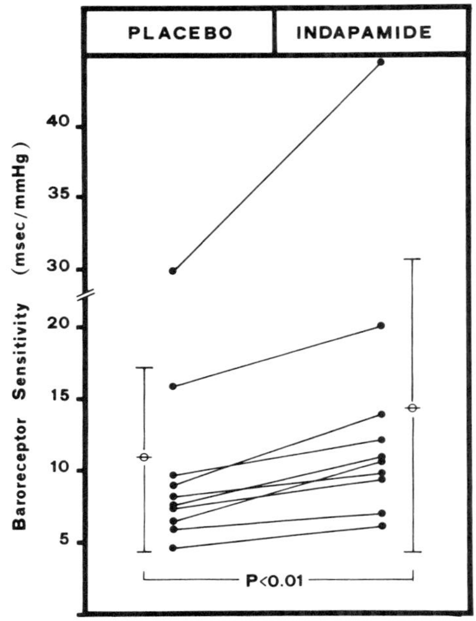

Figure 1

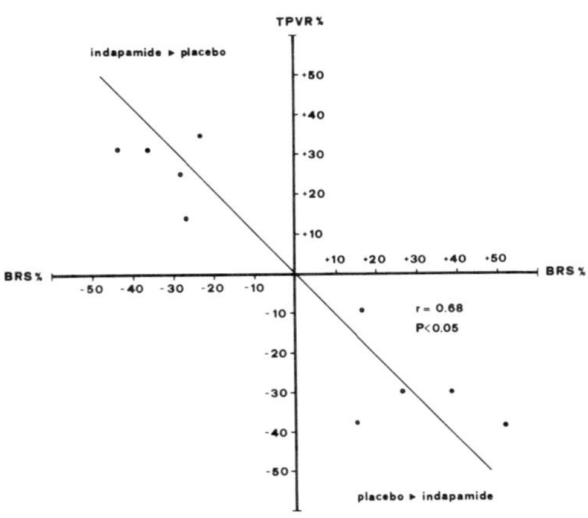

Figure 2

DISCUSSION

The changes in baroreceptor sensitivity, determined by chronic treatment with same antihypertensive drug, is achieved through different mechanisms. Clonidine, for instance, increases baroreceptor sensitivity through an action on central nervous system (2). Indapamide, as shown by the present and one of our previous studies (1), also increases baroreceptor sensitivity while it decreases vascular reactivity to pressor doses of noradrenaline. Therefore, it seems likely than this drug interferes with blood vessel contractility. Support to this hypothesis comes from the present study, in which we have shown that chronic treatment with indapamide increases the cardiac index and reduces total peripheral resistances. Although total peripheral resistances could not give information on districtual resistances, namely in the carotid and aortic arch district, the correlation that we found between reduction in vascular resistances and increase in baroreceptor sensitivity, after successful treatment with indapamide, suggests that the drug interferes with baroreceptor function through changes in vascular tone.

In conclusion, these data show that indapamide hemodynamic effects are different from those of the other diuretics and imply an action of the drug on blood vessels.

REFERENCES

1. Carretta, R. et al. Eur. J. Clin. Pharmacol. 24: 579-583, 1983
2. Sleight, P. et al. Proc. Inter. Sump. Turnbridge Wells, p. 291, 1975

COMPARISON OF LONG TERM METABOLIC EFFECTS OF MUZOLIMINE AND CHLORTHALIDONE IN PATIENTS WITH ARTERIAL HYPERTENSION.

F. GALLETTI, P. STRAZZULLO, G. BARBA, R. IACONE,*R.GAGLIARDI M. TREVISAN & M. MANCINI.

Institute of Internal Medicine & Metabolic Diseases
2nd Medical School, University of Naples, Italy.
* Medical Department, Bayer, Italy.

INTRODUCTION

The value of diuretics as a first step treatment of hypertension has been questioned on the basis of the occurrence of untoward metabolic side effects (1-4).On the other hand, previous studies showed no significant decrease in serum potassium (K) levels during treatment with Muzolimine (MZ), at least in short term trials (5,6). Aims of this study were: i) to confirme the clinical efficacy of long term treatment with either a high-ceiling (MZ) or a low-ceiling diuretic (Chlorthalidone, CHL); ii) to evaluate possible metabolic side effects during chronic treatment with these two drugs; iii) to evaluate their effects on some aspects of sodium (Na) and K metabolism.

METHODS

The study was carried out with a single blind design. 20 untreated hypertensive subjects, WHO class I-II, aged 25-65 years, were randomized into two groups: a) MZ 30 mg once a day, for 16 weeks; b) CHL 25 mg once a day for 16 weeks. The following parameters were evaluated during the trial: supine and standing arterial blood pressure (BP) and heart rate; body weight; fasting blood glucose; oral glucose tolerance test (OGTT); creatinine clearance (GFR); serum uric acid; plasma renin activity (PRA); plasma and red blood cell (RBC) Na and K concentration; RBC Na-Li countertransport and Na-K cotransport. Statistical evaluation of results was done by Student's t-test or by one-way ANOVA.

RESULTS AND DISCUSSION

Both MZ and CHL had clinically meaningful and statistically significant BP lowering effect (supine mean BP, MZ: 117$\pm$3 vs 102$\pm$3 mmHg**, CHL: 123$\pm$3 vs 109$\pm$3 **; standing mean BP, MZ 119$\pm$2 vs 106$\pm$3 **, CHL: 122$\pm$4 vs 108$\pm$4 **; **=$p<0.01$) without changes in heart rate. Both drugs affected most metabolic parameters to a modest and similar degree (Tab.I). Table II summarizes the effects of MZ and CHL treatment on electrolyte metabolism. Both drugs significantly increased PRA. CHL therapy was associated with a slightly higher decrease of plasma K levels compared to MZ, and with a significant reduction in RBC K concentration. The investigation Na and K transport by RBCs, isolated at baseline and at the end of 16 week treatment period, did not show significant changes in ion fluxes (Na-K cotransport and Na-Li countertransport). This finding however, does not exclude the possibility of a direct effect of either drug on these transports systems in circulating erythrocyte in vivo. In conclusion diuretic monotherapy was well tolerated and proved to be effective in the hypertensive patients studied although it was associated with some metabolic side effects as previously described. Treatment with MZ seemed to have somewhat lower effects on K metabolism.

Table I. - METABOLIC PARAMETERS DURING DIURETIC TREATMENTS.

	MUZOLIMINE			CHLORTHALIDONE		
Weeks	0	8	16	0	8	16
Body Weight (Kg)	76	76	76	72	73	73
	5	5	5	5	6	6
GFR (ml/min)	100	/	97	104	/	•80
	13	/	9	10	/	7
Uric Acid (mg/100 ml)	5.0	5.0	••6.0	4.7	5.0	••5.2
	0.4	0.3	0.4	0.5	0.5	0.6
Glucose (mg/100 ml)	94	95	98	95	97	••104
	5	5	3	14	19	15
OGTT (g·min/100 ml)	12.0	/	13.2	14.4	/	14.9
	3.9	/	1.3	1.1	/	1.4

Data are expressed as MEAN±SEM. •p<0.05; ••p<0.01

Table II.- ELECTROLYTE METABOLISM DURING DIURETIC TREATMENTS

	MUZOLIMINE			CHLORTHALIDONE		
Weeks	0	8	16	0	8	16
Plasma Na (mmol/l)	143	143	144	142	142	144
	0.9	0.8	0.6	0.8	1.1	0.9
Plasma K (mmol/l)	4.1	4.1	3.9	4.3	•3.8	••3.7
	0.1	0.2	0.1	0.8	0.2	0.1
PRA (ng/100 ml/h)	0.7	/	••1.5	0.4	/	••0.9
	0.2	/	0.4	.07	/	0.2
RBC Na (mmol/l cells)	9.0	8.8	8.7	8.6	8.1	8.4
	0.5	0.7	0.5	0.5	0.4	0.3
RBC K (mmol/l cells)	98	103	98	104	103	••89
	3	8	4	3	3	2
RBC Na-Li Count.	.27	.27	.26	.36	.39	.45
(mmol/l cells/h)	.03	.04	.03	.04	.05	.07
RBC Na-K Cot.	.77	.79	.90	.75	.78	.77
(mmol/l cells/h)	.09	.09	.10	.07	.07	.08

Data are expressed as MEAN±SEM. •p<0.05; ••p<0.01

REFERENCES

1) Conn, J.W. N. Engl. Med. 273: 1135, 1965.
2) Ames, R.P. & Hill, P. Am. J. Med. 61: 748, 1976.
3) Breckenridge, A. Lancet I: 15, 1966.
4) James, P.K. Am. J. Med. 5: 18, 1984.
5) Loew, D. Curr. Med. Res. Opin.4: 455, 1976.
6) Strazzullo, P., Ferrara, L.A., Galletti, F., Mancini, Marcello, Mastranzo, P. & Mancini, M. In: Recent Advances In Diuretic Therapy (Ed V.E. Andreucci), Excerpta Medica, 1982,pp.328-334.

ETOZOLIN IN HYPERTENSION WITH RENAL FAILURE

F. QUARELLO, R. BOERO, C. GUARENA, G. GIRAUDO, G. BELTRAME, G. PICCOLI.

Cattedra di Nefrologia Medica dell'Università di Torino (Prof. A. Vercellone). Divisioni di Nefrologia e Dialisi. Ospedale S. Giovanni Battista, Torino. Italy.

INTRODUCTION

Etozolin is a diuretic and antihypertensive drug, recently proposed for the treatment of arterial hypertension. The molecule is a racemic mixture of two enantiomers: l-etozolin acts as loop diuretic, whereas the d(+) enantiomer has no natriuretic activity, but seems to provide vascular relaxation [1,2].

Little information is available on the efficacy and tolerability of this compound in patients with hypertension and renal failure [3].

The aim of this study is to evaluate the antihypertensive and humoral effects of etozolin in patients with renal insufficiency.

PATIENTS AND METHODS

Seven ambulatory patients (5 males, 2 females), 19 to 67 yr old (mean age 54.5 yr) with mild to moderate arterial hypertension and chronic renal failure, were studied. Creatinine clearance rates ranged from 15 to 50 ml/min. Three had chronic glomerulonephritis, three interstitial nephritis and one polycystic kidney disease. None of the patients have heart or hepatic failure and all were oedema free. All were at a constant dietary water and sodium intake, checked by 24 hr urine collections, and gave their informed consent.

After two weeks of placebo wash out, patients received etozolin 200 mg/daily by mouth in a single dose. If after the first 2 wk diastolic blood pressure was still > 95 mmHg etozolin was increased to 400 mg/daily.

The following parameters were evaluated at the start of the study and after 15 and 30 days: body weight, blood pressure and heart rate in sitting position, urea and creatinine clearance, serum and urinary sodium and potassium, serum calcium and uric acid, plasma renin activity.

Statistical evaluation was carried out with the Kruskall-Wallis ANOVA and the Wilcoxon matched pairs test. Data are expressed as means±SEM.

RESULTS

Main results are reported in Tables I,II,III and in Fig. 1.
In two patients drug dosage was increased to 400 mg/daily.

	CONTROL	15 days	30 days	p value
Systolic B.P. (mmHg)	156±4	145±7	137±3	0.07
Diastolic B.P. (mmHg)	101±2	89±5	82±4	0.02
Heart Rate (b/min)	70±5	73±5	73±4	n.s.
Boby weight (Kg)	65±4	65±3	65±4	n.s.

Tab. I. Effects of etozolin treatment on arterial pressure, heart rate and body weight.

DISCUSSION

Our results show that etozolin is an effective antihypertensive drug even in mild to moderate hypertensive patients with advanced renal failure [Tab. I, Fig. 1]. The antihypertensive effect was probably not secondary only to the diuretic and natriuretic action, since body weight and urinary sodium excretion did not change significantly [Tab . I, II], and could be related to the direct vasodilating effect of etozolin [1].

	CONTROL	15 days	30 days	p value
Plasma Sodium (mEq/l)	140±1	139±1	140±1	n.s.
Plasma Potassium (mEq/l)	4.5±0.1	4.3±0.2	4.2±0.1	n.s.
Plasma Calcium (mg/dl)	9.5±0.3	-	9.4±0.2	n.s.
Urinary Volume (ml/day)	2130±220	2380±215	2280±230	n.s.
Urinary Sodium (mEq/day)	127±16	167±15	137±13	n.s.
Urinary Potassium (mEq/day)	42±5	52±8	46±7	n.s.

Tab. II. Effects of etozolin treatment on plasma and urinary electrolytes.

The drug was well tolerated, and no adverse effect was seen as regards renal function and plasma urea, creatinine and uric acid concentration [Tab. III]. Interestingly, plasma potassium concentration fell slightly and non significantly during etozolin treatment [Tab. II], and plasma renin activity remained stable [Tab.III].

	CONTROL	15 days	30 days	p value
Urea (mg/dl)	122±15	124±12	135±16	n.s.
Creatinine (mg/dl)	4.0±0.4	4.4±0.4	4.1±0.4	n.s.
Creatinine clearance (ml/min)	26.5±5	22.5±5	23.5±4	n.s
Uric acid (mg/dl)	5.3±0.4	-	5.5±0.5	n.s.
Plasma Renin Activity (ng/AII/ml/h)	0.5±0.1	-	0.6±0.2	n.s.

Tab. III. Effects of etozolin treatment on renal function and plasma composition.

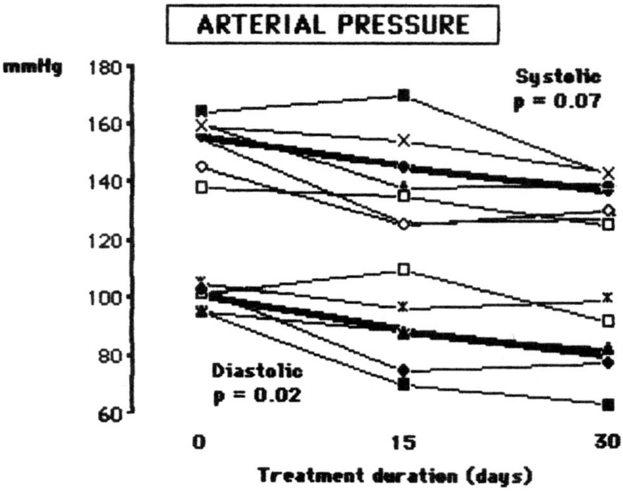

Fig. 1. Effects of etozolin treatment on arterial pressure. Bold lines represent mean values.

REFERENCES

1. Greven, J., Defrain, W., Glaser, K., et al. Europ. J. Physiol. 384: 57-68, 1980.
2. Greven, J., Heindereick, O. Arzneimittelforschung 27: 1755-1757, 1977.
3. Knauf, H., Liebig, R., Schollmeyer, P., Rosenthal, J., Koelle, E.U., Mutschler, E. Eur. J. Clin. Pharmacol. 26: 687-693, 1984.

EFFICACY AND TOLERABILITY OF MUZOLIMINE IN THE LONG-TERM TREATMENT OF ESSENTIAL HYPERTENSION

M. CARNOVALI, C. BORGNINO*, E. CRESPI, M. PANOZZO, A. MISSAGLIA, G. BANDERALI, AND G.B. PONTI

Hypertension Unit, Rho Hospital, Milan, Italy
* Medical Department, Bayer Italia, Milan, Italy

INTRODUCTION

Muzolimine (Edrul^{R}, Bayropharm Italiana) is a new high-ceiling long-acting loop diuretic (1-3). Its anti-hypertensive effect has been confirmed in several acute (4) and prolonged (5-8) clinical studies.

Aim of our study was to evaluate the long-term efficacy and tolerability of muzolimine in mild to moderate essential hypertension.

PATIENTS AND METHODS

Seventeen out-patients (14 females and 3 males), aged 51.2 ± 6.4 years (range 37-64 yrs) with mild to moderate essential hypertension (diastolic blood pressure between 100 and 115 mmHg), after a 2-week placebo period, were treated with 1 tablet (20 mg) of muzolimine q.d. for 1 year. Informed consent was obtained in all cases.

Systolic and diastolic blood pressure and heart rate were measured in sitting position at the end of the placebo period, every 15 days in the initial 6-week treatment period, and at the end of the 3rd, 6th, 9th and 12th month. After the initial 6 weeks a combination with other anti-hypertensive drugs was performed in not adequately controlled (diastolic blood pressure > 95 mmHg) patients.

Blood samples for evaluation of clinical chemistry parameters were collected after the placebo period and at the end of the 1st, 2nd, 6th and 12th month of treatment.

The results were analyzed by means of ANOVA test.

RESULTS

Mean systolic and diastolic blood pressure (BP) values during the initial 6 weeks of treatment are reported in Table 1. A significant decrease in systolic ($p < 0.001$) and diastolic ($p < 0.001$) BP values was detected. Systolic BP decreased from 168.2 $\pm$ 12.0 to 150.6 $\pm$ 10.1 mmHg and diastolic BP decreased from 105.0 $\pm$ 4.3 to 93.8 $\pm$ 5.7 mmHg.

After this period 11 patients satisfactorily controlled (diastolic BP $\leq$ 95 mmHg) continued monotherapy with muzolimine. Their mean BP values are shown on Table 2. During the long-term treatment a further significant ($p < 0.005$) reduction of diastolic BP was observed, without a further significant decrease in systolic BP. No changes in heart rate were observed throughout the treatment.

The other 6 patients were given a combination treatment with α-, β-blockers, or calcium antagonists, thus achieving a good BP control.

Laboratory parameters are listed in Table 3. Statistically significant changes were detected in serum uric acid, cholesterolemia, kaliemia and AST. Tolerability was good: in no case it was necessary to withdraw the treatment because of side effects.

CONCLUSION

These results show that muzolimine is highly effective in the long-term treatment of mild to moderate essential hypertension. A satisfactory reduction of BP (systolic and diastolic) was achieved in 11/17 ($\approx$ 65 %) patients with a single 20 mg daily administration of the drug. This hypotensive effect was nearly completely achieved during the very early phase of treatment; a slight further decrease in BP was noted from then on, but for diastolic values only.

The changes in laboratory parameters were clinically negligible, although some were statistically significant: the mean values did not exceed the normal range and actually the lowest potassium concentration measured was 3.4 mEq/l, in only one patient, once.

In conclusion, our data confirm the efficacy and safety of muzolimine in the treatment of essential hypertension.

Table 1 Systolic (SBP) and diastolic (DBP) blood pressure values at the end of the placebo period (bas) and during the initial 6 weeks of treatment with muzolimine in 17 patients (m ± SD)

	bas	2 wk	4 wk	6 wk
SBP	168.2 ± 12.0	157.1 ± 12.3	153.8 ± 13.2	150.6 ± 10.1
(mmHg)	(	$p < 0.001$		)
DBP	105.0 ± 4.3	96.2 ± 7.4	93.8 ± 4.2	93.8 ± 5.7
(mmHg)	(	$p < 0.001$		)

Table 2 Systolic (SBP) and diastolic (DBP) blood pressure values at the end of the placebo period (bas) and during long-term monotherapy with muzolimine in 11 patients (m ± SD)

	bas	6 wk	3 mo	6 mo	9 mo	12 mo
SBP	168.6	149.1	148.6	145.5	148.2	144.5
(mmHg)	±13.4	±11.1	±13.1	±14.4	±12.5	±11.1
	($p < 0.001$)	(		n.s.		)
DBP	103.6	91.8	92.3	89.1	89.1	86.4
(mmHg)	±3.2	±4.6	±6.5	±4.4	±5.8	±5.0
	($p < 0.001$)	(		$p < 0.005$		)

Table 3 Laboratory parameters before and after 12 months of treatment with muzolimine in 17 patients (m ± SD)

	before treatment	after treatment	p
Glicemia (mg/dl)	99.4 ± 11.2	98.8 ± 11.4	n.s.
Serum creatinine (mg/dl)	0.9 ± 0.1	0.9 ± 0.2	n.s.
Serum urea (mg/dl)	35.2 ± 7.6	33.8 ± 10.2	n.s.
Serum uric acid (mg/dl)	5.2 ± 0.8	6.0 ± 1.2	< 0.002
Cholesterolemia (mg/dl)	219.8 ± 44.6	239.6 ± 67.0	< 0.05
Serum triglycerides (mg/dl)	155.7 ± 93.5	154.9 ± 69.9	n.s.
Serum sodium (mEq/l)	141.2 ± 1.6	140.8 ± 3.1	n.s.
Serum potassium (mEq/l)	4.4 ± 0.4	4.1 ± 0.3	< 0.02
AST (U/l)	15.9 ± 5.2	21.4 ± 10.6	< 0.05
ALT (U/l)	17.5 ± 5.7	20.7 ± 7.8	n.s.

REFERENCES

1. Möller, E. et al., Experientia 33, 3, 382, 1977
2. Loew, D., Meng, K., Pharmatherapeutica 1, 333, 1977
3. Meng, K. et al., Curr. Med. Res. Opin. 4, 555, 1977
4. Ponti, G.B. et al., Curr. Ther. Res. 28, 520, 1980
5. Ponti, G.B. et al., Rev. Med. Pharm. Sci., 5, 569, 1983
6. Lucsko, M. et al., Z. Kardiol. 74 (2), 73, 1985
7. Ferrara, L.A. et al., Eur. J. Clin. Pharmacol. 28, 241, 1985
8. Kirsten, R. et al., Z. Kardiol. 74 (2), 66, 1985

MUZOLIMINE IN THE TREATMENT OF ARTERIAL HYPERTENSION IN THE ELDERLY.

L.S. MALATINO, C.E. FIORE, A. PETRALITO, M. LUNETTA (*), C. FARGETTA, R. FOTI, G. GRECO, F. GUZZARDI, C. LEONARDI, G. TAMBURINO

Istituto di Patologia Medica I and Cattedra di Malattie del Ricambio (*), University of Catania, Ospedale Garibaldi, 95124 Catania, Italy.

INTRODUCTION

Thiazide diuretics are often used in the treatment of arterial hypertension,although a number of side-effects,such as hypokalaemia,hyperglycaemia and hyperuricaemia,caused by its prolonged administration,may diminish the benefits of its hypotensive effect (1). Loop diuretics, on the other hand,have not so far been recommended in this indication because of either its sharp and short-term activity or its kaliuretic effect. Muzolimine, a new pyrazolinone derivative loop diuretic with high-ceiling activity and prolonged action (2), was shown in animal studies to cause a kaliuresis lower than that by Furosemide (2). Taking into account these features,the present open trial was designed to investigate the antihypertensive effect of a single oral dose (30 mg once a day) of Muzolimine in a group of overweight,elderly hypertensive patients who are more likely to develop metabolic side-effects on diuretic therapy.

MATERIALS AND METHODS

Study Population

Fifteen elderly patients (8 males,7 females)with mild to moderate hypertension (I-II WHO classes;mean age 67.3±8.2 SD yrs) were studied in an out-patient setting. Overweight was diagnosed by BMI nomograph. Each patient was kept on standard diet throughout the study. After a wash-out period (2 weeks),a run-in period (2 weeks) with placebo was allowed and then the patients were given Muzolimine 30 mg once a day (morning) for a period of 8 weeks.

Blood Pressure (BP), Heart Rate (HR) and Body Weight (BW)

BP was measured by an ordinary mercury sphygmomanometer both in supine and upright position and a mean of 3 consecutive measurements was used for statistical comparisons. Phase V was taken as diastolic reading. BP and HR were recorded weekly during the first 4 weeks and every 2 weeks for the remaining 4 weeks of treatment, 24 hours after the last dose of Muzolimine. BW was measured with light clothing and no shoes.

Biochemistry

Fasting plasma glucose, serum uric acid and creatinine, plasma K^+, total and HDL-cholesterol, triglycerides were assayed on placebo, at 2 and 8 weeks of Muzolimine, while plasma glucose and insulin (RIA) after OGTT were determined both on placebo and during Muzolimine (8 weeks) (Fig. 1). All the results are expressed as $\bar{x} \pm$ SD. Student's "t" test and Wilcoxon's rank sum test were used for statistical comparisons.

RESULTS

Blood Pressure (BP), Heart Rate (HR) and Body Weight (BW)

BP was lowered since 2 weeks (supine from 174/100±8/9 to 155/91±9/9; upright from 177/100±10/9 to 161/90±8/9 mm Hg) ($p<0.001$). A further decrease was observed at 8 weeks (supine: 147/88±10/9; upright: 150/87±9/8 mm Hg)

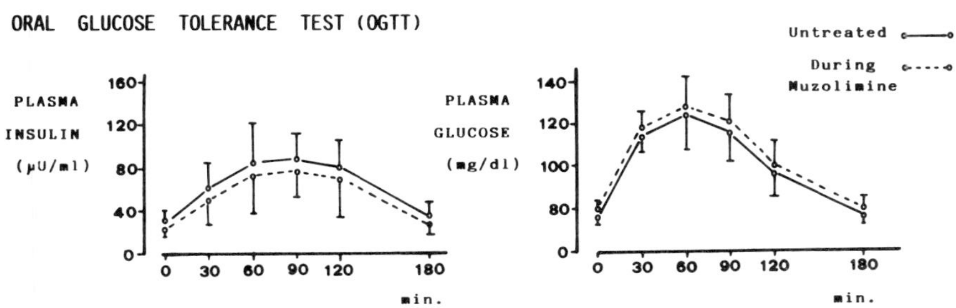

Fig. 1. OGTT on no treatment and during Muzolimine (8 weeks). $\bar{x} \pm$ SD.

($p < 0.01$). A slight but not significant increase in HR was seen at 2 weeks (supine from 68.8±6.5 to 69.5±7.3; upright from 73.2±7.2 to 75.1±8.1 b.p.m.). BW tended to fall at 2 weeks (from 71±10.9 to 70±10.7 Kg)($p < 0.01$).

Biochemistry

Fasting plasma glucose (placebo:93±0.1; 2 wks:95±0.1; 8 wks:92±0.1 mg/dl), serum creatinine (placebo:1±0.2; 2 wks:1±0.2; 8 wks:0.9±0.2 mg/dl), serum total cholesterol (placebo:240±10.5; 2 wks:243±11.4; 8 wks:245±11.7 mg/dl) and HDL-cholesterol (placebo:49±4.5; 2 wks:48±3.8; 8 wks:49±4 mg/dl), uric acid (placebo:5.9±3.1; 2 wks:6±3.1; 8 wks:5.4±2.3 mg/dl), plasma triglycerides (placebo:165±7.3; 2 wks:168±8.4; 8 wks:166±7.4 mg/dl) and K^+(placebo:4±0.4; 2 wks:4.1±0.3; 8 wks:4.1±0.3 mEq/l) did not change significantly on Muzolimine. No ECG-signs of K^+loss were recorded in the 2 strips performed during Muzolimine as well as no disturbance of glucose tolerance was shown after 8 weeks of treatment (Fig. 1).

DISCUSSION

No metabolic side-effects and a satisfactory BP control were shown during Muzolimine (30 mg o.d.) in elderly, overweight hypertensive patients. Given that the diuretic effect of Muzolimine is only elicited from the blood side and shown not to be dependent on the inhibition of the tubulo-glomerular feedback (3), that is, by contrast, a typical mechanism of the other loop diuretics, the possibility that not Muzolimine itself but rather one of its metabolites is the active agent cannot be ruled out (3). These features may account for some explanations for finding no signs of K^+ loss, thereby encouraging the use of Muzolimine long-term.

REFERENCES

1. Kaplan, N.M. Am. J. Cardiol. 51: 621-626, 1983.
2. Garthoff, B., Busse, W.D., Kazda, S., Luckhaus, G. In: Recent Advances in Diuretic Therapy. Excerpta Medica 1983, pp. 23-36.
3. Davis, J.M., Takabatake, T., Thurau, K., Haberle, D.A. Z. Kardiol. 74 (suppl. 2): 161-165, 1985.

LONG-TERM THERAPY WITH MUZOLIMINE IN PATIENTS WITH MILD TO MODERATE ESSENTIAL HYPERTENSION.

V.ORTALDA,E.VALVO,A.FABRIS,N.TESSITORE,L.OLDRIZZI,C.RUGIU,C.LOSCHIAVO,A.LUPO,L.GAMMARO,G.MASCHIO.
Cattedra Divisione di Nefrologia Medica-Istituti Ospitalieri,Verona(Italy)

INTRODUCTION

Diuretic therapy represents a first step in the treatment of hypertensive vascular disease.Its effectiveness is related to sodium and water loss and hence to a decrease in peripheral vascular resistance (1).
The Muzolimine is a loop of Henle diuretic able of an intense and prolonged natriuretic effect through a peculiar mechanism of action since it acts from the interstitial peritubular side.
Many studies have already shown an antihypertensive effect following a single dose of the drug, which is already evident at the end of the second week, and becomes even clearer after four to six week of treatment when blood pressure stabilizes.(2) Such antihypertensive effect seems to be stable with long term therapy during which a lower incidence of biochemical side effects as compared with other diuretics is reported.

AIM OF THE STUDY

1) To evaluate the antihypertensive activity and tolerability of the Muzolimine in the long-term treatment of patients with essential hypertension.

2) To study the effect of the diuretic treatment on serum and intracellular electrolytes, with particular references to the magnesium ions.

PATIENTS AND METHODS

Eighteen patients (11 m.- 7 f.)with mild-moderate essential hypertension and normal renal function were treated with Muzolimine (30 mg/24 h.) For 6 months. (Tab.1) Patients were hospitalized and submitted to a diagnostic work-up with a diet containing 120 mEq of Na^+ and 65 mEq of K^+;this regimen was also prescribed during outpatient treatment. The changes in blood pressure (BP),pulse rate (PR), plasma volume (PV),renal plasma flow (RPF), glomerular filtration rate (GFR), muscle electrolytes were evaluated.After a 2-week period, during which patients were given placebo,Muzolimine was administered.Patients were seen at bi-weely intervals in the first two months, then at monthly interval for 4 months.

Table 1 - General characteristics of the patients

Total number	18
Sex : males	11
females	7
Age	41.4 (Range 23-59)
Body weight (Kg)	72 ± 13
Plasma creatinine (mg/dl)	0.92 ± 0.9
Eye fundus	
grade 0	10
grade 1	8
Electrocardiogram	
normal	15
Left ventricular Hypertrophy	3

RESULTS

A significant and stable decrease in systolic and diastolic blood pressure was achieved; from 159 ± 9 to 139 ± 4 mmHg and 104 ± 5 to 88 ± 3 mmHg (Fig.1)

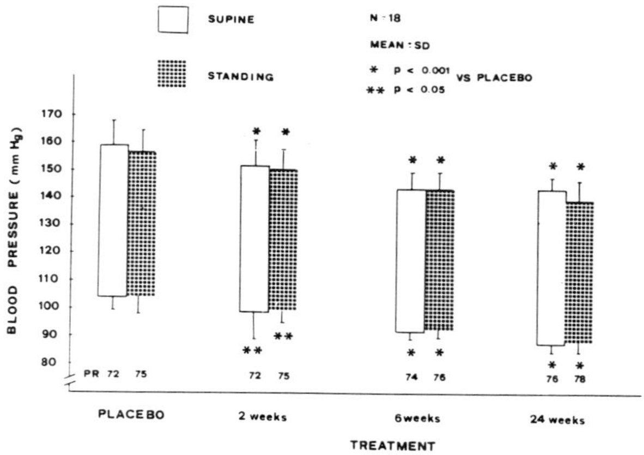

PV,RPF,GFR and intracellular skeletal muscle concentration of Na^+,K^+ and Mg^{++} were unchanged,compared to the pretreatment values (Tab.2)

Table 2 - Plasma volume (PV),renal plasma flow (RPF)glomerular filtration rate (GFR)and muscle eletrolytes before and after treatment with Muzolimine.

Parameters	Before Treatment	After Treatment	P Value
PV total (ml)	2660 ± 210	2591 ± 204	NS
RPF (ml/min/1.73 m^2)	451 ± 72	445 ± 61	NS
VFG (ml/min/1.73 m^2)	95.7 ± 10	93.4 ± 11	NS
MUSCLE ELECTROLYTES (mEq/100 g. FFS)			
Na^+	17.7 ± 4	16.6 ± 2.9	NS
K^+	32.2 ± 5.5	31.3 ± 4.8	NS
Mg^{++}	8.2 ± 0.9	8.1 ± 0.7	NS

The serum concentrations of Na^+ and K^+ decreased slightly;the mean values however stayed within the normal range. All the other plasma parameters studied did not show any significant variation.

There was a significant increase in the urinary excretion of Na^+; K^+ and PO_4^{--} at the end of the study. No important side effects were observed during the treatment.

CONCLUSIONS

Our results confirm that Muzolimine do not increase the urinary excretion nor modify the intramuscular concentration of magnesium even in the long term treatment. This latter effect may explain the lack of aritmic episodes during Muzolimine. Therefore Muzolimine seems to be a reasonably safe and well tolerated drug in the long-term treatment of mild to moderate hypertension.

REFERENCES

1)TOBIAN L. Annu.Rev.Pharmacol.,7,399 (1967).
2)O.de DIVITIIS et al. Recent Advances in diuretic therapy,315-320(1983)

HEMODYNAMIC CHANGES IN PATIENTS WITH ESSENTIAL HYPERTENSION AFTER THERAPY WITH MUZOLIMINE.

G.LICATA R.SCAGLIONE G.PARRINELLO G.CAPUANA N.ASTA

Institute of Clinical Medicine,Chair of Medical Therapy
University of Palermo.

INTRODUCTION

Muzolimine is a new nonsulfonamide diuretic belonging to the pyrazolinone group (1).It is a potent high-ceiling diuretic agent like furosemide and bumetanide with long duration of action like thiazides (1,2).

Studies in man and animals demonstrated that muzolimine has antihypertensive properties (3,4,5,6,7).

The present study was carried out to evaluate hemodynamic changes occurred in hypertensive patients (I° and II° WHO) after a month of treatment with muzolimine.

MATERIALS AND METHODS

20 subjects,12 males and 8 females from 22 to 64 years (mean age 44.96 $\pm$ 12.06 yr.) of which 11 with mild and 9 with moderate hypertension,have been consecutively examined.Subjects with severe concomitant diseases(cardiac,renal or hepatic) as well as patients with water-electrolytes imbalances were excluded.The patients were informed about the nature and purpose of the study and gave their consent.The following protocol has been used: -all the patients respected a wash-out time for 10 days;during wash-out time no antihypertensive drugs were administered but placebo and diet with free daily water intake and a costant $Na^+$and K^+content was started.

This dietetic treatment has been mantained also during the

study. - After wash-out time all the patients received a single daily oral dose of 30 mg of muzolimine for 30 days.During wash-out time and during and after treatment time,sistolic, diastolic and mean blood pressure (SBP,DBP,MBP)and heart rate (HR)were recorded daily in supine position.Moreover the last day of wash-out time and the next day after treatment time, computerized first-pass radionuclide angiography has been performed(8)and the following hemodynamic parameters have been evaluated:Cardiac Index(CI),Stroke Index(SI),End Diastolic Volume Index(EDVI),End Sistolic Volume Index(ESVI) and global left ventricular Ejection Fraction(EF).Systemic Vascular Resistance(SVR)by the formulaMBP x 60 x 1332/CI,Total Blood and Total Plasma Volume(TBV,TPV)by serum albumine diluted method (I^{125}SARI),were also measured(9).Student's test for paired data was used for the statistical analysis.P values below 0.05 were considered significant.

RESULTS AND DISCUSSION

After treatment with muzolimine (administered consecutively for 1 month) the following data have been found (Table I):

I- Increase of HR($P < 0.01$) and EF ($P < 0.02$);

II- Decrease of SBP,DBP,MBP ($P < 0.001$) and SVR,TBV and TPV ($P < 0.01$);

III- Unchanged values of CI,SI,EDVI and ESVI.

No relevant side effects have been observed.

Our study demonstrate a peculiar and known hemodynamic response to diuretic therapy in the essential hypertension(10, 11,12) and a mild but significative increment of left ventricular ejection fraction.This last finding,it's present in almost all hypertensive patients(18/20) and indicates the improvement of global left ventricular function.

We think that this interesting and unknown phenomenon is not due to the increase of miocardic contractility but it is sustained by reduction of sistemic vascular resistance and perhaps by volume depletion too.Therefore we can conclude that muzolimine is able to determine improvements of hemodynamic conditions of mild and moderate hypertensive patients.

Table I - HEMODYNAMIC PARAMETERS ON 20 HYPERTENSIVE PATIENTS BEFORE AND AFTER TREATMENT WITH MUZOLIMINE (30 mg/day)ADMINISTERED FOR ONE MONTH.

	BEFORE	AFTER	P<
H.R.	75.83 ± 9.25	80.16 ± 9.55	0.01
S.B.P.	177.95 ± 17.84	147.05 ± 12.18	0.001
D.B.P.	102.75 ± 8.89	87.63 ± 7.05	0.001
M.B.P.	127.69 ± 9.81	109.05 ± 7.12	0.001
C.I.	3757 ± 659	4030 ± 427	N.S.
S.I.	51.60 ± 10.27	51.80 ± 9.43	N.S.
E.D.V.I.	79.05 ± 14.55	77.12 ± 13.34	N.S.
E.S.V.I.	29.25 ± 6.36	26.73 ± 5.17	N.S.
E.F.	62.55 ± 4.40	65.16 ± 3.25	0.02
S.V.R.	2850 ± 510	2200 ± 271	0.01
T.B.V.	6282 ± 1280	5624 ± 1029	0.01
T.P.V.	3510 ± 725	3052 ± 701	0.01

REFERENCES

1) Horstman H;,Moeller E.,Wehinger E.,Meng K. In:Diuretic agents(Edr.E.J.Cragoe Jr) Am.Chem.Soc.,Washington,1978,p.8
2) Meng K.,Curr.Med.Res.Opin.,4,255,1977.
3) Wicher P.,Clementy J.,In:recent advances in diuteric therapy(Edr.Andreucci V.E.) Excerpta Medica,Amsterdam,1983,168.
4) Garthoff B.,Busse W.D.,Kazda S.,Luckaus G. In:recent advances in diuretic therapy(Edr.Andreucci V.E.)Excerpta Medica Amsterdam,1983,23.
5) Jabur P.,Ferreira S.In: recent advances in diuretic therapy(Edr.Andreucci V.E.)Excerpta Medica,Amsterdam,1983,119.
6) Nachev C.H.,Tomov I.L.,Vlaov V.In:recent advances in diuretic therapy(Edr.Andreucci V.E.)Excerpta Medica,Amsterdam, 1983,195.
7) Dal Canton A.In:recent advances in diuretic therapy(Edr.Andreucci V.E.)Excerpta Medica,Amsterdam,1983,156.
8) Licata G.,Indovina A.,Novo S.,Scaglione R.,Parrinello G., Capuana G. Cardiologia,XXIX,12,615,1984.

9) Licata G., Novo S. Atti II Congresso Internazionale di Cardiologia, Modena, Ottobre, 1980.

10) Lund-Johansen P. Acta Med. Scand. 187, 509, 1970.

11) Lund-Johansen P. Hypertension, Suppl. 3, 5, 49, 1983.

12) Andreucci V.E., Dal Canton A, Russo D., Veniero P., Oliva O., Cofelice E., Romano G. Z. Kardiol. 74, Suppl. 2, 43, 1985.

RELAXING ACTION OF MUZOLIMINE ON GUINEA-PIG ISOLATED AORTA

P. DORIGO, R.M. GAION, E. VALENTINI and I. MARAGNO

Department of Pharmacology, University of Padua, Largo E.Meneghetti 2, I-35131 Padua (Italy)

INTRODUCTION

Muzolimine, a pyrazolinone derivative (1) with high-ceiling activity (2) and a prolonged action, showed in preliminary studies a diuretic activity similar to that of furosemide (3) together with antihypertensive efficacy (4,5) similar to the thiazides (6). The aim of the present study was to investigate the influence of muzolimine on vascular smooth muscle and to compare vascular effect induced by muzolimine with those of furosemide whose vasodilatatory action is well known.

MATERIAL AND METHODS

Guinea-pig of either sex (300-500 g) were used. The toracic aorta was dissected free from connective tissue and helically cut into 20 mm long strips. Aortic strips were mounted in a 10 ml organ bath containing physiological salt solution of the following composition (mM) NaCl 120, KCl 2.7, $MgCl_2$ 0.9, NaK_2PO_4 0.4, $CaCl_2$ 1.37, $NaHCO_3$ 11.9, glucose 5.5. The solution was bubbled vigorously with a mixture of 95% oxygen on 5% carbon dioxide which produced a pH of 7.5. Changes in tension were recorded by means of E.C.T.A. isotonic transducer Watanabe Linearcorder Mark III. An initial tension of 1 g was applied to the strips. Drug were added to the perfusion medium as bolus of 10 µl. The tissue response to noradrenaline or to K^+ remained stable far at least 45 min (n=6). Muzolimine and furosemide were added cumulatively.

Drugs : muzolimine (Bayer), noradrenaline, furosemide (Sigma).

RESULTS AND CONCLUSION

Muzolimine relaxed preparations previously contracted with 10^{-7}M noradrenaline or 0.03 M K^+ (Tab. 1, 2). The relaxing effect was concentration -dependent. Nearly complete relaxation of contraction induced by noradrenaline was obtained with 3.10^{-4}M muzolimine (Tab. 1) while the same

Table 1. Effect of muzolimine on noradrenaline induced contraction in guinea-pig isolated aorta

Drugs (M)	Isotonic contraction (cm)		% inhib.
NA 10^{-7}	7.56 ± 0.25		
NA 10^{-7} + MUZ 4.10^{-5}	5.94 ± 0.18	P<0.001	-22
NA 10^{-7} + MUZ 8.10^{-5}	4.00 ± 0.30	P<0.001	-47
NA 10^{-7} + MUZ 10^{-4}	1.95 ± 0.41	P<0.001	-74
NA 10^{-7} + MUZ 3.10^{-4}	0.63 ± 0.10	P<0.001	-92

Each value is mean ± S.E. of four assays from four different experiments with four animals. The statistical significance of the difference from control (tissue samples incubated with noradrenaline alone) was calculated by the Student's t-test. NA = noradrenaline; MUZ = muzolimine.

Table 2. Effect of muzolimine on KCl induced contraction in guinea-pig isolated aorta

Drugs (M)	Isotonic contraction (cm)		% inhib.
KCl 0.03	7.56 ± 0.12		
KCl 0.03 + MUZ 4.10^{-5}	7.39 ± 0.11	n.s.	- 2
KCl 0.03 + MUZ 8.10^{-5}	6.49 ± 0.11	P<0.001	-24
KCl 0.03 + MUZ 10^{-4}	4.47 ± 0.43	P<0.001	-41
KCl 0.03 + MUZ 3.10^{-4}	2.55 ± 0.17	P<0.001	-66

Each value is mean ± S.E. of nine to twelve assays from twelve different experiments with twelve animals. The statistical significance of the differences from control (tissue samples incubated with KCl alone) was calculated by the Student's t-test. MUZ = muzolimine.

concentration inhibited by 66% the contraction induced by K^+ (Tab. 2). The relaxing effect induced by muzolimine on noradrenaline-evoked contraction in guinea-pig isolated aorta was not influenced by propranolol, atropine, promethazine, indomethacin, 8-phenyltheophylline or quinidine (data not shown). Muzolimine inhibited contractions induced by $CaCl_2$ in aorta strips depolarized by 40 mM K^+. The inhibition was concentration-dependent (Fig. 1). Analysis of the concentration response curves for Ca^{2+} shows that the antagonism by muzolimine is of competitive type. Furosemide, under the same experimental conditions, did not influence the noradrenaline or high K^+ induced contractions (Tab. 3).

These results indicate that in guinea-pig aorta muzolimine, but not furosemide, exerts a marked and dose-dependent relaxing activity.

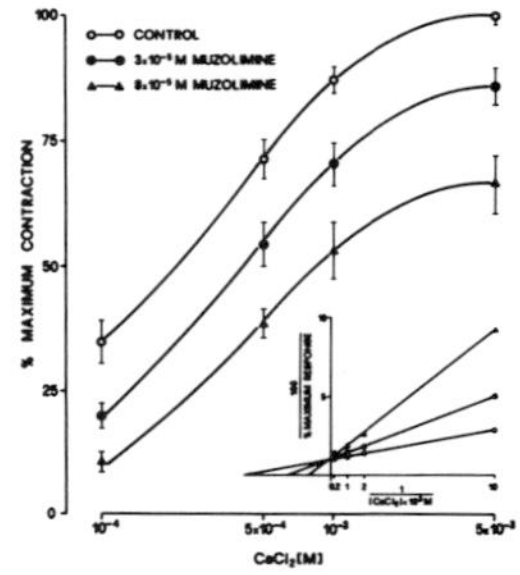

Fig. 1. Influence of muzolimine on the concentration-response curve to $CaCl_2$ in guinea-pig aorta depolarized with 40 mM KCl. The double reciprocal plot is inserted. Each point is the mean (± S.E.) of the data from 16 experiments.

Table 3. Lack of furosemide action on noradrenaline or K^+ induced contraction in guinea-pig isolated aorta

Drug (M)	Residual contraction (% of control) 10^{-7}M noradrenaline	0.03 M K^+
FUR 10^{-6}	96.75 ± 0.44	103.01 ± 0.57
FUR 10^{-5}	96.72 ± 0.82	105.15 ± 0.54
FUR 10^{-4}	98.12 ± 0.84	108.18 ± 0.62
FUR 3.10^{-4}	98.00 ± 1.05	107.98 ± 0.60

Each value is the mean ± S.E. of the data from eleven assays from different experiments with four animals.

Moreover data obtained in preparations depolarized by K^+ and contracted by $CaCl_2$ indicate that muzolimine relaxing effect is mediated by an inhibition of Ca^{2+} influx through voltage-sensitive channels.

REFERENCES

1. Moller, E., Horstmann, H. and Meng, K. Pharmaterapeutica 1:540-545, 1977.
2. Meng, K., Loew, D., Stoepel, K. and Hoffmeister Curr.Med.Res.Opin. 4:555-563, 1977.
3. Fauchald, P. and Lind, E. Pharmaterapeutica 1:409-414, 1977.
4. Bloem, Th., Lindner, P. and Braholte, J.M. Clin.Nephrology 19, suppl. 1:97-100, 1983.
5. Strazzullo, P., Ferrara, L.A., Galletti, F., Mancini, M., Mastranzo, P. and Mancini, M. In: Recent Advances in Diuretic Therapy (Ed. V.E. Andreucci), Excerpta Medica, Amsterdam, 1983.
6. Ferrara, L.A., Strazzullo, P., Scillitani, M., Mancini, M. and Gagliardi, R. Eur.J.Pharmacol. 28:241-244, 1985.

VIII. DIURETICS AND CARDIAC DISEASE

THE CARDIOVASCULAR EFFECTS OF DIURETICS

Heinrich Knauf, Gerd Hasenfuss, Hansjörg Just,
Medizinische-Universitätsklinik Freiburg/ Breisgau
Ernst Mutschler, Pharmakologisches Institut für
Naturwissenschaftler der Universität Frankfurt/Main

SUMMARY

In cases of chronic heart failure, diuretics are capable of reducing the usually increased preload. This effect may be limited in case of excessive edema causing a reduction of vascular distensibility. Nitrates are equally ineffective under these circumstances. It is possible to differentiate between so-called early and late effects. The so called early non-diuretic vascular effect depends on the endocrine activity of the kidney, i.e. on the activity of the RAA - system and the PG-synthesis, while the late preload -reducing effect entirely depends on the kidney's excretory functions. The changes in ventricular geometry resulting from the reduced preload improves cardiac function. This corresponds to a (pseudo-) inotropic effect of diuretic activity. When used in long- term therapy, diuretics also reduce the afterload of the heart. This effect is the result of a reduced pressor responsiveness (sensitivity) of the arterial system.

The indication for the use of diuretics in chronic heart failure should not be merely symptom-oriented; it should rather be based on the pathophysiological grounds of the disease. Therefore, a brief review is given first.

1. Pathophysiological Changes during Chronic Heart Failure

The pathophysiology of chronic heart failure is characterized by excessive ventricular filling pressure, and a cardiac output which is too small to meet organ requirements. In all cases of heart failure, compensatory mechanisms are activated which resemble in their effects those of hypovolemia.
The common denominator in both conditions is evidently the reduced circulating blood volume. The following circulatory adjustments as main compensation mechanisms are recognized:
1. Activation of the sympathetic nervous system
2. Stimulation of the renin-angiotensin-aldosterone system, and
3. the angiotensin-induced release of arginine-vasopressin.
4. Liberation of the atrial natriuretic factor (for details see special papers in this book).

It should be noted that when the sympathetic system is activated, the increased venous tone leads to an increase in the preload thereby augmenting ventricular filling, whilst vasoconstriction results in an increased afterload. These increases in load cause increased ventricular wall stress. The activation of the renin-angiotensin-aldosterone system usually occurs at the same time as the activation of the sympathetic nervous system. The effects are to enhance retention of salt and water, whereby ventricular filling is further increased. The increase in enddiastolic volume will raise the stroke volume according to the Frank-Starling Relation. The release of ADH is further enhanced by one of the central effects of angiotensin, thereby reducing the excretion of free water. The extracellular volume rises. These initially favourable compensation mechanisms can, however, increase to such an extent that they constitute the main manifestations of the heart failure and finally tend to worsen the situation by means of a vitious circle:

Increased preload may temporarily improve cardiac pumping, but the resulting increase in wall stress raises myocordial O_2-consumption. The raised venous tone leads to increased removal of fluid from the blood vessels, in turn leading to edema formation. The congestion in the lungs results in dyspnoe and the ob- struction of oxygen transport. Raised arterial vasoconstriction causes a reduced blood supply to the organs. Poor blood supply to the skin disturbs regulation of body temperature. Finally continuous activation of the sympathetic system leads to a down regulation of ß-receptors in the myocardium.

2. Influence of Diuretics on the Preload

2.1 "Early" effects of diuretics on the filling pressures of the heart.

Dikshit's investigations (1) demonstrate that within 15 minutes of i.v. administration of loop diuretics a distinct reduction of the filling pressures can occur before onset of any noticeable diuresis. This immediate fall in left ventricular filling pressure is described as an early vascular, non-diuretic effect of loop diuretics (2). Dikshit's investigations were carried out on patients with cardiac infarction. We could also demonstrate these effects in patients with heart failure but without severe edema.

Surprisingly, we arrived at quite different results with patients suffering from chronic edematous congestive heart failure (8). As shown in Fig. 1, patients with severe edema demonstrated no reduction in filling pressure within the first 15 minutes of i.v. administration of the loop diuretic Piretanide. Margini and co-workers likewise showed that no acute reduction of filling pressure could be seen after administration of nitrates to edematous patients (3).

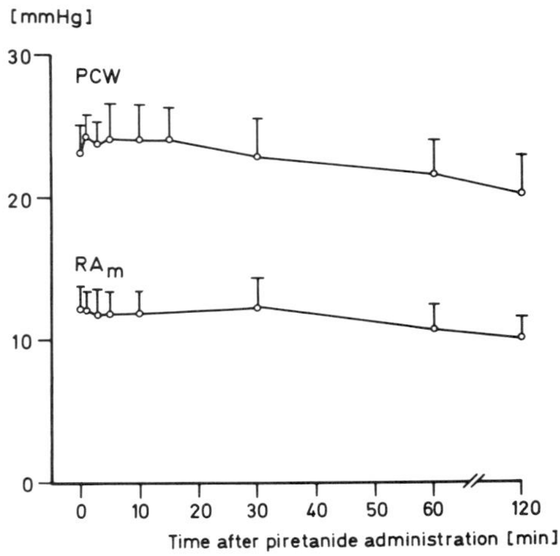

Fig.1 Changes in the mean pulmonary capillary pressure (PCW) and in the right aterial pressure (RA_m) after i.v. injection of 12 mg piretanide. (n=9, mean ± S.E.M.).

The most recent findings by Francis (4) should be cited in this context: he found that the treatment of patients with severe congestive heart failure with i.v. applications of loop diuretics could even have the opposite effect.

Francis observed a significant increase in the left ventricular filling pressures within 15 minutes of treatment with furosemide, together with a significant decrease in the cardiac index. There was a simultaneous rise in heart rate, in mean arterial pressure and in systemic vascular resistance. It took about one hour to regain the initial conditions. The i.v. administration of furosemide was temporally associated with acute neurohumoral changes: there was a rapid increase in plasma norepinephrine, plasma renin and arginine vasopressin activity. These findings are highly relevant, as they show that the desired reduction in preload is by no means demonstrable in all patients treated with loop diuretics, and that in cases of severe congestive heart failure they can in some circumstances even cause the adverse hemodynamic effect.

As a reduction of the ventricular filling pressures in edematous patients could neither be achieved with i.v. diuretics nor with nitrates, it can be assumed that the increased tissue pressure caused by the edema is responsible for this failure (5) by inhibition of venous dilatation.

The investigations by Johnston et al (2) yield further information about the so-called early vascular effect of diuretics. These authors used occlusion plethysmography to demonstrate that venous pooling only occurs under treatment with diuretics after low-salt nutrition. With a high-salt diet the effect was absent. When subjects on a low-salt diet had also been pretreated with indomethacin, beta blockers or ACE-inhibitors, they no longer reacted acutely to i.v. administration of diuretics with increased venous pooling. In nephrectomized patients, venous capacities remained unchanged after administration of furosemide.

The following conclusions may be drawn about the early vascular effect of diuretics:

Within the first 15 minutes after i.v. administration of a loop diuretic, a significant drop in filling pressures, i.e. a reduction in preload, may occur. However, this is only possible when kidney function is normal and when the renin-angiotensin system and the renal synthesis of prostaglandins is activated. The so-called early vascular effect is therefore mainly determined by the incretory function of the kidneys. Consequently, this response was not found in nephrectomised patients.

Patients with marked edema likewise do not demonstrate the early vascular effect. Neither does the effect appear in these patients after administration of nitrates, due to reduced vascular distensibility.

2.2 "Late" effects of diuretics on the filling pressures of the heart.

The drop in average pulmonary capillary wedge pressure within 2 hours after application of the diuretic varies markedly between patients. Mean pressure values for the right atrium behave similarly. As the kidney functions of the patients examined were all within the normal ranges kidney disorders cannot be held responsible for the differing reactions to the diuretic. The drop in the average pulmonary capillary pressure and the pressure of the right atrium were clearly correlated with the volume of urine excreted after 2 hours (Fig. 2). This indicates that the late effect on the filling pressures depends on the extent of diuresis.

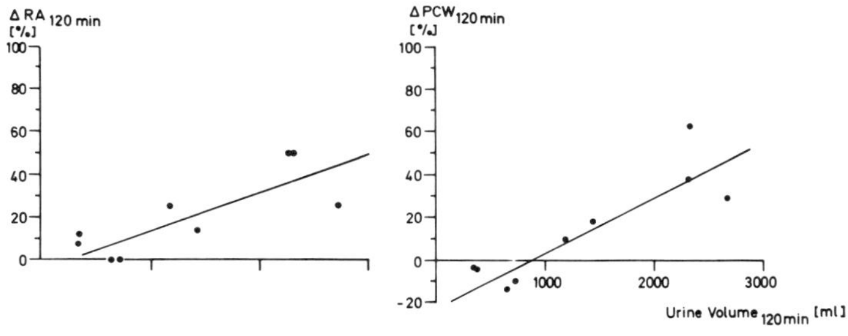

Fig.2 Percent reduction in the right aterial mean pressure (RA) and the mean pulmonary capillary pressure (PCW) 120 minutes after application of piretanid compared to the volume of urine excreted.

The large scatter in the diuretic response is in no way surprising. Brater(6) has already demonstrated that the amount of sodium excreted over time in relation to excretion of furosemide in the urine is extremely variable for cardiac patients. The dose-response curves of the patients with heart disease had comparable values on the abscissa to those of the control persons. However, the extent of sodium excretion is much less in the case of failure. In other words: the potency of furosemide is unaltered in patients with heart disease, but the intrinsic activity (i.e. the maximal possible effect) of the diuretic may be significantly reduced. The same characterics were observed with piretanide in these patients. It should also be noted that patients who, for other reasons, had a reduced circulating blood volume (e.g. nephrotic syndrome, liver cirrhosis with ascites), demonstrated fully analogous dose- response curves (7). It is clear that a further increase in the dose of the diuretic not only fails to enhance the effect, but it can also weaken it in some cases. This is of special clinical importance, as it demonstrates that raising the dose can have very serious consequences for the patient.

This pharmacological analysis shows that the mechanisms responsible for the altered dose-response relationships must be of a pharmacodynamic nature. Kinetic differences, such as changes in the volume of distribution, are insignificant. In an attempt to explain these changes in the dose-response curve and in order to analyse the scatter in the results, we compared the volume of urine excreted within the first 120 minutes after intravenous administration of Piretanide with the patients's cardiac index as determined before the onset of the experiment.There was a positive correlation between the volume excreted under influence of the diuretic and the cardiac index, i.e. patients with a low cardiac index showed a reduced response to loop diuretics. Patients with a low cardiac index also showed reduced fractional excretion of sodium (Fig. 3) (8).

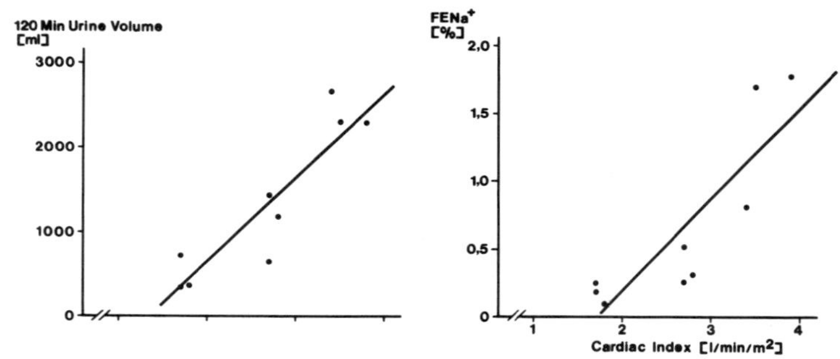

Fig.3 Relation between the response to the diuretic, i.e. the volume excreted, and the cardiac index (left). The right graph gives the relation between fractional sodium excretion (FE_{Na}) and cardiac index.

An explanation for these relationships can be found by considering the segmental transport processes along the nephron. With reduced circulating blood volume the percent of reabsorption of sodium chloride in each segment of the nephron is drastically altered in comparison to the healthy situation. Normally about one third of the filtered salt is reabsorbed from the segments of the proximal tubule. By comparison, the reabsorption rate in cases of volume depletion reaches 80% or more. The result is that relatively few sodium and chloride ions reach the distal segments of the nephron, which is where most diuretics exert their effect. The reduced effectiveness of the diuretics is thus a consequence of the low availability of substrate in the distal segments of the nephron. The cause of these altered segmental resorption rates is discussed by D.W. Seldin in this book. Skorecki and Brenner (10) pointed at humoral changes: In cases of volume depletion, circulating catecholamines and angiotensin II cause constriction of the vas efferens (11). In this way filtration can be maintained, but the effective filtration pressure in the vas efferens declines. The result is that the rate of passive backflux in the proximal tubule, from the intersititium to the lumen falls, and consequently only about 20% of the filtered material reaches the regions of the distal nephron, instead of the usual 40%. In other words: the influence of catecholamines and angiotensin result in hyperreabsorption from the proximal tubule.

Knowledge of these processes in cases of volume depletion or in contraction of the extracellular spaces allows access to appropriate therapeutic methods for correcting the pathophysiological changes. Proximal tubular hyperresorption can thus be reduced by treatment with carboanhydrase inhibitors, so that more sodium is available in the distal segments of the tubule. By combining a diuretic with a proximal tubular site of action with a diuretic active in the distal nephron, a patients's resistance to diuretic therapy can be overcome.

Krück and co-workers (12) have already demonstrated that hyperresorption can be halted in cases of cardiac failure by the administration of ACE-inhibitors, resulting in an increase in the cardiac index. The use of osmodiuretics on patients with congestive heart failure is of course out of question. They can, however, be used to treat patients with nephrotic syndrome or hepatic cirrhosis with ascites, who also have hyperresorption due to reduced circulating blood volume.

3. Effects of Diuretics on the Afterload

3.1. Acute hemodynamic effects of diuretics.

After administration of potent diuretics to patients without heart failure the blood pressure falls along with volume depletion of intra- and extravascular fluid. Thereby cardiac output decreases and systemic vascular resistance increases.

These diuretic-induced effects can completely be reversed by saline infusion. The early antihypertensive effect of diuretics is thus due to volume depletion. In other words, it is a renal effect.

In the state of heart failure the fall in aortic input impedance due to volume depletion may enhance cardiac output directly. Therefore the fall in blood pressure may not be seen. The thus improved working conditions of the failing heart may lessen sympathetic tone and thereby reduce systemic vascular resistance.

3.2. Long term effects of diuretics on the hemodynamics.

During long term treatment with diuretics in patients without heart failure the initially increased systemic vascular resistance falls again, and cardiac output increases towards normal. Typically, the responsiveness of the blood vessels of hypertensive patients to pressor agents (norepinephrine, angiotensin II) is changed by diuretics. Characteristically, essentially hypertensives exhibit a higher reagibility to pressor agents as compared to normotensives (13). Long term treatment of these patients with diuretics reduces and thus normalizes the reagibility of blood vessels to pressor agents (14). This causes the systemic vascular resistance of the patients to fall during diuretic treatment. Vascular tone, depending on cellular Na^{+} and Ca^{++} , and in turn the vascular reagibility to pressor agents is the target of long term treatment with diuretics.

REFERENCES

1. DIKSHIT K, VYDEN JK, FORRESTER JS, CHATTERJEE K, PRAKSHA R, SWAN HJC.
   N. Engl J Med 1973; 288:1087-1090
2. JOHNSTON GD, HIATT WR, NIES AS, PAYNE NA, MURPHY RC, GERBER IG.
   Circ Res. 1983; 53: 630-635
3. MARGINI F, NIARCHOS AP.
   Am Cardiol 1980; 45:841-847
4. FRANCIS GS, SIEGEL RM, GOLDSMITH SR, OLIVARI MT, LEVINE TB, COHN JN.
   Ann Intern Med 1985; 103:1-6
5. GUYTON AC.
   Circ Res 1965; 16:452-460
6. BRATER DC.
   Drugs 1981; 22: 477-494

7. KELLER E, HOPPE-SEYLER G, MUMM R, SCHOLLMEYER P.
Eur J Clin Pharmacol 1981; 20:27-33
8. HASENFUSS G, HOLUBARSCH CH, HERZOG CH, KNAUF H, SPAHN H, MUTSCHLER E, JUST H.
Clin Cardiol (1986) in press
9. LOPEZ-NOVAA JM, SANTOS JC, CARAMELO C, FERNANDEZ-MUNOZ D, BLANCHART A, HERNANDO L.
Hepatology 1984; 4:419-423
10. SKORECKI KL, BRENNER BM.
Am J Med 1982, 72:323-338
11. ICHIKAWA I, PFEFFER MA, HOSTETTER TH, BRENNER BM.
Circ Res 1984; 55:669-675
12. HECK I, KIKIS D, KNAUBER I, STUMPE KO, KRÜCK F.
Klin. Wochenschr. (1985), 63 (Suppl IV) 12
13. PHILIPP TH, DISTLER A, CORDES U.
Lancet 2 (1978) 959
14. WEIDMANN P.
Klin Wschr 58 (1980) 1971

ASPECTS OF THE MECHANISM OF ACTION OF DIURETICS IN HEART FAILURE

A.J. REYES

Departamento de Investigación Cardiovascular, Fundación Procardias, Holanda 1724, Montevideo, Uruguay

ABSTRACT

Chronic monotherapy of congestive heart failure with diuretics most frequently improves the functional class of patients. Diuretics rid the lungs of water and thus increase pulmonary compliance and diminish airway resistance to flow; a reduction in the work done by the respiratory muscles ensues, and the oxygen consumption by these muscles and the blood supply to them decrease. Arterial blood flow is redistributed in favour of territories other than the thoracic and abdominal walls.

Diuretic-induced Na^+ excretion opposes the action of the renin-angiotensin-aldosterone system and coincides with the effect of atrial natriuretic factor. The renin-angiotensin-aldosterone system and atrial natriuretic factor increase renal K^+ and Mg^{2+} outputs, as if reducing the somatic, and therefore the cardiac, concentrations of these cations were meant to help preserving myocardial contractility; K^+-loosing diuretics also augment the renal excretions of K^+ and Mg^{2+}. Notwithstanding, the effects of common diuretics on K^+ and Mg^{2+} turnovers may cause cardiac arrhythmias in patients whose myocardium is damaged and who suffer from congestive heart failure.

ACUTE EFFECTS OF DIURETICS IN HEART FAILURE

In vitro experiments in lung oedema have disclosed that furosemide vasodilates pulmonary vessels directly, but only in non-oedematous areas (1).

Diuretics reduce pulmonary vascular pressures before they exert their natriuretic effect; this acute vasodilatory action, which occurs in experimental animals (2), in healthy subjects

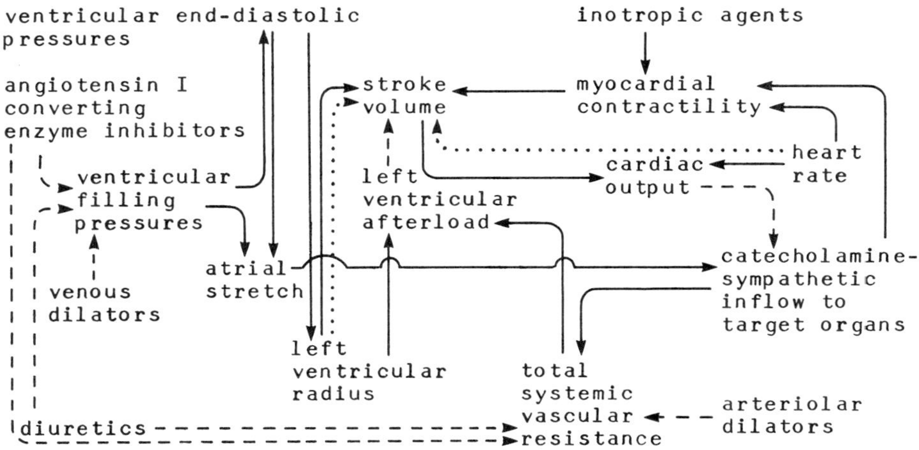

Fig. 1. Pathophysiological haemodynamic processes in congestive heart failure and principal mechanisms of action of various types of drugs used in the treatment of the condition. Each arrow depicts the directional change that an increase in the departing variable induces in the receiving variable; full arrows represent augmentations, dashed arrows represent diminutions, and dotted arrows represent diminutions elicited by extreme increases in the departing variable. An even number of dashed arrows connecting any two variables indicates that an increase in the departing variable causes an increase in the receiving variable; an odd number of dashed arrows connecting any two variables indicates that an increase in the departing variable causes a decrease in the receiving variable.

(3) and in patients with congestive heart failure (4-6), would be mediated by the kidney (2).

In patients with congestive heart failure it has been repeatedly confirmed that intravenously administered loop diuretics cause venodilation and decrease right atrial pressure, pulmonary arterial pressure and pulmonary wedge pressure (Fig. 1); cardiac output is also reduced, although slightly, in most cases (7). Unfortunately, the clinical correlation of these acute effects of loop diuretics has not deserved much attention.

In cases with pulmonary oedema furosemide has been found to significantly diminish pulmonary water 2-4 hr after intravenous administration (8). This time lag would appear

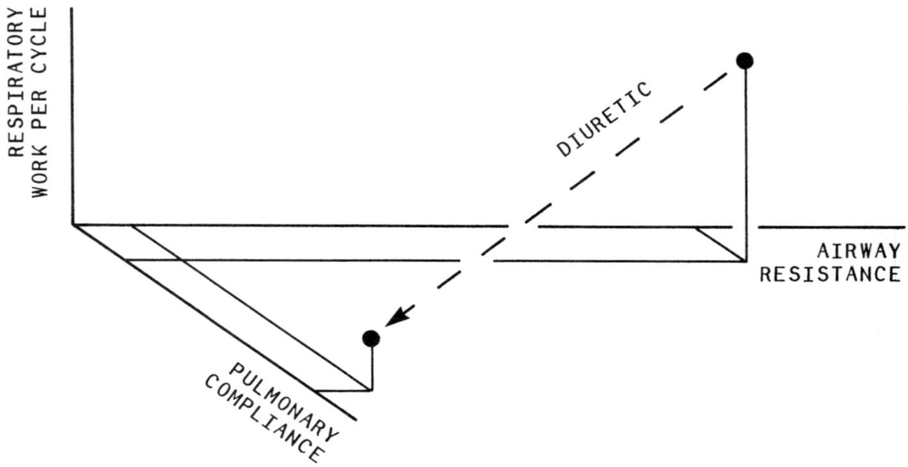

Fig. 2. Schematic representation of the effects of diuretics on pulmonary compliance, resistance to air flow and respiratory work per cycle in congestive heart failure.

to indicate that it is necessary for a diuretic to cause a significant loss of somatic fluid in order to reset the capillary pressure equilibrium in the lung and thus lower interstitial oedema.

CHRONIC HEART FAILURE

Beneficial effects of diuretics

When used as a chronic monotherapy diuretics improve the functional class of most patients with congestive heart failure (9-12). Cardiac output has been found to bear little change on average (9), though it may individually increase or decrease; the latter shift stems from the reduction in heart filling pressures induced by diuretics (Fig. 1). In cases in whom diuretics predominantly abate high blood pressure (13), or otherwise lower total systemic vascular resistance (14), the diminution in left ventricular afterload conduces to an elevation in cardiac output (Fig. 1).

The scheletal muscles whose activity accounts for the external respiration normally consume about 1% of the total bodily uptake of O_2. In congestive heart failure augmented pulmonary water decreases pulmonary compliance and increases

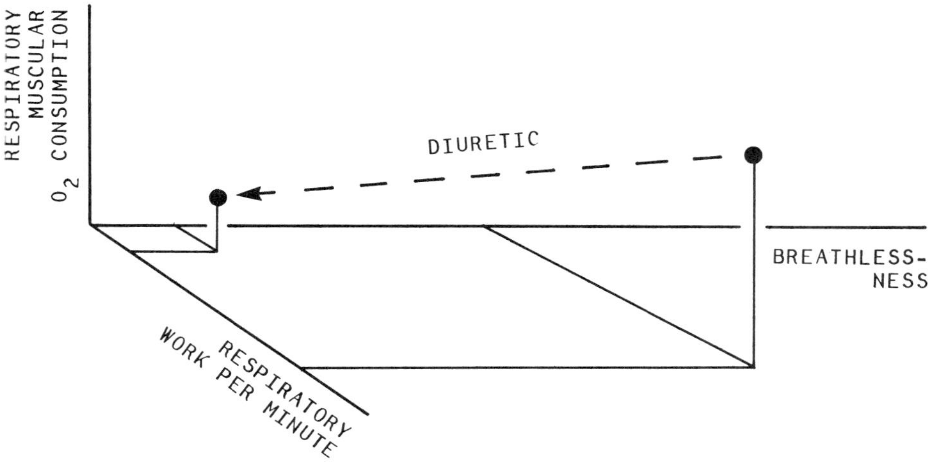

Fig. 3. Schematic representation of the effects of diuretics on respiratory work per minute, breathlessness and oxygen consumption by the respiratory muscles in congestive heart failure.

resistance to air flow (Fig. 2); these changes raise the work done by the respiratory muscles per respiratory cycle (15). Respiratory rate is elevated in cardiac insufficiency as a reflex result of the decrease in pulmonary compliance and as a response to the reduction that takes place in the blood supply to various structures that intervene in the control of respiratory activity. The rises in respiratory work per cycle and in respiratory rate augment the respiratory work per minute, thus conveying an increase in blood flow to the respiratory muscles and a diminution in the blood supply to other vascular beds. In severely decompensated congestive heart failure the respiratory muscles may consume as much as 40% of the corporal uptake of O_2. These functional shifts, which are perpetuated and aggravated by positive feedback processes, have increasing breathlessness and fatigue as their main clinical manifestations.

Diuretics increase diuresis and natriuresis and thus reduce pulmonary water; consequently pulmonary compliance is increased, airway resistance to flow is reduced, respiratory work per cycle is diminished (Fig. 2), O_2 consumption by the respiratory muscles falls (Fig. 3), blood flow is redistributed in favour

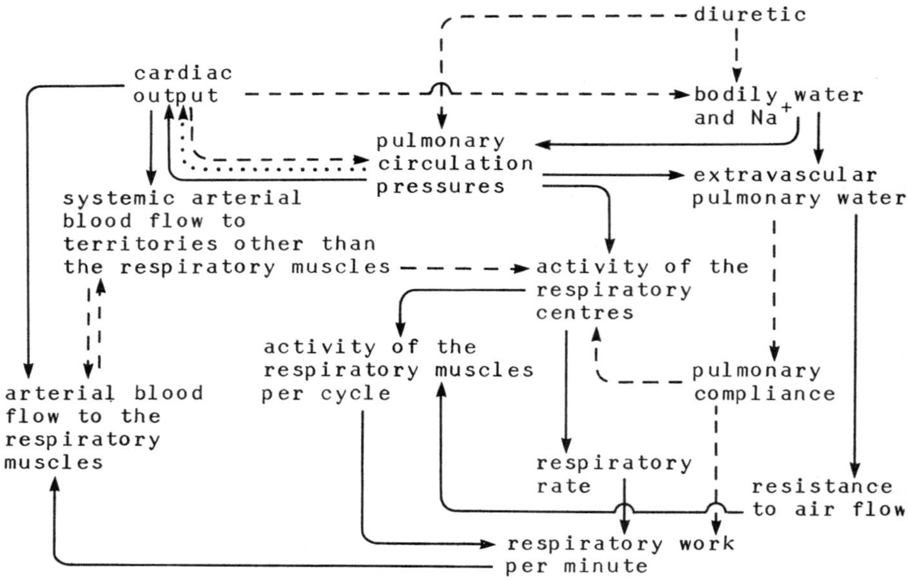

Fig. 4. Mechanisms of the beneficial action of diuretics in congestive heart failure. Each arrow depicts the directional change that an increase in the departing variable induces in the receiving variable; full arrows represent augmentations, dashed arrows represent diminutions, the dotted arrow represents diminutions elicited by extreme increases in the departing variable. An even number of dashed arrows connecting any two variables indicates that an increase in the departing variable causes an increase in the receiving variable; an odd number of dashed arrows connecting any two variables indicates that an increase in the departing variable causes a decrease in the receiving variable.

of territories other than the thoracic walls (Fig. 4), and the functional class of patients improves.

<u>Effects of diuretics which are not sought</u>

Diuretic-induced Na^+ excretion opposes the effect of the renin-angiotensin-aldosterone system and coincides with the action of atrial natriuretic factor (16) in congestive heart failure (17). Thus, diuretics would play an important role in the treatment of heart failure with significant atrial dilation. Nevertheless, the undue predominance of drug-induced natriuresis over the mechanisms regulating Na^+ and water turnovers may result in hyponatraemia.

Diuretics (18,19), the renin-angiotensin-aldosterone system (20) and atrial natriuretic factor (17) increase the renal outputs of K^+ and Mg^{2+}. Reductions in bodily K^+ and Mg^{2+} would contribute to preserve myocardial contractility, and therefore cardiac output, in congestive heart failure; overt K^+ and Mg^{2+} deficiencies may however induce cardiac arrhythmias in patients with an altered myocardium and heart failure.

REFERENCES

1. Ali, J., Unruh, H., Skoog, C. and Goldberg, H.S. J. Surg. Res. 35: 383-390, 1983.
2. Bourland, W.A., Day, D.K. and Williamson, H.E. J. Pharmacol. Exp. Ther. 202: 221-229, 1977.
3. Valette, H., Hebert, J.L., Raffestin, B., Lockhart, A. and Apoil, E. J. Cardiovasc. Pharmacol. 2: 103-111, 1980.
4. Dikshit, K., Vyden, J.K., Forrester, J.S., Chatterjee, K., Prakash, R. and Swan, H.J.C. N. Eng. J. Med. 288: 1087-1090, 1973.
5. Ikram, H., Chan, W., Espiner, E.A. and Nicholls, M.G. Clin. Sci. 59: 443-449, 1980.
6. Valette, H., Hebert, J.L. and Apoil, E. Eur. J. Clin. Pharmacol. 24: 163-167, 1984.
7. Taylor, S.H. Z. Kardiol. 74(Suppl. 2): 2-12, 1985.
8. Biddle, T.L. and Yu, P.N. Am. J. Cardiol. 43: 86-90, 1979.
9. Nishijima, H., Yasuda, H., Kazusuke, I., Murakami, R., Hayashi, K., Yamazaki, M. and Hattori, T. Jpn. Heart J. 25: 571-585, 1984.
10. Dixon, D.W., Barwolf-Gohlke, C. and Gunnar, R.M. J. Clin. Pharmacol. 21: 680-687, 1981.
11. Coodley, E.L., Nandi, P.S. and Chiotellis, P. J. Clin. Pharmacol. 19: 127-136, 1979.
12. Oversohl, K., Mehrabian, G., Hanisch, M. and Schmitz, H. Z. Kardiol. 74(Suppl. 2): 27-31, 1985.
13. Acosta-Barrios, T.N., Reyes, A.J., Leary, W.P. and van der Byl, K. Curr. Ther. Res. 33: 855-859, 1983.
14. Wilson, J.R., Reichek, N., Dunkman, W.B. and Goldberg, S. Am. J. Med. 70: 234-239, 1981.
15. Schlant, R.C. In: The Heart (Eds. J.W. Hurst and R.B. Logue), McGraw-Hill Book Company, New York, 1970, pp. 405-423.
16. Ishihara, T., Aisaka, K., Hattori, K., Hamashi, S., Morita, M., Noguchi, T., Kangawa, K. and Matsuo, H. Life Sci. 36: 1205-1215, 1985.
17. Tyckkanen, I., Metsärime, K., Fyhrquist, F. and Leidenius, R. Lancet 2: 66-69, 1985.
18. Reyes, A.J. and Leary, W.P. Human Toxicol. 3: 351-372, 1984.
19. Reyes, A.J. Prog. Pharmacol. 6: 51-87, 1985.
20. Reyes, A.J., Leary, W.P. and van der Byl, K. Magnesium-Bull. 7: 121-139, 1985.

TREATMENT OF CHRONIC NONHYDROPIC CONGESTIVE HEART FAILURE: EFFECT OF HYDROCHLOROTHIAZID AND TRIAMTEREN ON CARDIAC PERFORMANCE

G.E. SCHÄFER, H. SIEVERT

Medizinische Klinik III, Stadtkrankenhaus, Offenbach/M. (F.R.G.)

The term congestive heart failure (CHF) delineates a complex of symptoms characterized by the occurrence of shortness of breath, edema and reduction in performance. This syndrome is chiefly based on retention of sodium and fluid evoked by sympathetic and renin-angiotensin system activation. Congestive heart failure is thus characterized less by decline of cardiac output (CO) than by disturbance of feedback mechanisms. Since the underlying heart condition is mostly irreversible, diuretics appear to be a physiological approach in order to interrupt the frequently overshooting mechanisms of progressive congestion (1).

PATIENTS AND METHODS

So far, only occasional investigations have been communicated on the influence of long-term therapy with diuretics on hemodynamics in CHF (2). To assess the efficacy of diuretic treatment, hemodynamics have been evaluated in 8 patients before and 25 days after starting treatment with Hydrochlorothiazide (HCT) and Triamteren (T). All patients were normotensive and free of peripheral edema. A glycoside treatment was carried out for more than 6 weeks in all patients. The heart failure (stage III/IV according to NYHA) was caused in 5 cases by coronary heart disease and by aortic-mitral valvular defect in 3 cases. The dosage of HCT and T was carried out individually and varied in relation to the symptoms, results of investigations and weight fluctuations. On average, 30 mg HCT and 60 mg T were administered per day. The investigations were carried out by means of Swan-Ganz thermistor catheter.

RESULTS

After treatment for three weeks with HCT and T, an alleviation of the congestion symptoms and an improvement of exercise tolerance was reported by all patients corresponding to a regrouping by one stage of the NYHA classification. The body weight of the patients who were not edematous even before the beginning of treatment fell by an average of 1.1 kg. The pulse rate remained almost unchanged (87 ± 12/85 ± 15/min). In all patients investigated (Fig 1 a), the treatment led to a lowering of right atrial- (RA, from 10 ± 5 to 4 ± 3 mm Hg, $p < 0{,}01$) and pulmonary wedge pressure (PC, from 27 ± 8 to 16 ± 7 mm Hg, $p < 0.01$). The decline of afterload was also pronounced with a fall of the mean arterial pressure (MAP) from 107 ± 19 to 89 ± 7 mm Hg ($p < 0.01$) and the decline of the total peripheral resistance (TPR) by an average of 370 $dyn.s.cm^{-5}$. The pulmonary arteriolar resistance fell from 320 ± 152 to 267 ± 109 $dyn.s.cm^{-5}$ (n.s.). The cardiac output was 4.7 ± 0.9 l/min before institution of diuretic treatment and rose to 5.2 ± 1.0 l/min, stroke volume (SV) rose from 55 ± 15 to 65 ± 23 ml (n.s.).

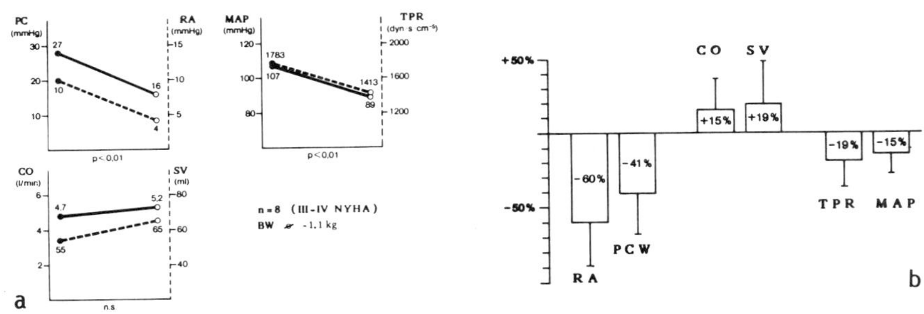

Fig 1. a) After 3 weeks of treatment with HCT + T reliable lowering of ventricular filling pressures and afterload, nonsignificant increase of cardiac output. b) Percentage deviation of the hemodynamic parameters from the initial finding after three weeks of diuretic treatment.

The hemodynamic alterations which have occurred under diuretic therapy are shown in Fig 1 b. Compared to the initial values, the pressures in the RA and in PC fell by an average of 60% and 41% respectively. On the other hand, stroke volume and cardiac output rose by 19% and 15% respectively, whereas peripheral resistance (-19%) and arterial pressure (-15%) fell to the same extent.

DISCUSSION

This study on the hemodynamic effects of chronic diuretic therapy shows that even in patients with nonhydropic chronic heart failure a distinct improvement in circulatory performance can be attained. The benefit associated with the systolic and diastolic relief of the myocardium evidently predominates over the disadvantage resulting from the lowering of ventricular filling pressures according to the FRANK-STARLING mechanism. Diuretics are thus not able only to flush out edema and alleviate the symptoms of congestion. They also bring about a lowering of high intracardiac pressures which have prognostically unfavorable effects on the cardiac patient endangered by acute decompensation and arrhythmias.

There is no doubt that the possible favorable effect of diuretics on well-being and hemodynamics can be abolished or reversed by an inappropriate dosage. The initial dose should be as low as possible (e.g.12.5 mg HCT/day) and can then be raised step by step depending on the clinical findings and the alteration in body weight. In CHF an individual and variable adaption of the diuretic dose is requested to maintain "dry weight" (3). Regular monitoring and self-control by the trained patient are the basis for management of treatment and prophylaxis. After clinical improvement and a hydratation balance have been attained, a "target weight" and a maintenance dose of the diuretic is to be laid down. In a further step, the cardiac patient is to be given an active and responsible role in the management of treatment.
The undramatic beginning of heart failure and the insidious course which frequently masks impending deteriorations require attention from the patient and the doctor. Long-term therapy of CHF thus does not only require a qualified physician, but also an informed patient prepared to collaborate under his own responsibility.

1. HAMER,J. The Modern Management of Congestive Heart Failure, LLOYD-LUKE LTD, London, 1982, pp 1-10
2. SCHÜREN,K.P. In: Therapie der Myokardinsuffizienz (Eds.W.SCHAPER and M.G.GOTTWIK), Steinkopff, Darmstadt, 1982,pp 124-138
3. ZATUCHNI,J. The Lancet, 1980, 746

COMPARISON OF THE EFFICACY AND SAFTEY OF 5 MG/ 10 MG TORASEMIDE (TO) IN PATIENTS WITH CHRONIC HEART FAILURE

I. ACHHAMMER, W. HÄCKER, M. GLOCKE,
Boehringer Mannheim GmbH

INTRODUCTION

Diuretics are one of the most important therapeutic agents in patients with congestive heart-failure. They increase elimination of water and sodium, accumulated in the organism, which leads to a decrease of the heart work and a considerable improvement of the symptoms.
The following study had been carried out to compare the efficacy and saftey of long-term treatment with 5 or 10 mg torasemide in patients with chronic heart-failure after pretreatment with furosemide 40 mg (switch over).

SUBJECTS AND METHODS

In a controlled double-blind multicentre study the patients were allocated in a randomized order to the 2 groups of either 5 or 10 mg torasemide. During the first 4 weeks of treatment the dose could once be doubled (and then maintained over the whole study), when the efficacy was considered to be not sufficient.
At the beginning, after 2, 4, 6, 8 and 12 weeks body-weight, blood pressure, pulse rate and status of oedema as well as serum-electrolytes, -uric acid, -creatinine and -glucose were recorded. Serum lipids and liver parameters were recorded in the beginning and after 6, 12 and 24 weeks.

RESULTS

115 patients with compensated chronic heart-failure after a pretreatment with furosemide 40 mg (minimum 4 weeks) had been included in the 6-month-lasting study.
111 patients completed it, one dropped out because of wrong dose adjustment (half a tablet of torasemide 5 mg), one because of intercurrent illness, one because of insufficiency of treatment, one didn't return to the centre. The patient description is shown in table I.
54 patients started with 5 mg (group 1), 35 remained on 5 mg (group 1.1) in 19 of them dose was doubled to 10 mg (group 1.2), 57 patients started with 10 mg (group 2), 42 remained on 10 mg (group 2.1), in 15 of them dose was doubled to 20 mg (group 2.2).
Main parameters for efficacy were decrease in body-weight and improvement in status of oedema. In group 1.1 body-weight dropped significantly from 80,4 to 78,4 kg, in group 1.2 significantly from 79,0 kg to 78,2 kg. In group 2.1 it decreased significantly from 79,2 to 77 kg, in group 2.2 significantly from 70,1 to 68,3 kg.
The change in body weight is shown in table II.

Table I

Patients description

	Torasemide 5 mg	Torasemide 10 mg
number of patients	54	57
male	27	29
female	27	28
age (years)	64.8 (49 – 86)	64,7 (45 – 78)
body weight (kg)	77.9	75.6
height (cm)	167.7	169.0

Table II

Change in body weight (Δ start – 6 month treatment)

groups	Δ bodyweight (kg)	
1.1	1.6	$p \leq 0.05$
1.2	1.2	$p \leq 0.05$
2.1	1.3	$p \leq 0.05$
2.2	1.2	$p \leq 0.05$

There was no significant difference between the groups. In each group there were patients with residual oedema (group 1: 16 of 54, group 2: 12 of 57) in the beginning of the study. During treatment, there was an improvement in the status of oedema. In group 1 only 3 patients had still oedema after 24 weeks. In group 2 there were only 2 patients with oedema at the end of the study.
A slight but significant fall in blood pressure and pulse rate was seen in both groups. The serum parameters didn't change relevantly in any group. The tolerance of torasemide was very good during the whole study, only mild and transient side-effects were recorded in 9 patients (mild cramps, dizziness, tiredness), which vanished during continuing therapy.

CONCLUSION

With the doses administered, all 111 patients, who were compensated under furosemide remained stable under torasemide. 1 patient dropped out because of insufficiency of therapy.
From the 28 patients with residual oedema 23 patients were further compensated under torasemide treatment. A drop in body-weight was significant in all groups, without significant difference between the groups. Serum parameters were not relevantly influenced. Therefore, we conclude that 5 mg torasemide in chronic treatment is sufficient to maintain patients with chronic heart-failure in a compensated state.

INFLUENCE ON WATER AND SOLUTES EXCRETION DETERMINED BY DIFFERENT ADMINISTRATIONS OF MUZOLIMINE AND FUROSEMIDE IN PATIENTS WITH CONGESTIVE HEART FAILURE.

F. TARTAGNI, D. DEGLI ESPOSTI, P. ORTOLANI, V. CERVI, E. ANTONELLI, B. MAGNANI

Cardiology Institute , University of Bologna, S.Orsola Hospital, 40138 Bologna, Italy

INTRODUCTION

A strong and prolonged diuresis in patients with severe heart failure may be obtained either with multiple doses or a single high dose of a loop diuretic or with administration of diuretics with different pharmacodynamic and pharmacokinetic properties (1-2). Nevertheless only a few works in literature have compared the differencies on water and solutes excretion determined by different drugs and different times of administration. The aim of our study was to evaluate the effects of muzolimine (M) and furosemide (F) in relation to their combined or sequential administration, since the different site of action and pharmacological properties might favourably influence the patient's water excretion and the quality of his life.

PATIENTS AND METHODS

Thirty patients (22 M and 8 F) with a mean age of 57 years (37-76 yrs), in II (n. 7) and III (n. 23) NYHA functional class, received 30 mg of M and 25 mg of F for three consecutive days. According to the three possible combinations (FM; M+F; F+M) and the times of drug administration (8 a.m., 4 p.m., for three days), six different sequences, were identified (Tab. I); each patient consecutively followed one treatment for a total of five patients for every therapeutical sequence. 40 mEq of KCl and 1000-1500 ml of water were also daily administered in order to prevent water and potassium depletion. The number of voids and the excretion of water, Na^+, K^+, Cl^-, Mg^{++}, Ca^{++}, uric acid and phosphate were measured each day, at the end of every eight hour period.

RESULTS

The values directly measured (*) or calculated (**) are shown in Table II. Hyperaldosteronism was found 20, 35 and 32 times following M, F and FM respectively.

CONCLUSIONS

Muzolimine induced a significantly greater ($p < 0.05$) diuresis and excretion of Na^+ and Cl^- either in the first or in the second period of the diuretic treatment. This accounts for similar results obtained after 24 hours with any drug combination. The daily calculated diuretic and saluretic effects are nevertheless significantly ($p < 0.05$) higher with the association of M administered at 8 a.m. and 4 p.m. rather than F at the same hours. The K^+, Mg^{++}, and Ca^{++} excretions resulted unaffected in the 24 hour period with any drug combination, and showed no correlations with the amount of diuresis. The more rapid effect evoked by F induced a higher number of hyperaldosteronisms and of bladder voids, in spite of a smaller quantity of water excretion and therefore F seems less tolerated by the patients with chronic heart failure. The association F+M determined, on the average, a more continuous diuresis on day time with reduced urine output at night. Regardless to the total amount of daily water excretion, that was uninfluenced by the drug combinations, a distribution of the bladder voids during the whole day was preferred by the patients and therefore the association F+M or M+M seem better tolerated by the patient with chronic heart failure who, after hospital discharge, wants to be reintegrated in his usual working life.

Table I. Sequence of treatments

Treatments	Day 1 Hour 8 am–4 pm	2 8 am–4 pm	3 8 am–4 pm
A	F + M	M + F	FM -
B	F + M	FM -	M + F
C	M + F	F + M	FM -
D	M + F	FM -	F + M
E	FM -	F + M	M + F
F	FM -	M + F	F + M

TABLE II. Excretion of water and solutes according to the different drugs and times of administration.

Period	8 a.m.-4 p.m.*			4 p.m.-12 p.m.*			24 hours*			24 hours**	
Drug	M	F	FM	M	F	FM	M+F	F+M	FM	M+M	F+F
H_2O	835±	770±	1108±	753±	563±	510±	1948±	1840±	1991±	2000±	1700±
ml	323	412	463	449	223	281	753	473	600	667	513
Na^+	71±	50±	110±	56±	43±	36±	132±	131±	165±	153±	112±
mEq/l	42	44	65	51	41	40	98	83	101	97	74
K^+	25±	23±	26±	23±	20±	19±	62±	59±	60±	64±	57±
mEq/l	16	12	10	12	10	14	19	26	25	27	21
Cl^-	117±	101±	160±	87±	77±	53±	235±	231±	238±	251±	215±
mEq/l	64	67	76	59	49	45	125	103	112	137	100
Ca^{++}	2.4±	2.4±	3.1±	2.0±	1.6±	1.0±	5.8±	5.3±	5.0±	5.8±	5.3±
mEq/l	1.6	1.8	1.9	1.7	1.2	1.1	3.9	3.8	3.4	3.9	4.0
Mg^{++}	3.0±	3.2±	3.5±	2.4±	1.9±	1.5±	7.3±	6.5±	6.3±	7.1±	6.7±
mEq/l	2.1	2.0	2.0	2.0	1.4	1.5	4.1	4.2	3.8	4.4	4.0
PO_4 mg	146±	207±	162±	155±	155±	190±	522±	487±	516±	461±	548±
	88	189	84	95	115	169	257	262	260	194	310
Uric	139±	179±	155±	108±	95±	99±	408±	344±	357±	368±	384±
Ac.mg	89	163	88	60	87	74	214	162	164	135	208

REFERENCES

1. Ziakas, G., Zioutas, G., Arvanitidis, T., and Zurukzoglu, W. Clin Nephrol 19: (Suppl 1) 85-91, 1983.
2. Stumpe, K.O., and Bartsch, B. Clin Nephrol 19: (Suppl 1) 92-96, 1983.
3. Kahles, H., Ertl, G., Riegger, G., Liebau, G. and Kochsier, K. Z Kardiol 74: (Suppl 2) 24-26, 1985

EVIDENCE OF IMPROVEMENT IN MYOCARDIAL CONTRACTILITY AFTER ACUTE ORALLY MUZOLIMINE ADMINISTRATION

R. SCOGNAMIGLIO, G. FASOLI and S. DALLA VOLTA

Cardiology Division, University of Padua, Padua, Italy

The drastic diuretics, such as muzolimine (M), because of their action on venous return and left ventricular (LV.) afterload, represent one of the therapeutical cornerstones in valvar heart disease with LV chronic severe volume overload. The study of LV pump function-afterload and LV pump function-myocardial contractility relations[1] showed that LV dysfunction depends on an afterload mismatch condition or on a severely depressed myocardial contractility. Thus, particular attention must be payed to drugs with a simultaneous unloading and positive inotropic action. In a recent work[2], it has been shown that M increases the LV pump function by decreasing the LV systolic wall stress and by increasing the LV myocardial contractility in pts. chronically treated with digoxin.

The goal of this study is to detect if M has an intrinsic positive inotropic action or if its action on myocardial contractility depends on an interaction with digoxin. Therefore, we studied LV function of pts. with severe chronic volume overload, wich have not been taking any cardiovascular drugs.

PATIENTS AND STUDY PROGRAM

The study group included 10 pts. (mean age 46 yrs.; range 36-52.): seven had severe chronic aortic regurgitation and three had severe chronic mitral regurgitation. LV function was studied by 2D guided M-mode and 2D quantitative echocardiography: end-diastolic (EDV.) and end-systolic volume (ESV.) was calculated by the Simpson's rule; ejection fraction (EF.) was derived as EDV-ESV/EDV; LV systolic wall stress was calculated as: $PAP.R/Th_{mean}$, where PAP is the peak arterial pressure (cuff method) and R/Th_{mean} is the ratio between the LV radius and the average of the septal and posterior wall thickness. As an index of myocardial contractility we used the PAP/ESV ratio.[3]

All therapy with cardioactive medications was tapered gradually and withdrawn completely before to introduce a patient into the study program. After a control LV echocardiogram, M (60 mg, orally.) was administered; then, echocardiograms were repeated after 1 hr., 2 and 24 hrs. During the study, the heart rate (HR) was monitored by an electrocardiographic tracing and the arterial systolic pressure was recorded by a mercury sphygmomanometry simultaneously with the echocardiographic examination of left ventricle.

CHANGES IN LEFT VENTRICULAR PERFORMANCE

The greatest changes on LV function occurred 2 hrs. after acute orally M administration. No significant modifications were present after 24 hrs. PAP and HR did not change significantly during the study.
The linear relation between control and after M values of EF differed from the identity line for control values greater than 48%. The myocardial contractility index (PAP/ESV.) increased after muzolimine and the linear relation between control and after drug values differed from the identity line (dashed line.) starting from control values greater than 2 (Fig-1.).

LV systolic wall stress did not change significantly during this acute study; moreover, the unloading action of M was previously demonstrated after protracted treatment.[1]

These data suggest an intrinsic mild-to-moderate positive inotropic action of muzolimine wich can improve LV function in pts. with a moderate depression of myocardial contractility.

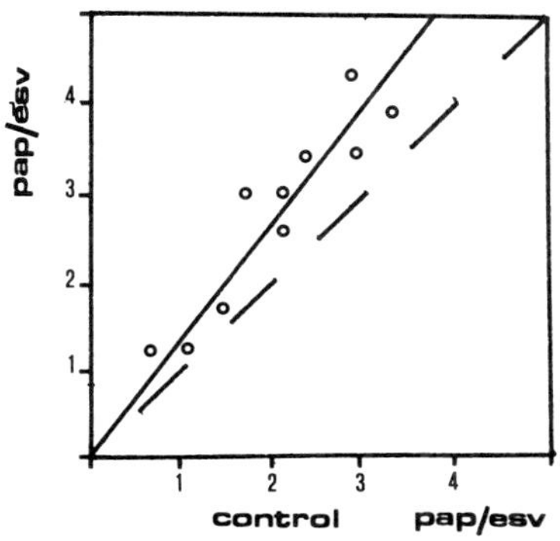

FIG-1: Relation between control and after M values of PAP/ESV ratio.

REFERENCES

1- Scognamiglio R, Roelandt J, Fasoli G: Relation between myocardial contractility, hypertrophy and pump performance in patients with chronic aortic regurgitation: an echocardiographic study.
Int. J. Cardiol. 6:473-484,1984.

2- Dalla Volta S, Scognamiglio R, Sorbo MD, Fasoli G, Maragno I: Effect of muzolimine in aortic insufficiency with different levels of left ventricular function.
Z. Kardiol. 74,suppl.2:13-18,1985.

3- Sagawa K: The end-systolic pressure-volume relation of the ventricle: definition, modification and clinical use.
Circulation 63:238-249,1981.

INTRAINDIVIDUAL COMPARISON OF EFFECTS OF PIRETANIDE, BUMETANIDE AND FUROSEMIDE IN CONGESTIVE HEART FAILURE

B.KRUEGER, R.THIEMANN

Medical Clinic, University of Erlangen-Nuernberg, D - 8520 Erlangen, FRG

The dose ratio between Furosemide (F), Piretanide (P) and Bumetanide (B) for equivalent diuretic and natriuretic action in healthy volunteers is reported as 40 mg F = 12 mg P = 1 mg B (1,2,3,4). Mean sodium excretionwithin four hours after application of 40 mg F - given intravenously - is of the order of 245 mVal sodium in healthy volunteers. It has been shown by Kamp et al. (5) that the dose ratio between F and B for equivalent diuretic action in healthy volunteers is different from patients with chronic renal insufficiency. The aim of our investigation was to study the dose ratio between the three loop diuretics Furosemide, Piretanide and Bumetanide, the most recently marketed loop diuretics, in patients with congestive heart failure.

PATIENTS AND METHODS

In 9 patients with decompensated congestive heart failure (NYHA III-IV) an intraindividual comparison of urine-, sodium-, potassium- and chloride-excretion between F (40 mg F), P (12mg and 6 mg P) and B (1 mg B) - given intravenously to avoid differences of resorption - was performed. Medication has not been changed the last 7 days before start of the study - with exception of F, given intravenously in addition in cases of clinical indication. All patients took Beta-Acetyldigoxin for at least 14 days before start of the study.

RESULTS

Excretion of sodium and potassium

Na	0 - 4 hrs	0 - 24 hrs	K 0 - 4 hrs	0 - 24 hrs	mVal
40 mg F	92.10	127.37	22.08	56.40	
12 mg P	100.89	136.80	21.70	51.93	
1 mg B	68.33	110.61	19.44	52.81	
6 mg P	45.84	93.32	13.55	49.38	

Na/K = Quotient of excreted sodium and potassium

	0 - 4 hrs	0 - 12 hrs	0 - 24 hrs
4o mg F	4.16	2.77	2.26
12 mg P	4.76	3.33	2.63
1 mg B	3.57	2.50	2.09
6 mg P	3.03	1.85	1.89

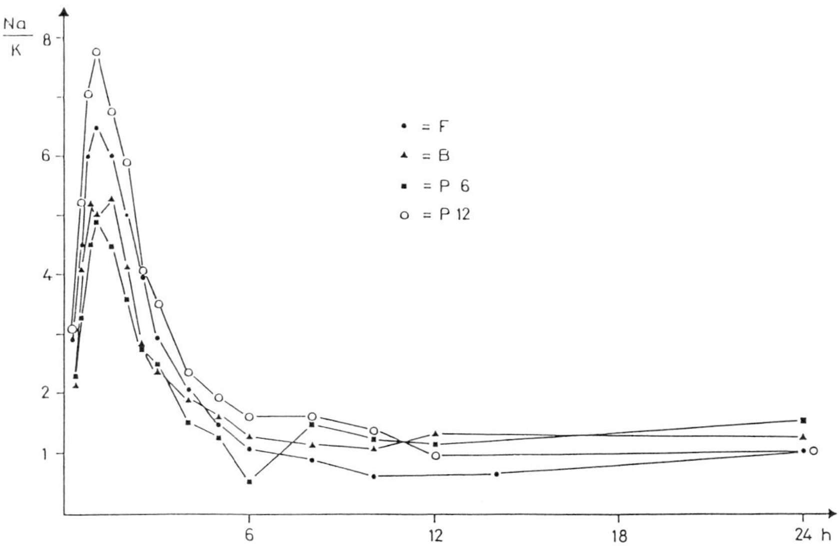

Maximal excretion of sodium and potassium per minute

	μVal Na/min	μVal K/min
4o mg F	759.37	158.05
12 mg P	886.27	133.08
1 mg B	646.98	125.85
6 mg P	503.75	117.52

Relative Natriuresis (F=100 percent)

%	0 - 4 hrs	0 - 12 hrs
40 mg F	**100**	**100**
12 mg P	109	119
1 mg B	73	96
6 mg P	50	67

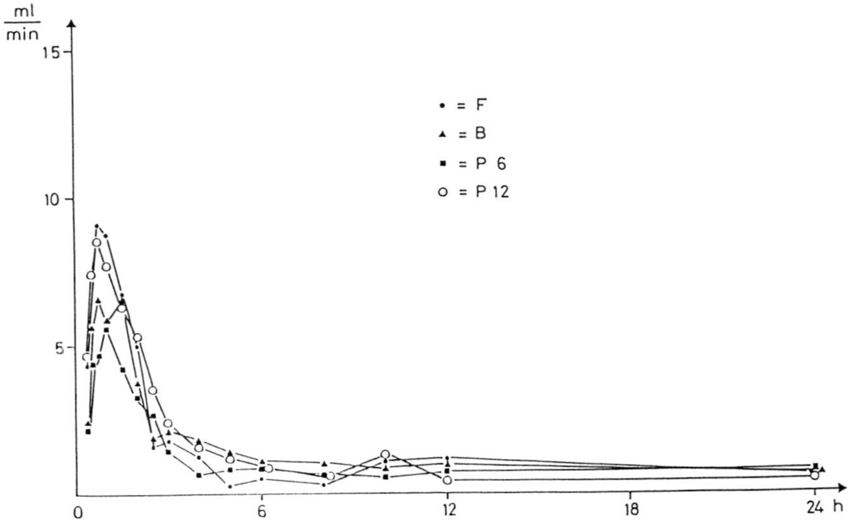

DISCUSSION

The dose ratio between Furosemide, Piretanide and Bumetanide for equivalent diuretic activity in patients with cardiac failure differs from that in healthy volunteers. During the first four hours after application 12 mg P showed the highest excretion of sodium, followed by 40 mg F, 1 mg B and 6 mg P. At the same time 12 mg P produced an potassium loss equal to 40 mg F, resulting in a significantly higher Na/K-Quotient after 12 mg P.

In comparison with the natriuretic activity in volunteers the natriuresis of the analysed diuretics is reduced on less by half the activity in patients with cardiac failure.

References

1. Roberts, C.J.C., Homeida, M., Roberts, F. Br.J.clin.Pharmac. 6: 129-133, 1978.
2. Murdoch, W.R., Auld, W.H.R. Postgrad.med.J. 51: 10-14, 1975.
3. Asbury, M.J., Gatenby, P.B.B., O'Sullivan, S., Bourke, E. Br.med.J. 1: 211-213 , 1972.

IX. DIURETICS AND RENAL DISEASE

PREVENTION OF ACUTE RENAL FAILURE (ARF) BY DIURETICS AND HYDRATION.

R. FAEDDA, A. SATTA, G.F. BRANCA, F. TURRINI, E. BARTOLI.

Istituto di Patologia Medica, University of Sassari, Viale San Pietro 12, 07100 Sassari, Italy.

INTRODUCTION

Although different pathogenetic factors are involved in the genesis of ARF (1), the morphological and functional modifications that occur are very similar and usually confined to the proximal tubule. There are modifications in active transport mechanisms, in permeability and a clear reduction of the mithocondrial cellular energy (2,3). The acute tubular damage, confirmed by the decreased activity of the correspondent enzyme markers, can be considered the common denominator of all the experimental models of ischemic ARF. Brush border and necrotic cells form casts that occlude the proximal and then the distal convoluted tubule (4). In these cases it was demonstrated that a large infusion of saline solution can prevent the oliguria, as does pretreatment with mannitol, vascular dilators and furosemide (5,6,7). The latters reduce the vascular resistances and increase the urinary excretion of solutes. Furosemide, on the other hand, inhibits the reabsorption of NaCl in the cells of Henle's loop, causing a drop in intracellular Na with inactivation of the Na-K-ATPase enzyme. Cells that are not using the residual ATP are therefore less exposed to the effects of the transitory ischemia. Finally a pretreatment with substances which inhibit xantine-oxidase was proposed. These substances block the production of superoxide radicals (7), decrease the vascular permeability, facilitating a quick functional recovery of the ischemic organ. The aim of our study is therefore to verify the importance of the volume load in the recovery of renal function during an experimental model of ischemic ARF. This was performed in the presence and in the absence of drugs and using different infusion rates.

MATERIAL AND METHODS

The experiments were performed on 36 Wistar rats weighing 250 to 400 g. After a 12 hour fast,they were anesthetized with Tiopenthal-Na (50 mg/ Kg). On a surgical table at 37° C, a tracheal tube was inserted and catheters placed in the jugular vein,femoral artery and ureters.The renal arteries were dissected free of the surrounding tissue and exposed.After quantitatively replacing the surgical losses, a maintenance infusion of an artificial isotonic solution containing normal concentrations of Na bicarbonate,NaCl, KCl and glucose was given. It contained ^{131}I-Hypaque in concentrations suitable for clearance measurements. The infusion of isotonic fluids was then set at one of the different rates (either 1-3-5-12 ml/hr) to achieve and maintain extracellular volume expansion. At steady state, two clearance periods were performed on both kidneys simultaneously. During the subsequent experimental period in the same animal one kidney served as control of the contralateral organ . In 7 rats (group I) the right renal artery was clamped for 20 minutes to induce ischemia. After the period of recovery during which 3 consecutive clearance periods were performed, superoxide-dismutase (30 mg/ Kg) was administered i.v. 30 min. before clamping the left renal artery.The same procedure was also followed for the left kidney. The maintenance infusion rate was 1 ml/hr to evaluate as much as possible the protective effect of the enzyme compared to saline expansion. In group II,dimethylsulphoxide (DMSO 200 mg/Kg) was administered shortly before and during the rehabitation of the left artery. The control right kidney was clamped and reperfused 5 min. after the contralateral organ,and could not be influenced by the residual drug. The infusion rate was 3 ml/hr. In group III the infusion rate was increased to 5 ml/hr and no drugs were given. Only one renal artery was clamped and the ischemia maintained for 20 min. In group IV (14 rats) the maintenance infusion rate was 12 ml/hr. At the end of the two basal clearance periods,the left ureter was connected to a H2O-manometer and a counterpressure of 60 cmH2O was maintained for 20 min. Then,in 4 animals placebo was injected,in 5 Furosemide (4 mg i.v.) and in the last 5 Muzolimine (1.2 mg i.v.).

After 3 min. ischemia was induced in the kidneys and maintained for 20'. The recovery was studied through clearance periods performed in the early phase. Once the experimental phase was over, the kidneys were removed and fixed in phormalin for histological examination. The biochemical study associated with the experimental study was performed by measuring GSH and ATP in a separate group of 23 animals. Similar procedures were followed but the kidneys were removed at the end of ischemia and after 2-5-15-30' from the rehabitation of the artery. The data were processed statistically, means and standard deviations of the mean calculated. Significance between means was tested by paired and unpaired "t" test between regression coefficients by covariance analysis.

RESULTS

After reperfusion the control kidney showed recovery of diuresis after 25.0±8.6 min. in group I, and 21.2±5.3 in group II. Four kidneys remained anuric. In the kidneys protected with DMSO and SOD recovery occurred respectively after 15.8±6.8 and 12.8±4.7 min, $P<.05$. In the recovery phase the initial GFR measured was not different between left and right kidneys, although it rose definitely faster in the treated kidneys (Fig.1)

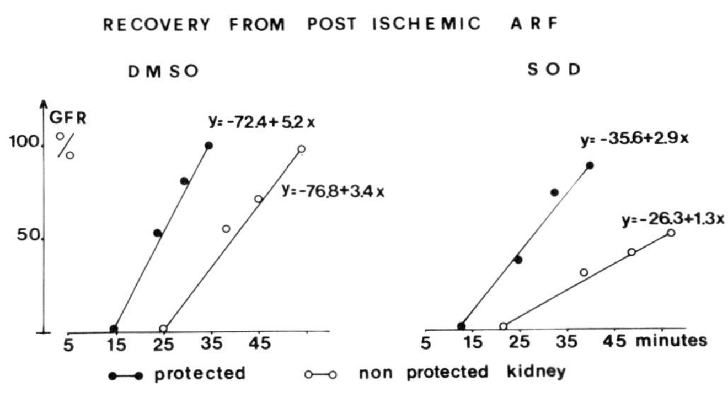

Fig 1. GFR, in the ordinate, is expressed as a percentage of the baseline preischemic value. The time after reperfusion is reported in abscissa. The closed circles refer to the protected, the open circles to the control kidney. Regression lines and equations were computed from mean values indicated by symbols.

Glutathion concentration increased progressively in the 20 minutes after reoxygenation,parallel to the physiological and hemodynamic recovery. In group III treated with a volume load of 5 ml/hr recovery occurred 20.7±8.2 min.after reperfusion. GFR,$\dot{V}$ and UNa $\dot{V}$ reached levels close to baseline in the 3rd clearance period,15 minutes from reperfusion. Finally in group IV, in which we induced hydronephrosis on the left side together with the ischemic insult,the saline infusion also showed protection.The recovery of diuresis in rats receiving placebo occurred after 22.3±13.3 min. on the right and after 19.0±11.5 min. on the left,while in animals pretreated with furosemide and muzolimine the recovery of the glomerular filtration occurred respectively after 10.2±5.0 min and after 15.4±9.7 min. In the control kidneys it occurred after 11.3±2.1 and 19.0±11.2 min. respectively.The functional recovery with time was not significantly different (Table 1) in pharmacologically treated as compared to untreated kidneys,thus demonstrating that the major protective effect was not due to the diuretic itself,but rather to volume expansion.

TABLE 1

Recovery of GFR expressed as percent of the control value

	GROUP III		GROUP IV					
			PLACEBO		FUROSEMIDE		MUZOLIMINE	
Infus.rates	5ml/hr		12ml/hr		12ml/hr		12ml/hr	
	L	R	L	R	L	R	L	R
B	100	100	100	100	100	100	100	100
1	102.5	18.5	7.7	10.9	16.4	20.0	15.9	18.2
2	100.1	39.8	32.5	53.1	29.9	22.6	41.2	39.2
3	102.3	60.3	47.4	58.4	37.4	39.3	47.0	49.6
4	-	-	62.0	78.2	39.2	60.2	48.6	75.6
5	-	-	61.5	82.1	39.0	63.5	58.8	88.4

R = right, L = left kidney. Horizontally are reported the data measured for 5 consecutive clearance periods during recovery. For further explanations see test. B indicates baseline values.

DISCUSSION

Complex alterations with different pathophysiology can occur in ARF (1).The tissue damage is more severe the longer is the time of ischemia.

Recently,experimental models of ARF were developed in animals to investigate the course of events and to elaborate effective therapeutic strategies. It was demonstrated that generous infusion of isotonic solutions (7) prevent the development of oliguria. Similar effects were recently described with substances capable of a "protective" action on the renal tissue in ischemic ARF models. If the volume load is administered before the ischemic insult and,more important,if it is combined with the infusion of a powerful diuretic, it maintains a high urinary flow by increasing the GFR and inhibiting the reabsorption of solutes. In this way the particulate matters deposited in the tubular lumen are washed away, preventing or eliminating the tubular obstruction. In our study we caused an ischemic damage and then assessed the importance of the volume load with and without association with protective drugs. SOD and DMSO either by preventing the production of superoxide radicals or by accelerating their removal had a protective effect on the kidney: they resulted in an early functional recovery,more evident in group II where the action of the drug was associated with a substained saline infusion (3 ml/hr) These results are supported by the GSH levels,which paralleled the functional recovery. In group III and IV , in which the infusion rate was 5 and 12 ml/hr respectively, the GFR reached the baseline levels at the 5th clearance time. Similar results were obtained after a pretreatment with furosemide (5 rats) and muzolimine (5 rats). Therefore,it is evident that the restauration of normal renal hemodynamics (2) is the basic factor in recovery of glomerular filtration and clearing of the intratubular debris. Furosemide,on the other side,induced a significant ATP saving by sparing the Na-K-ATPase (459 vs 300 nM/g, $P<.01$) and protecting in this way the tubular cell from the consequences of the ischemic damage. Since more than one factor is involved in the pathogenesis of ARF and in its self-maintenance, we conclude that a high urinary flow together with a high sodium excretion before the occurrance of the ischemic damage can have the best protective effect on the functional recovery of the organ,and that supportive drugs can definitely exert a favourable influence,if given in association.

REFERENCES

1. Levinsky,N.G. N.Engl.J.Med. 296: 1453-1458,1977
2. Myers,B.D.,Moran,S.M.N.Engl.J.Med. 314 : 97-105,1986
3. Kosower,N.S.,Kosower,E.M. Int.Rev.Cytol. 54 :109-160,1978
4. Donohoe,J.f.,Venkatachalan,M.A.,Bernard,D.B.,Levinsky,N.G. Kidney Intern. 13: 208-222,1978
5. Klein,L. Invest. Urol. 15 : 401-403,1968
6. Fujita,T.,Fujimoto,Y. Jpn.J.Pharmacol. 31 :795-800,1981
7. Burke,T.J.,Cronin,R.E.,Duchin,K.L.,Peterson,L.N.,Schrier,R.W. Am.J. Physiol. 238: F 305-314,1980
8. Ames,B.N.,Cathrat,R.,Schwiers,E.,Hochstein,P. Proc.Natl.Acad.Sci. USA 78: 6858,1981
9. Johnston,P.A.,Bernard,D.B.,Donohoe,J.F.,Perin,N.S.,Levinsky,N.G. J.Clin.Invest. 64 : 550-558,1964

COMPARISON OF DOSE-RELATED EFFICACY OF TORASEMIDE AND FUROSEMIDE IN PATIENTS WITH ADVANCED RENAL FAILURE

D. VERBEELEN, W. HACKER, J. ACHHAMMER, M. GLOCKE

Department of Medicine, Vrije Universiteit Brussel, Clinical Development and Department of Biostatic Boehringer Mannheim, Belgium

INTRODUCTION

Torasemide is a new loop diuretic with a linear dose response curve after administration of doses between 2.5 and 80 mg in subjects with normal renal function (1). In the present study, patients with advanced renal failure were studied because pharmacokinetics of potent diuretics are different under these conditions.

PATIENTS AND METHODS

Study-design :

Double-blind, completely randomized group comparative multicentre trial. Four different treatment groups were studied : Torasemide (T) 100 and 200 mg and Furosemide (F) 100 and 200 mg. Patients were eligable for this study on the following conditions, serum creatinine over 3.4 mg/dl, urine volume over 1000 ml/24 hrs, absence of hyponatremia or hypokalemia and informed written consent. The study period lasted three days as shown in fig 1.

Fig. 1.

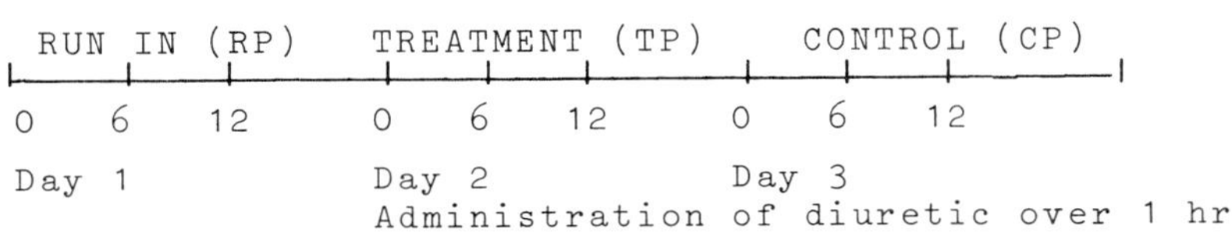

Statistics :

statistical analysis was performed using the BMPD-package (version 81/82 PSO modification). The non parametric H-test of Kruskal-Wallis and the U-test of Mann-Whitney-Wilcoxon with alpha = 0.05 were used for the comparison between the groups. All results are expressed as mean ± SD.

RESULTS AND DISCUSSION

95 patients entered the study. 5 patients were rejected because of drop-out, insufficient data or for not meeting the criteria. 90 remained for final evaluation.

Table 1. Summary of patient data.

Group	n	M/F	Age (yrs)	wt (kg)	creatinine clearance (ml/min.kg body wt)
1 (T100)	23	13/10	53±13	66.3±13.1	10.7±4.3
2 (T200)	20	12/8	56±9	68.7±17.3	14.0±7.4
3 (F100)	20	10/12	57±14	63.2±13.4	11.2±5.7
4 (F200)	25	15/10	55±13	72.1±13.6	13.3±6.8

Table 2. Summary of the effect on excretion of urinary volume, electrolytes and on creatinine clearance in the 4 groups

	DAY	100 TORA		200 TORA		100 FURO		200 FURO	
	RP	79.3	±38.8	91.2	±35.2	74.7	±28.8	86.0	±30.3
VOL	TP	107.0*	±36.1	118.1*	±38.8	104.5*	±27.4	118.9*	±36.0
(ml/hr)	CP	81.9	±31.4	79.4	±43.2	76.2	±31.3	86.1	±30.2
	RP	4.3	± 2.4	4.6	± 2.4	3.5	± 1.6	4.9	± 2.9
NA	TP	8.1*	± 4.1	9.0*	± 3.8	7.8*	± 5.9	9.7*	± 4.6
(mEq/hr)	CP	4.4	± 2.1	3.5*	± 1.3	2.9	± 1.4	4.0*	± 2.5
	RP	1.9	± 1.5	2.1	± 1.0	1.7	± 0.6	1.8	± 0.8
K	TP	1.9*	± 0.6	2.4	± 0.6	2.2*	± 0.8	2.4*	± 1.0
(mEq/hr)	CP	1.7	± 0.5	2.1	± 1.5	1.8	± 0.7	2.0	± 1.0
	RP	4.1	± 2.6	4.1	± 2.4	3.0	± 1.9	4.4	± 2.6
CL	TP	8.4*	± 4.7	10.0*	± 4.3	6.8*	± 2.2	9.6*	± 4.6
(mEq/hr)	CP	4.1	± 2.5	3.2	± 1.3	2.7	± 1.6	3.4	± 2.6
	RP	40.4	±16.0	51.5	±19.1	41.1	±16.2	44.7	±18.0
CREA	TP	40.0	±12.4	43.4*	±13.3	43.1	±16.0	38.6*	±17.2
(mg/hr)	CP	39.9	±16.4	47.5*	±26.0	38.8	±18.0	40.7	±16.9
	RP	10.7	± 4.3	14.0	± 7.4	11.2	± 5.7	13.3	± 6.8
C_{CREA}	TP	10.8	± 4.1	10.9*	± 4.4	11.4	± 4.8	11.4*	± 5.1
(ml/min)	CP	10.7	± 4.7	11.4*	± 8.0	10.7	± 5.3	12.3	± 6.8
	RP	5.8	± 4.5	4.3	± 2.2	4.2	± 2.3	5.3	± 3.8
FE_{NA}	TP	9.7*	± 4.4	10.5*	± 3.9	9.5*	± 8.1	12.2*	±10.3
(%)	CP	6.1	± 4.8	4.4	± 2.1	3.8	± 2.0	4.9	± 3.8

The excretion of volume and all electrolytes with exception of potassium increased in all groups within the 24 hours following the administration of the diuretic and was maximal within the first six hours. There was no statistical difference between the groups. K excretion is lower in the T 200 mg group. This finding confirms the observation made in animals, namely that T has less potent effect on K excretion (2). In groups 2 and 4 urinary excretion of creatinine decreased and serum creatinine increased. As a result there is a significant decrease of creatinine clearance. In advanced renal failure, urinary creatinine excretion depends on GFR and on tubular secretion. The latter may account for 40 % of creatinine excretion and can be inhibited by some drugs (e.g. cimetinine)(3). In this study, we cannot differentiate the origin of the decreased creatinine clearance in these groups of patients, but a real decrease of GFR cannot be excluded. It has been shown in rats that administration of high dose T (> 8 mg/kg bw) results in a dose dependent decrease of GFR (1). In the present study it is shown that there is a significant lowering of creatinine clearance in the F 200 group. Despite the lowering of creatinine clearance, Na excretion is of the same magnitude in the T 200 group and fractional excretion of Na is higher in T 200 than in the other groups.

It is concluded that T is a powerfull diuretic that remains effective even in high grade renal failure.

REFERENCES

1. Daragh A., Scully A., Lambe R. In : Documentation Part n° M 3 Boehringer Mannheim.
2. Roesch E. In : Documentation Part A 2. Boehringer Mannheim.
3. Shemesh O., Golbetz H., Kriss J.P., Meyers B.M. Kidney Int, 28, 1985, 830-838.

/namics and kinetics of torasemide and its metabolites in chro- (failure after i.v. administration of 20 mg torasemide

H. Spann, H. Knauf* and E. Mutschler

Pharmakologisches Institut für Naturwissenschaftler, Theodor-Stern-Kai 7, Geb. 75 A, D-6000 Frankfurt/Main, * Klinikum Dortmund, West-Germany

INTRODUCTION

Torasemide is a new loop diuretic with a similar pharmacodynamic action as furosemide. In contrast to furosemide, which is predominantly excreted unchanged, torasemide undergoes extensive oxidative biotransformation (Fig.1). From these metabolites M1 and M3 are biologically active.

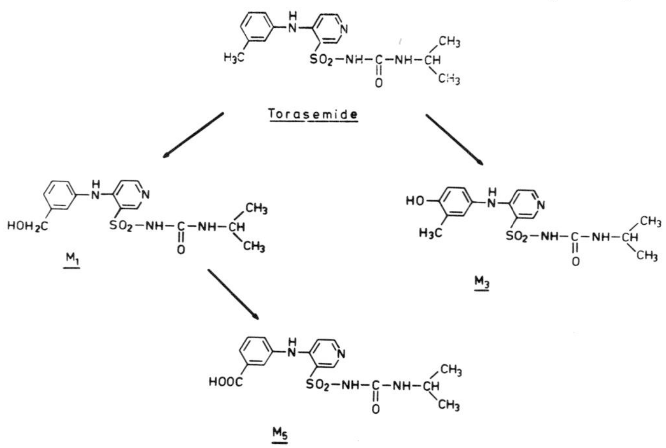

Fig. 1. Biotransformation scheme of torasemide

Since pharmacokinetic data of these metabolites in renal insufficiency were not available, the aim of the present study was to investigate the pharmacodynamics and pharmacokinetics of torasemide and its metabolites in healthy volunteers and in patients with renal failure.

PATIENTS AND METHODS

Torasemide (20 mg) was administered intravenously to 7 healthy volunteers (group A: mean creatinine clearance ± SD: 122.9 ± 22.6 ml/min; range 91 -148 ml/min) and to 9 patients with varying degrees of renal failure (group B: mean CL_{cr} ± SD: 19.9 ± 15.4 ml/min; range 2.8-48 ml/min).

The excretion of electrolytes and of urine volume was measured during 24h after administration and compared to the control period. The plasma concentrations of torasemide and its metabolites were determined by HPLC over a period of 48 h.
Rate constants, half-lives, the maximum concentrations (C_{max}), the AUC values (log-trapezoidal rule; AUC(0-∞)) and the mean residence times (MRT) of torasemide and its metabolites were determined (arithmetical means ± SD).

RESULTS

Pharmacodynamics

Torasemide did not influence the CL_{cr} significantly neither in healthy volunteers nor in patients with renal failure. The duration of action (τ) was independent of CL_{cr}, whereas the electrolyte excretion was correlated with CL_{cr}. Furthermore a good correlation was found between the sodium and calcium excretion. Within 24 h there was a drug-induced extra-excretion of electrolytes, which means that the rebound does not completely blunt the drug effect.

Pharmacokinetics of torasemide and its metabolites

Torasemide. For the parent compound no difference could be detected between the plasma concentrations (and half-lives) of healthy volunteers and of patients with renal failure (Fig. 2).
The mean half-life ($t_{1/2}$) was 5.1 ± 4.2 h for the healthy volunteers and 4.6 ± 2.2 h for the patients with renal failure. The AUC values were 10.5 ± 6.2 for group A and 9.5 ± 3.6 µg ml^{-1} h for group B. The MRTs were 6.6 ± 7.3 h in group A and 5.4 ± 2.6 h in group B.
M1. The plasma concentrations of this (active) metabolite were higher in the patients with renal failure. C_{max} was 137 ng/ml in group A and 297 ng/ml in group B. The mean AUC value was also higher in the patients (group A: 333 ± 373, group B: 563 ± 449 ng ml^{-1} h).
M3. M3 - which is as active as torasemide itself - was detectable over a short period of time only. Thus only C_{max} could be determined, which did not differ significantly between the two groups (group A: 215 ± 112 ng/ml; group B: 203 ± 192).
M5. Within 9 to 24 h the plasma concentrations of this metabolite were significantly higher in patients with renal insufficiency than in healthy

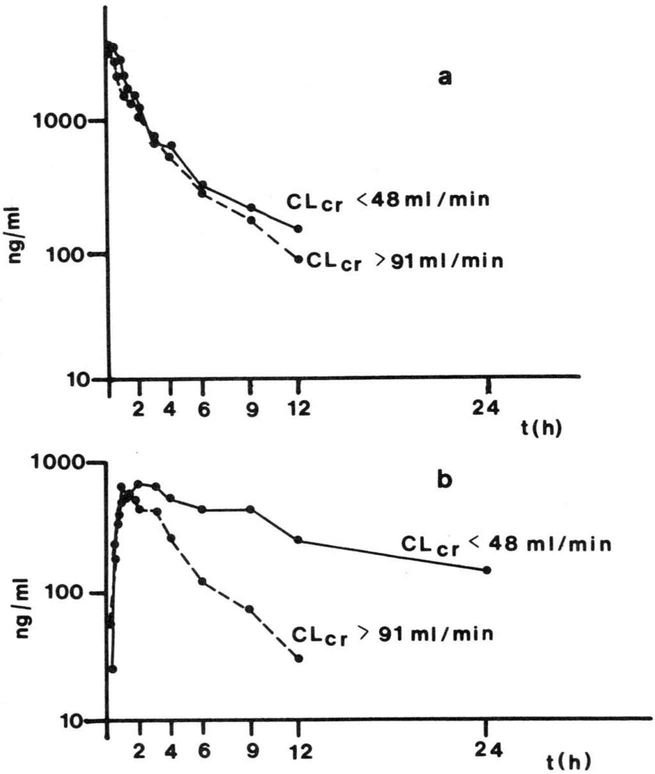

Fig. 2. Median plasma concentration curves of torasemide (a) and M5 (b).

volunteers. Even 36 h after administration this compound was still measurable in 2 patients (group B). $T_{1/2app}$ was 3.1 ± 1.0 h in group A, but 7.3 ± 4.3 h in group B. AUC(0-∞) and MRT were also increased in renal failure.

CONCLUSIONS

Our data with non-metabolised torasemide confirm those of a previous investigation. Concerning the metabolites, alterations were only detected for M1 and especially for M5, which was found to have no diuretic activity.

The results from the pharmacokinetic investigation are confirmed by those from the pharmacodynamic studies, which demonstrate that the duration of action is not prolonged in patients with renal failure. On the other hand, electrolyte excretion decreases with decreasing CL_{cr}.

MUZOLIMINE IN THE TREATMENT OF ACUTE TUBULAR NECROSIS FOLLOWING RENAL TRANSPLANTATION

G. Orsoni, A. Di Felice, G. Liviano D'Arcangelo, M.P. Scolari, S. Stefoni and V. Bonomini

Department of Nephrology and Dialysis, St. Orsola University Hospital, Bologna, Italy

INTRODUCTION

Despite the advances of intensive-care and surgical management, a substantial ischemia of the graft can still occur during every renal transplantation from cadaver donor. The ensuing tubular damage can lead to acute, oliguric graft failure, whereupon the recovery of renal function is deferred in such patients (1, 2). Moreover, long-term survival of the graft is believed by some (3), though not all (4) authors, to be shorter in patients with post-transplant acute tubular necrosis (ATN).

The overall experience of our transplant center encompasses 62 cases of ATN out of 322 renal transplantations from 1967 to late 1985. Although controlled studies are not available in this field, most nephrologists, and we among them, often employ diuretic agents in the treatment of post-transplant ATN in order to increase the daily urine output, prevent fluid overload, delay the individual dialysis needs and maybe reverse the glomerulo-tubular imbalance in the vascular supply and ultimately hasten the recovery of graft function. To our knowledge, a comparison between the effects of different diuretic drugs or different schedules of treatment, e.g. intravenous or oral route, high or low dose, short or long-term, has never been performed. To supply the omission, we underwent a blind, controlled study regarding the effect of muzolimine, furosemide or placebo in the treatment of ATN following renal transplantation. The present paper deals with the first year results of the trial.

STUDY DESIGN

Twenty-eight consecutive patients with acute oliguria (daily diuresis lower than 500 ml) in the first days following cadaver-donor renal transplantation were originally considered. Proper evaluation (diagnostic imaging, immunological monitoring, clinical and bioptical criteria) established that in 10 cases the oliguria was due to hemodinamically-mediated renal failure, graft artery thrombosis or stenosis, rejection or urinary tract obstruction. The remaining 18 patients were diagnosed as suffering from post-transplant ATN. They were assigned randomly to blind treatment with muzolimine (240 mg/day - 6 pts.), furosemide (500 mg/day - 6 pts.) or placebo (6 pts), by mouth, for 4 to 6 consecutive days. Monitoring of diuresis, body weight, blood pressure, graft function, blood and urine chemistry was performed daily.

RESULTS

Table I

	days	-1	1	2	3	4	5	6	+1
Urine output (ml/24h)*	M	350± 68	740± 85	1070± 115	1980± 353	2250± 442	2850± 519	2167± 249	1750± 274
	F	296± 97	596± 227	920± 239	1280± 298	1425± 411	1830± 381	1970± 298	1550± 251
	P	114± 59	117± 48	175± 75	178± 78	234± 112	204± 60	249± 60	672± 197
Urine Sodium (mmol/l)	M	10± 3	46± 22	65± 26	90± 28	99± 35	161± 33	149± 36	80± 8
	F	37± 14	64± 13	88± 6	138± 17	167± 38	232± 32	199± 39	67± 16
	P	4± 2	4± 1	8± 4	8± 3	9± 4	6± 1	8± 1	23± 6
Urine Potassium (mmol/l)	M	7± 3	14± 5	18± 5	25± 6	29± 9	27± 8	26± 8	25± 7
	F	21± 5	26± 6	39± 7	67± 21	87± 27	114± 29	37± 5	39± 6
	P	6± 2	8± 3	9± 4	10± 4	13± 6	9± 2	10± 3	25± 7

* mean ± SEM

M = Muzolimine F = Furosemide P = Placebo

Table II

	MUZOLIMINE (No 6)	FUROSEMIDE (No 6)	PLACEBO (No 6)
Oliguria time (days)	6.0 ± 4.5*	7.2 ± 6.3	7.8 ± 0.8
Dialysis (hr/days of graft failure)	0.63±0.35	0.88±0.21	1.01±0.27
Recovery time (days)	17.4±4.4	21.6±8.3	22.8±5.0

* mean ± SD

CONCLUSIONS

The present results, though largely preliminary, demonstrate that the short-term, high-dose diuretic treatment of post-transplant ATN is effective and safe. Compared to the placebo group, the two diuretic-treated groups exhibited a shorter oliguria time, required less substitutive dialysis and recovered a normal graft function in a shorter period. Moreover, no noteworthy untoward effects were observed, even in the few patients on simultaneous cyclosporin therapy.

Despite some suggestion of a greater effect of muzolimine compared to furosemide, the number of patients was too small for us to draw any definitive conclusions. However, the overall effects of the two drugs on water and salt balances show considerable differences, probably because each drug has a different site of action on the renal tubular cell.

REFERENCES

1. Sheil, A.G.R., Stewart, J.H., Johnson, J.R. et al. Transplant Proc. 3: 347-351, 1971
2. Whittaker, J.R., Veith, F.J., Soberman, R. et al. Surg. Gynecol. Obstet. 136: 919-921, 1973
3. Baxby, K., Taylor, R.M.R., Anderson, M. et al. Lancet 2: 977-979, 1974
4. Brophy, D., Najarian, J.S., Kjellstrand, C.M. Transplantation 29: 245-248, 1980

Torasemide in chronic renal failure

O.Ickrath, T.Risler

Torasemide is a new diuretic acting at the loop of Henle.

As far as known torasemide has a different mode of action compared to furosemide or muzolimine.

According to results of GREGER et al. (1) torasemide inhibits the sodium-chloride-potassium-carrier system at the luminal side of Henle´s loop cells. It also impairs the chloride permeability at the serosal border of these cells.

Referring to LESNE et al. (2) the pharmacokinetic data of torasemide are characterised by a bioavailibility of more than 90 %, a ß-half live of about 3 hours and a protein binding of 98-99 %.

Loop diuretics are the drugs of choice in the management of patients suffering from chronic renal failure. To compare the effect of 100 and 200 mg of torasemide with 100 and 200 mg of furosemide a multicenter controlled randomised double blind study was performed.

92 patients (51 male, 41 female) were enclosed into this study. On an average the patients were 55 years. Renal failure resulted from glomerulonephritis, pyelonephritis, diabetic nephropathy as well as nephrosclerosis. In all patients renal function was characterised by serum creatinine levels higher than 3.4 mg %, creatinine clearances of less than 30 ml/h as well as more than 1000 ml of daily urine volumes.

Diuretic drugs used were withdrawn at least 36 hours before the beginning of the trial.

During the first twenty-four hours of the study, the run in period, blood samples were drawn and urine samples were collected in three portions while the patients still received no diuretic. The second day, called therapy period, the diuretic was infused over 1 hour; afterwards blood and urine samples were drawn again in the same manner as the day before. The study was completed by controls on the third day, when patients received no diuretic again.

The results of our study show that urine volume in our patients significantly increased due to 100 respectively 200 mg furosemide and torasemide. While this increase due to 100 mg of torasemide was 24 %, after 100 mg of furosemide urine volume increased by 51 %. Doubling the dose of torasemide or furosemide did not induce a further significant increase in the urine volume.

Sodium excretion per hour increased after 100 mg torasemide by 55 % compared to 81 % in 100 mg furosemide. 200 mg of torasemide induced a rise of 82 %, while the increase of sodium excretion due to 200 mg furosemide by another 10 % was not significant always compared to the run in period.

Potassium excretion per hour increased by 11 % due to 100 mg torasemide; in contrast to this 200 mg torasemide did not influence potassium excretion. In comparison to torasemide, 100 mg of furosemide induced a significantly higher increase in potassium excretion by 37 %, while potassium excretion merely rose by 9 % due to 200 mg furosemide.

100 and 200 mg torasemide induced an increase in renal calcium excretion by 133 and 168 % per hour. Calcium excretion increased by 150 % after 100 mg furosemide, while an increase in the dosage of furosemide did not affect a further increase in renal calcium excretion.

Excretion of chloride increased by 98 % due to 100 mg torasemide and furosemide. Higher dosages of torasemide and furosemide resulted in a further rise of chloride excretion to 146 and 126 % compared to the run in period.

References:

1. Wittner, M., Greger, R. Nieren- und Hochdruckkrankheiten 14: 376-377, 1985

2. Lesne, M., van Ypersele, C., Arch. int. Pharmacodyn. 249: 322-325, 1981

MUZOLIMINE vs FRUSEMIDE IN CHRONIC RENAL FAILURE: SHORT TERM EFFECT IN DOUBLE-BLIND STUDY

G. PASSAVANTI, M. GIANNATTASIO, G. MAZZIA, P. CORATELLI

Institute of Nephrology, University of Bari, Italy

INTRODUCTION

Muzolimine is a new loop diuretic of the pyrazolinone series, which contains no sulfonamide radical in its structure and has a longer half-life and duration of action than frusemide (1), bumetanide (2) or ethacrynic acid (3).

In this study the diuretic response to muzolimine was compared with that to frusemide in patients with renal failure of varying degree.

PATIENTS AND METHODS

16 patients(pts),aged 27-60 years,with chronic renal failure were studied with frusemide (A) and muzolimine (B). More detailed information on the pts is given in Table 1.

Table 1. Clinical data on patients in whom muzolimine was compared with frusemide.

Patients number (sex)	Age (yrs)	Renal disease and associated conditions	Creatinine clearance (ml/min)	Body weight (Kg)	Blood pressure (mmHg)	Oedema
1 (M)	57	Pyelonephritis	39	51	190/120	+
2 (F)	46	Hypertension	40	58	180/110	-
3 (F)	59	Glomerulonephritis	74	79	120/70	++
4 (M)	59	Glomerulonephritis	28	55	180/100	-
5 (F)	51	Nephrosclerosis, cardiac failure	29	52	120/70	+++
6 (F)	57	Glomerulonephritis	76	77	140/80	++
7 (M)	27	Glomerulonephritis	29	66	170/110	+
8 (F)	70	Nephrosclerosis	10	65	170/100	-
9 (F)	49	Pyelonephritis, cardiac failure	35	51	110/70	++
10(M)	31	Glomerulonephritis	31	65	160/110	+
11(M)	76	Kimmestiel-Wilson, diabetes	29	62	180/110	+++
12(F)	51	Nephrolithiasis	16	61	140/90	-
13(M)	64	Nephrosclerosis	5	80	150/90	+
14(M)	37	Glomerulonephritis	3	54	160/95	+++
15(M)	66	Nephrosclerosis	7	76	160/80	-
16(F)	68	Nephrosclerosis	12	63	190/90	-

Drugs were administered in the random patterns ABBA or BAAB following the procedure recommended by Gold et al(4)in order to eliminate a source of bias that is possible when a drug always precedes or follows the other in paired response comparison.

The study was performed in double-blind and planned through 24 hrs urine collection as follows : day 1(control),day 2(diuretic A or B),day 3(wash-out),day 4(diuretic B or A),day 5(wash-out),day 6(diuretic B or A),day 7(wash-out),day 8(diuretic A or B),day 9(final control).

The dose employed was 25 mg (A) and 30 mg (B) in pts with creatinine clearance(CrCl) higher than 40 ml/min, 50 mg (A)and 60 mg(B)in pts with CrCl from 40 to 20 ml/min, 125 mg (A) and 120 mg (B)in pts with CrCl from 20 to 10 ml/min,500 mg (A) and 480 mg (B) in pts with CrCl lower than 10 ml/min.

The increment in excretion of urine volume, sodium, potassium and chloride was calculated substracting the control daily excretion (determined by adding the control days 1,3,5,7,9 and taking the average) from the mean daily excretion for each drug. All results are expressed as the mean ± standard error of the mean (S.E.M.). Analysis of significance was performed with the Student t-test for pair samples.

RESULTS

The effects of muzolimine and frusemide on urine volume, sodium, chloride and potassium excretion are presented in Fig.1.

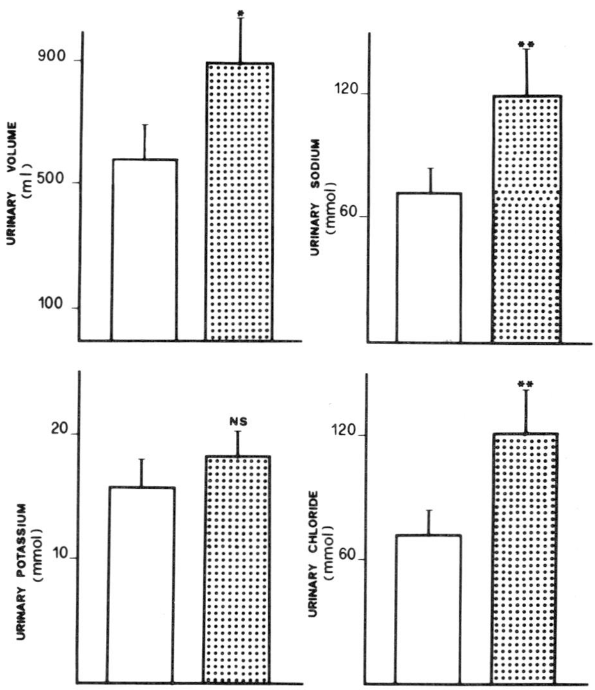

Fig. 1. Effects of muzolimine(dotted areas) and frusemide(open areas) on urine output (* = p/0.02), sodium and chloride (* * = p/0.01)potassium excretion(not significant)expressed as increments per 24 hrs.

Muzolimine induces higher statistically significant increment than frusemide in excretion of urine volume (902 ± 168 vs 574 ± 108 ml; p/0.02),of urinary sodium(121.3 ± 22 vs 69.7 ± 12 mmol; p/0.01) and of urinary chloride (124 ± 26 vs 73.4 ± 14 mmol; p/0.01); no difference in increment of potassium excretion was found(18 ± 4.7 vs 16 ± 5.5 mmol).

Besides, no percent change in plasma electrolytes, urea,uric acid and CrCl was observed between muzolimine and frusemide.

DISCUSSION AND CONCLUSIONS

Hypertension,nephrotic syndrome,cardiac failure,chronic renal failure are all conditions responsible for salt retention and oedema requiring diuretic treatment.

Our double-blind study demonstrates that muzolimine at the dose levels used produces a significantly greater urine volume,sodium and chloride excretion than frusemide;no significant change in increment of urinary potassium excretion rate was demonstrated.

In conclusion,our data emphasize that muzolimine,despite a greater increase in sodium urinary excretion than frusemide,did not induce a more pronounced excretion of potassium. Therefore,muzolimine provides certain advances to other high-ceiling diuretic drugs in treatment of salt retention in all various degrees of chronic renal failure (5,6).

REFERENCES

1. Hoppe-Seyler,G.,Heissler,A.,Coppencastrop,M.,Schindler,M.,Schollmeyer, P.and Ritter W. Pharmatherapeutica 1:422-429,1977.
2. Davies,D.L.,Lant,A.F.,Millard,N.R.,Smith,A.J.,Ward,J.W.and Wilson,G. M. Clin.Pharmacol.Ther.15:141-155,1974.
3. Goldberg,M.,Mc Curdy,D.K.,Foltz,E.L.and Bluemle,L.W. J.Clin.Invest. 43:201-216,1964.
4. Gold,H.,Kwit,N.T.,Messeloff,C.R.,Kramer,M.L.,Golfins,A.J.,Greiner,T.H. Goessel,E.A.,Hughes,J.H.and Warshaw,L. J.Am.Med.Ass.173:745-752,1960
5. Dal Canton,A.,Russo,D.,Gallo,R.,Conte,G. and Andreucci,V.E. Br.Med.J. 283:595-598,1981.
6. Schmidt,P.,Loew,D.,Dycka,J.,Kopsa,H.,Balcke,P.,Zazgornik,J. and Deut sh,E. Eur.J.Clin.Pharmacol. 14:399-403,1978.

Reprint requests to :
Dott. G. Passavanti
Institute of Nephrology
University of Bari
Piazza G. Cesare n°11
70124 BARI(Italy)

EFFECTS OF ETOZOLIN IN UREMIC PATIENTS ON DIALYSIS WITH RESIDUAL RENAL FUNCTION

G. GIORCELLI, G.M. VACHA, G.P. ICARDI

Department of Nephrology and Dialysis, Ospedale Mauriziano Umberto I°, Torino, Italy

INTRODUCTION

In the last ten years hemodialysis has been employed on a greater number of aged patients suffering from various diseases, most of them being of cardiovascular nature. Today, an ever increasing number of Dialysis Centers employ Bicarbonate-buffered dialysate in order to achieve a better dialytic tolerance with high efficiency dialyzers.

As a result, the acid-base status of the patients may change too suddenly, and consequently a rapid displacement of Potassium from the extra- to the intracellular space may occur. This consequence is even more serious for those patients giving digitalis and for those still keeping a residual renal function, with a significant daily electrolytes loss.

On one hand, the maintenance of a residual GFR may be useful in the management of these aged patients, because they show less interdialytic weight gain (therefore there will be no need of a strict control of the fluid introduction); prescription of a loop diuretic may contribute to obtain an appropriate daily urinary output.

On the other hand the patients will be more sensitive to variations of the intra- and extracellular Potassium concentration, due to rapid changes of the acid-base status in the course of the dialysis. In some case severe arrhitmy can occur during dialysis.

Being in these particular conditions, these patients could benefit by the use of a diuretic drug showing the following properties: the drug shall assure a Sodium and water elimination similar to those obtained using others loop diuretics; it shall avoid excessive Potassium loss, but its use shall be more safe and reliable than that of the true Potassium-sparing diuretics,and it shall have no adverse effects on the carbohydrates and and lipids metabolism.

In view of these main characteristics, we have chosen Etozolin, because some data in literature showed its safety and effectiveness in chronic renal failure (1) and its lower potassiuric effect (2, 3).

MATERIALS AND METHODS

We have carried out a study on 12 uremic patients suffering from heart diseases, on regular bicarbonate dialysis, with a residual GFR ranging from 10.2 to 14.7 ml/'. The age was ranging from 67 to 79. The patients were all giving digoxin. All of them had been previously treated with Furosemide for at least 6 months; they were then given Etozolin (400-800 mg/day) for 6 months, and then they went back to the first treatment. ECG, Urea and Creatinine clearances, urinary Na^+, K^+ and Cl^- evaluations were performed on a monthly base. Blood samples were taken weekly, before and after dialysis, for monitoring the electrolytes and digoxin levels and the acid-base status.

RESULTS

The data are summarized in the following Table.

	A: Furosemide	B: Etozolin	C: Furosemide
Urine output (ml/24 hrs):	2170 $\pm$ 776	1610 $\pm$ 481	1950 $\pm$ 322
UNa^+ (mEq/24 hrs):	138 $\pm$ 24	167 $\pm$ 34	141 $\pm$ 31
UK^+ (mEq/24 hrs):	32.2 $\pm$ 11.3	23.8 $\pm$ 7.0	30.7 $\pm$ 6.1
UCl^- (mEq/24 hrs):	190 $\pm$ 46	156 $\pm$ 35	198 $\pm$ 53
UNa^+/Cl^- ratio:	0.72 $\pm$ 0.25	1.07 $\pm$ 0.19	0.75 $\pm$ 0.13
UNa^+/K^+ ratio:	4.31 $\pm$ 1.3	6.19 $\pm$ 1.2	4.96 $\pm$ 1.5
Mean Arterial Pressure (mmHg):	121.7 $\pm$ 16.3	108.4 $\pm$ 10.1	107.9 $\pm$ 21.1

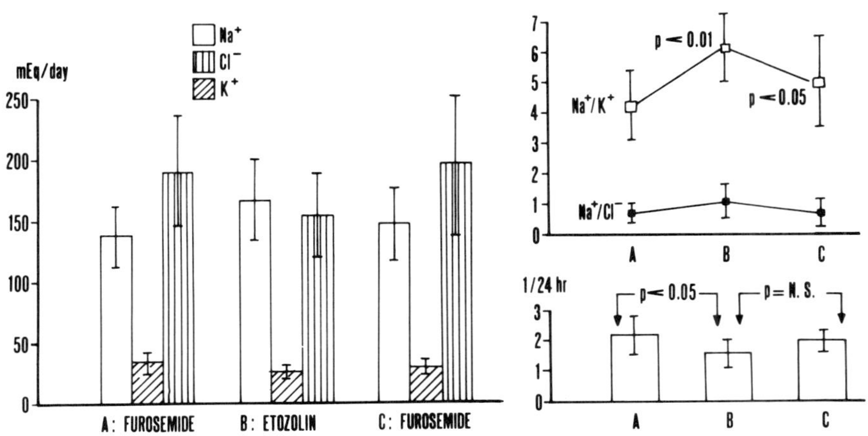

The Figure shows on the left the daily urinary Na^+, K^+ and Cl^- elimination, and, on the right, the urinary Na^+/K^+ and Na^+/Cl^- ratios (top), and the daily urine output (bottom).

Only two cases of intradialytic hypokalemia have been observed with Etozolin, instead of 12 observed during the previous period, and 7 of the subsequent treatment. The cases of arrhythmy were: 3 with Etozolin, 8 and 5 respectively with Furosemide. Two patients,assuming 800 mg/day of Etozolin suffered from myalgias: in these patients neither electromyographic alterations nor changes in serum CPK levels have been observed These effects ceased by temporarily suspending the use of Etozolin and did not appeared with a new prescription of 600 mg/day.

DISCUSSION

In our experience, the administration of 400 to 800 mg/day of Etozolin to uremic patients has given good results. Our data seem consistent with those referred in literature (1, 4, 5). In our opinion this drug could be especially useful when the following conditions shall occur.

- Patients suffering from heart diseases, subjected to digitalis treatment.
- Patients to be treated with bicarbonate dialysis, wich may induce sudden variations in the acid-base status and in serum Potassium levels.
- Patients with residual GFR and residual and residual urine output leading to significant losses of electrolytes.

In these particular cases other loop diuretics might be used with similar results, the only difference being a significant Potassium depletion. The muscular pain - disappearing with the temporary suspension of the drug, or with a reduction of dosage - is difficult to explain; some other Authors (7, 8, 9) have observed this symptom using other loop diuretics. In order to avoid this effect, we point out that daily dosage exceeding 600 mg must be employed very cautiously in uremic patients.

REFERENCES

1. Knauf, H., Liebig, R., Schollmeyer, P., Rosenthal, J., Koelle, E.U. and Mutschler,E. Eur. J. Clin. Pharmacol. 26:687-693, 1984.
2. Greven, J. and Heidenreich, O. Arzneimittelforschung 27:1755-1757, 1977.
3. Merzweiler, G.A. and Gladigau, V. Terapiewoche 28:9972-9980, 1978.
4. Kindler, J. and Schulz, V. Internist 22:615-697, 1981.
5. Coratelli, P., Rizzi, R., Corciulo, R. and Amerio, A. Farmaci 3(Supp.3):226-231, 1979.
6. Hropot, M., Fowler, N., Karlmark, B. and Giebisch, G. Kidney Int. 28:477-489, 1985.
7. Stefoni, S., Orsoni, G., Perini, L., Raimondi, A. and Bonomini, V. Farmaci 3(Supp.3): 232-236, 1979.
8. Lynggaard, F. Farmaci 3(Supp.3):216-220, 1979.
9. Hettiarachi, J. Br. J. Clin. Pharmacol. 4:644-651, 1977.

CAN HIGH-DOSE DIURETIC THERAPY REDUCE THE FREQUENCY OF HEMODIALYTIC TREATMENT?

N.E. MONTEMURRO, R. GIORDANO, F. GODINO, C. GROSSI

Servizio Nefrologia e Dialisi, Ospedale Civile, Martina Franca (Taranto), Italy

In order to reduce the frequency of hemodialytic treatment (and so to permit more people to be treated), we're giving high-dose diuretics to all new hemodialyzed patients.

For the last 22 months, 17 patients underwent hemodialysis in our Center. All patients began hemodialysis 3 time a week (on the whole 6 - 9 hours weekly) and in the meantime they were orally treated by frusemide (F) 10 mg/Kg/die (10 patients) or muzolimine (M) 5 mg/Kg/die (7 patients), according to the drug used during conservative stage. Patients aged from 40 to 69 years (mean 56.8 $\pm$ 8.1): n. 4 suffered from chronic glomerulonephritis (CGN), n. 2 chronic pyelonephritis (CPN), n. 4 nephroangiosclerosis (NAS), n. 2 interstitial nephritis (IN), n. 2 polycystic Kidney (PK), n. 2 sistemic lupus erythematosus (SLE) and n. 1 tubercular nephritis.

In spite of diuretics, diuresis decreased in 5 patients, all treated with frusemide (2 CGN and 3 NAS): drug was dismissed and patients kept on with the tri-weekly hemodialysis (12 - 14 hours weekly). Other 3 patients were intolerant to drug (nausea, gastric pain) and stopped diuretic therapy; 2 patients were treated with muzolimine and 1 with frusemide.

In the last 9 patients, diuresis remained or increased: so, after 2 months, we reduced hemodialysis frequency from 3 to 2 times weekly (8 - 9 hours weekly); from these, 2 patients deteriorated with own hematochemical values in spite of increased diuresis, so they went back to tri-weekly hemodialysis. The last 7 patients (40%) are following up bi-weekly treatment and high-dose diuretic therapy from 9 to 22 months without, at present, significant deteriorations of clinical and/or laboratory findings; interdialytic body weight increase is kept under 3%; all patients showed increases of uricoemia well controllated with allopurinol. These 7 patients are suffering from n. 1 IN, n. 1 NAS, n. 1 TBC, n. 1 CPN, n. 1 PK, n. 1 SLE and n. 1 CGN. 3 patients are treated with frusemide and 4 with muzolimine.

Use of high-dose diuretics seems to be encouraging in reducing the frequency of hemodialytic treatment. Muzolimine seems to be better than frusemide in mantaining diuresis in hemodialyzed patients. Surprisingly there are no difference among base nephropaty in the response to drugs, but our experience is too little to come to significant conclusions.

PATIENTS	SEX	AGE	DIAGNOSIS	BASE DATA DIURESIS ml/die	HTC %	CREAT. mg/dl	WEIGHT Kg	DRUG	AFTER 2 MONTHS TRI-WEEKLY DIALYSIS DIURESIS	HTC	CREAT.	interdialytic weightincrease %	FOLLOW-UP IN BI-WEEKLY DIALYSIS	DIURESIS	HTC	CREAT.	interdial. weight incr.	Notes
1	m	40	PK	2500	31	9.3	74	F	3000	32	10.0	0.5%	after 9 months	2000	30	10.1	1.0%	on in bi-weekly hemodialysis
2	f	49	TBC	1800	29	9.7	54	F	1800	27	10.3	1.0%	" 10 "	1800	27	9.6	1.0%	
3	m	69	NAS	2000	31	9.4	55	M	2400	36	9.7	0	" 15 "	2000	32	9.2	1.0%	
4	f	57	CGN	2000	41	6.4	42	F	2400	40	6.8	0	" 16 "	2400	40	7.2	0	
5	m	48	SLE	2000	22	13.0	85	M	1500	22	12.6	1.5%	" 18 "	1500	23	13.1	2.0%	
6	f	46	IN	1500	31	11.1	43	M	1700	26	11.7	1.0%	" 20 "	2000	25	10.8	0.5%	
7	m	54	CPN	2000	31	7.5	46	M	1800	28	6.9	0	" 22 "	1800	28	7.9	1.0%	
8	f	67	CPN	1800	20	10.0	62	F	1800	22	10.9	1.5%	" 3 "	1800	18	13.2	2.0%	back to tri-weekly dialysis
9	f	54	IN	1500	22	11.3	60	M	1800	22	12.5	2.0%	" 4 "	2000	17	15.1	3.0%	
10	m	60	CGN	2000	20	10.6	80	F	<500	21	10.8	3.0%						on in tri-weekly hemodialysis
11	f	65	NAS	2000	24	9.1	53	F	<500	17	8.9	4.0%						
12	f	68	NAS	1400	21	10.2	61	F	600	22	9.6	2.0%						
13	m	61	CGN	1800	29	8.5	57	F	800	30	8.8	3.0%						
14	m	62	NAS	2000	26	11.4	58	F	<500	27	14.2	4.0%						
15	f	55	SLE	1300	24	11.0	65	F										intolerant to drug
16	m	55	CGN	2500	26	13.0	58	M										
17	f	56	PK	1700	30	12.1	69	M										

USE OF HIGH DOSE OF MUZOLIMINE IN ACUTE FLUID RETENTION IN PATIENTS UNDERGOING CONTINUOUS AMBULATORY PERITONEAL DIALYSIS (CAPD).

G. BANDIANI, E. CAMAIORA, M.A. NICOLINI, U. PEROTTA

Servizio di Nefrologia e Dialisi - Ospedale Civile San Andrea
La Spezia - Italy.

INTRODUCTION

Recurrent peritonitis remains the most frequent complication of CAPD and produces a rapid temporary loss of peritoneal ultrafiltration required in order to maintain an adequate body fluid balance.

Symptoms are water retention, oedema and in some patients congestive heart failure, despite the reduction of fluid and Na intake and sometimes require temporary transfer to hemodialysis or extracorporeal ultrafiltration for fluid removal.

Previous report have showed that low (1) and high (2) doses of muzolimine produce a significant increase in daily urine volume in patients undergoing CAPD.

Therefore we studied the possibility of increasing the residual diuresis in patients on CAPD during recurrent peritonitis by the administration of a high dose of muzolimine.

PATIENTS AND METHODS

The study was carried out in 20 episodes of peritonitis occurred in the last 4 years in our dialysis unit in 8 patients (6 male and 2 female), 53 to 75 years old, who had been on CAPD for 10 to 48 months. The patients suffered form chronic glomerulonephritis (3 pts.), polycystic renal disease (1 pt.), nephrocalcinosis (1 pt.) and chronic pielonephitis (3 pts.). No patients were nephrectomized.

During recurrent peritonitis no hypertonic CAPD solutions were used in order to remove fluid excess.

Patients were treated by high daily dose of muzolimine (240-480 mg).

In each patient the body weight, the 24 hrs urine volume and the urine excretion of Na and K were daily determined. Moreover all drainage bags were collected and their volume was measured.

Results were compared with the data obtained in 18 previous episodes of peritonitis occurred in a second group of 7 patients well matched for age, sex, etiology of renal disease and residual renal function and not treated by diuretic agents.

The data were analyzed by the Student's t test.

RESULTS

During muzolimine treatment all patients showed a significant increase in daily urine volume compared either to basal value (from 215 ± 56 ml/24 hrs to 784 ± 195 ml/24 hrs) or to untreated group of patients (228 ± 60 ml/24 hrs) ($p < .001$) (Fig. 1).

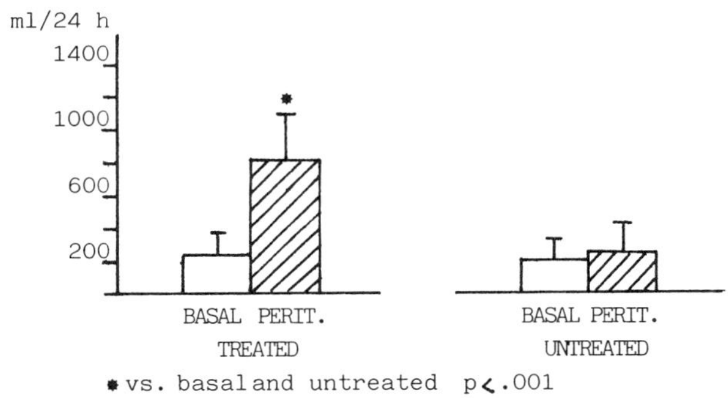

Fig. 1. Basal diuresis in treated and untreated patients and during recurrent peritonitis.

Basal urinary excretion of Na resulted 30 ± 12.2 mEq/24 hrs in treated group and 31.6 ± 16.2 mEq/24 hrs in untreated group. Muzolimine significantly increased natriuresis in the first group to 65.7 ± 18.4 mEq/24 hrs ($p < .001$).

No significant change was observed in daily urine output of K.

In the treated group weight gain did not occur (Δ b.w.= 0.7 ± 0.4 kg) while in the untreated group body weight significantly increased because of water retention (Δ b.w.= 5.1 $\pm$ 1.2 kg) ($p < .001$).

Both groups of patients showed a significant reduction in daily excess drainage volume: in first group the daily ultrafiltration volume decreased from 1180 $\pm$ 308 ml/24 hrs to 487 $\pm$ 195 ml/24 hrs, in second group from 1095 $\pm$ 380 ml/24 hrs to 409 $\pm$ 205 ml/24 hrs.

DISCUSSION

Uremic patients undergoing CAPD show a significant loss of peritoneal ultrafiltration during recurrent peritonitis and a rapid increase in water retention. The administration of daily dose of 240-480 mg of muzolimine produced a significant increase in residual diuresis and urinary Na excretion, preventing weight gain. None of treated patients needed extracorporeal treatment for fluid removal.

No toxic side effects have been observed.

REFERENCES

1. Bandiani G., Camaiora E., Nicolini M.A., Perotta U.: Muzolimine in patients on chronic hemodialysis (HD) and continuous ambulatory peritoneal dialysis (CAPD). Z. Kardiol 74, suppl. 2: 84-87, 1985.
2. Scarpioni L., Ballocchi S., Bergonzi G., Fontana F., Poisetti P.G., Zanassi M.A.: High-dose diuretics in continuous ambulatory peritoneal dialysis. Perit. Bial. Bull. 2, 4: 177-178, 1982.

DOUBLE BLIND CROSS-OVER COMPARISON OF MUZOLIMINE AND PLACEBO IN PATIENTS ON MAINTENANCE HEMODIALYSIS

M. PALESTINI, A. MESSINA, M. CAROSI*, C. BORGNINO*
Hemodialysis Service, 1st Institute of Surgical Clinic, University "La Sapienza", Rome, Italy
* Medical Department, Bayer Italia, Milan, Italy

INTRODUCTION

Recently, positive results have been achieved with muzolimine (Edrul^R, Bayropharm Italiana), a new high ceiling diuretic (1), even in patients with advanced renal failure (2,3,4).

Aim of this study was to evaluate the effects of muzolimine (M)in non anuric patients on maintenance hemodialysis.

PATIENTS AND METHODS

The study was designed as a double blind, placebo (P) controlled, completely randomized cross-over trial (Fig.1). Sixteen patients (8 males, 8 females) aged 32-68 years (m$\pm$SD 51.9$\pm$10.4) on maintenance hemodialysis were enrolled. All had a residual diuresis$\geq$300 ml/24h.

Renal disease was due to polycystic kidney (n=5), chronic pyelonephritis (n=3), gouty nephropathy (n=2), renovascular disease by arterial hypertension (n=2), microcystic dysplasia (n=1), hepatorenal syndrome in chronic hepatitis B with IgA glomerulonephritis and mixed cryoglobulinemia (n=1). In two cases the etiology was not defined. The patients had been on maintenance hemodialysis for 2-76 months (m 21.8). They were dialyzed 3 times weekly for about 4 hours, using a cuprophan dialyzer. Patients with congestive heart failure (NYHA III-IV classes), massive fluid retention or insuline dependent diabetes mellitus were excluded. Informed consent was obtained in all cases.

After a 7-day wash-out period with progressive withdrawal of all *drugs affecting hydroelectrolytic homeostasis, the patients underwent a 5-day diuretic free run-in, during which basal controls were performed. The treatment consisted of two 7-day periods separated by an intermediate 5-day wash-out phase. The patients were randomly allocated to either M (240 mg tablets, 1 tablet o.d. in the morning) or P. For each half group (HG) the measurements of daily urinary volume (DUV) were performed 3 times during the run-in as well as during the two treatment periods. Body weight was recorded before (PBW) and at the end of each dialysis; afterwards, the increase in interdialytic body weight (IBWI) was calculated. The patients were maintained on a constant dietary regimen throughout the study. The results were analyzed by means of ANOVA and Wilcoxon test.*

RESULTS

The results are reported in Table I. Significant differences were observed between M and P on DUV (ANOVA $p < .001$), IBWI ($p < .05$) and PBW ($p < .02$). Conversely, there were no significant differences between the two HGs and between the cross-over phases. During M the increase in DUV (Wilcoxon test, HG1: $p = .005$; HG2: $p = .05$) as well as the decrease in IBWI (HG1: $p = .05$; HG2: $p < .01$) and PBW (HG1: $p = .01$; HG2: $p = .05$) were significant in both HGs. On the contrary, P did not produce any significant change. Under M the average increase in DUV was ≈60 % in HG1 and ≈ 80 % in HG2. Subjective short-lasting dizziness (n=2), dyspepsia (n=1), occasional hypotensive episodes (n=2) were reported under M treatment, whereas during P single complaints of aerophagy and nausea were collected.

CONCLUSION

Previous controlled studies in patients on maintenance dialysis have shown a more pronounced diuretic and natriuretic effect of M in comparison with furosemide (5-6). The results of this study do confirm the considerable diuretic action of M in hemodialysis patients with residual urinary flow. This effect appears to be important in order to improve the quality of life and the compliance to hemodialysis of non anuric patients.

Our results strongly support the feasibility of high M doses in the treatment of non anuric uremic subjects because of the remarkable diuretic effect and of the satisfactory tolerability.

Figure 1 Study design
(↓ hemodialysis sessions - *daily urinary collections)

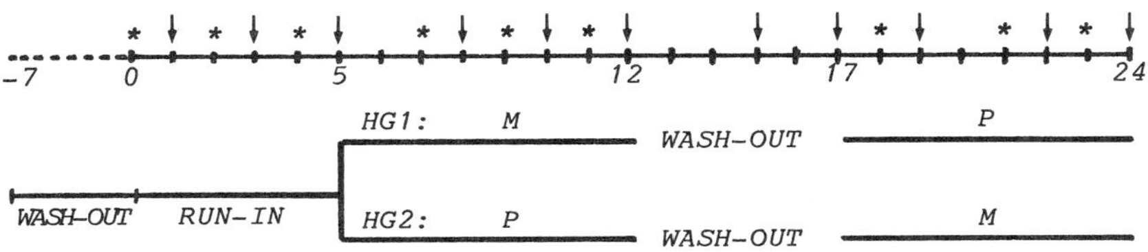

Table 1 DUV, IBWI and PBW during run-in and each treatment period (m ± SD)

	HG1			HG2			Comparison between treatments◊
	Run-in	M	P	Run-in	P	M	
DUV (ml/24h)	591 ±406	947*** ±488	610 ±438	455 ±215	428 ±199	821* ±515	$p < 0.001$
IBWI (mg)	1712 ±823	1434* ±908	1762 ±894	2457 ±889	2259 ±921	2039** ±887	$p < 0.05$
PWG (kg)	63.96 ±9.20	63.41** ±8.98	64.07 ±9.15	68.54 ±13.18	68.42 ±12.83	68.19* ±13.08	$p < 0.02$

Ante-post comparison carried out with Wilcoxon test
* $p = 0.05$, ** $p \leq 0.01$, *** $p = 0.005$

◊ Performed by means of ANOVA cross-over, referring to the differences between baseline and post-treatment (i.e. baseline-M versus baseline-P)

ACKNOWLEDGEMENTS

We thank Prof. M. Mancuso, Prof. S. Persichetti, Dr. F. Ciaraffo and Dr.D.Romoli for their support, advice and encouragement.

REFERENCES

1. Berg, K.Y. et al., Pharmatherapeutica 1, 5, 319-332, 1976
2. Röckel, A., Curr. Med. Res. Opin. 4, 574-579, 1977
3. Dal Canton, A. et al., Br. Med. J. 283, 595-598, 1981
4. Schmidt, P. et al., Clin. Nephrol. 19, Suppl. 1, 45-49, 1983
5. Weisschedel, E. et al., Clin. Nephrol. 19, Suppl. 1, 50-53, 1983
6. Schmidt, P. et al., Eur. J. Clin. Pharmacol. 20, 23-26, 1981

EFFECTS OF THE LOOP-DIURETIC MUZOLIMINE IN RATS WITH $HgCl_2$-INDUCED ACUTE RENAL FAILURE (ARF).

C.ESPOSITO, M. SABBATINI, M. ALTOMONTE, G. ROMANO, F. UCCELLO, P. VENIERO, A. DAL CANTON, V.E. ANDREUCCI.

Department of Nephrology, 2nd Faculty of Medicine, University of Naples (Italy).

INTRODUCTION

Pre-treatment with diuretics (D) can prevent the onset or shorten the course of many models of experimental ARF (1). It is not clear, however, whether D can improve renal function when administered after ARF has estabilished. The aim of our study was to investigate the effects of Muzolimine (M) in $HgCl_2$ induced ARF.

METHODS

Our study was carried out in 60 male Wistar rats, housed in individual metabolic cages, fed a constant Na^+ diet and offered a choice of tap water and hypotonic saline (70 mmol/l) to drink. After a three-day control period, 50 rats were injected s.c. $HgCl_2$ (4 mg/kg bw). 30 out of these 50 rats were used as $HgCl_2$ group ($HgCl_2$); the remaining 20 were treated daily with M (100 mg/kg bw, by gavage), starting 24 hrs after $HgCl_2$ injection ($HgCl_2$+M). The last 10 rats were given only M at the same dosage (group M). Rats were sacrificed on day 2 and 5 in group $HgCl_2$ and $HgCl_2$+M, and on day 5 in group M. Metabolic studies consisted of daily determination of bw, BP (tail-cuff), and daily measurements of Na^+, K^+, and water intake and excretion. Serum creatinine (S_{Cr}), Na^+, K^+(K_S^+), and BUN were measured at time of sacrifice in blood collected by decapitation.

RESULTS

Bw and BP were similar in the three groups of rats during

both control and experimental period. Despite the administration of D in group $HgCl_2$+M, urinary volume (V) was similar as in $HgCl_2$ (Fig.1). In group M, V was strikingly increased. Sodium handling was similar in the three groups during control period (Fig. 2). $HgCl_2$ administration induced a statistically significant decrease of Na^+ excretion, paralleled by a significantly lower intake. In group $HgCl_2$+M both Na^+_E and Na^+_I fell similarly and Na^+ was unchanged. In group M, diuretic effect was evident: Na^+_E was greatly increased and was well counterbalanced by higher intake. K^+ excretion is represented in Fig.3. In both groups with ARF, K^+_E was significantly lower than in control period, and more markedly in group $HgCl_2$+M than in $HgCl_2$. In group M, K^+_E was normal when compared to control period. Finally, data of renal function are shown in Table I. It is noteworth that no data are available in group $HgCl_2$+M on day 5, as all the rats died before time of sacrifice.

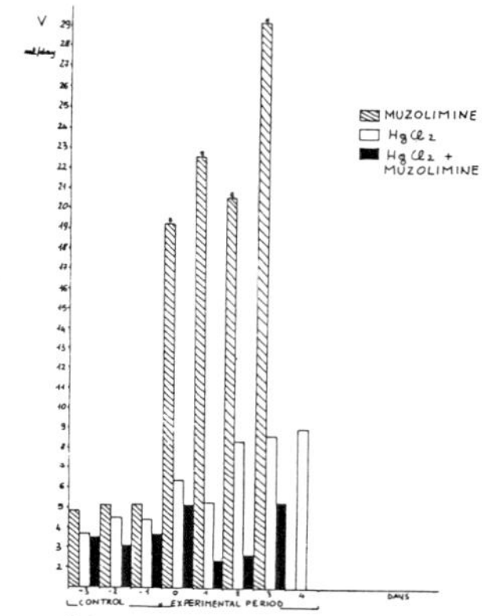

Fig 1 URINARY VOLUME   * p < 0.005 vs control period

DISCUSSION

The pathogenesis of $HgCl_2$-induced ARF is still unclear in rats. Probably, the main event leading to renal insufficiency is an early renal vasoconstriction (2), followed by a prompt return of renal blood flow toward normal values within 24 hrs, in spite of severely reduced GFR (3). The rationale of our study was, therefore, to use M, a diuretic acting from vascular

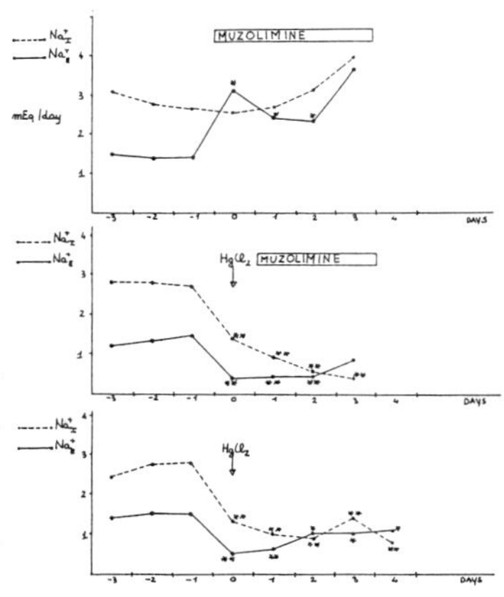

Fig 2: SODIUM INTAKE (Na_I) and EXCRETION (Na_E)
* p < 0.05 vs control period
** p < 0.001 vs control period

site of tubular cells, requiring preserved RBF, but not GFR to be effective (4).

M administration had no beneficial effect on ARF. Neither urinary volume, nor Na^+ balance, nor S_{Cr} and BUN, were modified by such treatment.

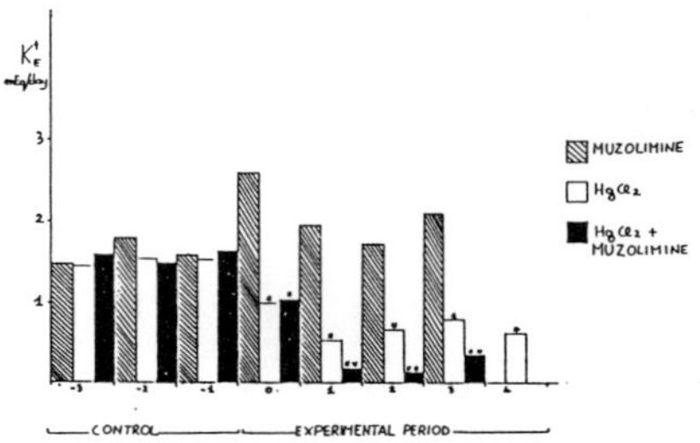

Fig. 3 : POTASSIUM EXCRETION
* $p < 0.005$
** $p < 0.001$

Moreover, M administration was associated with higher mortality in group $HgCl_2$+M: none of these rats survived on day 5 after M. This may be accounted for by decreased K^+ excretion, with consequent hyperkalemia, in $HgCl_2$+M rats. Even if unable to ameliorate ARF, M administered at this dosage was not toxic in normal rats, nor caused volume depletion because our rats had free access to unlimited Na^+ amount (in saline offered to drink).

REFERENCES

1. A. Dal Canton,V.E. Andreucci. In: Acute Renal Failure (V.E. Andreucci Ed.), Martinus Nijhoff, Boston, 1984, p119-147.
2. Baheler RW,Kothcen TA,Burke JA,Galla JA,Bathena JA. L Lab Clin Med 90:330-340,1977.
3. CH Hsu,TW Kurtz,JM Weller. Nephron 18:326-332,1977.
4. R Faedda,A Satta,GF Branca,B Contu,E Bartoli. Z. Kardiol. 74 (suppl. 2), 166-171,1985.

Table I. Data of renal function (mean ± SD).

	S_{Cr} (mg%)		BUN 4mg%)		K^+_S (mEq/l)	
$HgCl_2$	5.63 ±1.5	9.48 ±5.2	175.1 ±37.1	271.1 ±91.4	5.72 ±1.2	8.37 ±2.3
$HgCl_2$+M	5.29 ±1.2	--	203.7 ±44.7	--	7.65* ±1.3	--
M		0.35** ±0.1		26.1** ±7.6		4.96** ±0.7
	48 hrs	5 days	48 hrs	5 days	48 hrs	5 days

*, ** : $p<0.05$ and $p<0.001$, respectively, vs. $HgCl_2$ group.

EFFECTS OF MUZOLIMINE ON EXPERIMENTAL ACUTE RENAL FAILURE (ARF).

M. SABBATINI, C. ESPOSITO, M. ALTOMONTE, G. ROMANO, F. UCCELLO, P. VENIERO, A. DAL CANTON, V.E. ANDREUCCI.

Department of Nephrology, 2nd Faculty of Medicine, University of Naples, Italy.

INTRODUCTION

Experimental ischemic-ARF has been widely studied because of its pathogenic similarity to human ARF. Administration of loop diuretics immediately after the ischemic insult is of no benefit to renal function (1). This study was carried out to evaluate the effects of a new loop diuretic, Muzolimine (M), active from the peritubular site.

METHODS

18 female Münich-Wistar rats were anesthetized and prepared for renal micropuncture (2). Through the abdominal incision both renal arteries were gently isolated at their origin from aorta. ARF was induced by clamping these arteries for 60 min, with a small vascular clamp. Thirty min after release of vascular clamps, 7 rats were given i.v. M (25 mg/kg bw, group M) dissolved in polyethileneglycol and then diluted in one ml of saline; 7 rats received an equal amount of saline (control, C). A third group of sham-operated normal rats (n=4, N) was studied to estabilish normal values. 30 min after M administration, the following measurements were performed: hydrostatic pressures (ITP= intratubular pressure; EAP= efferent arteriole pressure; GCP= glomerular capillary pressure) recorded by a servo-nulling measuring system; single-nephron GFR (SNGFR), by timed collections of tubular fluid; total kidney urine output and GFR.

RESULTS

BP and Ht were statistically similar in all groups of rats. Hydrostatic pressures and SNGFRs are shown in Table I. No statistically significant difference between M and C group was found; both M and C were highly significantly different when compared to N group, with the unique exception of GCP, which was similar in all the rats.

Table I. Hydrostatic pressures (mm Hg) and SNGFR (nl/min). Data are expressed as means ± SD.

	ITP	EAP	GCP	SNGFR
C	33.4±14.9	22.8±8.4	44.2±7.6	20.1±6.8
(n)	(39)	(25)	(6)	(17)
M	33.7±13.6	20.0±6.1	49.3±3.9	17.2±8.6
(n)	(48)	(29)	(11)	(18)
N	13.5±1.7*	14.6±4.8*	47.7±4.8	28.4±8.2*
(n)	(24)	(13)	(8)	(12)

* = $p<0.005$ when compared to both C and M group.

One rat in M group and two in group C were anuric. Even if urinary output was greatly increased in M group, when compared to both C and N, the difference was at the limit of significance ($0.06<p<0.05$). Total kidney GFR was less depressed (vs normal values) in M group than in C group. All these data are summarized in Table II.

M administration, finally, was associated with a greater mortality of rats (ratio: 3:1 vs C group).

DISCUSSION

Tubular obstruction seems to play a major role in the pathogenesis of ischemic-ARF. Therefore, the maintainance of high tubular flow rate induced by diuretics could interfere with formation of tubular casts and improve renal function.

Table II. Urinary output (V, ul/min) and total kidney GFR (GFR, ml/min). Data are expressed as means ± SD.

	C	M	N
V	4.16±7.18	16.13±15.9	8.05±6.26
(n)	(5)	(11)	(8)
GFR	0.02±0.003	0.13±0.11	0.45±0.11*
(n)	(5)	(7)	(8)

* = $p<0.001$ when compared to both group M and C.

Our preliminary data show that M administration has determined a consistent increase of urinary volume associated with an improvment in renal function. The micropuncture results show a relatively well preserved function of superficial nephrons; this may explain why M does not appear to have any benefit on them. This does not exclude that M may act on deeper nephrons, not accessible to micropuncture, where glomerular blood flow has been shown to be depressed (3) and where tubular obstruction is quantitatively important (4).

REFERENCES

1. J. Mason,H. Koin,J. Welsh,J. Schnermann. Pflügers Arch. 392:125-133,1981.
2. V.E. Andreucci. In: Manual of Renal Micropuncture. (V.E. Andreucci Ed.). Idelson, Naples, 1978; p. 50-86.
3. J. Mason,J. Welsh,T. Takabatake. Kidney Int, 24:27-36, 1983.
4. J.F. Donohe,M.A. Venkatachalam,D.B. Bernard,N.G. Levinsky. Kidney Int, 13:208-222,1978.

ENHANCED RECOVERY OF ACUTE RENAL FAILURE WITH DOPAMINE + MUZOLIMINE.

B.MEMOLI, S.FEDERICO, A.PAPA, M.SABBATINI, G.CONTE, R.M.GAZZOTTI, G.PACCHIANO, T.RAMPINO, R.IANDOLO, A.TESTA, A.DAL CANTON and V.E.ANDREUCCI.
Dept. of Nephrology, II Faculty of Medicine, University of Naples, Italy.

INTRODUCTION.

Diuretic treatment in oliguric "organic" Acute Renal Failure (ARF) is commonly used in order to increase urine output and improve the course of the disease (1). Muzolimine is a new high-ceiling loop diuretic acting from the serosal side of tubular cells (2), indipendently on the rate of glomerular filtration. Dopamine, a splanchnic vasodilating agent, appears to have a direct action on renal vasculature (3).

The aim of our study was to evaluate the combined effect of Muzolimine + Dopamine administration in human ARF.

PATIENTS AND METHODS.

Six patients (3 males and 3 females), admitted to our unit with clinical diagnosis of oliguric "organic" Acute Renal Failure, were included in the study. Dopamine (1-3 μg/Kg b.w./min in continuous i.v. infusion) and Muzolimine (480+240 mg per os in the first day and 240 mg b.i.d. in the following ones) were administered until urinary volume was greater than 3500 ml/24 hrs or for a maximum of 6 days. Serum creatinine (Cr_s), urea, Na^+ and K^+ concentrations were determined daily; 24 hrs urine collections, for determinations of Na^+, K^+, creatinine, were performed daily.

RESULTS.

Four "responder" patients shown a marked increase of urine output in a few hours after Dopamine + Muzolimine administration. In these patients the therapy induced a marked increase of FE_{Na^+} (38.25%) and a tenfold increase of urine output which attained its maximum in four days (Fig.1). Serum concentrations of creatinine and urea, after a light raise, slowly fell toward normal values (Fig.2). The remainder "irresponsive" two patients showed only a light increase of urine output and underwent hemodialytic treatment.

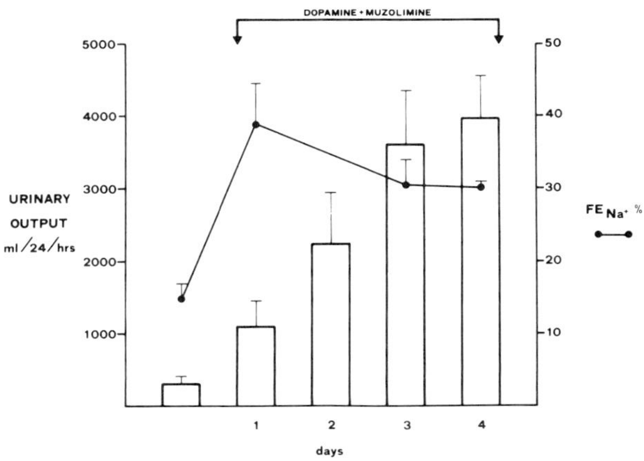

Figure 1: Effects of Dopamine + Muzolimine on urine output and FE_{Na^+} (Mean ∓ SE).

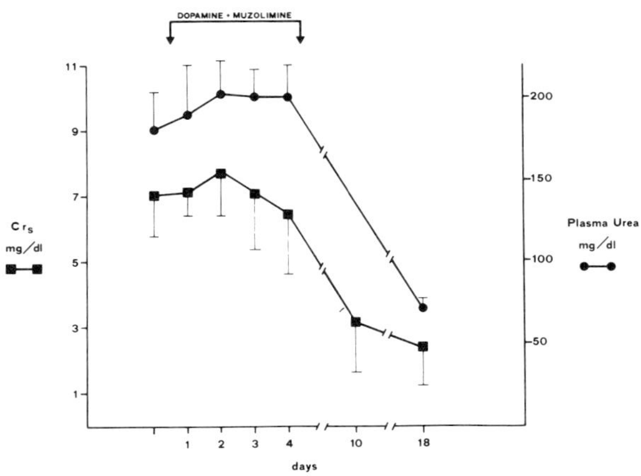

Figure 2: Effects of Dopamine + Muzolimine on serum creatinine and urea (Mean ∓ SE).

DISCUSSION.

The primary event leading to human Acute Renal Failure is commonly believed to be a vasomotor change followed by tubular cells damage and tubular lumen obstruction (4). In our study, Muzolimine + Dopamine administration resulted in a early recovery from ARF in four out of six patients.This effect may be accounted for by a direct renal vasodilating action of Dopamine which would improve renal perfusion and may allow Muzolimine to act in high concentration. The inhibition of NaCl reabsorption by muzolimine would increase tubular flow and favor the wash-out of cellular debris occluding tubular lumen. Another possible effect of the diuretic might be the inhibition of NaCl reabsorption at Macula Densa level thereby interrupting the negative tubulo-glomerular feedback mechanism responsible for the afferent arteriole constriction (5). The latter effect, however, would occur in the early phase of Acute Renal Failure.

REFERENCES.

1. Epstein M., Schneider N.S., Befeler B. Am.J.Med. 58:510-516, 1975.
2. Faedda R., Satta A., Branca G.F., Contu B., Bartoli E. Z.Kardiol. 74, Suppl.2, 166-170, 1985.
3. Goldberg L.I. Pharmacol. Rev. 24:1-29, 1972.
4. Tanner G.A. Kidney Int. (Suppl.12):S213-S218, 1982.
5. Mason J., Tekabatake T., Olbricht C., Thurau K. Pfügers Arch. 373:69-76, 1978.

THE USE OF MUZOLIMINE IN NEPHROTIC SYNDROME: DIURETIC EFFECT AND TUBULAR FUNCTIONS.

M. BRUNO, C. MARTINI, M. MARANGELLA, B. FRUTTERO, A. TRICERRI, G. SEBASTIANI, F. LINARI.

Department of Nephrology, Mauriziano Umberto I Hospital, 10128 Turin, Italy.

INTRODUCTION

Muzolimine (M) is a potent diuretic drug recently introduced into clinical use, which shows both high cieling and long acting properties (1,2). It has been held effective in hypertension and in oedematous syndromes from cardiac, hepatic and renal aetiology (3,4,5). This study was designed to evaluate the diuretic or any other effect on tubular transport in patients (pts) with oedema from nephrotic syndrome in course of diverse renal diseases.

PATIENTS AND METHODS

Fifteen nephrotic pts, aged 43M ± 17SD years, with various degree of renal failure (Creat. Cl. 83 ± 32 ml/min) and hypertension (Sist. Blood Pressure 168 ± 28 mm Hg) were given M 60 mg once a day.

Following parameters have been investigated:

Clinical parameters (days 0-1-7-14-28): diuresis, body weight, blood pressure, heart rate.

Urinary parameters (days 0-1-7):

1) Net Acid Excretion (NAE) as estimated by pH, Ammonium, Titratable Acid and Bicarbonate.
2) Cations (Na, K, Ca, Mg, Zn); inorganic (Chloride, Phosphate, Sulfate) and organic (Citrate) anions.
3) Urine excretion of 24 Aminoacids (8 pts).

Blood chemistries (days 0-28): Glucose, Urea, Creatinine, Uric Acid, Thriglycerides, Cholesterol, Sodium, Potassium and plasma proteins.

Results are expressed as means ± SD; significances of differences assessed by the paired and unpaired Wilcoxon's tests.

RESULTS

Clinical (Fig. 1):

diuresis rose significantly ($p<0.01$) by the first day and kept high thereafter; loss of body weight attained 6.8% after a week reaching 10% after a month ($p<0.01$); both diastolic and sistolic blood pressure showed a significant reduction during the first week ($p<0.01$); heart rate did not change.

Urine (Tab. I)

NAE did not differ cumulatively from basal values, as both Titratable Acid and Bicarbonate increased.

Fig. 1 - Clinical parameters in 15 pts on M therapy.

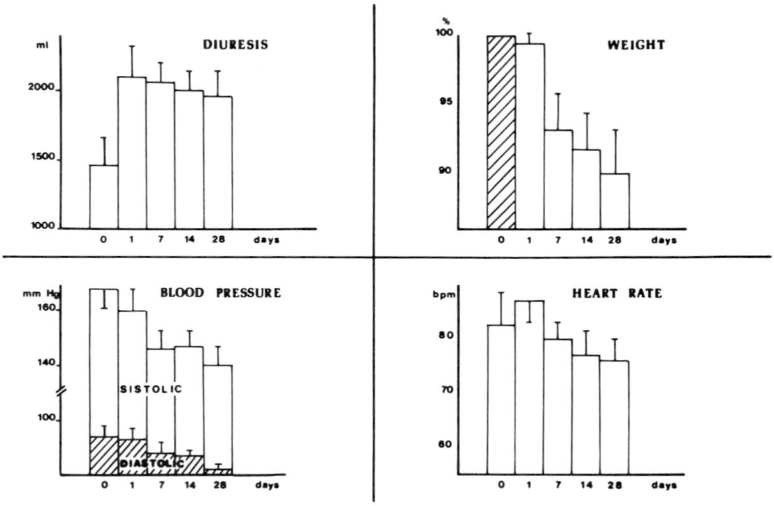

Tab. I - Urine parameters

H^+ Excretion	Basal	1st day	7th day
pH	6.33	6.27	6.47
NH_4 (umol/min)	20.8	24	23.1
A.T. (uEq/min)	11	21.8*	12.7
HCO_3 (uEq/min)	1.5	8 *	5.6
NAE (uEq/min)	31	36	33
Cations			
Na (mEq/24 hr)	116	301 *	127
FE_{Na} (%)	0.7	1.9**	0.8
K (mEq/24 hr)	54	71	57
Ca (mmol/24 hr)	4.2	7.3*	9 **
Zn (mmol/min)	0.9	1.1	1.4
Anions			
Cl (mEq/24 hr)	101	287 **	100
FE_{Cl} (%)	0.8	2.4**	0.9
Phosphate (mmol/24 hr)	23	26	25
$TmPO_4$ (mg % ml GFR)	2.7	2.7	2.5
Citrate (mmol/24 hr)	3.7	4.3	2.4
Sulfate (mmol/24 hr)	17	20	19

* $p<0.05$, ** $p<0.02$ vs basal values.

Sodium and chloride excretions rose up 2.5 times in the first day; afterwards they decreased, but their fractional excretions (FE) remained mildly higher. Urinary Ca was persistently increased.

Basal aminoacid excretion, cheked in 8 pts (Tab. II), differed from normal subjects with respect to Phosphoethanolamine, Ornitine and Lysine which were increased, and with Glycine and Glutamine which were decreased ($p<0.001$); after 7 day M therapy, only Glicine showed further reduction.

No significant change in the other considered parameters was found. Blood: a slight statistically unsignificant increase in nitrogenous compounds and plasma proteins was observed as a likely consequence of haemoconcentration.

Tab. II - Urine Aminoacid Excretion in 18 Normal Subjects and in 8 pts on Muzolimine Therapy (umol/24 hr).

	Normal		Before		After	
	M	SD	M	SD	M	SD
PSER	86	29	129	65	102	42
TAU	522	401	413	211	455	357
PETH	44	38	98*	21	100*	29
ASP	69	15	61	28	57	30
THR	166	68	100	32	73	20
SER	391	123	265	130	212	100
ASN	190	80	119	35	127	120
GLN	592	191	276°	155	209°	135
GLY	1732	935	865°	519	503°	122
ALA	298	110	216	87	152	41
VAL	59	18	65	33	46	27
CYS	64	22	65	12	61	18
MET	46	34	68	35	56	24
ILEU	52	26	46	20	50	24
LEU	93	30	103	36	77	51
TYR	122	40	123	41	117	65
PHE	84	17	74	29	62	14
ORN	29	16	89*	36	116*	88
LYS	167	54	321*	160	310*	155
1M-HIS	663	489	782	746	1199	914
HIS	1031	782	638	434	908	904
3M-HIS	347	202	500	282	489	247
ARG	15	13	9	10	8	12

*=increased, °= decreased, $p<0.001$

CONCLUSIONS

In our pts with nephrotic syndrome and various degree of renal failure and hypertension M has displayed a high diuretic potency, leading to resolution of oedema and reduction of hypertension.

Concerning to tubular functions, M seemed not to alter proximal tubular transports, as no change in Tm PO_4 and aa excretion occurred; some interferences on distal tubule might be suggested by the increased Ca and, to a lesser extent, Zn, K and bicarbonate excretions.

Noteworthy M did not induce Mg nor K wasting, as stressed by other Authors (5).

In conclusion M has proved to be a potent and safe diuretic drug in pts with oedema from kidney disease.

REFERENCES

1) Berg KJ, Jørstad S, Tromsdal A. Pharmaterapeutica, 1: 319-32, 1976.
2) Dal Canton A, Russo D, Gallo R, Conte G, Andreucci V. Brit Med J, 282: 595-8, 1981.
3) Heinrich F, Loew D, Dycka J. Curr Med Res Opin, 4: 706-11, 1977.
4) Brørs O, Fauchald P, Jacobsen S. Curr Med Res Opin, 6:431-36, 1980.
5) Weisscheld E, Russendorf MG, Ritz E. Clin Nephrol, Vol 19, Suppl. No.1: S 50-3, 1983.

FAVOURABLE EFFECTS OF MUZOLIMINE ON UREA PLASMA LEVELS IN CHRONIC RENAL FAILURE

F. MASTRANGELO, M. NAPOLI, C. CORLIANO', V. DE BLASI, S. RIZZELLI, L. ALFONSO, A.M. MONTINARO, M. APRILE, P. PATRUNO

Department of Nephrology and Dialysis, "V. Fazzi" Hospital, Lecce (Italy)

In chronic uremia a diuresis of more than 2 ml/min has been generally considered to be of little value regarding to urea elimination (1). In previous studies (2) we found that the combination of diuretic and reinfusion measures may lead to a rather quick decrease in blood urea in some pts with GFR of less than 20 ml/min. An inverse relation between blood urea and diuresis during treatment with Muzolimine was seen. To clarify this phenomenon, the urea excretion studies were performed in non oedematous pts with advanced CFR. The pts were treated by Muzolimine (240 mg) and saline infusion, in order to avoid the "braking phenomenon" (3) and the depletion of Extracellular Fluid Volume.

MATERIALS AND METHODS

20 pts with a GFR of 9.6$\pm$4.4 ml/min, age 57$\pm$6.3 yrs, body weight Kg 59$\pm$7.4 were studied. The underlying nephropathies were chronic glomerulonephritis (n=9), nephrosclerosis (n=10), hepato-renal syndrome (n=1). They were selected from a group of 30 pts becouse of their respondiveness to Muzolimina. The pts have been on low protein diet (25-35 g/day) for 1 mo. During a 2 wks period, the pts had a "wash-out" period of 5 days (control period). Subsequently they received a 240 mg single oral dose of Muzolimine for 8-15 days. They also were daily refilled with saline solution in order to replace urinary losses of H_2O, Na, K, Ca, and to maintain normal extracellular fluid volume. Nitrogen balance (protein catabolic rate) and urinary excretion of creatinine, urea, Na, K, Ca, Cl, were daily measured. Blood urea and creatinine were measured every other day.

RESULTS

Urine vol (UV) rose in all pts (min 57% and max 182%). This increase was steady and lasting during the treatment time and the braking phenomenon was lacking, probably owing to fluids and electrolytes replacement. Plasma creatinine levels did non change (6.8±1.6 → 7±1.4 mg/dl). The blood urea fell in 15 pts (178±35 → 139±31 mg/dl) and did not change in 5 pts (127±19 → 125±23). According to blood urea levels the pts were divided in 3 groups (tab. I):

1) Group A: In 5 pts with a catabolic state (nitrogen catabolism = 36±7 g/day of protein). Blood urea levels increased during the control period and decreased during the treatment period. Urea excretion increased to 47 %. This rise is 31 %, if urea excreted is related to renal load of urea expressed by body urea (Urinary urea / Body urea ratio).

2) Group B: In 10 pts a fall of blood urea levels was seen during control period as well as during treatment. Absolute urea excretion did not change (+ 0.005%). But the renal load of urea changed. An 35 % increase of urea excretion could be found, if the urinary urea / body urea ratio were considered.

3) Group C: In 5 pts blod urea did not change, but urea excretion rose 46.7 %. Nitrogen catabolism was increased during the treatment period becouse of the rise of the protein diet (2 pts) and the little duodenal bleeding (2pts).

Our study shown that in CRF an increase of diuresis after Muzolimine effects an enhancement of the fractional as well as the absolute urea excretion. This enhancement may be steady and lasting, if the "braking phenomenon" and the volume depletion are avoided. The effect on urea excretion depends on the changes in urea concentration and contact time in distal convolutions and collecting ducts, with a decrease of urea reabsorption: an inverse relationship between the creatinine U/P ratio and fractional urea excretion was observed, in fact (fig. 1).

REFERENCES

1. Reubi, F. Intern. Symp. Fealdafing. Springer Verlag Berlin 1969, p. 381.
2. Mastrangelo, F. et al. Z. Kardiol. 74, Suppl. 2 : 109-114, 1985.
3. Grantham, J.J. and Chonco, A.M. In: Sodium and Water Homeostasis (Eds B.M. Brenner and J.H. Stein), Churchill Livingstone, N.Y. 1978, p. 178.

	GROUP A (5 pts)			GROUP B (10 pts)			GROUP C (5 pts)		
	control 5 gg (**)	treatment 8 gg (**)	changes % (*)	control 5 gg (**)	treatment 8 gg (**)	changes % (*)	control 5 gg (**)	treatment 8 gg (**)	changes % (*)
Blood urea mg/dl	200±10 ↗ 117±9	210±8 ↘ 162±12	17.3	199±31 ↘ 161±18	161±18 ↘ 122±19	-21.4	127±19 ↗ 125±20	127±19 ↘ 125±23	-.007
Urine vol l	1770±250	3600±700	103	1500±207	3816±610	154	1250±160	2180±445	74
Urin urea g/day	9.4±2.1	13.8±2.9	47	11±2	11.55±2.4	.05	3.25±0.7	4.77±0.7	46.7
Body urea g	54.36±9	60.8±4.4	11.9	64.9±10	50.5±8	-22	46.87±3.3	46.95±2.7	.001
$U_{urea}/Body_{urea}$ %	17.3	22.7	31	16.9	22.8	35	6.9	10.1	46
Body weight Kg	57.17±4.5	54.5±4	-4.6	60.15±5.1	59.6±4.6	.009	62±4	62.6±3.9	.009
Nitrogen catab. g	36	37	2	23	24	4	18	26	44
GFR ml/min	9.7±1.6	9±2		10±4.1	10.2±3		8.1±3	9±3.1	

TABLE I

(*) $\frac{\text{treatment - control}}{\text{control}} \times 100$

(**) valori medi per 5 gg e per 8 gg

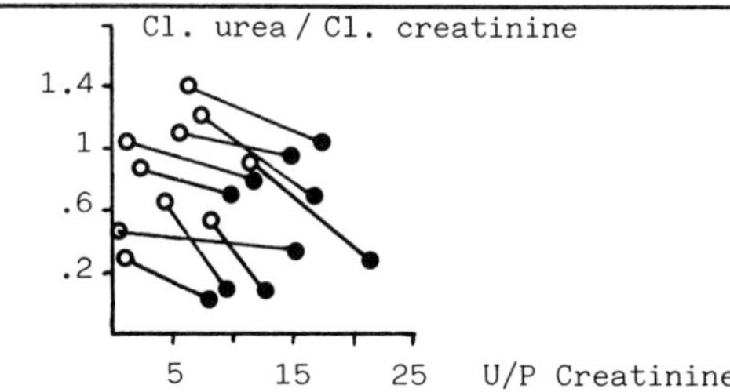

Fig. 1 : CORRELATION BETWEEN UREA EXCRETION FRACTION AND U/P RATIO OF CREATININE (● before; ⊙ 2nd day of treatment)

FUROSEMIDE AS AN AGENT ENHANCING PERITONEAL DIALYSIS EFFICIENCY

A.Grzegorzewska, K.Bączyk

Department of Nephrology, Academy of Medicine, Poznań, Poland

INTRODUCTION

Beneficial effect of furosemide /F/ on peritoneal sodium removal was reported by Giordano et al. /1/. Further publications show differences in evaluation of F action on peritoneal transfer of water, electrolytes and low molecular weight substances /2-6/. Thus, we decided to determine which way of F administration - intraperitoneal or intravenous - is more useful for augmenting peritoneal dialysis /PD/ efficiency.

METHODS

Our examinations were performed in 3 groups of patients with terminal uraemia regularly treated with intermittent PD. In group I /5 patients/ F was added to PD fluid /40 mg/l/ during 3 dialysate exchanges which were preceded and followed by 3 exchanges without F. PD fluid osmolality was 369 mOsm/kg H_2O, dialysate flow rate - 2,4 l/hr. In group II each of the 15 patients had 2 dialyses: the first PD was without F and the second one with the addition of F /40 mg/l/ to every exchange. In both dialyses was the same PD fluid osmolality /431 mOsm/kg H_2O/, flow rate /1,8 l/hr/ and number of exchanges /16 - 24/. Seven patients of group III were given 80 mg of F intravenously at the beginning of 3 consecutive exchanges which were preceded and followed by 3 exchanges without F administration. During all exchanges dwell time was 20 min and PD fluid volume was 2 l/exchange. In groups I and III dialysate samples for biochemical determinations were taken from every exchange; in group II dialysate from 2 exchanges was collected and analysed. In groups I and III

Table 1. Ultrafiltration and peritoneal transfer of some solutes mean ± SEM during dialyses with the use of furosemide /F/

	Group I			Group II		Group III		
	before F	with F	after F	without F	with F	before F	with F	after F
ultrafiltration /ml/min/	4,6 0,6	4,1 0,3	5,7 0,5	3,5 0,4	3,4 0,4	2,6 0,7	3,5 0,8	2,6 0,6
sodium balance /mmol/hr/	10,6 1,5	14,9 1,6	15,6 2,6	12,6 1,6	19,3 2,0	10,0 2,4	19,7 3,7	9,1 1,8
clearance /ml/min/ of:								
potassium	19,4 1,5	19,2 1,6	19,3 1,6	18,4 1,3	18,1 1,0	14,3 1,1	15,0 0,8	14,2 1,5
urea	17,4 1,6	19,3 1,5	17,7 1,7	18,0 0,4	19,0 0,4	17,5 0,2	18,3 0,2	17,4 0,2
creatinine	14,6 1,0	16,8 1,2	14,7 1,1	15,0 0,2	15,9 0,1	14,0 0,2	14,1 0,2	14,0 0,2
uric acid	12,6 0,8	15,2 1,4	14,1 0,3	15,1 0,2	17,1 0,7	12,5 0,8	13,3 0,8	13,0 0,8
protein excretion /mg/min/	15,4 2,2	13,5 1,1	13,5 1,0	17,1 0,4	17,1 0,4	14,9 0,4	14,9 0,4	14,8 0,4

blood samples were obtained at the beginning of PD and after every 3 exchanges. In group II blood was taken at the beginning and at the end of PD.

Ultrafiltration, peritoneal sodium balance, peritoneal clearances of potassium, urea, creatinine and uric acid as well as protein excretion were calculated for every exchange /or 2 exchanges/ and then mean values of these parameters for the whole of PD were determined. In each group of patients results were expressed as mean ± SEM and analysed statistically.

RESULTS

Mean values of peritoneal transfer coefficients are summarized in Table 1.

Intraperitoneal F administration resulted in significant increase of sodium balance and clearances of urea, creatinine and uric acid without effect on potassium clearance and protein excretion. This was observed during both used osmolalities and flow rates, however, F-induced changes were more evident with lower osmolality of PD fluid.

F given intravenously enhanced ultrafiltration and sodium balance with no significant effect on clearance of potassium, urea, creatinine and uric acid as well as protein excretion.

Thus, for PD treatment we recommend the intraperitoneal F administration which is superior to the intravenous one because the former results in augmenting the removal of sodium and also of low molecular weight substances.

REFERENCES

1. Giordano, C., De Santo, N.G., Capasso, G. and Papa, A. Trans. Am. Soc. Artif. Intern. Organs. 4:10, 1975.
2. Grzegorzewska, A. and Bączyk, K. Perit. Dial. Bull. 3: 160-161, 1983.
3. Grzegorzewska, A. and Bączyk, K. Artif. Organs. 6:220-224, 1982.
4. Maher, J.F., Hohnadel, D.C., Shea, C., DiSanzo, F. and Cassetta, M. Clin. Nephrol. 7:96-100, 1977.
5. Scarpioni, L., Ballocchi, S., Bergonzi, G., Fontana, F., Poisetti, P. and Zanazzi, M. Perit. Dial. Bull. 2:177-178, 1982.
6. Treviño-Becerra, A. XVI Congr. E.D.T.A. 8, 1979.

FUROSEMIDE AND PERITONEAL TRANSPORT OF URIC ACID - EXPERIMENTAL STUDIES

J. Knapowski, A. Bręborowicz and K. Czyżewska

Department of Pathophysiology, University Medical School, 60-781 Poznań, Poland

INTRODUCTION

Application of Furosemide /F/ into dialysate,during peritoneal dialysis, had been proposed for enlargement of peritoneal excretion of uric acid /UA/ /1/, however, localization and mechanism of this action remained uncertain. We want to present in this paper some experimental data which on one hand confirm that the diuretic can change peritoneal transport of UA, but at the same time show that the mechanism of this action is more complicated than it had been expected.

MATERIALS AND METHODS

Experiments were performed in vitro on fragments of mesentery /ileal region/ and parietal peritoneum /middle part of anterior abdominal wall/ taken from New Zealand rabbits immediately after they were killed. A careful preparation was used to obtain the membranes covered with intact, single layer of mesothelium on one side only, and as few of the tissue underneath as possible. The procedures had been described in details before /2,3/. The membranes were mounted between two halves of a lucite chamber with special measures to diminish the edge damage of the membrane. Both semi-chambers were filled with Hanks solution which was being bubbled continuously with O_2+CO_2 gas mixture. The experiments were performed at 37° C.

UA /pure, Ubichem Ltd, Middlesex, England/ was added into the medium bathing the contra-mesothelial /"vascular"/ side of the membrane to obtain its final concentration of 0.9-1.1 mmol/l. In the experiments carried out on the mesentery radiolabelled /14C/ UA /Amersham,England/ was also added to the solution on the same side. Samples of the fluid from both sides of the membranes were taken throughout the experiments, lasting 100 /mesentery/ or 120 /parietal peritoneum/ minutes, in consecutive intervals of 10 or 15 minutes, respectively. After a control period involving 3 intervals of the fluid sampling F /Polfa, Poland/ was added up to final conc. of 10^{-4} M into the medium bathing either sides of the membranes, and the sampling was being continued. UA concentration in the samples was estimated either enzymatically /Urica-Quant, Boehringer-Mannheim, GFR/ or by measuring the ^{14}C radioactivity in a β-counter /LS 100C, Beckman, USA/.

Transmesothelial flux of UA was estimated from differences between its concentration in the consecutive samples of the fluid taken from the mesothelial side of the membranes, considering the declining concentration gradient, volume change after sampling, time, and the membrane area. The results, expressed as mean, were analysed statistically using nonparametric test of Wilcoxon. $P > 0.05$ was assumed as non-significant.

RESULTS

Furosemide induced divergent changes of transperitoneal UA flux, depending on the type of the peritoneum, used in experiments as well as on the side of the membrane to which the drug was applied: a/ in the mesentery /Fig. 1-I/ the effects were bi-phasal, the second phase being rather stable, while in the parietal peritoneum /Fig. 1-II/ only one and transient phase of changes was observed. These effects were statistically significant when compared with control periods; the respective mean values in the Figure were marked by S.

b/ The direction of the observed changes /stimulation or inhibition/ was opposite when the diuretic was applied either to the mesothelial /Part A of Fig.1/ or to the vascular /Part B of Fig.1/ side of the membrane.

The results show that in peritoneum, presumably in the mesothelium, there are some mechanisms responsible for regulation of UA transport through this membrane. The mechanisms are furosemide-dependent, however, the divergent reactions for the drug reveal inhomogeneity of the membrane lining different

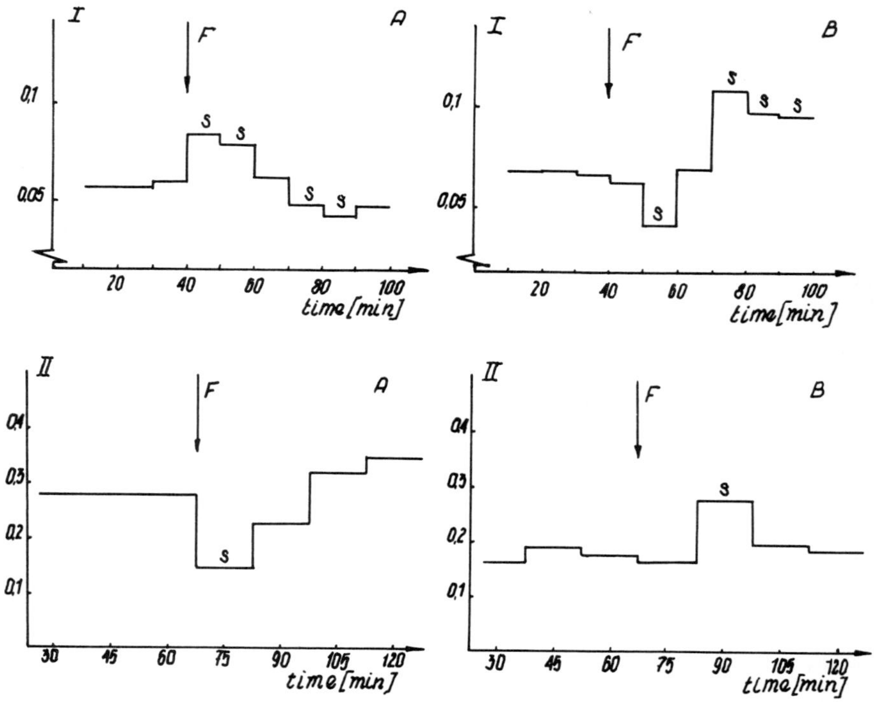

Fig.1 In vitro transperitoneal UA flux /mmol·cm^{-2}·sec^{-1}/ before and after /arrow/ application of F /10^{-4} M/ to medium bathing mesothelial /A/ or vascular /B/ side of mesentery /I/ or parietal peritoneum /II/.

parts of the peritoneal cavity as far as pharmacological susceptibility is concerned. This confirms our previous suggestions concerning the functional topographic differentiation of the peritoneal membrane /4,5/.

REFERENCES

1. Grzegorzewska A., Bączyk K.: Perit. Dial. Bull. 3: 160, 1983.
2. Knapowski J., Feder E., Simon M., Zabel M.: Proc. E.D.T.A. 16:, 155-164, 1979.
3. Bręborowicz A., Janecki A., Bręborowicz G., Knapowski J.: Perit. Dial. Bull. 5: 96-100, 1985.
4. Bręborowicz A., Knapowski J.: Acta Med. Pol. 25: 1-4, 1984.
5. Feder E., Knapowski J. In: Adv. Physiol.Sci. vol. 3, Physiology of non-excitable cells /Ed.: Salánki J./ Pergamon Press Academiai Kiado, Budapest 1981.

X. DIURETICS IN CIRRHOSIS

COMPARISON OF PHARMACODYNAMICS AND PHARMACOKINETICS OF TORASEMIDE AND FURODEMIDE IN PATIENTS WITH ASCITES DUE TO CIRRHOSIS OF THE LIVER

K. von Bergmann[1] G. Brunner[2] W. Haecker[3] and E. von Moellendorff[3]
Department of Medicine University of Bonn[1] and Hannover[2], and Clinical and Pharmacological Development of Boehringer Mannheim[3], FRG.

Introduction

Development of ascites in patients with cirrhosis of the liver is due to several pathophysiological mechanisms. One pathophysiological mechanisms in sustaining ascites is an increased sodium and water reabsorption in the nephron of both proximal and distal sites. Thus, strict dietary sodium and fluid restriction is the first therapeutic approach in these patients. Despite this dietary regiments satisfactory lose of ascites is often unsuccessful and treatment with diuretics is essential.

The present study was performed to compare in a double-blind, randomized order the effect of torasemide, a new saluretic agent, with furosemide on electrolyte and water excretion in patients with ascites due to cirrhosis of the liver. In addition, pharmacokinetics of the two loop-diuretics were measured, and the results of torasemide were compared with those obtained in healthy control subjects.

Methods

Nineteen patients with cirrhosis of the liver and ascites participated in the study. All patients were treated with 40 mg/day of furosemide at least 1 to 8 days prior to the study. Thereafter torasemide (20 mg: n = 10) or furosemide (40 mg; n = 9) were administered as a single dose in the morning after an overnight fast in a double-blind, randomized order. Urine was collected from 0-4, 4-6, 6-8, 8-10, 10-12, and 12-24 hourly fractions. Volume, sodium, potassium, and chloride were measured on every sample. Cumulative excretion (0-24 h) and for assessing the duration of diuretic activity the filtration related excretions (FE) were calculated.

Drug concentrations were measured in all urine samples and in plasma specimens obtained before and after 0.5, 1, 2, 3, 4, 6, 8, 10, and 24 hours after dosing in both groups of patients and in 9 healthy volunteers receiving an identical dose of torasemide. Measurements of torasemide and its major metabolites in man (M1, M3, and M5) and of furosemide were performed by high pressure liquid chromatography.

Both diuretics were well-tolerated and no obvious side effects could be observed. The study was conducted in accordance with the Declaration of Helsinki and consent was obtained from every subject.

For statistical comparisons of the results in the different groups the non-parametic U-test and for individual comparisons the Wilcoxon's signed rank test were used (2-tailed).

Results

No difference in the cumulative urinary excretion (0-24 h) of volume, sodium, potassium or chloride could be observed between patients treated with torasemide or furosemide (Table 1).

Table 1 Cumulative renal excretion

Treatment	Volume (ml/24 h)	Sodium	Potassium (mval/24 h)	Chloride
Torasemide	2159	142	49	231
Furosemide	1740	196	83	200

None of the parameters were significantly different

FE of volume during the first two collection periods (0-2 and 2-4 h) were also not different. During collection period 4-6 hours, the FE of volume after furosemide administration had almost reached values measured in the later periods. In contrast, the FE after administration of torasemide was distinctly higher during this period (p between 0.05 and 0.1) and significantly higher between 6-8 hours ($p < 0.02$) when compared to furosemide.

The FE of sodium was greater during 4-6 and 8-10 hours in patients treated with torasemide, but this difference did not reach statistical significance.

Pharmacokinetic parameters in both groups of patients and healthy volunteers are summarized in Table 2.

Table 2 Pharmacokinetic parameters (median) of torasemide and furosemide in patients with cirrhosis of the liver and healthy controls.

Treatment		C_{max} (ug/l)	t_{max} (h)	AUC_{0-oo} (ug x h/l)	$t_{1/2}$ (h)	Bioavailability (%)
Torasemide	Patients	3074	1.0	15621	4.81	88
	Controls	2722	1.0	6292	3.16	73
Furosemide		876	1.0	2380	2.16	36

The area under the curve ($AUC_{0-\infty}$) of torasemide was 2.5 fold greater in the patients with cirrhosis of the liver than in healthy controls and the half life was prolonged. Total urinary excretion (bioavailability) of torasemide and its metabolites (date not given) was not different.

Discussion

Diuretics are often used in the treatment of ascites in patients with cirrhosis of the liver when dietary restrictions of sodium and fluid are unsuccessful. Therefore, the present study was conducted to compare the diuretic activity of torasemide with furosemide in patients with cirrhosis of the liver.

Although, the number of patients was relatively small, the diuretic and saluretic activity of 20 mg of torasemide was comparable to 40 mg of furosemide. The time curve of the FE of volume after administration of torasemide, however, was different from furosemide, showing a longer duration of action. This is in accordance with the longer half life of torasemide, and might be of benefit in the treatment of ascites where strict diuresis is often followed by impaired renal function.

The comparison of the pharmacokinetic parameters between patients with cirrhosis of the liver and healthy controls revealed an unexpected higher area under the curve. The bioavailability was on the average slightly higher in patients with cirrhosis but could not account for the great difference in the area under the curve. Thus, the results indicate that a decreased first pass metabolism in the patients might be responsible for this difference. This is in line with the possibility that the metabolic sequence from the metabolite M1 to M5 could be slowed down without altering total urinary excretion of M5 (data not shown).

In conclusion, the present results demonstrate that the diuretic action of oral administration of 20 mg of torasemide is comparable with 40 mg of furosemide in patients with ascites due to cirrhosis of the liver. Therefore, torasemide might be an useful alternative diuretic for treatment of patients with ascites, especially, because of its longer duration of action.

COMPARATIVE EVALUATION OF MUZOLIMINE AND FUROSEMIDE IN HEALTHY SUBJECTS AND IN LIVER CIRRHOSIS.

G. Crippa, L. Scarpioni

Department of Internal Medicine and Renal Unit, Piacenza, Italy.

INTRODUCTION

In this study we have evaluated the effect of muzolimine (M), a diuretic drug acting on the ascending limb of Henle's loop. We chose as comparison drugs, piretanide (P), azosemide (A) and furosemide (F) in healthy subjects, and furosemide (F) in patients with liver cirrhosis.

PATIENTS AND METHODS

Ten healthy young volunteers were treated with a single dose of M (90 mg), F (100 mg), P (24 mg) and A (320 mg), with 6-7 day intervals to evaluate the time-response curve.

M and F activity were compared in 44 cirrhotic patients with ascites and oedemas (25 males and 19 females; aged between 38 and 71, 22 treated with M 90 mg/day, 22 with F 100 mg/day in single dose orally given) during 10 days of treatment. In the week before the treatment, all the diuretic drugs were withdrawm and a diet with a fixed sodium (80 mEq/day), potassium (45 mEq/day) and water (600 ml/day) intake was given.

Before and after the treatment, BUN, creatinine, ammonia, Cl^-, Na^+, K^+, Ca^{++}, Mg^{++}, and uric acid in blood samples were determined.

Furthermore the acid-base balance, creatinine clearance and uric acid clearance were evaluated. During the 4 days before the diuretic administration and throughout the treatment period, urinary Na^+, Cl^-, K^+, uric acid, Ca^{++}, and Mg^{++} excretion were evaluated together with the body weight and urine volume.

The statistical analysis of the differences, between the groups was performed with the Student's t-test for unpaired data.

RESULTS

Study on healthy subjects:

DIURETICS	CASES NUMBER	URINE VOLUME ml/day	Na mEq/day	K mEq/day	URIC ACID mg/day
PIRETANIDE 24 mg/day	10	2592±369	282.3±55.0	63.8±9.1	445.1±42.1
FUROSEMIDE 100 mg/day	10	2800±193	315.5±20.6	61.7±7.3	334.8±48.2
MUZOLIMINE 90 mg/day	10	2952±252	348.8±36.2	54.4±5.8	243.3±26.6
AZOSEMIDE 320 mg/day	10	3076±196	337.4±25.4	73.9±4.9	369.0±40.0

Tab. I: Effect of piretanide, furosemide, muzolimine and azosemide on urine volume, urinary sodium, potassium and uric acid excretion (MEAN ± SEM) in healthy volunteers.

In ten healthy volunteers treated with the four different diuretics, we did not observe significant differences in diuresis and in urinary sodium excretion between M and F curves, while P showed the most rapid onset of action and the shortest duration of action; A showed the slowest and most lasting effect.

In Table I, daily urine volume, urinary sodium, potassium and uric acid excretion are reported. The differences between the groups did not result statistically significant.

Study on cirrhotic patients:

For both drugs we observed the highest diuretic action during the first two days of treatment. M showed a slightly more intense diuretic effect than F, although such a difference was not statistically significant (Fig. 2). No significant difference was found in urinary K^+ excretion between the two groups (Fig. 3).

Plasma potassium levels decrease likewise and significantly in both groups (Table II), and no changes were found in plasma sodium levels.

Urinary sodium/potassium excretion ratio increased after both treatments, and no differences were observed between M and F curves.

Urinary calcium excretion was slightly higher in patients treated with F than in those treated with M, but without statistically significant differences between the two groups.

POTASSIUM mEq/l

DIURETIC	CASES NUMBER	CONTROL	END OF TREATMENT	p
MUZOLIMINE 90 mg/day	22	4.01±0.09	2.97±0.10	<0.0025
FUROSEMIDE 100 mg/day	22	3.98±0.08	3.03±0.05	<0.0025

Tab. II: Plasma potassium levels (MEAN± SEM) before and at the end of diuretic administration.

MAGNESIUM mg/dl

DIURETIC	CASES NUMBER	CONTROL	END OF TREATMENT	p
MUZOLIMINE 90 mg/day	22	2.30±0.13	2.15±0.12	N.S.
FUROSEMIDE 100 mg/day	22	2.23±0.15	2.14±0.12	N.S.

Tab. III: Serum calcium levels (MEAN±SEM) before and at the end of diuretic administration.

Fig. 4 shows the changes induced on urinary magnesium excretion: F cause a significant higher urinary magnesium loss than M, but without evident changes in serum magnesium levels at the end of treatment (Table III).

Serum creatinine levels and endogenous creatinine clearance were not significantly modified at the end of diuretic treatment.

In both groups we observed an increase in plasma uric acid levels, due to the reduction of urates renal clearance and extracellular volume contraction.

After treatment with M and F, the patients showed rise of blood bicarbonates values and moderate reduction of plasma chloride levels.

COMMENTS AND CONCLUSIONS

Our data confirm that in patients suffering from liver cirrhosis with water-salt retention, M is an effective, diuretic agent. The urinary potassium loss in cirrohotic patients and in healthy volunteers did not turn out different from that due to F. (1,2)

Also the decrease of plasma potassium levels induced by M did not result significantly different from that observed after F. [3,4]

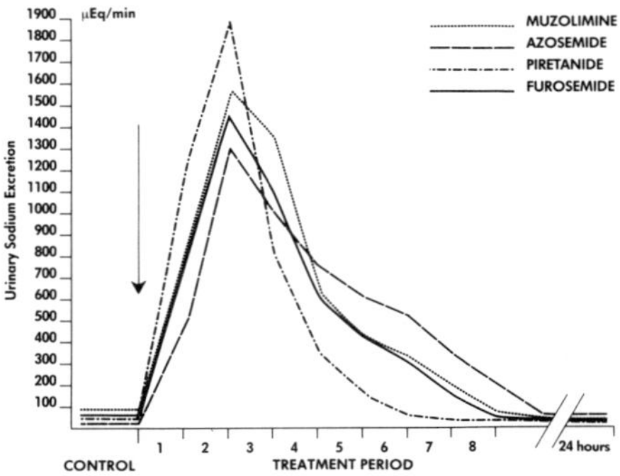

Fig. 1: Urinary sodium excretion (µEq/min) after a single dose of piretanide (24 mg), furosemide (100 mg) muzolimine (90 mg) and azosemide (320 mg) in ten healthy volunteers.

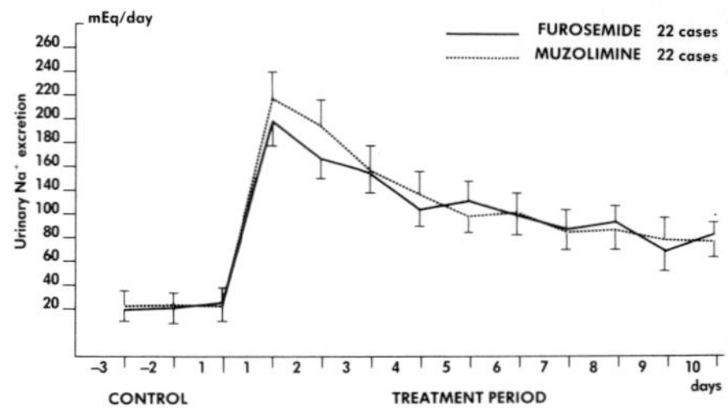

Fig. 2: Urinary sodium excretion (mEq/day, MEAN ± SEM) during treatment with furosemide (100 mg/day) and muzolimine (90 mg/day) in liver cirrhosis.

Both drugs determined evident changes in plasma uric acid and in acid-base balance.

In the group of healthy subjects treated with M, we did not observe a longer duration and a slower onset of action than F. In patients affected with cirrhosis, the urinary magnesium excretion resulted significantly higher than in the control period for both drugs, but in the group treated with M it was significantly lower than in the group treated with F. This observation is certainly interesting since it is well known that magnesium depletion, caused by prolonged diuretic treatments, can induce arrhythmias and lower effectiveness of antihypertensive drugs. (5)

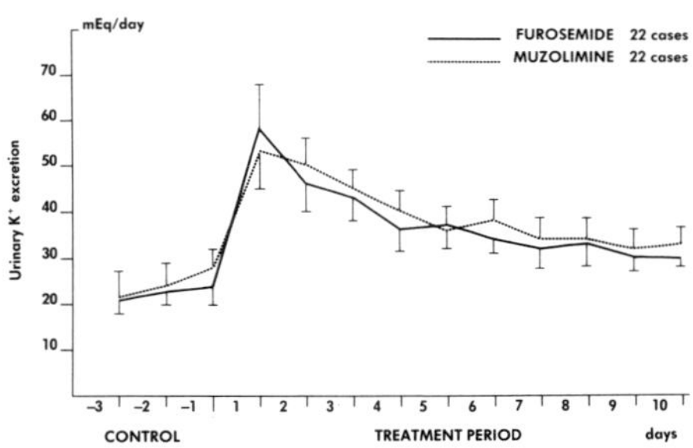

Fig. 3: Urinary potassium excretion (mEq/day, MEAN ± SEM) during treatment with furosemide (100 mg/day) and muzolimine (90 mg/day) in liver cirrhosis.

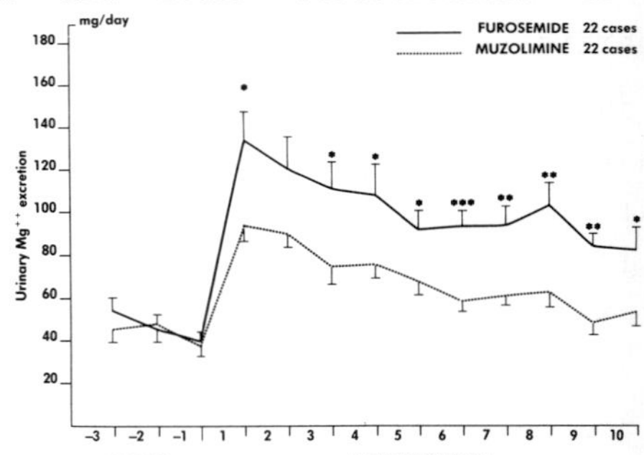

Fig. 4: Urinary magnesium excretion (mg/day, MEAN ± SEM) during treatment with furosemide (100 mg/day) and muzolimine (90 mg/day) in liver cirrhosis.
* $p < 0,025$, ** $p < 0,005$, *** $p < 0,001$: significant differences between the two groups.

REFERENCES

1. Garthoff B. Niere-und Hochdruckkrankheiten, 10:79, 1981.
2. Ritter W. Curr. Med. Res. Opin. 4: 564:573, 1977
3. Dal Canton A., Russo D., Gallo R., Conte G. and Andreucci V.E. Brit. Med. J. 282:595-598, 1981
4. Meng K., Loew D., Stoepel K and Hohhmeister F. Curr.Med. Res. Opin 4, 555, 1977.
5. Leary W.P., Reyes A.J. and Van Der Byl K., Z. Kardiol. 74, Suppl. 2, 135-140, 1985

RESTORATION OF RESPONSE TO DIURETICS WITH PLASMA EXPANDERS AND AMINOPHYLLINE IN ASCITIC CIRRHOSIS OF LIVER.

D. S. BAKHLE*, C.J. MISTRY*, L.M. PINTO PEREIRA**, R. D. KULKARNI*

* Division of Clinical Pharmacology
Grant Medical College, Bombay, India

** Hoechst India Limited, Bombay, India

INTRODUCTION

Liver cirrhotics with ascites respond poorly to diuretics (1) including aldosterone antagonists like spironolactone (2). Decreased central blood volume due to impaired albumin synthesis causes sodium retention (3) and reduced renal blood flow (RBF) (4) in liver cirrhosis.

We attempted to enhance response to furosemide (F) by giving plasma expanders (modified gelatin and dextran 40) and aminophylline i.v. Diuresis was restored in 3 cases of "diuretic resistant" ascites with dextran 40 infusion and aminophylline alternately.

MATERIALS AND METHODS

RBF was estimated in 6 cirrhotics (biopsy confirmed) with ascites using shadow shield whole body counter for determining renal elimination of Hippuran (^{131}I).

12 ascitic patients with histologically proven liver cirrhosis and serum albumin $<$ 3 gm%, without hypertension, primary renal disease or diabetes mellitus entered the study. 3 days prior diuretics were stopped. 20 mg F i.v. was given as control. Subsequently they received these 4 treatments. (1) 100 mg spironolactone orally. (2) 500 ml Haemaccel (modified gelatin) infused for 4 hours. (3) 540 ml Lomodex (dextran 40) infused for 4 hours. (4) 250 mg aminophylline (in 10 ml) injected intravenously for 30 min. Treatments 2 to 4 were followed by 20 mg F i.v. 2 hours after commencing treatment.

Cirrhotics with ascites who failed to respond to an average daily dose of 300 mg F also entered the study. 40 mg F i.v. was the control treatment. Dextran 40 infusion and i.v. aminophylline were then alternately given for 15 days, followed by 40 mg F i.v. 2 hours after commencing treatment.

Evaluation of Parameters : (1) 6 hour urine vol.

(2) Urinary sodium by flame photometry.

RESULTS

Mean elimination of Hippuran was significantly reduced in 6 cirrhotics (53.53±4.075%) as compared to normal value (70±5%). In these patients 6 hr urine vol and sodium excretion respectively was significantly lower with spironolactone 100 mg (230.83±44.99 ml and 3.35±0.94 meq) ($P < 0.05$) as compared to that with F (627.5±123.23 ml and 31.78±7.84 meq) ($P < 0.05$).

Mean 6 hour urine vol and sodium with other treatments

TREATMENTS	MEAN 6 hr vol (ml)	MEAN 6 hr SODIUM EXCRETION (meq)
I (12 patients)		
F 20 mg i.v.	721.25±103.12	39.26± 6.05
F 20 mg i.v. + plasma expanders°	1264.17±146.21 ($P < 0.001$)	91.79±15.49 ($P < 0.001$)
II (5 patients)		
F 20 mg i.v.	902.0 ±176.7	46.9 ±10.75
F 20 mg i.v. + 250 mg Aminophylline i.v.	1316.0 ±231.18 ($P < 0.05$)	129.94±24.33 ($P < 0.01$)
III (3 "diuretic resistant" patients)		
F 40 mg i.v.	260.0 ± 50.33	11.02± 2.94
F 40 mg i.v. + alternate regimen°°	731.91± 44.79 ($P < 0.01$)	57.44± 9.56 ($P < 0.05$)

o 500 ml HAEMACCEL or 540 ml DEXTRAN 40.
00 DEXTRAN 40 or AMINOPHYLLINE 250 mg i.v. alternately for 15 days.

DISCUSSION

Our study confirms reduction in RBF in cirrhotics (4). Increasing the central blood vol with "head out water immerssion" produces spontaneous natriuresis in such patients (2), confirming the importance of low central blood vol in sodium retention of cirrhosis.

We adapted a pharmacological manouevre to increase central blood vol and renal perfusion with plasma expanders restoring diuretic efficacy.

Aminophylline, which increases RBF in cirrhotics (5) enhanced diuresis in our study. Thus low RBF seems to be causative in limiting diuresis in cirrhotics with ascites.

"Diuretic resistant" cases of ascites have grossly impaired renal perfusion (6). Diuretic response was restored in 3 such cases with alternate plasma expander infusion and i.v. aminophylline. This regimen while maintaining central blood vol prevents diuretic induced renal failure despite profuse diuresis.

Plasma vol expansion releases Atrial Natriuretic Peptides (ANP) in circulation (7). The probable link between ANP levels and diuresis restored by plasma expanders need to be explored.

REFERENCES

(1) Arroya V., Bosch J., Casamitjana R., Rivera F. and Rodes J. Gut 21: 855, 1980.
(2) Epstein M., Pins D.S., Schneider N. and Levinson R. J. Lab. Clin. Med. 87: 822, 1976.
(3) Epstein M., Levinson R., Sancho J. et al Circulation Research, 41: 818, 1977.
(4) Kew M.C., Brunt P.W., Varma R.R. and Sherlock S. Lancet, 2: 504, 1971.
(5) Milani L., Merkel C. and Gatta A. Eur. J. Clin. Pharmacol, 24: 757, 1983.
(6) Baldus W.P., Feichter R.N., Summerskill W.H.J., Hunt J.C., and Wakim K.G., Ann. Intern. Med. 60: 366, 1964.
(7) Lang R.E., Thoelken H., Ganten D., Luft F.C., Ruskoaho H. and Unger Th. Nature, 314: 264, 1985.

BEHAVIOUR OF RED BLOOD CELL POTASSIUM AND OF OTHER HYDRO-ELECTROLYTE PARAMETERS DURING SPIRONALACTONE TREATMENT IN PATIENTS WITH NON COMPENSATED LIVER CIRRHOSIS.

Di Sciacca A., Durante F., Di Piazza R.M., Cucchiara G., Frontini A., Ingrassia A., Barbagallo Sangiorgi G.

Institute of Internal Medicine and Geriatrics held by Prof. Giuseppe Barbagallo Sangiorgi. Chair of Systematic Medical Therapy held by Prof. Arnaldo Di Sciacca, Palermo, Italy.

INTRODUCTION

The purpose of this research was to stress the importance of the treatment of water-salt decompensation in the cirrhotic patient with antagonists of aldosterone and in particular of spironolactone.

The possible untoward effects of this therapy and the clinical and laboratory methodology to be adopted in the course of treatment are indicated. We paid special attention to the water-salt situation, particularly with regard to variations in cell potassium calculated on the basis of red blood cell potassium; we also considered parameters that must be monitored in order to avoid the various untoward effects of a usually long-term therapy. These effects include hyponatremia, isotonic dehydration and hyperkaliemia.

CASES, MATERIALS AND METHODS

10 patients suffering from liver cirrhosis with water-salt decompensation and hyperaldostronism, after drug wash out for 10 days, were monitored electrolytically to assess the behaviour of certain parameters: daily diuresis, ratio between urinary sodium and potassium excretion (Na_U/K_U), serum sodium (Na_S), serum potassium (K_S), and in particular red blood cell potassium (K_{RBC}) as an indication of the amount of potassium in the cells, before and after 30 days of treatment with spironolactone at 200 mg/day, administered twice daily. The patients were kept on a steady dietetic water salt intake (400 ml water per day, sodium and potassium equivalent to the amount excreted in the urine daily) (Tab. 1).

RESULTS

The results show: a) increase of diuresis; b) gradual increase of urinary sodium tending towards optimal Na_U/K_U ratio; c) decrease of Na_S ; d) increase of K_S; e) progressive decrease of K_{RBC}.

These changes were statistically significant (Tab. 2).

Tab. 1 –

CASES	Age	W.O. Diuresis ml/24h	T. Diuresis ml/24h	W.O. Na_S	T Na_S	W.O. K_S	T K_S	W.O. K_{RBC}	T. K_{RBC}	W.O. Na_U/K_U ratio	T. Na_U/K_U ratio
C. Rosa	55	500	1.400	139	132	4,0	5,1	98,11	89,6	1,417	3,433
D.M. Antonino	82	500	1.900	140	130	4,3	6,1	94,0	86,9	1,08	4,666
D.T. Francesco	50	650	1.100	138	130	3,8	4,4	96,8	87,5	1,627	1,805
F. Rosario	69	700	1.000	139	138	3,8	4,6	101,8	94,5	1,119	1,52
C.B. Domenico	64	700	1.650	139	131	4,4	5,1	101,0	93,0	1,000	2,970
F. Giuseppa	71	500	1.300	139	135	4,6	6,0	103,9	93,2	1,444	2,837
M. Rosaria	58	800	1.600	140	130	4,2	5,0	107,0	100,0	0,441	3,384
O. Angela	57	500	1.400	144	136	4,0	5,2	97,5	90,8	0,75	1,888
R. Antonino	57	700	1.600	152	134	4,3	5,1	103,0	84,0	0,660	4,027
T. Calogero	44	600	1.500	135	135	3,3	4,5	104,0	93,0	0,75	1,620

Diagnosis = Non compensated liver cirrhosis
Treatment time = 30 days
Daily dose = 200 mg/day

W.O. = Wash Out
T. = Therapy

Tab. 2 – STATISTIC SIGNIFICANCE

1)	Daily diuresis	W. O. 625	T. 1445	$p <$	0,001
2)	K_S	W. O. 4,07	T. 5,11	$p <$	0,001
3)	K_{RBC}	W. O. 100,80	T. 91,25	$p <$	0,001
4)	Na_S	W. O. 140,5	T. 133,1	$p <$	0,01
5)	Na_U/K_U ratio	W. O. 1,032	T. 2,880	$p <$	0,001

CONCLUSIONS

- Treatment with diuretics requires continuous control of the water-salt situation.
- Spironolactone affects the potassium pool by means of a displacing mechanism on the peripheral receptors (distal tubule).
- The increase of K_S and vice versa the decrease of K_{RBC} probably reflect the effect of a transfer of cell potassium from the intracellular to the extracellular compartment due to the action of the antialdosterone drug on the Na-K-ATPase-dependent pump.

REFERENCES:

1. Astrup J., Thomsen A. C., Westrup M.: Red cell sodium and potassium contents in liver cirrhosis. Gastrenterology 78, 530-534, 1980.
2. Barbagallo Sangiorgi G., Di Sciacca A., Pardo A.: Potassium depletion in aged patients: an evaluation through red-cell potassium determination. Age and Ageing 8, 190-195, 1980.
3. Barbagallo Sangiorgi G., Di Sciacca A., Fradà G. jr., Cupidi G., Barbagallo M.: Il danno jatrogenico da farmaci in geriatria. Nuovo Boll. Farmacol. Clinica, Napoli, 1981, 3, 157-168.
4. Barbagallo Sangiorgi G., Fradà G. jr., Di Sciacca A., Cupidi G., Affronti M., Costanza G., Putignano E., Barbagallo M.: Turbe del ricambio idroelettrico come causa di encefalopatia metabolica nell'anziano. Giorn. Geront. 30, 199-202, 1982.
5. Barbagallo Sangiorgi G., Di Sciacca A., Durante F., Fradà G. jr., Costanza G., Cupidi G.: La terapia diuretica e la terapia antiipertensiva nell'anziano. Giorn. Geront. 30, 749-774, 1982.
6. Black D.A.K.: Potassium metabolism. In: Clinical Disorders of Fluid and Electrolyte Metabolism, 2nd ed. M.H. Maxwell, C.R. Kleeman (eds.). New York, McGraw-Hill, 1972, pp. 121-149.
7. Greemblatt D.J., Koch-Weser J.: Adverse reactions to spironolactone. Jama 225, 40-43; 1973.
8. Hochs H.R., Greemblatt D.J., Bodeng: Spironolactone. Am. Heart J. 90, 389, 1978.
9. Ibsen: Red blood cell potassium as a measure of body potassium. Scand. J. Clin. Lab. Invest. 34, 161-165, 1974.
10. Soler N.G., Jain S., James H., Paton A.: Potassium status of patients with cirrhosis. Gut 17, 152-157, 1976.

MUZOLIMINE AS TREATMENT OF ASCITES FROM HEPATIC CHIRROSIS.

A. AJELLO, A. SPADARO, M.A. FRENI, I. CALAPRISTI, A. FAVA, A. CAPPELLO, and O. FERRAU' *.

Istituto di Clinica Medica, * Cattedra di Patologia Medica III, Messina University.

INTRODUCTION

The antagonists of Aldosterone are considered the first choice diuretics in the treatment of ascites from liver cirrhosis. They are able to induce a slow and progressive weight loss without potassium depletion(1). Their long term use causes anyway hyperkalaemia and hyperchloraemic acidosis (2) and their efficacy is reduced in long lasting ascites. In such a case the more drastic loop diuretics are required. These have however serious side effects in cirrhotics more than in other patients (hypokalaemia, encephalopathy, hepatorenal syndrome) (3).

Aim of this study was to evaluate the efficacy of a new loop diuretic, Muzolimine, on ascites secondary to hepatic cirrhosis.

PATIENTS AND METHODS

Forty patients with ascites from hepatic cirrhosis entered this study. Patients with encephalopathy, renal failure and serious electrolyte desorder were excluded. The patients studied were on diet (2.000 Kcal/day, $<$ 1 l/day water intake and $<$ 50 mEq/day sodium intake). After a 4 day wash-out they were given 60 mg/day of Muzolimine. The drug dose was gradually increased (30 mg/day) in non responder patients until the right diuretic effect was achieved. Blood glucose and ammonia, azotaemia, serum and urinary Na^+ and K^+, creatinine clearance were periodically tested. Patients with hypokalaemia ($K^+ <$ 3.8 mEq/l) were given since the beginning also a potassium sparing diuretic (K^+ canreonate 200 mg/day). Patients who during treatment developed hypokalaemia ($K^+ <$ 3.4 mEq/l) were given per os potassium chloride supplement

(16 mEq/day). Muzolimine treatment was temporarily stopped in the patients with severe hypokalaemia ($<$ 3.2 mEq/l).

RESULTS

Ascites disappeared in all the patients during a treatment period ranging from 5 to 28 days (13 ± 5). The mean weight loss was Kg 6.8 ± 4.33 (range (Kg 2.1 - 19.2). 60 mg/day of Muzolimine were efficient in 22/40 patients; 90 mg/day were necessary in 12 patients, while in the other 6 more than 90 mg/day were requested. Out of the 40 patients admitted to the study, 20 were given muzolimine only at start and 20 were given Muzolimine + potassium sparing diuretic since the beginning because of hypokalaemia ($<$ 3.8 mEq/l). Ten patients from the first group who presented hypokalaemia during the treatment were given also K^+ canreonate. Oral potassium supplements were necessary in 10/40 patients.

The drug was efficient since the first day of treatment in all the patients, causing marked natriuresis and urinary volume increase which persisted until ascites disappeared (Fig. 1). The efficacy was greater in the patients with satisfactory basal natriuresis and normal kalaemia (Fig. 2): in such group, where ascites was less important and recently appeared, K^+ canreonate was not required and ascites disappeared more rapidly than in the other two groups. In the patients with low basal natriuresis, more important diuresis contraction and tendency to hypokalaemia Muzolimine had to be administered for longer and often ad higher doses. Muzolimine did not cause significant alterations of the parameters tested, except a modest increase of kaliuresis in the patients on monotherapy. Some of such subjects showed hypokalaemia easily corrected by oral administration of K^+ canreonate and/or potassium supplements. Reduction of creatinine clearance with moderate increase of azotaemia was sometimes present at the end of therapy in those patients who had been treated for longer time (Table 1).

CONCLUSIONS

From our data, Muzolimine is able to remove ascites in short time and without important side effects: in particular no patients presented hepatic encephalopathy or severe renal failure.

Constant association with antagonists of aldosterone is anyway suggested by the frequent hypokalaemia in the patients with liver cirrhosis.

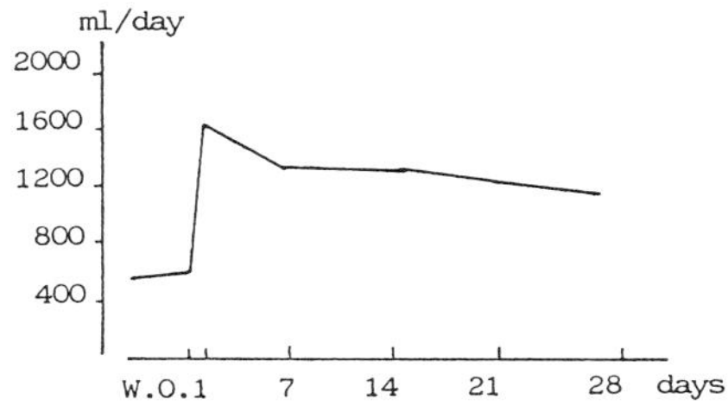

Fig.1. Effect of Muzolimine on urinary volume

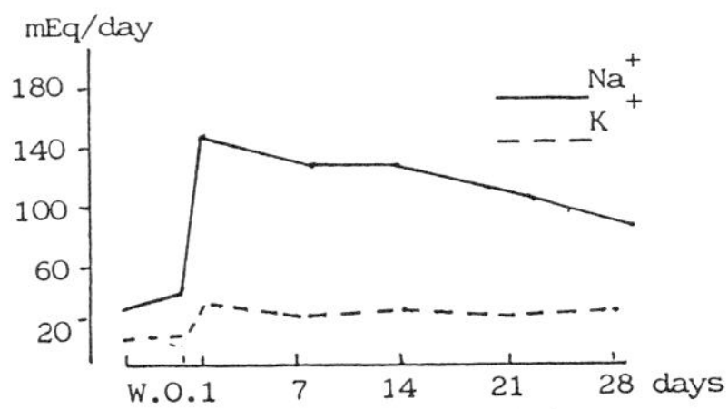

Fig.2. Effect of Muzolimine on urinary excretion of Na^+ and K^+

Table 1. Plasmatic changes during Muzolimine treatment (40 patients).

		before	after
azotaemia	> 60 mg%	3	7
creat. clear.	< 60 ml/m'	2	8
blood ammonia	> 100 mcg%	5	8
kalaemia	< 3.8 mEq/l	9	5

REFERENCES

1. Eggert, R.C.: Br. Med. J. 4: 401-403, 1970
2. Gabow, P.A., Moore, S., Schrier, R.W.: Ann. Intern. Med. 90: 338-340, 1979
3. Sherlock, S.: Scand. J. Gastroenterol. 7 (Suppl.): 9-15, 1970

XI. DIURETICS AND STONE FORMATION

EXTRARENAL EFFECTS OF HYDROCHLOROTHIAZIDE IN HYPERCALCIURIC STONE FORMERS.

P.Messa,G.Mioni,L.Paganin°,Lo Greco P.°°,Enzmann G.,Montanaro D.,Adorati M.,Antonucci F.,Favazza A.,Messa M.,Gropuzzo M.

Division of Nephrology,°Division of Urology,°°Clinical Chemistry Laboratory-City Hospital Udine-ITALY.

INTRODUCTION

The anticalciuric effect of thiazide diuretics is well known to be due to an increased Ca reabsorption by the distal tubule(1).However the maintenance of hypocalciuria cannot occur without a reduction of intestinal absorption and/or bone resorption of Ca.In humans,Int. Ca Abs. has been reported to remain unchanged(2),to fall(3) of to rise(4) with thiazide administration.Recently an increased bone mineral content(5) and a reduced bone resorption(6) have been reported in patients treated with Hydrochlorothiazide(HTZ).The present study was undertaken to evaluate the effects of HTZ on bone and intestine,in relation to its anticalciuric activity,in a group of Hypercalciuric Stone Formers(HSF).

PATIENTS AND METHODS

We studied 13 stone formers (7 M,6 F),aged 20-44,with normal renal function(Cr.Cl. 98-154 ml/min).They all were hypercalciuric(u-Ca>4 mg/kg//day,on free diet) and 10 of them had also fasting hypercalciuria(fast u-Ca//Cr>.11 mg/mg).They were firstly evaluated while on their free diet;then a Low Ca Diet(LCD)(400 mg/day) was started.After 10 days of LCD,a first evaluation was performed;then HTZ(50 mg/day) was added to the diet and after 30 days of treatment a further evaluation was performed.The parameters evaluated were:Ca,Mg,phosphate,Na,Creatinine in 24 hr urine(2 repeated samples)and inplasma;fasting urinary excretion of Ca,phosphate,Na,Creatinine, hydroxyproline(OHP) and c-AMP;serum PTH(-COOh);Fract.Int.Ca Abs. and Ca Pool at 24th hr(kinetic methodology).The methods employed for analysis and calculations were described elsewhere(7).The resulte are expressed as mean ± sd.Statistics were performed using variance analysis and linear regression.

RESULTS

The effects of LCD and LCD+HTZ on daily and fasting Ca excretions are shown in the Table 1.:

TABLE 1.	Free Diet	LCD	LCD+HTZ
u-Ca/day	352	207°°	202°°
mg/day	±86	±70	±88
u-Ca/Cr(fast)	.141	.137	.097§°
mg/mg	±.045	±.030	±.039

°=p<.01, °°=p<.001 vs Free Diet; §=p<.01 vs LCD.

LCD resulted in a striking reduction of u-Ca/day,though 8 pat. remained hypercalciuric(u-Ca>200 mg/day on LCD);no effect of LCD was evident on fast Ca excretion.HTZ did not result in any significant reduction of the mean u-Ca/day,when compaired with LCD:however a wide range of the individual responses to the drug was seen,with 6 pat. clearly reducing,4 showing little changes and 3 presenting a paradoxical increase of u-Ca/day.On the contrary HTZ markedly reduced fast u-Ca.The effects of HTZ on the parameters related to osseous and intestinal activity are shown in Table 2.:

TABLE 2.	Ca Pool at 24th hr	OHP/Cr	%Int.Ca Abs.
	l	mg/g	%
LCD	42.1	28.6	60
	±12.9	±8.5	±15
LCD+HTZ	35.4°	20.0°°	58
	± 8.4	±9.9	±13

°=p<.05; °°=p<.001

It is evident that HTZ resulted in a significant decrease of bone indices. Furthermore the variations of these parameters were well correlated with the changes of fast Ca excretion:

1. Δ fast u-Ca/Cr = 0.085 + 0.063 Δ OHP/Cr;r=.929,p <.001;

2. Δ fastu-Ca/Cr =-11.22 + 3.77 ΔPool ;r=.674,p< .05.

The effects of HTZ on Int.Ca Abs. was apparently null:as a matter of fact a great variability in the individual responses was evident.It is worth noting that the changes in Int.Ca Abs. resulted correlated with the variations of u-Ca/day at a highly significant level:

3. Δ u-Ca/day= -12.8 + 5.95 Δ % Int.Ca Abs. ;r=.945,p <.001.

The effects of HTZ on the other parameters are shown in Table 3.:

TABLE 3.

	Cr.Cl. ml/min	u-Na mEq/l	diuresis ml/day	s-Ca mg/dl	TTiP mg/dl	u-cAMP nmol/dlGFR	s-PTH ng/ml
LCD	120	124	1681	9.4	3.5	3.9	.62
	± 9	±42	±545	±.6	±.5	±2.0	±.19
LCD+HTZ	118	155	2125°	9.7°	3.2°	4.6	.52
	±10	±100	±608	±.3	±.5	±2.1	±.52

°= $p < .05$.

A mild but significant increase of diuresis and s-Ca and a decrease of Tm Pi/GFR were noted.

DISCUSSION

The patients we studied did not show any significant variation in u-Ca/ day after HTZ:this finding is in apparent contrast with previous data of the literature.It may be explained in part because our patients started HTZ after a period at a LCD.Moreover,we did not prescribe any Na restriction and so the hypocalciuric component due to volume depletion was not present.Furthermore the dose of HTZ was half of that used in most studies(but this is the most widely utilized dose in our country).The apparent lack of anticalciuric effect was also due to different individual responses to HTZ,the variations of u-Ca/day resulting strictly correlated to the changes of Int.Ca Abs.On the contrary the anticalciuric effect of HTZ during fast was constant and sigificant.This effect appeared closely dependent on the reduction of bone turnover. Our data are in agreement with other reports(5,6).We can conclude that dietary Ca restriction plays a major role in reducing u-Ca/day;HTZ,when given on a LCD,without Na restriction,has a variable and not predictable effect on u-Ca/day,depending on changes of Int.Ca Abs.HTZ,by reducing Bone turnover rate,did result in a significant decrease in fasting Calcium excretion.

REFERENCES

1.Costanzo ls,Windhager e.Am.J.Physiol.235:F492,1978.
2.Harrison AR,Rose GA.Clin.Sci.34:343,1978.
3.Barilla DE,Tolentino R.et Al.Metabolism.27:125,1978.
4.Yendt ER,Cohanim M.Kidney Internat.13:397,1978.
5.Wasnich RD,Benfante RJ,et Al.New.Eng J.Med.309:344,1983.
6.Lemann J.,Gray RW,et Al.Kidney Internat.28:951,1985.
7.Messa P.,Mioni G.,et Al.In"Diuretics"ed.J.Puschett,pg.491,1984.

CAUSES OF FAILURE IN THIAZIDE DIURETIC THERAPY OF HYPERCALCIURIC NEPHROLITHIASIS

K.MATSUSHITA, K.TANIKAWA, N.KAWAMURA

Department of Urology, Tokai University School of Medicine, Isehara, Kanagawa, Japan

INTRODUCTION

It is well established that thiazide diuretics can prevent a new stone formation in patients with a history of recurrent idiopathic calcium nephrolithiasis. However, in our recent study of the 49 patients who received a long-term thiazide therapy, 17 (34.7 %) developed recurrent calcium stones. We analyzed the causes of that rather high recurrent incidence.

MATERIALS AND METHODS

For the past 3 yrs we followed 342 patients with urolithiasis. Of those, 109 were hypercalciuric (32 %). 49 hypercalciuric patients with a history of recurrent stone disease were selected as candidates for thiazide diuretic therapy. According to oral calcium load tests, 10 patients were categorized as renal hypercalciuria and the remaining 39, as type 1 absorptive hypercalciuria. Trichlormethiazide 4 mg/day was prescribed to all the subjects. Treatment period ranged from 4 to 43 months. During therapy all had repeated examinations of urine and blood chemistry. Urinary oxalate was measured by gas chromatography, citrate by enzymatic analysis. The state of urinary saturation with respect to calcium oxalate was examined by measuring concentration product ratios of this substance before and after incubation of single-voided urine samples mixed with calcium oxalate monohydrate as seeding crystals. Relative supersaturation of urine with calcium oxalate (CaOX) was quickly obtained on the nomogram of Robertson et al.(1). The patients were allowed to take their ordinary diet and fluid, without sodium or calcium restriction. Thiazide-induced hypokalemia was corrected by supplementary potassium.

RESULTS

Evaluation of effectiveness of the therapy was based on new stone formation rate and urinary calcium excretion. The outcome was subdivided into 3 categories. 15 patients were defined as success because new stone formation rate as well as urinary calcium excretion was significantly reduced. 17 failed because new stone formation rate was not reduced by treatment. In the remaining 17 patients new stone formation rate was suppressed, but hypercalciuria was not completely eradicated by the drug and so they were defined as indeterminate.

Various factors were compared between success and failure groups (Table 1). In the failure group urinary oxalate and uric acid were elevated during treatment whereas citrate was lower as compared with pretreatment values.

In a limited number of thiazide-treated patients regardless of outcomes of the medication we studied relationship between urinary calcium excretion and concentration product ratios as well as relative supersaturation with respect to calcium oxalate, and we found a negative correlation between them ($p<0.01$, see Fig.1 and 2). In the same subjects we observed a positive correlation between urinary citrate and oxalate excretion (both, to creatinine ratio, mg/dl/mg/dl, Fig.3).

DISCUSSION

The first report that demonstrated hypocalciuric action of thiazide diuretics appeared in 1959 (2). Based on htis observation, Yendt et al. attempted to prevent kidney stone with the use of thiazide diuretics and their successful results were published in 1970 (3). In our recent study, however, we observed a rather high percentage of treatment failure. But if only the new stone formation rate is taken into account, our success rate was 65 % which is clinically acceptable.

There is a little possibility that subclinical hyperparathyroidism was included in the failure group because transient elevation of serum calcium was noted in a few patients although the PTH-C remained normal throughout the treatment.

Reduction in urinary calcium excretion was observed in a majority of the studied patients. However, in the failure group urinary oxalate level was elevated as compared with pretreatment value. Since the randomly chosen subjects having thiazides had a negative correlation between urinary calcium excretion and state of saturation with respect to CaOX, it may be that in the failure group despite of diminished calcium excretion, increased urinary oxalate level was such that urinary saturation with respect to CaOX exceeded its formation product ratio, resulting in spontaneous crystallization of that substance and new stone formation (Fig.1,2). According to our observation (Fig.3), urinary citrate is expected to be higher as urinary oxalate increases. However, in the failure group the citrate level was low (Table 1). Possibly, this hypocitraturia was another cause of the unfavorable results. Why not all the subjects having thiazide diuretics develop hypocitraturia remains to be solved.

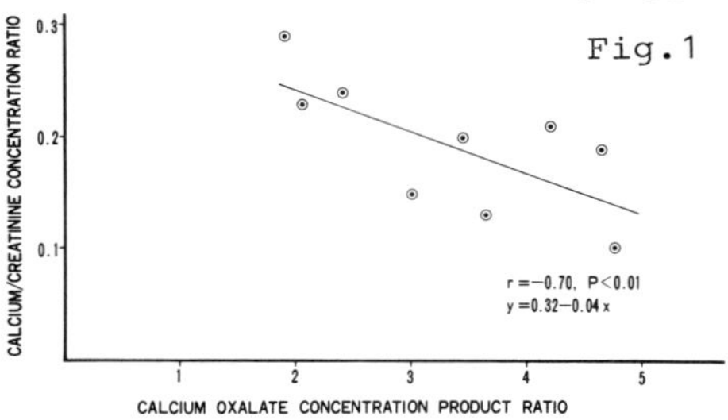

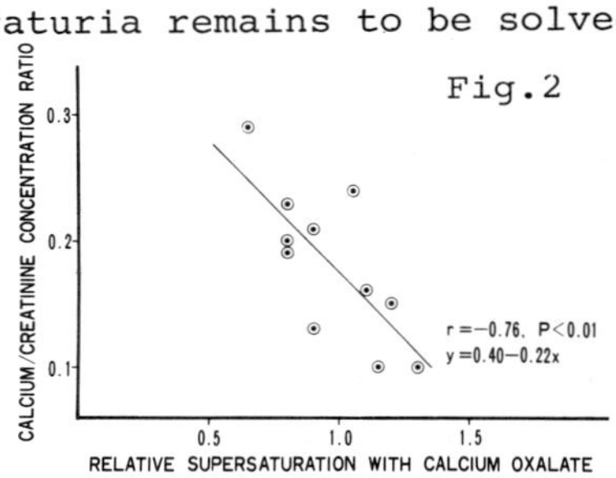

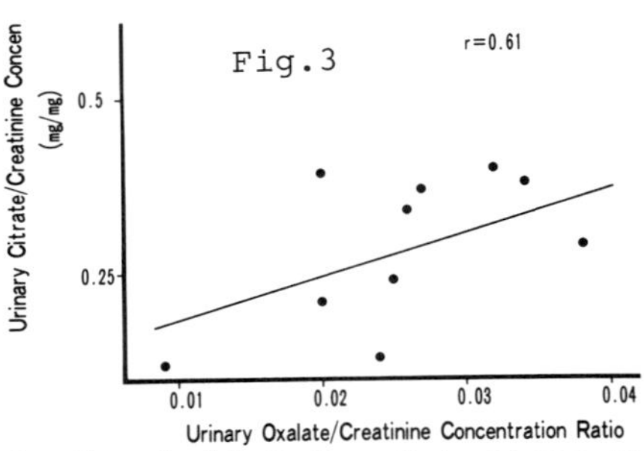

Table 1
Outcomes of Thiazide Diuretic Therapy of Idiopathic Calcium Nephrolithiasis in Success and Failure Groups(mean±S.D.)

	Before Treatment		During Treatment	
	Success	Failure	Success	Failure
No. of cases	15	17	15	17
Stone formation rate (no./patient/year)	3.4±1.1	2.5±2.0	0.8±0.2*	1.9±1.0
	In the 24-hour urine specimen			
URINE Urinary volume (ml/day)	1530±120	1300±150	1710±180	1690±150
URINE Calcium (mg/day)	298±52	271±65	175±30*	192±43*
URINE Magnesium (〃)	85±11	90±22	74±18	92±10
URINE Uric acid (〃)	433±74	501±80	440±56	550±61**
URINE Oxalate (〃)	44±8.0	42±10	41±8.5	49±9.3**
URINE Citrate (〃)	353±25	384±43	347±30	311±25*

* $p<0.01$ versus pretreatment values
** $p<0.05$ versus pretreatment values

1. Marshall,R.W., Robertson,W.G. Clin.Chim.Acta 72:253-260, 1976
2. Lamberg,B.A., Kuhlback,B. Scand.J.Clin.Lab.Invest. 2:351-357, 1959
3. Yendt,E.R. Can.Med.Assoc.J. 102:479-489, 1970

COMPARISON OF TWO DIFFERENT ASSOCIATION OF DIURETICS IN REDUCING HYPERCALCIURIA IN RECURRENT CALCIUM STONE FORMERS

M.A. LEONE, N. VIGGIANI, G. DIMONA, F.P. SCHENA

Chair of Medical Therapy, University of Bari, Polyclinic, Bari, Italy

INTRODUCTION

Idiopathic hypercalciuria is thought to be one of the most important determining factors in the pathogenesis of stone formation. Many studies (1-3) have demonstrated the efficacy of thiazide diuretics in reducing urinary calcium excretion and in preventing recurrent nephrolithiasis.

In this paper we report our experience on the metabolic effects of patients (pts) with calcium stones.

PATIENTS AND METHODS

Twenty-three randomized out-patients suffering from recurrent calcium stones were put on a diuretic therapy. No patient had primary hyperparathyroidism or urinary tract infections. The subjects were divided into 3 groups. Group A: 8 pts (5 F and 3 M) treated with hydroclorothiazide (HCT) 25 mg/day + amiloride (A) 2.5 mg/day. Group B: 10 pts (5 F and 5 M) treated with HCT 50 mg/day + A 5 mg/day. Group C: 5 pts (3 F and 2 M) treated with butizide (B) 5 mg + canreonate-potassium (CRK) 50 mg/day.

The mean age was similar for all groups.

Urinary calcium, phosphorus, uric acid and magnesium were measured before and after 3 and 6 months of diuretic treatment.

Thirteen pts were studied for a period of 6 months, whereas the remaining 10 were followed for over 1 year.

Statistical analysis: Data from groups of pts have been given as the mean ± standard error mean (SEM). The values were compared by the Wilcoxon test for paired data and the Kruskal-Wallis test.

RESULTS

The metabolic effects of the therapy are represented in figure 1.

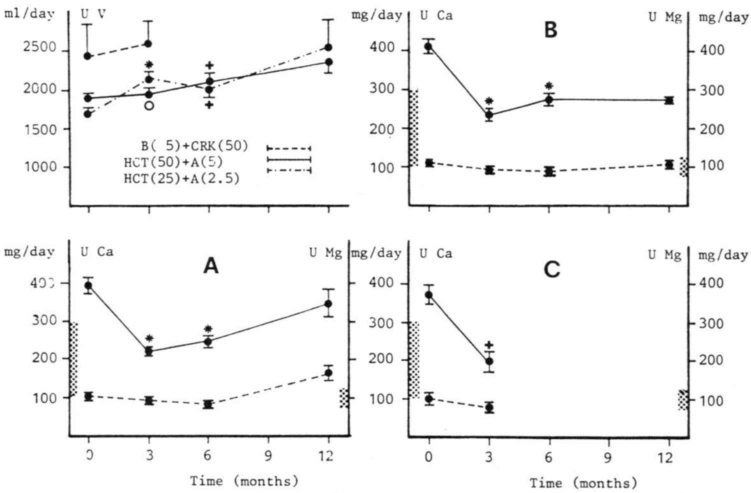

Figure 1: Follow-up of daily diuresis, urinary calcium and magnesium in recurrent calcium stone formers who had been treated with HCT (25mg/day) + A (2.5mg/day) [A],HCT (50mg/day) + A (5mg/day) [B],B (5mg/day) + CRK (50mg/day) [C]. The values are expressed as mean ± SEM.
The normal range of urinary solutes is expressed by the dotted column.
✱ $p<0.005$ ✚ $p<0.05$ o $p<0.025$

1. The values of hypercalciuria before treatment did not differ in the three groups.
2. Urine volume increased after 3 months in group A ($p<0.005$) and B ($p<0.025$) while urine output did not increase significantly in group C ($p<0.1$).
3. Urinary calcium decreased significantly reaching the normal range in all groups (group A: $p<0.005$; group B: $p<0.005$; group C: $p<0.05$). The reduction persisted after 6 months of therapy in groups A and B; nevertheless, no statistical difference in urinary calcium excretion was observed when the values at the third and sixth month were compared.
4. Urinary magnesium values did not change in any of the groups.
5. In the third month the percentage of reduction of urinary calcium excretion reached the value of 40% in group A, 36% in group B and 46% in group C. The comparison among the three groups showed no significant difference (H=0.99;DF=2).
6. There was no modification in phosphorus excretion, while we observed a decrease in urinary excretion of uric acid ($p<0.05$).

7. Four pts of group A and 6 pts of group B were followed for 1 year; in these pts calcium excretion remained similar to the values measured at the sixth month.

Treated pts did not show side effects on the metabolism of glucose and serum potassium levels; nevertheless, 2/10 pts developed hypotension.

DISCUSSION

Previous reports (1-3,6,7) have shown that diuretic treatment with thiazide in calcium stone formers with evidence of hypercalciuria, drastically reduces the incidence of stone relapses. This is due to the reduction of urinary calcium which persists throughout treatment. Our data confirm previous findings reported by Maschio et al. (2) who treated stone formers by associating HCT (50mg/day) and A (5mg/day).

We have administred in a group of 5 pts a new association of diuretics (B 5mg/day + CRK 50mg/day) and we have obtained the reduction of the urinary calcium levels within 3 months of treatment.This reduction did not differ significantly from that of pts receiving HCT + A. The decrease of the urinary calcium level was equal in all the groups and did not differ significantly. In contrast to the findings of other investigators (4,6,7) we did not observe any increase of magnesium excretion but,rather,as in agreement with Scholz (5), a slight reduction of the magnesiuria.

We did not observe any modification of the excretion of the phosphorus but there was a decrease in urinary excretion of uric acid probably due to the association with allopurinol in some cases.

In conclusion, our data show that a low dose of a new association of diuretics (B+CRK) is able to reduce hypercalciuria in calcium stone formers. Nevertheless, we are not able in this preliminary study to give definite data on the prevention of stone recurrence, even though in 2 pts suffering from frequent relapses of nephrolithiasis (2/3 stones/year) we observed a reduced number of episodes of stone formation.

REFERENCES

1. Yendt E.R. and Cohaim M. Kid. Inter. 13:397-409,1978.
2. Maschio G. et al. Am. J. Med. 71:623-626,1981.
3. Barilla D.E. et al. Metabolism Clin. Exp. 27:125-131,1978.
4. Pak C.Y.C. et al. Clin. Pharmacol. Therap. 14:209-217,1972.
5. Scholz D. et al. in Urolithiasis Clin. Basic Res.(Eds Smith, Robertson, Finlayson),Plenum Press New York 1981, pp 249-252.
6. Ljunghall S. et al. in Urolith. Clin. Bas. Res.,Plenum Press NY 1981,pp245-248
7. Ahlstrand C. et al. in Urolithiasis and Related Clin.Res.(Eds Schwille, Smith,Robertson,Vahlensieck),Plenum Press New York 1985,pp471-473.

MEDICAL TREATMENT OF IDIOPATHIC CALCIUM NEPHROLITHIASIS: THIAZIDE (T) VS STONE CLINIC EFFECT.

M.E. DE FERRARI, G. COLUSSI, G. ROMBOLA', E. BENAZZI, M. SURIAN, F. MALBERTI, L. MINETTI.

Renal Unit, Niguarda Ca'Granda Hospital, Milan, Italy.

INTRODUCTION

The efficacy of T in the treatment of idiopathic calcium nephrolithiasis has been recently questioned (1) both in randomized and non randomized clinical trials. Moreover, the positive effect in preventing Ca stone recurrences so far reported might be due at least in part to dietary advice and close clinical supervision ("stone clinic effect")(2). The purpose of our study was to investigate the effects of T vs non medical treatment in idiopathic calcium stone formers (CSF).

MATERIALS AND METHODS

Among 984 stone formers in file at our department since 1976 we have retrospectively evaluated 87 CSF selected for having formed at least 2 stones, of which one in the last year, and with a follow up on treatment of at least one year. Patients were excluded who had systemic diseases, urological abnormalities, urinary tract infection or chronic renal failure (GFR > 80 ml/min).

Clinical, radiological and biochemical parameters were recorded before treatment and every 6 months during the follow up. All the patients were advised to increase their fluid intake, mainly water, and to avoid dietary calcium, oxalate and salt excess, with reduction of caloric intake when needed. Forty-five patients were treated with fluid and diet alone (D), while to 42 T (hydrochlorothiazide 25-50 mg plus amiloride 2.5-5 mg/day) was added (D + T). The treatment was chosen for pts with recent surgery, stone recurrences on D, hypertension requiring drugs. Allopurinol was added to T if hyperuricosuria was present.

RESULTS

D and D + T pts had formed respectively 209 and 256 stones, with a follow up of 453 and 383 pt-yr (table 1); stone activity was slightly lower in D (0.46 stone/pt-yr vs 0.67: $p < 0.02$). Mean follow up on treatment was 2.07 and 2.31 yr/pt (ranges 1-5) in D and D + T. During a total of 93.1 and 97.2 pt-yr respectively of follow up on treatment, stone events significantly fell to 25 in D and 39 in D + T (0.27 and 0.4 stone/pt-yr: $p < 0.05$), but with no significative difference between the 2 groups.

Considering separately only the pts with hypercalciuria (27 pts in D and 29 pts in D + T), stone recurrence rate was lower in D than D+T (0.27 vs 0.56 stone pt-yr, $p < 0.05$).

In both groups, recurrent pts did not differ from non recurrent pts during treatment for calcium, oxalate and uric acid excretion, while only in D recurrent pts had lower urine volume than non recurrent pts (1612 ± 827 ml/day vs 2237 ± 882, $p < 0.05$).

DISCUSSION

Our study indicates that thiazide therapy of idiopathic calcium nephrolithiasis does not offer better results than diet and fluid recommandations alone and this is in line with recent controlled clinical trials (3,4). Both groups show a reduced stone activity along the follow up when compared to pre-treatment data as a positive result of the stone clinic effect or a natural fading of the activity of stone disease. From our data, it would appear that the presence of a metabolic derangement such as hypercalciuria is not determinant for the effects of either diet or drug treatment. In fact, T therapy was not more effective than diet and fluids alone in reducing stone formation rate in selected hypercalciuric pts. Moreover, calcium excretion along treatment was not different in recurring or non recurring pts.

The efficacy of T in calcium stone disease is still an open question (1-6); we feel, on the basis of our results, that the efficacy of dietary advice, increased fluid intake and close clinical supervision, should be evaluated in every patient before prescribing any drug therapy.

Table 1. Clinical activity of stone disease before and during therapy.

		D	D+T	
	n =	45	42	p<
Pre-treatment:				
patient-year		453	383	NS
no. stones		209	256	NS
no. stones/year		.83±.93	1.1±1.2	NS
no. stones/pt-year		0.46	0.67	0.02
Post-treatment:				
patient-year		93.1	97.2	NS
no. stones		25	39	NS
no. stones/year		.33±.52°°	.34±.56*	NS
no. stones/pt-year		0.27°°	0.40°	NS

vs pre-treatment p : °= 0.05, °°= 0.02, *= 0.001

REFERENCES

1. Churchill, D. and Taylor, W. J.Urol. 133: 749-751, 1985.
2. Hosking, D.H., Erickson, S.B., Van Den Berg, C.J., Wilson, D.M. and Smith, L.H. J.Urol. 130:1115-1118, 1983.
3. Brocks, P., Dahl, C. and Wolf, H. Lancet 2:124-125, 1981.
4. Scholz, D., Schwille P.O. and Sigel, A. J.Urol. 128:903-907, 1982.
5. Laerum, E. and Larsen, S. Acta Med.Scand. 215:383-389, 1984.
6. Yendt, E.R. and Cohanim, M. In: Urolithiasis and Related Clinical Research (Eds. P.O. Schwille, L.H. Smith, W.G. Robertson and W. Vahlensieck), Plenum, New York, 1985, pp. 463-470.

EFFECT OF THIAZIDE DIURETICS ON HYPERCALCIURIA INDUCED BY ACTIVE VITAMIN D METABOLITES.

FERNANDO SANTOS and JAMES C.M. CHAN

Sections of Pediatric Nephrology, N.S.Covadonga Hospital, Oviedo, Spain, and Medical College of Virginia, Richmond, VA, USA

Active metabolites of vitamin D have been successfully used in the treatment of children undergoing endocrine and renal disorders in which mineral metabolism is impaired. Adequate therapy with vitamin D metabolites will produce increased intestinal absorption of calcium and phosphorus giving rise to beneficial effects on bone mineralization and growth. Chan et al (1) demonstrated accelerated height velocity in uremic children, younger than 12 years, after starting calcitriol administration. Similar growth enhancement and improvement of skeletal deformities have also been showed (2) in patients with hypophosphatemic rickets as a result of long-term treatment with active vitamin D metabolites and phosphate supplementation. In a similar fashion, effectiveness of prolonged calcitriol administration has been demonstrated (3) in children with abnormal parathyroid function.

Concurrently with these favorable actions on growth and mineral metabolism, administration of highly potent vitamin D metabolites may bring about harmful side effects such as hypercalcemia and hypercalciuria. One episode of hypercalcemia every 13 months was documented in 29 uremic children taking calcitriol at maintenance dose of 20-40 ng/kg/day (4). Otherwise, significant increase of urinary calcium excretion has been shown (5) in patients undergoing renal hypophosphatemic rickets after therapy with high doses of calcitriol (Fig. 1). Due to the relatively short half-lives of most potent vitamin D metabolites, 1 alpha hydroxyvitamin D and 1,25 dihydroxyvitamin D, rapid reversal of their toxic effects is usually achieved by temporary interruption of their administration (6).

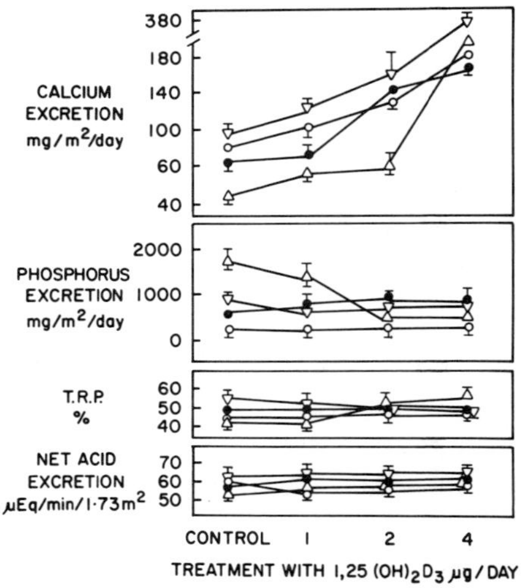

Fig. 1. Hypercalciuric effect of calcitriol in four children with renal hypophosphatemic rickets. From reference (2). By permission.

From 1959 (7) the anticalciuric action of thiazides has been widely recognized. It is known (8) that thiazides directly stimulate the distal tubular reabsorption of calcium by dissociating calcium and sodium transports. Thus, thiazides are natriuretic and hypocalciuric. This hypocalciuric effect is not usually observed until three or four days after starting drug administration.

The hypercalciuric effect of calcitriol therapy has been showed (9) in 19 children undergoing chronic renal failure, renal hypophosphatemic rickets or hypoparathyroidism. Addition of hydrochlorothiazide, at dosage of 1 to 2 mg/kg/day, to maintenance dose of calcitriol (31 ng/kg/day) brought about significant decrease of urine calcium excretion (Fig. 2). Moreover, the hypocalciuric action of thiazides may be enhanced by simultaneous amiloride administration (10). Combined diuretic regimen provides a sooner and larger reduction in the urinary excretion of calcium and prevents the hypokalemic effect of thiazides.

Interestingly, we have also observed (9) slight increment of serum calcium concentration following short-term thiazide therapy. Hypercalcemia seems to be related to volume contraction and is very uncommon in patients receiving prolonged thiazide treatment (11). Nonetheless, this potential complication should be taken into account.

In conclusion, thiazide administration, alone or combined with amiloride should be considered as an efficient form of therapy to counteract or prevent episodes of hypercalciuria in children who require continuous supplements of active vitamin D metabolites provided serum calcium and potassium concentrations are closely monitored.

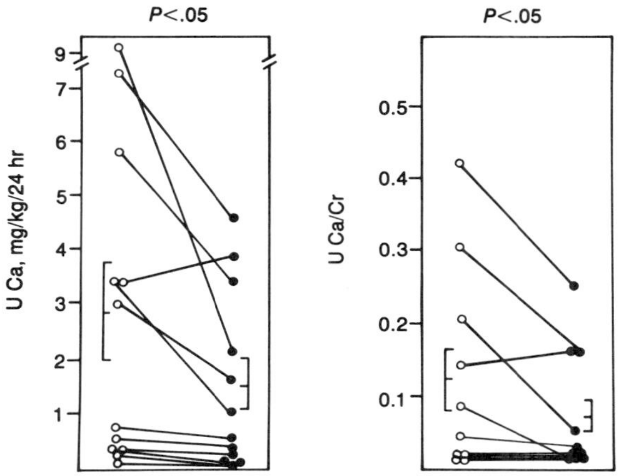

Fig. 2. Reduction in urine calcium excretion after hydrochlorothiazide therapy in children taking chronic supplements of 1,25 dihydroxyvitamin D.

REFERENCES

1. Chan, J.C.M., Kodroff, M.B. and Landwehr, D.M. Pediatrics 68: 559-571, 1981.
2. Chan, J.C.M., Lovinger, R.D. and Mamunes, P. Pediatrics 66: 445-454, 1980.
3. Chan, J.C.M., Young, R.B., Hartenberg, M.A. and Chinchilli, V.M. J Pediatr 106: 421-426, 1985.
4. Chan, J.C.M., Young, R.B., Alon, U. and Mamunes, P. Pediatrics 72: 225-233, 1983.
5. Chan, J.C.M. Int J Pediatr Nephrol 3: 305-310, 1982.
6. Santos, F., Friedman, B.I. and Chan, J.C.M. Curr Probl Pediatr 16: 237-301, 1986.
7. Lamberg, B.A. and Kuhlback, B. Scand J Lab Clin Invest 11: 351-357, 1959.
8. Costanzo, L.S. and Weiner, I.M. Am J Physiol 230: 67-73, 1976.
9. Santos, F., Vernon Smith, M.J. and Chan, J.C.M. AJDC 140: 139-142, 1986.
10. Alon, U., Costanzo, L.S. and Chan, J.C.M. Miner Electrolyte Metab 10: 379-386, 1984.
11. Yendt, E.R. and Cohanim, M. Kidney Int 13: 397-409, 1978.

XII. SIDE EFFECTS OF DIURETIC THERAPY

CAPTOPRIL PROTECTS AGAINST METABOLIC EFFECTS OF CHRONIC HYDROCHLOROTHIAZIDE THERAPY

F.V.Costa, C.Borghi, A.Mussi & E.Ambrosioni

Cattedra e Servizio di Farmacologia Clinica.Policlinico S.Orsola. Università di Bologna.ITALY.

INTRODUCTION

Many studies have shown that antihypertensive treatment with diuretics often induces several unwanted metabolic effects which could partially counteract the favourable effects (in terms of reduction in cardiovascular risk) obtained by decreasing blood pressure (1) . In a previous report, we observed that in hypertensive patients, the administration of the combination of hydrochlorothiazide (HCT) + captopril (CPT)does not cause after a 10 month treatment, any unwanted metabolic effect (2).
In the present study, we compared the long-term metabolic effects induced in hypertensive patients by HCT alone and by the combination HCT+CPT.

PATIENTS AND METHODS

Two groups of patients were studied. patients of Group 1 had,at the end of a two week placebo run-in ,a diastolic blood pressure >90≤105 mmHg. Patients of Group 2 had diastolic blood pressure values ≥105≤125 mmHg. The first group was treated with HCT, 25 mg o.i.d., the second group with HCT 25 mg o.i.d.+CPT 50 mg b.i.d. After three months of treatment,subjects having a satisfactory blood pressure reduction (diastolic blood pressure <90 mmHg in the first group and <95 mmHg in the second group) entered the long-term study and were re-checked after 6 and 12 months. Patients receiving HCT+CPT were recontrolled also after 24 months. At the end of placebo run-in, after 3,6 and 12 months (and after 24 months in the HCT+CPT group)the following biochemical variables were measured : serum glucose, uric acid,BUN,creatinine, Na^+,K^+,triglycerides,cholesterol. Clinical controls,blood pressure and body weight measurements were performed at 3 month intervals.

The comparison between basal values of the two groups was performed by means of Student's T test for unpaired data whereas within-group changes induced by therapy were assessed by means of analysis of variance.

RESULTS

Forty-six patients were enrolled in the HCT group and 43 in the HCT+CPT group. Their sex distribution (26 male,21 female in the HCT group and 22 male,19 female in the HCT+CPT group) and their age (53±11 years and 52±9 years respectively, were not different. Subjects treated with HCT had lower blood pressure values during placebo than those treated with HCT+CPT (163/96 mmHg vs.171/106 mmHg;p<0.001 for both systolic and diastolic blood pressure). After 3 months of therapy 41 patients of the HCT group and 38 of the HCT+CPT group had a satisfactory blood pressure control (diastolic blood pressure <90 mmHg in the HCT group and <95 mmHg in the HCT+CPT group)and therefore enterd the long-term study and were re-checked after 12 months.Subjects of the HCT+CPT group having a normal blood pressure after 1 year (n.27) were re-checked also after 24 months. Some of the biochemical variables recorded in the two group during placebo and during therapy are shown in Table 1.

TABLE 1	Glucose mg%	Uric acid mg%	Triglycerides mg%	Cholesterol mg%	K^+ mmol/1
Placebo	92±10	5.0±1.4	148±82	218±35	4.2±.3
HCT 3 months	96± 9*	5.4±1.6*	161±89**	222±41	3.8±.4***
HCT 12 months	99±11*	5.9±2.1**	166±90***	228±47**	3.7±.4***
Placebo	91±8	4.8±1.3	152±86	227±27	4.3±.3
HCT+CPT 3 months	92±9	4.9±1.0	140±60	213±28	4.1±.3
HCT+CPT 12 months	92±8	5.0±1.1	134±39*	208±29**	4.0±.4
HCT+CPT 24 months	93±10	4.9±1.0	121±39**	195±17***	4.1±.2

* p<0.05 ** p<0.005 *** p<0.001 in comparison with placebo

Treatment with HCT induced the typical metabolic effects of diuretic therapy whereas the combination of HCT+CPT caused no unwanted metabolic effect. Triglycerides had a slight but significant decrease after 12 months and an even greater fall after 24 months.Cholesterol too had a decrease from the 12th month on. The separate analysis of patients having during placebo cholesterol values <200 MG% (n.13) or >200 mg% (n.25) showed that HCT+CPT induced a significant decrease only in those subjects whose basal values were >200 mg% (from 242±43 to 216±20 mg% after 12 months;$p<0.005$) while no change was observed in subjects having basal values <200 mg% (from 190±10 to 187±21 mg%). The same trend was observed in the 27 subjects who continued HCT+CPT treatment for 24 months: cholesterol decreased from 242±34 to 198±15 mg% ($p<0.001$) and remaijned unchanged in the other subjects (from 190±11 to 187±19). The other variables we measured (BUN,creatinine,Na^+) had no changes with both treatments.

DISCUSSION

The results of the present study have shown that the combination of HCT+CPT is a safe and highly effective treatment for moderate-to-severe hypertension, the percentage of patients achieving normotension with this treatment being very high (92% after one year,71% after two years). Furthermore the unwanted metabolic effects observed in the HCT group were not observed in the HCT+CPT group. Other studies have demonstrated that CPT counteracts the hypokalaemic and hyperuricemic actions of diuretics and blunts their hypercholesterolemic and hyperglicemic action (3). The reduction in triglicerydes and in cholesterol we observed cannot be attributed to changes in dietary habits since in the HCT group they had an increase and dietary habits of patients remained unchanged during all the study. The mechanism leading to the decrease in serum cholesterol is at present unknown, but this effect could be important for a further reduction of cardiovascular risk in treated hypertensive patients.

REFERENCES

1)Ames P.R.:Negative effects of diuretic drugs on metabolic risk factors for coronary heart disease: possible alternative drugs. Am J Cardiol,51:633,1983

2)Costa F.V.,Borghi C.,Boschi S.,Ambrosioni E.:Differing dosages of captopril and hydrochlorothiazide in the treatment of hypertension:long-term effects on metabolic values and intracellular electrolytes.J Crdiovasc Pharmacol,7:70s,1985.

3)Weinberger M.H.:Comparison of captopril and hydrochlorothiazide in essential hypertension. Br J Clin Pharmacol;14:127s,1982.

GYNECOMASTIA AND MASTODYNIA AFTER SPIRONOLACTONE AND POTASSIUM CANRENOATE

G. BELLATI, C. PEVERELLI, A. SIRONI and G. IDEO
Department of Internal Medicine A, St'Anna's Hospital, 22100 Como,Italy

Spironolactone,a competitive antagonist of aldosterone, is widely used as a diuretic and anthypertensive agent. However, long term use may be restricted by a decrease in libido, gynecomastia and impotence, likely related to the antiandrogenic effect of the drug (1). Disappearance of spironolactone-induced gynecomastia has been reported during treatment with potassium canrenoate (2), which structuraly resembles spironolactone, but is more polar, and it seems to have different metabolites (3). Moreover gynecomastia is rare after potassium canrenoate or canrenone (4,5), while 30-62% of patients on long term spironolactone experience this side-effect (4,7). However, these studies were retrospective and were in patients with arterial hypertension or heart failure or in normal males. To clarify the exact frequency of gynecomastia and mastodynia also in cirrhotics with ascites after treatment with spironolactone or potassium canrenoate we have done a prospective clinical trial.

MATERIALS AND METHODS

From September 1983 to March 1985, 144 patients (90 males), affected by liver cirrhosis with ascites, heart failure or arterial hypertension were considered for this study. Criteria for patient selection were the necessity of diuretics, absence of gynecomastia, normal levels of plasma urea, creatinine, sodium and potassium.

Patients were randomized to have a ratio 2:1 in favour of treatment with potassium canrenoate. One group of 96 patients (56 males) received potassium canrenoate, 100 mg once or twice a day for six months; a second group of 48 patients (34 males) were treated with spironolactone 100 or 200 mg a day for six months. No other drugs were used.

All the patients were monthly checked from clinical and laboratorial point of view. Six male patients (three in the potassium canrenoate group and three in the spironolactone group) were lost to follow up and were not considered in the results.

Gynecomastia was defined as a palpable discrete button of firm subareolar breast tissue at least 2 cm in diameter, according to Niewoehner and Nuttal (8). The examining physician did not know to which group any subject belonged until all the data were collected and analyzed.

RESULTS

Gynecomastia and mastodynia appeared more frequently during treatment with spironolactone than potassium canrenoate, the difference being statistically significant (table 1 and 2)

Table 1.
Number of subjects in which gynecomastia appeared during treatment

GYNECOMASTIA (males)

	Spironolactone	K-Canrenoate
All	21/31 (67.7%)	22/53 (41.5%)*
Cirrhotics	14/14 (100.0%)	16/30 (53.3%)**
Non cirrhotics	7/17 (41.1%)	6/23 (26.0%)

* $p < 0.05$
** $p < 0.01$

Table 2.
Number of subjects in which mastodynia appeared during treatment

MASTODYNIA (males and females)

	Spironolactone	K-Canrenoate
All	24/45 (51.1%)	11/93 (11.8%)**
Cirrhotics	11/14 (78.5%)	7/42 (16.7%)**
Non cirrhotics	13/31 (41.9%)	4/51 (7.8%)*

*$p < 0.05$
**$p < 0.01$

On the contrary the effects of both traetments were similar in respect of the amount of the drugs, of diuresis, body weight, plasma and urine sodium and potassium, and plasma sugar, urea creatinine and uric acid.

DISCUSSION

Gynecomastia and mastodynia appeared more frequently during treatment with spironolactone than with potassium canrenoate. These results suggest that potassium canrenoate may be less antiandrogenic then spironolactone.

Gardiner (9) has claimed that the renal antimineral corticoid potency of potassium canrenoate is only one-third that of spironolactone, but this does not seem a likely explanation for the reduced toxicity of canrenoate, because the therapeutic effects of the two drugs at the same dosage were similar, as we show here and elsewere (10).

Spironolactone exerts its antiandrogenic effect by a direct action on the target tissue, as well as by reducing androgen biosythesis via in inhibition of cytochrome P-450 (11). The enzyme inhibition is not mediated by canrenone (12), which is an active metabolite of both spironolactone and potassium canrenoate.

Metabolites of spironolactone other than canrenoate may contribute to the anti-androgenic effect of this drug. In fact cytochrome P-450 showed a dose-related decrease more pronounced after methyl-thio and mercapto-derivatives of spironolactone than with canrenone or spironolactone itself (13). Moreover Armanini et al. (14) have reported that spironolactone produces a sgnificantly higher androgen antagonism than potassium canrenoate in the castrated mouse.

In conclusion, the use of potassium canrenoate rather than spironolactone may carry a reduced risk of gynecomastia and mastodynia, particularly in cirrhotic patients.

REFERENCES

1. Rose, I.J., Underwood, R.H., Newmark, S.R., Kisk, E.S. and Williams, G.H. Ann. Intern. 87:398,1977.
2. Dupont, A. The Lancet ii: 731, 1985.
3. Karim, A. Proceedings of the Searle Symposium, Excepta Medica, pag. 115, 1978.
4. Marco, J., Constans, R., Alibelli, M.J. Baradat, G. and Dardenne, P. Nouv. Presse Med. 7: 3668, 1978.
5. Fromantin, M. Mises Jour Cardiol. 19: 95,1980
6. Greenblatt, D.J. and Koch-Weser, J. J.A.M.A. 225: 40 1973.
7. Huffman, D.H., Kampmann, J.P., Hignite, C.E. and Azarnoff, D.L. Clin. Pharm. Ther. 24: 465, 1978
8. Niewoehner, C.B. and Nuttal, F.Q. Amer.J.Med. 77: 633, 1984
9. Gardiner, P.The Lancet ii:1432, 1985
10. Tempini, S., Bellati, G. and , Idéo, G. Minerva Diet. Gastroenterol. 29: 1 1983.
11. Loriaux D.L., Menard, R., Taylor, A.Pita, J.C. and Santen, R. Ann. Intern. Med. 85: 630 1976
12. Greiner, J.W., Rumbaugh, R.C., Kramer, R.E. and Colby, H.D. Endocrinology 103: 1313, 1978.
13. Ricci, G.L. Baldassarre, V.Zanninelli, G. and Cuppone, R.Ital. J.Gastroenterol. 18: 73, 1986
14. Armanini, D., Karbowiak, I., Goi, A. and Mantero, F. J. Endocrinol. Invest. 6 (suppl 1): 115,1983.

SIDE EFFECTS FROM DIURETICS IN HOSPITALIZED PATIENTS

A.ILIOPOULOU,D.KONTOYANNIS,P.ZIROYANIS,S.KONTOYANIS,M.MAVRIKAKIS and S.MOULOPOULOS

Dept.of Clin.Therapeutics,Univ.of Athens,"Alexandra"Hospital, Greece.

INTRODUCTION

Many methods are available for gathering information about adverse drug effects for either drugs which have been used for a long time and those newly marketed. Whilst anecdotal reports provide inexpensive and immediate data,the formal intensive hospital monitoring studies,though more expensive,provide much better quantification and documentation of information.The adverse effects from diuretics are presented,which were recorded during the last four years in a teaching department of medicine as part of a hospital monitoring programme of adverse drug effects.

MATERIAL AND METHODS

During the past four years a simple hospital monitoring programme for adverse drug effects was operating in a teaching department of medicine. The programme monitored all adverse drug effects (including those from diuretics) in 15.505 consecutively admitted patients.The characteristics of patients who manifested adverse effects were recorded including age,sex, weight,medical history,results of routine,blood-urine tests and blood levels for a number of drugs. The final judgement concerning the existence of a connection between the drug and the adverse event was made by an adverse effects committee on the basis of a detailed review of all relevant facts including :1) time-relation of drug exposure to the appearance of the event,2) improvement or disappearance of the side-effect on drug discontinuation,3) relation of high blood-levels of the drug to the event and 4)confirmation of the event by the physician in charge. This judgement was expressed in terms of "definite" and "probable" events. "Doubtful" events were not recorded.

RESULTS

The total number and the percentage of the adverse drug effects classified according to in hospital or out of hospital onset of manifestation are presented in Table 1.The corresponding values of the adverse effects related to the administration of diuretics in particular are also shown in Table 1. The eight diuretics or combination of diuretics most frequently associated with adverse reactions are given in Table 2. The eleven most often reported adverse effects are listed in Table 3.

Table 1. Adverse drug effects(AE) in hospital patients (PS)

PS (total)	15.505 (%)		
PS with AE	912(5,88)	PS with AE from diuretics	108
" " on admission	393(2,53)	" " " " on admission	78
" " in hospital	519(3,34)	" " " " in hospital	30
" "aged>60 yrs.	564(3,63)	" " " " aged > 60 yrs.	75

Table 2. List of diuretics associated with adverse reactions

DIURETIC OR COMBINATION	PERCENTAGE OF ADVERSE EFFECTS FROM DIURETICS(%)
1. Frusemide	29.30
2. Amiloride-hydrocholothiazide	24.07
3. Chlorthalidone	22.20
4. Spironolactone	9.26
5. Spironolactone-frusemide	8.33
6. Butametanide	3.70
7. Hydrochlorothiazide	1.85
8. Chlorthalidone-enalapril	0.92

Table 3. List of adverse effects due to diuretics

ADVERSE EVENTS FROM DIURETICS	PERCENTAGE OF ADVERSE EFFECTS FROM DIURETICS(%)
1. Electrolyte changes :	
Hypokalaemia (< 3 mEq/l)	23.15
Hyponatraemia(< 125 mEq/l)	12.03
Hyperkalaemia(> 5,5 mEq/l)	1.85
2. Blood urea rise(>80 mg%)	32.50
3. Blood pressure fall	11.10
4. Neurological events	7.40
5. Hyperuricaemia(>10 ng%)	3.70
6. Blood glucose rise	2.80
7. Rash	1.85
8. Ventricular ectopic beats	0.92
9. Thrombosis	0.92
10. Gynecomastia	0.92
11. Exacerbation of gout	0.92

DISCUSSION

Although the results reported here do not express the frequency of adverse effects,since the total number of patients taking these drugs was not recorded,they are indicative of the problem.

It was found that 5,88% of the admitted patients suffered some adverse effect because of their drug treatment,which started before admission or during their hospitalization(ratio 0,75). Diuretics were responsible for 11,8% of the total adverse effects and the ratio of out of hospital to in hospital onset of effect was 2.60 for diuretics. The ratio of adverse effects in patients over 60 years old to total adverse effects was 0.61 similar to the ratio of adverse effects from diuretics in patients over 60 years old to total adverse effects from diuretics (0,69). The most common reactions related to diuretics were found to be electrolyte changes, blood urea levels rise and blood pressure fall. The most often reported drugs were frusemide,amiloride plus hydrochlorothiazide and chlothalidone. There appears to be an agreement with other reports on the list of manifested reactions from diuretics (1,2,3,4). In contrast, the list of the drugs most often involved varies with local prescribing habbits.

From the two recorded cases of fatal reactions from diuretics (1,8%), one was hyponatraemic coma due to frusemide and the other was cerebral thrombotic incidence due to chlorthalidone. From the rest cerebral incidents,two were also related to the use of chlorthalidone and left permanent deficit.

Although most reactions from diuretics were minor,their contribution to the total number of the out of hospital total adverse effects,especially in aged patients was high, reflecting the high frequency of administration of these drugs in general practice. This could be avoided if diuretics were used appropriately in our patients, especially those of old age.

REFERENCES

1. Morgan,D.B., Davidson,C. Br. Med. J. 280 : 905-908, 1980.
2. Fichman,H.P., Vorherr,H., Kleeman,C.R., Telfer,N. Ann. Intern. Med. 75 : 853-863, 1971.
3. Cogan,E., Abramow,M. Lancet ii :1249, 1983.
4. Freis, E.D., Papademetriou,V. Drugs 30 : 469-474, 1985.

DIURETIC-ASSOCIATED HYPOKALEMIA:A PREVALENT AND EXPENSIVE DISEASE?

G.R.FITZGERALD,E.DELANEY,M.CUSHEN,M.J.KENNEDY,A.KENNY,J.MURPHY,
D.GILLIGAN,M.G.FITZGERALD.

Department of Medicine, Waterford Regional Hospital, Ireland.

INTRODUCTION

Diuretic drugs are widely used in heart failure and hypertension. Recent discussion has concentrated on likely importance of diuretic-associated hypokalemia (DAH) in the genesis of cardiac dysrhythmia.Less attention has recently been directed to other morbidity of DAH (1, 2). This communication addresses DAH sufficiently severe to warrant hospital admission.

PATIENTS AND METHODS

All acute admissions (n=3042) from Sept.1983 to Oct.1985 into an internal medicine unit,serving a population of 66,000 had serum K^+ estimated on fresh samples within eight hours of admission.Comprehensive relevant clinical details were recorded and subsequently analysed in 103(3.4%) patients with DAH ($K^+ \leq 3.4$ mmol/l). Hypokalemia in the absence of diuretic therapy was present in a further 46 cases(1.5%).

RESULTS

DAH could be allocated to 3 groupings i.e.,a) Isolated DAH;symptoms due solely to low K^+ and reversed by KCl administration b) Contributory DAH;non-hypokalemic symptoms aggravated or precipitated by low K^+ and c) Incidential DAH; symptoms unrelated to low K^+.Age (mean 61 yr.),sex (F= 58 %) and indication for diuretic therapy (hypertension-68%; failure-21%; other-11%) were similar in all 3 groups.Diuretics responsible for DAH likely reflected their relative frequency of prescription in the region, with the possible exception of metolazone,which is traditionally used without K^+ supplements. Lower mean K^+ values in metolazone DAH were noted. (Table 1).

Symptoms in isolated DAH were typically hypokalemic,muscular and neurologic in type,with an unexpected high incidence (32%) of chest pain.

Table 1. Diuretics prescribed in DAH .(Diuretic-associated hypokalemia)

	Isolated DAH (n=59)		All DAH (n=103)	
	% cases	K^+(mean)	% cases	K^+(mean)
Thiazide $\pm K^+$	30	3.1	31	3.1
Frusemide $\pm K^+$	23	3.1	24	3.1
Metolazone	20	2.7	19	2.9
Combinations	20	3.1	22	3.2
Other	7	3.1	4	3.2
All	-	3.0	-	3.1

Costs amounted to U.S.$0.85m (Isolated DAH) and $1.2m (Isolated+Contributory), when projected to the State (pop. 3,000,000).For the U.K.and Ireland,these costs would be $21m and $30m approx.,given similar prescribing patterns.

Detailed analysis of pre-admission medication in DAH patients indicated that a majority of hypokalemic admissions might be avoided,if a change in physician prescribing habits were achieved (Table 2).

Table 2. Avoidable and unavoidable DAH

	Isolated DAH		All DAH	
	no.	%	no.	%
Inappropriate drug/dose	31	53	40	39
Incorrect indication	10	17	17	17
Predictable interaction	7	12	20	19
Unavoidable	11	18	26	25

We attempted to reduce DAH admissions by alerting physicians (by mail Sept.1984),by changing hospital diuretic policy (May 1985),and by encouraging a more alert prescribing attitude in relation to diuretics at doctors› regional clinical meetings (Oct.1984,May,Nov.1985). This education program was followed by an impressive reduction in DAH admissions from 3.6% in July 1985,to 3.3% in Oct.1985,to 1.4% in Jan.1986 and 0.7% by May 1986.

CONCLUSION

In our practice,DAH is an important contributor to hospital admissions and costs.It is avoidable in the majority of instances.Education of physician prescribing habits may achieve a substantial reduction in morbid diuretic-associated hypokalemia.This identification of prevalent ill-effects followed by prescribing re-education may be applicable to other iatrogenic illnesses.

REFERENCES

1. Ramsay,L.E. and Toner J.M. In Diuretics in Heart Failure (Ed.L.E.Ramsay) Royal Society of Medicine International Congress and Symposium Series No.83,Royal Society of Medicine,1985,pp 67-75.
2. Poole-Wilson,P.A.,Postgraduate Medical Journal,1983,59 (Suppl.3), 137-139.

EFFECTS OF MUZOLIMINE ON FREE-WATER EXCRETION IN EDEMATOUS AND HYPONATREMIC PATIENTS.

Conte G, •Satta A, Aucella F, Imperatore P, Russo D, DelloRusso A, •Branca G, •Faedda R, Dal Canton A, Bartoli E;

Department of Nephrology, Second Faculty of Medicine of Naples; •Institute of Medical Pathology of Sassari; Italy.

INTRODUCTION

Muzolimine (M) is a new Henle's loop diuretic with no structural similarity to currently available diuretics. M is characterized by high-ceiling activity, long duration of action and absence of the 'rebound phenomenon' (1) and therefore may be more advantageous than the other diuretics in the treatment of renal, cardiac or epatic edema, generally associated with antidiuresis and hyponatremia. Several reports of life-threatening hyponatremia associated with thiazide administration have recently appeared in the literature (2,3). The administration of Henle's loop diuretic may, in fact, impair the capacity to excrete dilute urine by inhibiting NaCl reabsorption in the distal diluting segments. Yet, the effect of M on free-water excretion has not been investigated in edematous patients with hyponatremia.

METHODS

Patients with cirrhosis (n=3) or nephrotic syndrome (n=3) were selected for the study because of peripheral edema and serum sodium concentration below 135 mEq/l. The protocol was as follows: at 8.00 a.m. an infusion containing paraaminohippurate (PAH) was started. After one hour the patient emptied his bladder and then two 60' control urine collections were made by spontaneous voiding. Blood samples were collected at the mid-point of each clearance period. After the two control periods muzolimine (2 mg/Kg of body wt) was administered orally. After one hr from the administration of the diuretic, two 60' clearance periods were performed with the same modalities as the control period. Urine and plasma samples were analyzed for creatinine, PAH, potassium and osmolality.

RESULTS

During M, there were no significant changes in creatinine and PAH clearance in any of the patients. As expected, during M, urine output and urinary sodium excretion increased markedly. As shown in table 1, it is important to observe that in all patients who excreted hypertonic urine (UOsm/POsm>1) in control period (n=5), the urinary osmolality fell during M: in three patients, isotonic urine was excreted during M and in the other two urinary osmolality became hypotonic. In the remaining one patient isotonic urinary osmolality was not changed by M.

Table 1. Effect of M on C_{H_2O} in edematous and hyponatremic patients

	Case n°	P_{Na} mEq/l	U_{Osm} mOsm/Kg	U/P_{Osm}	C_{Osm} ml/min	C_{H_2O} ml/min
Basal values:						
	1	134	624	2.31	0.94	-0.53
	2	131	400	1.51	1.90	-0.65
	3	135	808	2.80	2.71	-1.7
	4	132	544	1.84	0.6	-0.27
	5	120	252	0.92	0.55	+0.05
	6	130	470	1.63	1.47	-0.57
	MEAN	130.3	516.3	1.83	1.36	-0.61
	±SD	5.3	151.3	0.50	0.04	0.59
With muzolimine:						
	1	135	193	0.71	1.66	+0.62
	2	129	222	0.85	5.11	+1.05
	3	135	291	1.03	7.94	+0.90
	4	130	287	1.0	10.2	0.00
	5	125	283	1.0	10.3	-0.03
	6	134	284	0.99	9.46	+0.04
	MEAN	131.3	260	0.93	7.42	+0.43
	±SD	4.0	41.7	0.09	3.46	0.49
	p<	NS	0.01	0.01	0.001	0.05

COMMENTS

M improved the excretion of free-water in edematous and hyponatremic patients in antidiuresis. In such patients (n=5) there was a relative increase in free-water clearance with the excretion of distinctly hypotonic urine in two of them. This effect is very important because it allows to increase the ability to excrete water in antidiuretic patients with hyperidratation. We suggest two possible explanations for the excretion of solute-free water during M:

1) Incomplete osmotic equilibration during high flow rates through collecting ducts associated with reduced interstitial tonicity due to medullary 'wash-out' and to inhibition of NaCl reabsorption in the medullary ascending limb of Henle's loop.
2) Increased secretion of prostaglandin which antagonize the effects of ADH on collecting ducts(5).

REFERENCES

1. Dal Canton A., Russo D., Gallo R.,Conte G., Andreucci V.E. 'Muzolimine: a new high-ceiling diuretic suitable for patients with advanced renal disease'. Brit. Med. J. 282: 595-598, 1981.
2. Ayus J.C., Olivero J.J. and Frammer J.P.:'Rapid correction of severe hyponatremia with intravenous hypertonic saline solution'. Am. J. Med. 72: 43-48, 1982.
3. Ashraf N., Locksley R. and Arieff A.I.:'Thiazide-induced hyponatremia with death or neurological damage in outpatients'. Am. J. Med. 70: 1163-1168, 1981.
4. Berg K.J., Jorstad S., Tromsdal A.: 'Studies on the clinical pharmacology of a new potent diuretic, Bay g 2821'. Pharmatherapeutica 1: 319-321, 1972.
5. Bandiera F., Dessi-Fulgheri P., Madeddu P., Cocco F., Oppes M., Glorioso N., Spanedda M., Rappelli A.: 'Role of renal prostaglandins in mediating the activity of muzolimine'. Proceedings of the International Meeting on Diuretics. Sorrento, 1986. In press. Martinus Nijhoff Publ. Andreucci V.E. and Dal Canton A. Ed. 1986.

IRREVERSIBLE HYPONATREMIA DUE TO INCONGRUOUS SPIRONOLACTONE TREATMENT

Di Sciacca A., Durante F., Frontini A., Ingrassia A., Di Piazza R.M., Cucchiara G., Mira G., Barbagallo Sangiorgi G.

Institute of Internal Medicine and Geriatrics held by Prof. Giuseppe Barbagallo Sangiorgi Chair of Systematic Medical Therapy held by Prof. Arnaldo Di Sciacca -Palermo, Italy

INTRODUCTION

A patient suffering from non compensated liver cirrhosis and hyperaldosteronism was treated with spironolactone (SP). Severe irreversible hyponatremia developed with severe clinical and symptomatic manifestations documented by laboratory test. Death of the patient ensued.

ANAMNESIS

The patient emigrated to Belgium at the age of 30 and began to drink 150 gm per day of ethyl alcohol. Painful dyspepsia at age 38. At age 44, jaundice, hyperchromic urine and acholic faeces.

First admission: general condition fair, sensorium normal; jaundice and free pouring in the peritoneal cavity; liver enlarged, cutting edge, hard-fibrous consistency, not painful. Normal pressure values in supine and upright position. Weight 68 Kg.

Laboratory data: Na_S 142, K_S 3,9, K_{RBC} 97,1, mEq/l; Ht 43% ; Na_U/K_U 17,6/26, 1 = 0,67; average daily diuresis 400 ml; serum osmolarity 272 mOsm/Kg.

SP treatment began at a dose of 200 mg per day with a congruous diet (sodium intake equivalent to that excreted in urine and water intake not greater than 400/500 ml per day). Clinical parameters and laboratory data were kept under constant control. The patient's general condition improved, his weight dropped (64 Kg.) and ascites disappeared.

Laboratory data: Na_S 136, K_S 4,7, K_{RBC} 90,1 mEq/l; Ht 49%, Na_U/K_U 190/35 = 5,42; average daily diuresis 1500 ml; serum osmolarity 269 mOsm/Kg.

The patient was discharged with maintenance therapy (SP 100 mg per day) and congruous diet. He continued well for about 15 days until, at home, because of reduction of diuresis and the reappearance of ascites and oedemas, the dose of SP was increased to 400 mg daily and a strictly sodium-less diet was prescribed. After about 20 days the patient was mentally confused, unable to stand up his general condition had deteriorated.

Second admission: general condition poor, with mental confusion; arterial blood pressure 90/70 mmHg supine, 70/50 mmHg upright. Abdomen globose with abundant peritoneal pouring, liver unexceptional. Weight 68 Kg.

Laboratory data: Na_S 116, K_S 5,4, K_{RBC} 86 mEq/l; Ht 45% ; Na_U/K_U 101/27,2 = 3,71; average daily diuresis 700 ml; serum osmolarity 257 mOsm/Kg; urine osmolarity 626 mOsm/Kg.

SP therapy was suspended and liquid intake reduced. NaCl was administered in equivalent amount to the sodium excreted: average daily diuresis increased to 1500 ml, but the electrolytic picture scarcelly changed. The patient died after a few days.

CASE: *A. ANTONINO, aged 44, from Aragona, Sicily.*

- At age 30 daily intake of 150 gm ethyl alcohol
- At age 44 jaundice and ascites. Diagnosis of non compensated liver cirrhosis.
- Treatment with spironolactone (SP) at daily dose of 200 mg and congrous diet, with clinical and laboratory parameters under control.
- Improvement of general condition, disappearance of ascites.
- Discharge on maintenance therapy of daily dose of 100 mg SP.
- Fair condition for about 15 days followed by reappearance of oedemas and ascites, and reduction of diuresis.
- Drastic reduction of sodium intake and increase of SP to 400 mg daily.
- Severe mental confusion, inability to stand up, severe neuromuscolar asthenia.
- Readmission.
- Severe clinical and symptomatic picture due to hyponatremia confirmed by laboratory data.
- Death of patient.

CONCLUSIONS

In all patients with severe water-salt non compensation treated with diuretics, certain parameters must be kept under constant control (Tables 1 and 2):

- water-salt monitoring, both clinical (variations of body weight, appearance of the skin and mucosae, plicometry, arterial blood pressure in supine and upright position, heart frequency, venous blood pressure, sensorium, bone and tendon reflexes) and laboratory (ratio between daily fluid intake and diuresis, Na/K ratio in daily urine, serum Na and K levels, red blood cell potassium, serum and urine osmolarity, hematocrit value, serum protein values, blood nitrogen and creatinin levels);
- fluid intake should be limited to 400 ml per day, while sodium intake should balance urinary sodium excretion.

Pharmacological therapy must therefore be applied with caution and on an individual basis in order to avoid further alterations of water and salt balance that are often irreversible and fatal, as in the case reported here.

Table 1 . Clinical parameters in Hyponatremia

- Pharmacological case history
- Variations of body weight
- Plicometry
- Appearance of skin and mucosae
- Cardiovascular system: arterial hypotension in upright position, venous blood hypertension, lung stasis with possible lung oedema
- Neuromuscolar system: asthenia, bone and tendon hyporeflexes, muscular cramp,
- Convulsions, lethargy, Cheyne-Stokes breathing, hypothermia, coma.
- Alimentary system: nausea, vomiting, adbominal pain, paralytic ileum.

Table 2 . The laboratory in Hyponatremia

▪ Liquids taken	▪ K_S
▪ Liquids excreted	▪ K_{RBC}
▪ Blood nitrogen	▪ Na_U/K_U ratio
▪ Hematocrit	▪ Serum osmolarity
▪ Serum protein	▪ Urine osmolarity
▪ Na_S	▪ Creatinine clearance

REFERENCES

1. Barbagallo Sangiorgi G., Di Sciacca A., Fradà G. jr., Cupidi G., Barbagallo M.: Il danno jatrogenico da farmaci in geriatria. Nuovo Boll. Farmacol. Clin., Napoli, 3, 157-168, 1981.
2. Barbagallo Sangiorgi G., Fradà G. jr., Di Sciacca A., Cupidi G., Costanza G., Affronti M., Putignano E., Barbagallo M.: Turbe del ricambio idroelettrolitico come causa di encefalopatia metabolica nell'anziano. Giorn. Geront. 30, 199-202, 1982.
3. Barbagallo Sangiorgi G., Di Sciacca A., Durante F. Fradà G. Jr., Costanza G., Cupidi G.: La terapia diuretica e la terapia antiipertensiva nell'anziano. Giorn. Geront. 30, 749-774, 1982.
4. Barbagallo Sangiorgi G., Exton-Smith A.N.: General symptomathology of pathogenic drug usuge in old patients. In: Barbagallo Sangiorgi G. and Exton-Smith: Aging and drug therapy. Plenum Press. New York - London, 31 - 40, 1984.
5. Bartter F.G., Schwartz W.B.: The syndrome of inappropriate secretion of anti-diuretic hormone. Am. J. Med. 42, 790-806, 1967.
6. Berl T., Schrier R.W.: Water metabolism and the hypo-osmolar syndromes. In: Brenner B.M., Stein J.H. (eds): Sodium and water Homeostasis. Edinburgh, Churchill Livingstone, 1978.
7. Caird F.I.: Postural hypotension in the elderly. Drug and the elderly. Mac Millan Press LTD, London 1979.
8. Flear C.T,G., Gill G.V., Burn J.: Hyponatremia: Mechanism and management. Lancet 2, 26-31, 1981.
9. Cupidi G., Affronti M., Di Sciacca A., Costanza G. Gaglio M., Maggio F.P.: L'iponatriemia nell'anziano. Atti del XXIX Congr. Naz. Soc. It., Geront. Ger., Bari, 32, 10, 765-766, 1984.
10. Morton H., Maxwell-Kleeman C.R.: Clinical Disorders of fluid and electrolyte metabolism. McGraw-Hill, Book Company, 1979.

THE DIURETIC EFFECTS OF LITHIUM SALTS. ABSENCE OF SIDE EFFECTS.

L. CARRERAS, J. RIERA, A.M. AMENOS, T. PORTIS, H. RAMA, M. ROMERO, X. SARRIAS, and J. ALSINA.
Departments of Nephrology, Biochemistry and Cardiology, Hospital de Bellvitge, "Princeps d'Espanya", Barcelona, SPAIN.

INTRODUCTION

Lithium salts are known to posses antidiuretic properties as antidiuretic hormone antagonists affecting adenyl cyclase and may be considered collecting duct diuretics.(1) Nevertheless, fear of potential nephrotoxicity(2) has limited their use in clinical practice and they have been used almost esclusively as antidepressants. The strict monitorization of psychiatric patients undergoing long term treatment with lithium carbonate enabled us to evaluate the diuretic properties and secondary effects of lithium salts.

MATERIAL AND METHODS

This prospective study was started in March 1980.

Patients:58 psychiatric outpatients with a normosodium diet and normal renal function. CO_3Li_2 doses: 1.104± 2.36 mg/day Mean follow-up: 4.34 years. Laboratory determinations: every 6 months. Plasma and urine urea, creatinine, uric acid, Na+, Ka+, Cl^-, Ca++, $Po_4^=$, Mg++, and osmolality. Plasma total cholesterol, triglycerides, glycemia and basal acid balance. Urine pH, titerable acids, amoniogenesis, bicarbonates and proteinuria. Concentration test by 18 hour water restriction and oral $ClNH_4$ for acidification.

Statistical analysis

Students test for paired values for distribution of differences:

$$t = \frac{/\bar{d}/}{(\sigma_n - 1/\sqrt{n}}$$

RESULTS

There were no significant variations in the following parameters ($p<0.001$):

BLOOD	$\bar{d}$	t		URINE	$\bar{d}$	t	
CH_2O.........	-0.20	1.113	ns.	K+.........	-7.41	1.30	ns
Creatinine....	-1.97	0.66	ns.	Na++........	9.60	0.64	ns.
K+...........	0.01	0.17	ns.	Ca++......	0.31	0.74	ns.
Ca++........	+0.033	1.61	ns.	Mg++........	0.28	0.76	ns.
Mg++.........	0.02	0.18	ns.	Uric acid..	-0.21	0.48	ns.
Urates......	-15.9	1.65	ns.	Proteinuria	-0.25	1.38	ns.
Glycemia.....	0.64	1.33	ns.				
Total cholest.	0.11	0.59	ns.				
Triglycerides	-0.03	0.24	ns.				

The "t" value for plasma Na++ was significant ($\bar{d}$= 1.94 and t=3.48, for $p<0.01$). There was no increase in the urate values for 7 hyperuricemic patients and values went from $\bar{x}=437.85 \pm 33.73$ to 338.25 ± 38.36 mmol/l. At the start of the study 11 patients were hypercholesterolemic and during treatment values changed from $\bar{x}= 6.95 \pm 0.054$ to 6.33 ± 0.74 mmol/l. Six diabetic patients, 4 with type II and 2 with type I, did not show any alterations in glycemia values. Because of the low number of these patients, the different insulin doses and dietary variations could not be statistically evaluated. Incomplete distal tubule acidosis was detected in 6 patients which remitted two months after suspension of the treatment. Only one patient presented an episode of insipid nephrogenic diabetes which regressed when the CO_3Li_2 was suspended. One patient with accidental lithium intoxication (lithemia=1.95 mmol/l) recovered spontaneusly.

CONCLUSIONS

Co_3Li_2 administration caused marked aqueous diuresis without provoking severe complications in spite of the type of patients under study.[3] In none of the patients receiving prolonged treatment was there worsening in renal function.[4] No variations were seen in the ionogram and the expected increase in natriuresis due to direct competition was not seen. Neither in the parameters usually altered by diuretic treatment. We feel that the possible use of Co_3Li_2 for states of edema requiring hydric diuresis or in patients with diabetes, hyperuricemia, dyslipemia or hyponatremia should be reconsidered.

REFERENCES

1.Singer I, Kidney Int., 19:374-387, 1981.
2.Hansen H.E., Hestbech J, Sorensen J.L., Norgaarel K., Heilskov J. and Amdisen A.,Q. J. Med. New Series, 192:577-591,1979.
3.Bone S., Roose S.P., Dunner D.L. and Fieve R.R. Am. J. Psychiatry, 137: 103-104, 1980.
4.Wallin L., Alling C. and Aurell M. Clin. Nephrol, 18:23-28, 1982.

RENAL FAILURE DUE TO DIURETICS

A.M. Castelao, S. Gil-Vernet, J. Torras, E. Andrés, J.M. Griñó, J.M. Mauri, J. Alsina.
Nephrology Department. Hospital de Bellvitge. Barcelona.Spain

INTRODUCTION

Among the possible secondary effects of diuretics, hydroelectrolyte disturbances are the most frequent (hyponatremia, hypo-or hyperkalaemia, hypocalcemia, metabolic alkalosis, hyperglycemia, hyperuricemia) (1,2). Skin rashes, ototoxicity, gynecomasty, false SLE phenomena or increased gestational myopia are produced only rarely. One of the most frequent adverse effects of diuretics is renal insufficiency (RI) which, although often without serious consequences for the patient, may on occasion worsen preexisting RI and turn it irreversible.

This type of RI is usually attributed to a reduction in glomerular filtration and in the filtrate fraction due to decreasing volemia (3-5). Bus this is not always the case and with proximal diuretics direct tubular toxicity may develop while on occasion a hypersensitivity reaction may give rise to acute tubulointerstitial nephritis (6). In this paper the experience of a nephrology service in a general hospital with diuretics induced RI, is reviewed.

MATERIAL AND METHODS

Between June 1982 and March 1986, 57 patients presented RI. The mean age of the patients was 62.5 years and there were 37 males and 20 females. The reasons for diuretic treatment included hypertension (24 patients), cardiac insufficiency (14), other cardiac disorders (5), chronic cor pulmonale (5), edema from a variety of causes (5) and cirrhosis of the liver with ascitis (5). Sixteen patients received proximal diuretics (frusemide, thiazide), eight were given distal diuretics (spironolactone, triamterene) and thirty-three a combination of the two.

Smac (Smac Technicon System) was used for biochemical determinations. Statistical calculation was done using the Mann-Whitney U test for non-parametric independent data.

RESULTS

Table 1 expresses the diuretics administered together with the daily dosages and length of treatment when RI was detected. The patients were divided into two groups according to whether the diuretic was the only evident cause of RI (group I, 35 patients) or whether there were other possible associated factors such as hypotension, low heart rate, infection of the ascitic fluid (group II, 22 patients).

Table 2 shows the age of the patients, plasma urea and creatinine levels and the number of patients with pre-existing RI or hypertension.

Besides worsening of renal function, there were other secondary effects: hyponatremia in 23 patients, hypokalaemia in 5, hyperkalaemia in 28, hypocalcemia in 12, hyperuricemia in 36 and hyperphosphatemia in 27. Oliguria was present in 33 patients (57,9 %) during RI.

A 62-year-old man with pre-existing RI on outpatient treatment with frusemide (20 mg/day) who was switched to thiazide - amyloride for 21 days, was admitted to our hospital because of worsening of the RI and general condition. He presented generalized skin rash which was classified as toxicodermia. Proteinuria was 0.80 mg/day. Because of suspected acute interstitial nephritis the diuretic was suspended and prednisone 1 mg/Kg/day started. The skin rash improved after 7 days and creatinine values returned to previous value 3 weeks later.

Five patients, one of which with pre-existing RI, required hemodialysis because of hyperkalaemia (2 patients), anasarca (1), and severe RI with hyperkalaemia (1). Nine patients (15.8 %) died because of RI (1) or complications: respiratory insuffiency (2 patients), hepatic encephalopathy (2), digestive tract hemorrhage (1) and other causes (3). Two of the nine had cirrhosis of the liver. In the remaining patients renal function returned to normal or regressed to previous levels.

Mean recovery time for renal function was similar in both groups (Group I, 15.2 ± 8.3 days; Group II, 12.1 ± 8.6 days.)

Table 1.

DIURETIC	MEAN DAILY DOSAGE	MEAN TREATMENT LENGTH
Thiazide	75 mg/d	11 ± 3.7 days
Clortalidone	50 "	22.8 ± 27.6 "
Furosemide	62 ± 42 "	23.9 ± 26 "
Spironolactone	195 ± 82 "	34.6 ± 39.1 "
Triamterene	333 ±137 "	5.3 ± 1.2 "
Thiazide	67 ± 23.5 "	48.1 ± 75.9 "
+ Amiloride	6.7 ± 3.5 "	48.1 ± 75.9 "

Table 2

	Group I	Group II
Age	60.1 y	65.1 y
Plasma urea	34.8 mmol/l	40.6 mmol/l
Plasma creatinine	316.7 umol/l	469 umol/l
Previous RI	7 p	9 p

Previous Hy	18	p	8		p

RI: Renal Insufficience. Hy: Arterial Hypertension
p: patients

CONCLUSIONS

1. Treatment with distal diuretics may cause irreversible RI in patients with decompensated hepatic disease or pre-existing RI.
2. Diuretic treatment for high risk patients (aged 60 years, severe cardiopathy, decompensated hepatic cirrhosis, pre-existing RI), must be carefully adapted to the patient, using the most appropriate diuretic for each case.
3. During treatment of such patients, renal function must be evaluated through seried monitorization.

REFERENCES

1. Fichman M.P., Vorherr H., Kleeman C.R. and Telfer N. Ann. Intern. Med. 69: 249-863, 1971.
2. Leth A. Circulation 42: 479-485, 1970.
3. Epstein M., Schneider N.S. and Befeler B. Am. J. Med. 58: 510-516, 1975.
4. Kaufman A.M. and Levitt M.F. Am. J. Kidney Dis. 5: 71-78, 1985.
5. Muth R.G. Ann. Intern. Med. 69: 249-261, 1968.
6. Linton A.M., Clark W.F., Driedger A.A., Turnbull D.I. and Lindsay R.M. Ann. Intern. Med. 93: 735-741, 1980.

THE EFFECTS OF SPIRONOLACTONE AND AMILORIDE ON PLASMA ELECTROLYTES IN THIAZIDE TREATED SUBJECTS

G. T. McINNES AND D.L. DAVIES

University Department of Medicine, Gardiner Institute, Western Infirmary, Glasgow G11 6NT, Scotland

INTRODUCTION

Spironolactone and amiloride are distal tubular diuretics widely used for their potassium sparing properties. The potency of spironolactone relative to amiloride in reducing urine potassium is approximately 0.04 on a weight basis (1) while, in clinical studies, estimates of relative potency have varied between 0.10 and 0.36 (2-4). The major objective of this study was to make a precise quantitative comparison of the two agents in attenuating thiazide induced hypokalaemia. The effects on plasma magnesium were also assessed since correction of potassium deficiency may depend in part on maintaining levels of this cation (5).

MATERIALS AND METHODS

Subjects

12 healthy males (mean age 33 yr, range 25-43) gave written informed consent for the study which had ethical committee approval.

Study design

The study was in 2 parts. In part 1, all subjects received hydrochlorothiazide 100 mg daily for 7 days. Part 2 was a randomised, balanced, crossover comparison of spironolactone (25 mg and 100 mg) and amiloride (5 mg and 20 mg) in combination with hydrochlorothiazide 100 mg. Treatments were taken for 8 days, sufficient for the maximum effect of diuretics and potassium sparing agents on plasma potassium (6-9). Study periods were separated by drug free intervals of at least 2 weeks.

Procedure

Drugs were administered once daily at 0900 hr. In part 1, subjects were studied on day 0 (day before drug) and on day 7; in part 2, subjects were studied on day 8. Venous blood for plasma electrolyte concentrations was sampled at 0900 hr and hourly until 1700 hr, to allow for intraindividual variability in potassium levels (9,10). Forearm exercise was avoided to minimise sampling error in potassium estimation (6).

Measurements

Sodium and potassium concentrations were measured by flame photometry using lithium as internal standard. Magnesium concentrations were assayed by atomic absorption spectrophotometry.

Statistical analysis

Plasma levels before and after hydrochlorothiazide were compared by Student's t-test for paired data. Analysis of variance was employed to test the difference between spironolactone and amiloride, the significance of the average slope and the parallelism of the slopes for the two compounds. If the average slope was significant and there was no contraindication to parallelism, the potency of spironolactone relative to amiloride was calculated with 95% confidence limits.

RESULTS

The results for each subject on each study day were averaged and the day mean results are presented in Table 1. Hydrochlorothiazide led to significant falls in plasma sodium and potassium ($p < 0.001$ in each case) but no change in plasma magnesium. Spironolactone and amiloride produced highly significant, parallel log dose-response relationships ($p < 0.001$ in each case), negative for plasma sodium and positive for plasma potassium. Relative potency estimates (95% confidence limits) spironolactone : amiloride were 0.10 (0.04-0.16) for plasma sodium and 0.10 (0.06-0.16) for plasma potassium. Plasma magnesium concentrations after amiloride were greater than those after spironolactone ($p = 0.003$) and the log amiloride dose-response relationship was significant ($p = 0.006$). This relationship was significantly non-parallel to that for spironolactone ($p = 0.007$), precluding estimation of relative potency.

Table 1. Mean (s.d.) results for plasma electrolytes (mmol/l)

Variable	Hydrochlorothiazide		+ spironolactone		+ amiloride	
	Before	After	25mg	100mg	5mg	20mg
Sodium	139.5 (1.0)	137.2 (1.2)	136.6 (1.6)	135.5 (1.6)	136.2 (1.1)	134.5 (1.7)
Potassium	4.08 (0.13)	3.30 (0.19)	3.46 (0.19)	3.70 (0.11)	3.56 (0.16)	3.85 (0.17)
Magnesium	0.802 (0.050)	0.806 (0.052)	0.802 (0.054)	0.789 (0.040)	0.804 (0.057)	0.837 (0.053)

DISCUSSION

Our estimate of the potassium sparing potency of spironolactone relative to amiloride was similar to that noted in hypertensive patients (3), although amiloride's advantage may wane with prolonged treatment (3). Quantitative differences between the drugs may also be influenced by whether they are used to correct hypokalaemia as in this study or to prevent its development (10). In the latter circumstance (4), relative potency spironolactone : amiloride was significantly greater than in the present study. However, in that and in other comparisons, plasma potassium was measured at only one time point after drug administration. Since plasma potassium concentrations fluctuate considerably throughout the day (9,10), repeated measurements are likely to improve greatly the precision of the comparison. Relative potency for plasma sodium was the same as that for plasma potassium indicating that at doses provoking equivalent hyponatraemia (equivalent diuretic doses), the potassium sparing effects of spironolactone and amiloride are identical.

Amiloride induced a dose related increase in plasma magnesium concentration while the reverse was the case for spironolactone. The absence of a hydrochlorothiazide effect on plasma magnesium together with the considerable evidence that thiazides increase urine magnesium excretion (11) suggests efflux of the cation from the intracellular pool. Amiloride may maintain extracellular levels at the expense of cellular concentrations while spironolactone may have the opposite effect.

REFERENCES

1. McInnes, G.T. Clin. Pharmacol. Ther. 31: 472-477, 1982.
2. Bull, M.V. and Laragh, J.H. Circulation 37: 45-53, 1968.
3. George, C.F., Breckenridge, A.M. and Dollery, C.T. Lancet 2: 1288-1291, 1973.
4. Ramsay, L.E., Hettiarachchi, J., Fraser, R. and Morton, J.J. Clin. Pharmacol. Ther. 27: 533-543, 1980.
5. Dyckner, T. and Wester, P.O. Royal Soc. Med.: Int. Congr. Symp. Ser. 44: 43-46, 1981.
6. Bergstrom, J. Acta Cardiol. (suppl.17): 15-24, 1973.
7. McInnes, G.T., Shelton, J.R., Harrison, I.R., Clarke, J.M. and Perkins, R.M. Pharm. Med. 1: 17-25, 1984.
8. Maronde, R.F., Milgrom, M. and Dickey, J.M. Am. Heart J. 78: 16-21, 1969.
9. Morgan, D.B. and Davidson, C. Br. Med. J. 1: 905-908, 1980.
10. Morgan, D.B. Royal Soc. Med.: Int. Congr. Symp. Ser. 44, 3-8, 1981.
11. Swales, J.D. Br. Med. J. 285: 1377-1378, 1982.

HEMORHEOLOGICAL EFFECTS OF DIURETICS

A. MATRAI and E. ERNST

Hemorheology Research Laboratory, Clinic for Physical Medicine, University of Munich, 8000 Munchen 2, Ziemssenstr. 1, FRG

INTRODUCTION

Flow properties of blood affect tissue perfusion, especially when vascular regulation reserves are exhausted, or vascular regulation is disturbed. A common effect of diuretics is the loss of body water. This may decrease intravascular volume and consequently increase blood viscosity. Since the latter is an exponential function of hematocrit (1), relatively small plasma volume variations may result in physiologically significant changes. Diuretical treatment is frequently applied to patients with vascular diseases, already burdened by deteriorated blood rheology. Therefore, the effects of such treatment on blood rheology may be clinically relevant and were investigated in this study.

SUBJECTS AND METHODS

Two groups of subjects were studied:

Group I: 15 healthy male volunteers (age 23-28 yr). These were given three Furosemide doses of 30, 30 and 40 mg, at 10 a.m., 8 p.m. and 7 a.m. next day, respectively. Venous blood samples were taken before the first dose, and at 10 a.m. next day.

Group II: 23 previously untreated hypertensive patients (12 male, 11 female, age 26-69 yr). These were treated by Hydrochlorothiazide (individual dosages of 25-50 mg/die), as required to normalize their blood pressure.

Venous blood was taken before starting the treatment, and after 3 weeks. The following variables were measured: whole blood viscosity at 37 ^{o}C at native and standard (0.45) hematocrits, at low (0.7 s^{-1}) and high (95 s^{-1}) shear rates: LS-BV, HS-BV, LS-BV45 and HS-BV45, respectively. Plasma viscosity (at 37 ^{o}C,

PV), red cell aggregation (RCA) and filterability (RCF), red and white blood cell counts (RCC, WCC), serum protein concentration (SEPR), systolic and diastolic blood pressures (RR-sys, RR-dia). The applied methods were described and validated earlier (2). Statistics: Mann-Whitney U-test for paired data.

RESULTS

In Group I, treatment resulted in an apparent hemoconcentration, with significant increase of HCT, PV, SEPR, LS-BV, HS-BV and HS-BV45 (Table I).
In contrast to this, Group II presented no hemoconcentration, but significant decrease of (the pathologically high) LS-BV, LS-BV45 and RCF. However, RCF did not reach normal values (Table I).

Table 1. Effects of diuretical treatment (*): $p<0.05$

Parameter	Group I before	Group I after		Group II before	Group II after	
LS-BV (mPas)	26.8±4.6	33.0±4.9	(*)	33.1±5.5	27.9±5.1	(*)
HS-BV (mPas)	4.7±0.36	5.2±0.44	(*)	5.1±0.49	4.9±0.37	
LS-BV45 (mPas)	27.3±2.6	28.6±3.3		32.6±4.0	28.7±3.5	(*)
HS-BV45 (mPas)	4.7±0.21	4.9±0.24	(*)	5.2±0.29	5.0±0.27	
HCT (l/l)	46±2	48±3	(*)	44±4	43±4	
PV (mPas)	1.20±0.03	1.25±0.04	(*)	1.25±0.06	1.22±0.05	
RCA (-)	11.4±2.8	10.7±3.0		17.9±5.2	17.2±6.4	
RCD (ml/min)	0.76±0.10	0.77±0.08		0.55±0.13	0.59±0.11	(*)
RCC $(10^{12}/l)$	5.47±0.42	5.89±0.47	(*)	5.20±0.51	5.30±0.53	
WCC $(10^{9}/l)$	6.0±1.0	6.4±2.0		6.8±2.3	6.3±1.7	
SEPR (g/l)	70±3	76±3	(*)	68±4	69±3	
RR-sys (mmHg)	120± 8	122±11		164±17	125±12	(*)
RR-dia (mmHg)	84±5	81±4		97±14	85±6	(*)

DISCUSSION

Blood rheology is determined by plasma viscosity, hematocrit, red cell aggregability and deformability (3). Alterations of intravascular volume certainly affect the first two components. Excretion of water and salts induced by diuretics may result in decreased blood volume and consequent increase in blood viscosity. In epidemiological studies, increased cardiovascular mortality was observed among patients treated with diuretics, and a possible role of blood viscosity increase was suggested (4). However, vascular effects of diuretics (5) may increase intravascular volume, and effective treatment of the disease may result in improved intrinsic rheological properties of blood. As a consequence, blood rheology may improve, despite decreased total body water content. In the present study, short term, high dose Furosemid treatment of volunteers caused hemoconcentration and elevated blood viscosity. Long term treatment of mild hypertensives with Hydrochlorothiazide did not result in hemoconcentration, but normalized red cell deformability and low shear blood viscosity. The latter changes may be related to normalized blood pressure, rather than direct effect on erythrocytes.

These results suggest, that different diuretics may have diverse effect on blood volume and blood viscosity. Alternatively the hemorheologic reaction to diuretics in healthy volunteers could differ from that seen in hypertensives. Finally, acute effects may be not identical to alterations due to long term medication. Hemorheological "side-efects" of diuretics are of possible clinical significance, needing more detailed investigations.

REFERENCES

1. Matrai, A., Skalak, R. and Whittingtom R.B. In: Clinical Hemorheology (Eds. S. Chien, J. Dormandy, E. Ernst and A. Matrai), Martinus Nijhoff, Dordrecht, 1986.

2. Ernst, E., Matrai, A., Scherer, A., Schmidlechner, Ch. and Monshausen, Ch. Clin. Hemorheol. 5: 511-514, 1985.

3. Chien, S. In: The red Blood Cell, Vol. II. (Ed. D.M. Surgenor), Academic Press, New York, 1975.

4. Ernst, E. and Matrai, A. Clin. Hemorheol. 4: 589-590, 1984.

5. Mukherjee, S.K., Katz, M.A., Michael, U.F. and Ogden, D.A. Amer. Heart J. 101: 307-318, 1981.

DIURETIC EFFECT AND ELECTROLYTE CHANGES CAUSED BY ORAL PEG 200 IN RAT

S. SONKODI, B. TICHY, *W. BROWN, *J.I.S. ROBERTSON

First Department of Internal Medicine, Szeged University Medical School, Hungary and *MRC Blood Pressure Unit, Western Infirmary, Glasgow, Great Britain.

INTRODUCTION

Polyethylene glycol (PEG 200) is a useful vehicle for the administration of drugs (1). In an earlier investigation when PEG 200 was administered to rats by gavage, we observed changes in sodium and water metabolism (2). The aim of the present work was to obtain further data in connection with this phenomenon.

MATERIALS AND METHODS

Male Wistar rats weighing 220-250 g were used. For 6-hour experiments the rats were placed in mesh-wire metabolic cages, and no food was provided. Urine was collected in an Erlenmayer flask placed directly under the funnel, in an ice bath. One group of eight animals received 1 ml PEG 200 per 100 g body weight, and the second group of eight 1 ml tap water by gavage. At the end of the experiment the animals were lightly anaesthetized with ether, and blood was taken by puncture of the abdominal aorta.

In the first and second experiments, tap water was available ad libitum.

In the first experiment the packed cell volume (PCV), plasma renin activity (PRA), serum and urine Na and K, and osmotic and free water clearance were measured, and in the second experiment the endogenous creatinine clearance was determined. In the third experiment, in which the animals did not receive drinking water the PCV, PRA and serum and urine Na and K were determined. PCV was measured with a micromethod, the electrolytes, osmolality and creatinine by standard laboratory methods, and the PRA with a New England Nuclear (Chicago) kit.

RESULTS

The results of the first experiment are shown in Table 1. PEG 200 given orally by gavage caused significant increases in PCV, PRA, urine volume, and osmotic and free water clearance, Na loss and K loss. The urine Na/K ratio was significantly higher in the PEG 200-treated group than in the controls. There was no significant change in serum electrolytes.

In the second experiment the endogenous creatinine clearance was significantly higher in the PEG 200-treated (0.60 ± 0.22 ml/min) than in the control group (0.19 ± 0.09 ml/min; $p<0.001$).

The results of the third experiment are presented in Table 2. When the drinking water was withdrawn, the PEG 200 treatment was found to cause significant increases in the PCV, PRA, serum Na and in urine volume, with decreases in serum K and in urinary Na and K output as compared to the controls. We did not find a significant difference in the urinary Na/K ratio between the two groups.

DISCUSSION

Our results showed that PEG 200 administered by gavage leads to diuresis in the rat. This can not be a secondary consequence of a higher fluid intake resulting from enhanced drinking, as it was confirmed by the elevated water diuresis that developed when the animals were deprived of their drinking water.

When we previously used PEG 200 as a vehicle, this was done in the belief that this substance is not absorbed or reabsorbed. The higher serum and urine osmolality in our experiments indicates absorption of PEG 200, which was found earlier (3). The elevated serum and urine osmolality raises the possibility that the mechanism of the diuretic effect of PEG 200 is osmotic. This is supported by our other findings of increases in urinary Na output in free water clearance; which indicates that PEG 200 inhibits Na and water reabsorption from renal tubules. It is important to note that osmotic diuretics, such as mannitol (4), decrease the PCV. In our PEG 200-treated animals we found an increased PCV, suggesting the possibility of a decreased plasma volume. Osmotic diuretics usually decrease PRA (5); we found PRA to be higher in our PEG-treated animals.

Further investigations are necessary to clarify the mechanism of the diuretic effect of PEG 200.

SUMMARY

PEG 200, which has been suggested for use as an inert vehicle for drug administration, has a diuretic effect in rat. Treatment with this substance increases packed cell volume, decreases plasma renin activity and enhances urinary sodium output, osmotic and free water clearance.

REFERENCES

1. MARTINDALE: Extra Pharmacopoeia 27, 630-632. Pharmaceutical Press, London 1977.
2. SONKODI, S., TICHY, B., *BROWN, W.B., *ROBERTSON, J.I.S. Clinical Science (1986) in press.
3. SMYTH, H.F., CARPENTER, C.P., and Well, C.S. The chronic oral toxicology of the polyethylene glycols.
4. WARREN, S.E., BLANTZ, R.C. Mannitol. Arch. Intern. Med. 141, 493-497, 1981.
5. CHURCHILL, P.C., CHURCHILL, M.C., and McDONALD, F.C. Effects of saline and mannitol on renin and distal tubule Na in rats. Circ. Res. 45, 786-791, (1979)

Table 1.

Group	n	PCV	Serum K mmol/l	Serum Na mmol/l	Serum osmol mosm/l	Urine volume ml/100g	Urine K-loss µmol/min/ /100g	Urine Na-loss µmol/min/ /100g	Urine Na/K	Urine osmol mosm/l	C_{H_2O} ml/min	C_{Osm} ml/min	PRA ng/ml/h
PEG 200 treated	8	49,1 ± 1,o8	4,98 ± o,17	144,8 ± o,7	333,2 ± 2,6	7,54 ± o,37	o,75 ± o,o4	1,54 ± o,1o	2,o5 ± o,14	999,9 ± 26,7	o,137 ± o,oo7	o,2o6 ± o,o10	3,51 ± o,37
CONTROL	8	43,1 ± 1,16	5,35 ± o,13	142,9 ± o,7	3o9,4 ± 3,1	2,o6 ± o,24	o,19 ± o,o2	o,16 ± o,o3	o,84 ± o,11	75o,3 ± 5o,9	o,o23 ± o,oo3	o,o39 ± o,oo5	2,11 ± o,22
p <		.o1	n.s.	n.s.	.ooo1	.ooo1	.ooo1	.ooo1	.ooo1	.oo1	.oo1	.oo1	.o1

Table 2.

Group	n	PCV	Serum K mmol/l	Serum Na mmol/l	Urine volume ml/loog	Urine K-loss μM/min/ /loog	Urine Na-loss μM/min/ /loog	Urine Na/K	PRA ng/ml/h
PEG 200 treated	8	49,oo o,41	4,75 ±o,o7	153,8 ±1,43	6,18 ±o,16	o,874 ±o,o44	1,764 ±o,o73	2,oo ±o,o6	6,45 ±o,56
Control	8	44,94 ±o,59	5,46 ±o,14	143,3 ±1,o9	o,87 ±o,14	o,2o4 ±o,o4o	o,29o ±o,o4o	1,5o ±o,128	2,9o ±o,35
$p <$		.ol	.ol	.ol	.ool	.ool	.ool	n.s.	.ol

XIII. EFFECTS OF DIURETICS ON WATER AND ELECTROLYTE EXCRETION

CHANGES IN KINETICS OF ELECTROLYTE EXCRETIONS INDUCED BY ADDING TRIAMTERENE TO THIAZIDE

N.POZET,M.LABEEUW,A.HADJ AISSA,J.SASSARD,P.ZECH.

Clinic of Nephrology,INSERM U 80,E.Herriot Hospital,Lyon, France

Diuretics acting on the distal tubule show some magnesium sparing activity (1) which might be particularly relevant in long term diuretic therapy of hypertension or renal stone disease, given the potential magnesium depletion induced by thiazides (2).

MATERIALS AND METHODS

This study evaluates the short term effect on sodium (Nae), magnesium (Mge),calcium (Cae),and potassium (Ke) excretions in eight normal volunteers (age:32.5±4.6) given, in random order, at two weeks interval: Placebo (P), Methyclothiazide (MCT 2 mg), and MCT + triamterene (T, 25 or 75 mg) at 7 am for four days. Urine was collected every twelve hours and blood was drawn at day 1 and day 5.

RESULTS

On the twelwe hours following the first dose of diuretic Nae increased significantly and similarly with all diuretics. MCT increased Ke and this change was lessened by T, in a dose dependent manner.Although the rise in Mge following MCT was not significant, T reduced the MCT induced magnesuria.

On four days,all treatments decreased Cae to a similar extent. As expected in these non sodium loaded subjects, the effect on natriuresis was moderate and significant only with MCT+75mg which induced larger natriuresis and aldosterone stimulation than

MCT and MCT+25mg. A significant increase in Ke was evident with all treatments but the K sparing effect of T was obvious only during the daytime, leaving unaffected the nocturnal MCT increase in Ke. Mge followed the same pattern. However it can be seen from Table 1 that while the Mg sparing activity was evident with 25 mg of T, 75 mg did not oppose the MCT increase in Mge

Table 1.Excretions(micromol min-1,mean±SD).p vs P :*:<.05,#:<.01
vs MCT § _ *f* _

	First 12 hours		Mean of four days					
	Mge	Ke	Mge			Ke		
			24h	day	night	24h	day	night
P	2.90	45	2.88	2.69	3.03	47	60	34
	±0.98	±12	±.76	±.82	±.82	± 9	±11	±11
MCT	3.26	74#	3.31#	3.15#	3.59#	56#	71#	41*
	±.73	±24	±.43	±.51	±.78	±11	±15	± 8
MCT+25	2.66§	69#	2.99§	2.71§	3.30§	52*§	66*§	38
	±.94	±23	±.46	±.47	±.59	±20	±16	±11
MCT+75	2.45§	57*f*	3.26*	2.87	3.63*	52*§	62§	41*
	±.63	±19	±.52	±.53	±.85	±12	±15	±12

Table 2.Excretions as in 1.PRA(ng.l-1.min-1).Aldost(pmol.l-1)

	Mean of four days		Blood values on the last day			
	Nae	Cae	PRA	ALDOST	Mg	K
P	109	3.86	59	91	.88	3.80
	±25	±1.30	±22	± 23	±.06	± .28
MCT	117	2.81#	248#	307#	.90	3.41#
	±34	±1.26	±93	±164	±.08	± .34
MCT+25	131*	2.97#	242#	279#	.85	3.52*
	±15	± .79	±79	±150	±.06	± .14
MCT+75	139**f*	2.91#	251	367#§	.87	3.58
	±22	±1.12	±85	±161	±.06	± .31

COMMENTS

The magnesuric effect of thiazides has been recently emphasized as it may lead to some degree of magnesium depletion(1-3). It is related to a direct effect on magnesium reabsorption and perhaps worsened by a secondary hyperaldosteronism.In the present study,MCT produced only a mild increase in Mge following the first dose,while,over four days,magnesuria exceeded the placebo value by an average of 0.6 mmol/day. This depended on both the increased diurnal and nocturnal Mge,extending beyond the natriuretic effect .

Ours results show that the Mg sparing activity of distally acting diuretics occurs within the twelve hours following the first dose, which suggests that T acts directly on the thiazide induced changes in magnesium reabsorption.This effect appears dose-dependent and tends to decrease at night, in accordance with the pharmacokinetics of T.

The Mg sparing activity of T is also obvious on the four days period in keeping with its opposite effect on aldosterone action. Its is obtained with low dose of T;75 mg produced no beneficial effect since magnesuria reached the value obtained with thiazide. This was associated with a larger increase in plasma aldosterone due to the improved natriuretic activity: although a Mg sparing activity was present during the day,this effect was cancelled by the nocturnal increase in Mge. Ke followed the same pattern.

In conclusion, magnesium and potassium sparing effects of adding triamterene to methyclothiazide are optimal for low doses of triamterene. Howewer, they do not extend beyond twelwe hours. Increasing the dose of triamterene, through increased natriuretic efficacy may jeopardize this beneficial effect. This might be worth considering during long term therapy.

REFERENCES

1 Bellorin-Font,E,Weisinger,J,Paz Martinez,V.In:Diuretics, Elsevier,New York,1984,pp174-181

2 Mountokalakis,T.D.Magnesium 2,2,57-61,1983

3 Leary,W.P,Reyes,A.J.In:Diuretics,Elsevier,New York,1984, pp494-496

BENEFICIAL EFFECTS OF IBOPAMINE IN IDIOPATHIC EDEMA

C.CAMPIERI, R.PRANDINI, A.TERNI, S.STEFONI, A.VANGELISTA and V.BONOMINI

Institute of Nephrology, S.Orsola University Hospital,
Via Massarenti 9, 40138 Bologna - Italy.

INTRODUCTION

The main clinical feature of idiopathic edema is an excessive fluid retention aggravated by orthostatism. Several mechanism have been proposed to explain this pathophysiological event. An abnormal capillary permeability to albumin with secondary volume depletion and renal hypoperfusion (1); a secondary form hyperaldosteronism due to an overactive Renin-Angiotensin-Aldosterone System (RAAS); an abnormal regulation of ADH release (2) and a possible suppression of the renal dopaminergic system (3). Different therapeutical approaches have been tried with incostant results. Antialdosterone drugs and beta-blockers to interfere with the overactive Renin-Angiotensin-Aldosterone-System (RAAS); Bromocriptine with its dopaminergic activity (4); Captopril to block Angiotensin II production and with some intrinsic natriuretic properties (5). Diet with sodium and carbohydrates reduction has been also suggested (6). Diuretics, however, are the most frequently used drugs but, despite a quick symptomatic benefit due to a rapid fluid removal, they can worsen the clinical profile of the syndrome in a long-term follow-up (6).

MATERIALS AND METHODS

We have selected 5 symptomatic women suffering from idiopathic edema. After 4 weeks of diuretic wash-out we administered, in an open study, 200 mg of IBOPAMINE p.o. in the morning for 2 months. IBOPAMINE (N-methil-dopamine di-isobutyric ester) is a dopaminergic agonist with β adrenergic activity, that improves the renal blood flow by reducing renal vessel resistance and exerts a natriuretic action. Diurnal weight gain (between

7 a.m. and 7 p.m.), daily diuresis and sodium excretion have been evaluated before and after 30 and 60 days of treatment. All patients have been followed up for 5 months.

RESULTS

In all patients a significative decrease in diurnal weight gain and an increase in daily urine output and Na^+ excretion has been detected after 30 and 60 days of treatment (Fig.1).

	Age	Diurnal weight gain (g)			Daily urine out put (ml)			Daily Na^+ escretion (mEq)		
		Before	30d.	60d.	Before	30d.	60d.	Before	30d.	60d.
M.V.	47	1100	400	380	150	1100	980	73	120	115
R.G.	50	1400	350	460	200	1000	1150	10	78	85
M.G.	28	1250	200	210	350	1250	1120	95	146	138
C.L.	38	1100	350	280	400	1350	1020	53	138	154
M.A.	35	1150	150	220	400	1400	1380	75	135	127
		1200	290	310	300	1220	1130	61	127	123
		±127	±108	±107	±117	±168	±156	±32	±270	±26
			p<0,001	n.s.		p<0,001	n.s.		p<0,001	n.s.

Fig. 1. Clinical parameters of patients on IBOPAMINE

From the 3d month up to the end of the 5th month of follow-up, these patients have been evaluated to establish the persistence of clinical benefits. In this interval no recurrence of the symptoms was detected and IBOPAMINE was tapered down in all patients and discontinued in two of them (Fig.2).

CONCLUSIONS

IBOPAMINE exerts some beneficial effects on the clinical symptoms of idiopathic edema. It improves also daily urine output and Na^+ excretion and reduces diurnal weight gain.

Its influence in the pathophysiological mechanisms of the syndrome may be related to its dopaminergic activity.

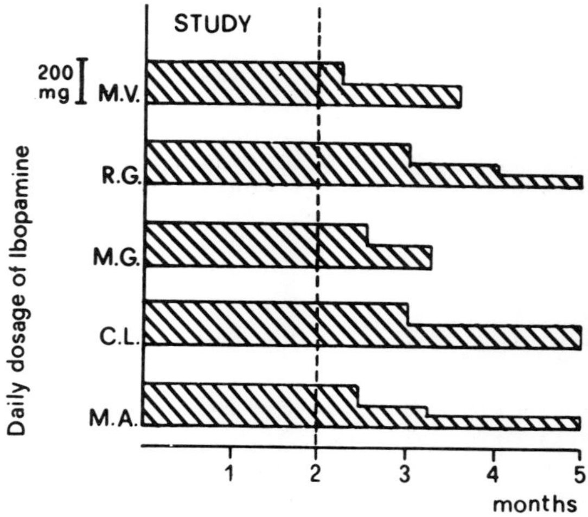

Fig. 2. IBOPAMINE dosage in the follow-up

Its dosage can be reduced and discontinued without rebound effects and with stable clinical results in the short term follow-up.

REFERENCES

1. De Wardener, H.E. Kidney International 19 : 881-892, 1981
2. Thibonnier, M., Marchetti, J., Corvol, P., Menard, J., Milliez, P. Am.J.Med. 67 : 67-73, 1979
3. Kuchel, O., Cuche J.L., Buu, N.T., Guthrie, G.P. Jr., Unger, T., Nowaczynski, W., Boucher, R., Genest, J. J.C.E. & M. 4 : 639-646, 1977
4. Edwards, C.R.W., Besser, G.M., Thorner, M.O. Lancet ii 94, 1979
5. Mimran, A., Targhetta, R. N.Engl.J.Med. 301 : 1289-1290, 1979
6. Mac Gregor, G.A., Markandu, N.D., Roulston, J.E., Jones, J.C. Lancet i : 397-399, 1979

KALIURESIS INDUCED BY VARIOUS DIURETICS

W.P. LEARY* AND A.J. REYES**

*Department of Experimental and Clinical Pharmacology, University of Natal, P.O. Box 17039, Congella 4013, Durban, South Africa, and **Departamento de Investigación Cardiovascular, Fundación Procardias, Montevideo, Uruguay

ABSTRACT

Single doses of placebo and of various commonly used K^+-loosing diuretic formulations were randomly and double blind administered to healthy volunteers kept in a metabolic ward. All studied formulations increased mean 24-hr natriuresis significantly; early distal tubular diuretics increased mean 24-hr urinary Na^+ and K^+ outputs more than loop diuretics. Both types of diuretic yielded undistinguishable ranges of mean 24-hr urinary K^+/Na^+ ratio. Diuretic-induced 24-hr natriuresis, in subjects with normal Na^+ turnover, would depend on the type of substance used (loop or early distal tubular diuretic) for a given Na^+ and K^+ diet. In the same circumstances urinary K^+ losses would depend more on the absolute amount of Na^+ mobilized by a diuretic than on the drug specimen used.

INTRODUCTION

Diuretic-induced kaliuresis has been studied in laboratory animals, healthy volunteers and patients. The likelihood of K^+ deficiency developing in patients treated with K^+-loosing diuretics principally depends upon the functional status of the subjects and upon factors other than the diuretic used. However it is in order to evaluate the kaliuretic effects of diuretics in clinical use and under investigation. These assessments must be carried out in normal volunteers for reasons of biological homogeneity.

SUBJECTS AND METHODS

Experiments were carried out in biologically equivalent

healthy volunteers confined to a metabolic ward. Similar standard procedures (1,2) were followed throughout this long experimental series.

A tablet containing placebo or a diuretic formulation was administered to volunteer subjects randomly and in double-blind manner at hr 08.00 (hr 0 of the experiments). Urine voided in the 24-hr after dosing was collected and analysed by flame photometry for its K^+ and Na^+ contents. The paired t test was used for contrasting mean values.

RESULTS

The mean 24-hr urinary outputs of K^+ and Na^+ and the corresponding mean K^+/Na^+ ratios after the administration of placebo, the percentage changes in mean 24-hr urinary K^+ and Na^+ excretions induced by the studied diuretics and the post-diuretic mean urinary K^+/Na^+ ratios are depicted in Table 1.

Loop diuretics (LD), including furosemide 40 and 80 mg,

Table 1. Effects of the administration of single doses of various diuretic formulations on mean 24-hr urinary Na^+ and K^+ output and on mean K^+/Na^+ ratio in healthy volunteers.

n	Diuretic and dose (mg)	placebo			post-diuretic		
		K^+ (mmol/24 hr)	Na^+ (mmol/24 hr)	$\frac{K^+}{Na^+}$	$\%\Delta K^+$	$\%\Delta Na^+$	$\frac{K^+}{Na^+}$
9	clopamide 5	61	154	0.40	26*	85***	0.27
14	furosemide 40	44	147	0.30	7	51***	0.21
16	furosemide 80	39	148	0.26	38***	51**	0.24
14	HCTZ 25	44	147	0.30	26*	85***	0.20
10	HCTZ 50	56	133	0.42	41	109***	0.28
19	HCTZ 50	48	177	0.27	31*	60***	0.22
10	muzolimine 30	54	186	0.29	20	33**	0.26
10	muzolimine 40	49	225	0.22	24*	17*	0.23
16	piretanide 12	39	148	0.26	33*	39*	0.25
13	xipamide 5	42	151	0.28	40**	46**	0.27
13	xipamide 10	42	151	0.28	55**	120***	0.20
13	xipamide 20	42	151	0.28	79***	110***	0.24
13	xipamide 40	42	151	0.28	69**	115***	0.22

n = number of subjects. HCTZ = hydrochlorothiazide.
Significances of the differences between mean 24-hr post-diuretic and mean 24-hr post-placebo outputs: *$p < 0.05$; **$p < 0.01$; ***$p < 0.001$.

muzolimine 30 and 40 mg and piretanide 12 mg, increased mean 24-hr urinary K^+ and Na^+ outputs from 7 to 38% and 17 to 51% respectively. Early distal tubular diuretics (DTD), including clopamide 5 mg, hydrochlorothiazide 25 and 50 mg and xipamide 5, 10, 20 and 40 mg, raised mean 24-hr urinary K^+ and Na^+ outputs by 26 to 79% and 46 to 120% respectively.

The mean 24-hr urinary K^+/Na^+ ratio after placebo ranged from 0.22 to 0.42. After dosing with diuretics, the mean 24-hr urinary K^+/Na^+ ratio generally decreased; the variable ranged 0.21-0.26 after LD and 0.20-0.28 after DTD.

DISCUSSION AND CONCLUSIONS

The 24-hr urinary K^+ excretion that followed the administration of a diuretic formulation in the present study would indicate the potential of such formulation for provoking K^+ deficiency. Loop diuretics caused less kaliuresis than DTD, a fact that is readily explained by the lower 24-hr natriuretic effect of LD. These relatively weak actions of loop-acting substances are due to undershoots in the urinary flows of K^+ and Na^+ that follow the early post-dosing excretory effects of LD (A.J. Reyes and W.P. Leary, unpublished).

Diuretic formulations causing higher urinary Na^+ excretions tended to elicit higher K^+ outputs. The presently evaluated urinary K^+/Na^+ ratios, which express the amount of K^+ lost per unit of Na^+ excreted under the conditions of this investigation, would not provide an important guideline for selecting a K^+-loosing diuretic; diet and other factors affecting bodily Na^+ and K^+ turnovers physiologically and/or pathophysiologically would be more important determinants of diuretic-induced natriuresis-related kaliuresis than the particular pharmacological properties of any of the studied formulations.

REFERENCES

1. Reyes, A.J. and Leary, W.P. Curr. Ther. Res. 30: 227-235, 1981.
2. Roberts, C.J.C. and Daneshmend, T.K. Br. J. Clin. Pharmacol. 12: 465-474, 1981.

NATRIURETIC POTENCY OF VARIOUS DIURETICS

A.J. REYES* AND W.P. LEARY**

*Departamento de Investigación Cardiovascular, Fundación Procardias, Holanda 1724, Montevideo, Uruguay, and
**Department of Experimental and Clinical Pharmacology, University of Natal, Durban, South Africa

ABSTRACT

Single doses of various commonly used diuretic formulations and of placebo were randomly and double blind administered to healthy volunteers kept in a metabolic ward. All studied formulations increased mean 24-hr natriuresis significantly. Early distal tubular diuretics elevated urinary Na^+ flow over the 24-hr period that followed medication; loop-diuretic formulations raised urinary Na^+ output strikingly in the 0-3-hr period after dosing, but invariably caused an undershoot in urinary Na^+ flow in the 6-24-hr post-dosing interval. As a consequence, loop diuretics induced lower increases in mean 24-hr urinary Na^+ output than early distal tubular substances. When monodoses are given to healthy individuals, loop-diuretic formulations in current use generally elicit lower 24-hr natriuretic effects than commonly employed early distal tubular diuretic formulations.

INTRODUCTION

In experimental pharmacology the natriuretic potency of diuretics is usually described on the basis of the increase in the urinary fractional excretion of Na^+ determined by single doses of the drug formulations under consideration. The time after dosing which should be taken into account in terms of the above description has not been standardized, and most frequently it has been limited to less than 8 hr.

In clinical pharmacology natriuretic potency should be defined in normal volunteers, for reasons of biological homogeneity, under strictly controlled conditions; since diuretics are most frequently prescribed once daily, natriuretic potency should be assessed on the basis of the 24-hr natriuretic effects of single doses of the diuretic formulations investigated.

SUBJECTS AND METHODS

Experiments were carried out in biologically equivalent healthy volunteers who were confined to a metabolic ward. Similar standard procedures (1,2) were followed throughout this series.

A tablet containing placebo or a diuretic formulation was administered to volunteer subjects randomly and in double-blind manner at hr 08.00 (hr 0 of each experiment). Urine was collected during the post-dosing intervals 0-3, 3-6, 6-12 and 12-24 hr. Urinary Na^+ concentration was assessed by flame photometry.

RESULTS

Results are depicted in Table 1. All studied formulations

Table 1. Effects of the administration of single doses of various diuretic formulations on urinary Na^+ output in healthy volunteers. Hour 0 of the experiments corresponds to hr 08.00.

n	Diuretic and dose (mg)	Post-placebo urinary Na^+ output (mmol)					Post-diuretic % change of urinary Na^+ output				
		—Hours after dosing—					—Hours after dosing—				
		0-3	3-6	6-12	12-24	0-24	0-3	3-6	6-12	12-24	0-24
13	amiloride 5	17	19	27	58	121	76	37	70	14	39*
13	amiloride 10	17	19	27	58	121	100	74	126	28	67***
9	clopamide 5	25	27	49	53	154	124	133	106	23	85***
14	furosemide 40	24	26	52	46	147	385	35	-16	-35	51***
16	furosemide 80	16	30	54	48	148	594	87	-39	-50	51**
14	HCTZ 25	24	26	52	46	147	172	170	69	11	85***
10	HCTZ 50	17	23	51	42	133	218	204	78	50	109***
19	HCTZ 50	24	21	57	75	177	100	205	53	13	60***
10	muzolimine 30	31	26	71	58	186	213	85	-10	-33	33**
10	muzolimine 40	31	29	101	64	225	229	93	-37	-34	17*
16	piretanide 12	16	30	54	48	148	681	33	-61	-60	39*
13	xipamide 5	22	21	39	69	151	95	95	38	19	46**
13	xipamide 10	22	21	39	69	151	136	248	110	81	120***
13	xipamide 20	22	21	39	69	151	155	124	97	99	110***
13	xipamide 40	22	21	39	69	151	159	157	105	94	115***

n = number of subjects. HCTZ = hydrochlorothiazide.
Significances of the differences between mean 24-hr post-diuretic and mean 24-hr post-placebo outputs (paired t test): *$p < 0.05$; **$p < 0.01$; ***$p < 0.001$.

increased 24-hr urinary Na^+ output significantly.

Loop diuretics (LD), including furosemide 40 and 80 mg, muzolimine 30 and 40 mg and piretanide 12 mg, increased mean 24-hr urinary Na^+ output in the range of 17-51% with respect to excretion after placebo; early distal tubular diuretics (DTD), including clopamide 5 mg, hydrochlorothiazide 25 and 50 mg and xipamide 5, 10, 20 and 40 mg, increased mean 24-hr urinary Na^+ excretion 46-120% with respect to post-placebo output; amiloride 5 and 10 mg increased mean urinary Na^+ excretion 39-67% with respect to post-placebo output.

In the post-dosing period 0-3-hr, LD increased mean urinary Na^+ output 213-681%, DTD raised mean excretion by 95-218%, and amiloride provoked a 76-100% augmentation in mean Na^+ output. During the intervals 6-12 and 12-24 hr after dosing, LD reduced mean renal Na^+ excretion below post-placebo levels. This undershoot of urinary Na^+ flow, which invariably followed the natriuretic action of LD, explains why the mean 24-hr natriuretic effects of LD were lower than those of DTD.

CONCLUSIONS

The present findings support the view that time should be taken into account as a critical variable when diuretic potency is defined (3).

Diuretics may be classified into two groups on the basis of the 24-hr natriuresis elicited by single doses of commonly used formulations when administered to healthy subjects: (A) low-potency natriuretics, which include LD and amiloride; (B) high-potency natriuretics, which include DTD.

REFERENCES

1. Reyes, A.J. and Leary, W.P. Curr. Ther. Res. 30: 227-235, 1981.
2. Roberts, C.J.C. and Daneshmend, T.K. Br. J. Clin. Pharmacol. 12: 465-474, 1981.
3. Hamdy, R.C., Vinson, M., Robbins, A.D., Struthers, L.P.L., Chapman, S.F., Norris, R.J. and Shaw, H.L. In: Diuretics (Ed. J.B. Puschett), Elsevier, New York Amsterdam Oxford, 1984, pp. 403-406.

SHORT TERM EFFECTS OF MUZOLIMINE ON ELECTROLYTES AND ACID-BASE BALANCE

Boschetti E., Minestrini C., Scortecci A., Cipolloni S., Istituto di Semeiotica Medica, Università di Perugia (I).

INTRODUCTION

The present study was undertaken to assess the short term effects of Muzolimine a new powerful loop diuretic on electrolytes and acid-base balance in normal subjects and mild hypertensives.

MATERIAL AND METHODS

Five subjects (3 healthy and 2 with mild hypertension) were admitted to our clinical research center and started on a standard Na-K diet (100 and 80 mEq per day). After a few days (3 to 5) all patiens underwent the following measurements: body weight, diuresis, arterial pressure, blood gases, BUN, plasma uric acid, Na-K, glucose and creatinine, urinary excretion of Na, K, ammonia and tritratable acid. Appropriate preservatives avoided gas loss during urine collection and HCO_3^- was thus indirectly calculated from pH and pCO_2. Urinary ammonia was determined by a colorimetric method and tritratable acid was measured according to the established technique of tritratation with NaOH. The net renal acid excretion was calculated employing the usual formula:

Net acid excretion=Ammonia+tritratable acid-HCO_3^-.

Following the basal assessment every subject was started on Muzolimine, 30 mg a day by mouth. All the above measures were repeatedly done over a 7-day period treatment, with a variable intermittence, depending upon the ease of the procedure. Data were evaluated by analysis of variance for repeated measures (2). In the case of significance ($p < 0.05$) at the F test, each group mean, corresponding to a given day of treatment, was compared with the control mean using a modified t-test.

RESULTS

A significant decrease in body weight was observed along with a rise in urinary sodium excretion (Fig.1), most evident in the first three days of treatment. Net acid excretion significantly changed as well, showing a progressive increase throughout the study (Fig. 2). Plasma K was decreased by Muzolimine, but it was still normal at the end of the study. No significant changes were observed in the other parameters used for analysis; acid-base balance, in particular, did not undergo any changes.

DISCUSSION

The increase in diuresis with Muzolimine is prompt and sustained and is accompanied by a signicant decrease in body weight, which is the landmark of a true contraction of the extracellular fluid volume (3). The fact that sodium excretion went back to the basal values, after an initial rise, might be expression of a new balance in total body sodium, which appears, therefore, not to be impaired by Muzolimine. The drug caused a mild decrease in plasma potassium concentration, that was still normal at the end of the treatment. In fact a clear hypokaliemia is more likely to occurr with loop diureticts either when the Renin-Angiotensin System is stimulated by a greater sodium loss than the one observed in our patients or when the potassium intake is not maintained at a suffi-

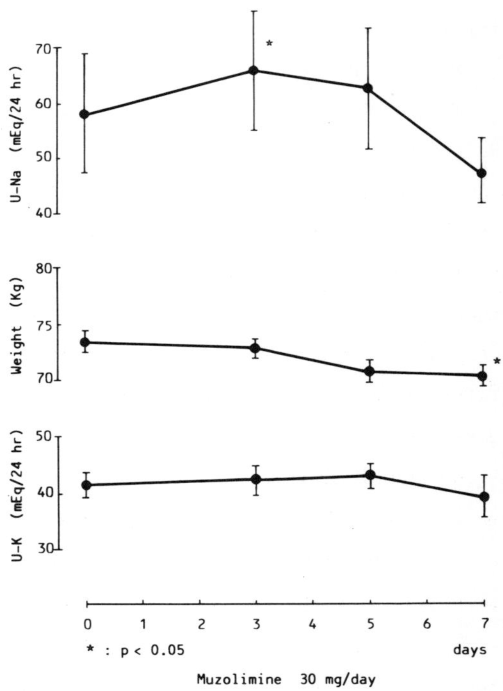

Fig. 1

cient level (4). The acid -base balance was not affected by this short course with Muzolimine for the potassium defiency, if any, was very small. The progressive increase in urinary net acid excretion can be explained solely by the high urinary flow maintained by Muzolimine for the whole period of observation. In conclusion Muzolimine appears to be a phisiologically acting diuretic drug that needs, however, a wider evaluation in long term treatment.

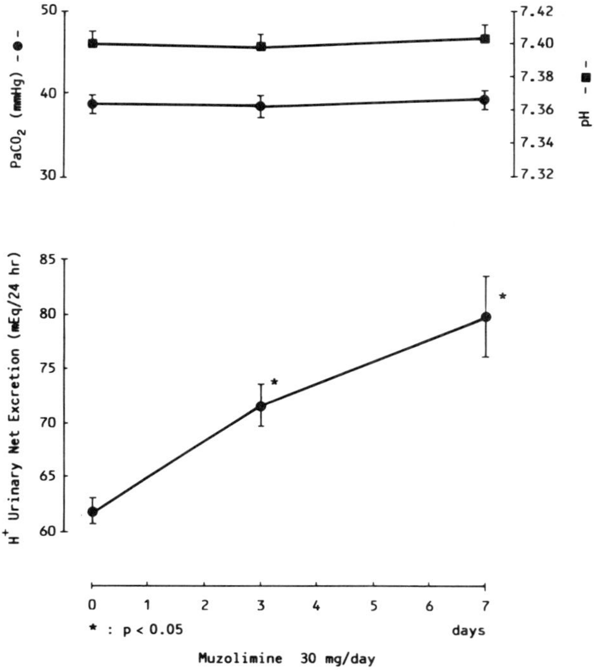

Fig. 2

REFERENCES

1)-Branco de Araũjo, E.,Faccioli,R., Mandarano F.,Proenca.

In:Recent advances in diuretic therapy (Ed.V.E.Andreucci) Excerpta medica, Amsterdam, 1983, pp.65-72.

2)-Winer B.J.

Statistical principles in experimental design, Mc Graw Hill, New York, 1971.

3)-Kokko J.P., Tannen R.L.

Fluids and electrolytes saunders, Philadelphia, 1986.

4)-Seldin D.W.

In: Recent advances in diuretic therapy (Ed. V.E. Andreucci) Excerpta medica, Amsterdam, 1983, pp. 9-20.

EFFECTS OF TORASEMIDE'S METABOLITES ON WATER AND ELECTROLYTE EXCRETION IN THE RAT

J. GENARD, R. PENNINCKX, B. CAPEL, R. LENOIR and R. KRAMP

Service de Physiologie, Université de Mons, B-7000 Mons, Belgium

INTRODUCTION

Several metabolites of torasemide appear in the urine of the rat (1). The efficacy of two metabolites, C3534 and C3535, was tested in the present study. Their effects upon urine flow ($\dot{V}$), sodium ($U_{Na}.\dot{V}$), chloride ($U_{Cl}.\dot{V}$) and potassium ($U_K.\dot{V}$) were studied after application of the metabolites upon the left renal capsule or after i.v. injection.

METHODS AND CALCULATIONS

Anesthetized male Wistar rats weighing between 240 and 320 g were prepared as previously described with the left kidney exposed through an abdominal incision and each ureter catheterised (2). A solution of 5 % mannitol in isotonic saline was infused in order to maintain a control urine flow rate of approximately 40 ul/min/kidney.

Test solutions were prepared as 200 ul of isotonic saline containing 10^{-4} or 10^{-3} M C3534 or C3535. Following baseline determinations (control period), a test solution was either applied upon the left renal capsule (A.L.R.C.) or i.v. injected (I.V.). Urine was then rapidly and serially collected from the left and the right kidney (experimental period).

Net effects of the metabolites were calculated separately for the left and the right kidney by substracting the effects due to the mannitol infusion as well as the average of baseline measurements from urine flow and electrolyte excretion rates determined in each urine sample collected during the experimental period. Peak and cumulated (15, 30 and 60 min after start of treatment) effects are presented.

Statistical significance was evaluated by variance and Student paired and unpaired t-test, as appropriate.

RESULTS

Overall effects.

Experiments were satisfactorily carried out in 34 rats. C3534 only had minor effects at the highest concentration tested. To the converse, C3535 induced major diuretic effects, especially so after i.v. injection. Its onset of action was rapid, peak effect occurred within minutes and the diuretic effect lasted approximately 45 min.

Peak and cumulated effects.

Peak excretion (highest excretion rate in an urine collection) and cumulated outputs (60 min. after treatment) of $\dot{V}$ and $U_{Na}.\dot{V}$ from the left kidney are presented as net effects in the following table.

	$\dot{V}$	$U_{Na}.\dot{V}$	$\dot{V}$	$U_{Na}.\dot{V}$
	A.L.R.C.		I.V.	
peak*				
C3534 10^{-3} M	8 ± 5	2 ± 1	54 ± 31	9 ± 4
C3535 10^{-4} M	18 ± 4	3 ± 1	83 ± 3	12 ± 1
C3535 10^{-3} M	108 ± 12	15 ± 2	144 ± 24	19 ± 2
cumulated* (60 min.)				
C3534 10^{-3} M	199 ± 334	54 ± 73	728 ± 172	118 ± 83
C3535 10^{-4} M	452 ± 128	76 ± 25	1233 ± 340	205 ± 46
C3535 10^{-3} M	2741 ± 724	392 ± 86	4469 ± 556	534 ± 121

Results are presented as mean values ± S.D.

Results from the right kidney were almost similar.

COMMENTS

The results show that the metabolite C3535, but not 3534, has highly potent diuretic effects. The diuretic potency of C3535 is greatly enhanced after i.v. injections as compared to capsular applications suggesting that the renal capsule is a barrier to the transfer of C3535 to the tubular site(s) of action.

Compared to torasemide and furosemide, the order of diuretic potency in the rat is the following

C3535 > torasemide > furosemide ≫ C3534.

*peak units : $\dot{V}$ = ul/min and $U_{Na}.\dot{V}$ = uEq/min ; cumulated units : $\dot{V}$ = ul/hr and $U_{Na}.\dot{V}$ = uEq/hr.

REFERENCES

1. Ghys, A., Denef, J., de Suray, J.M., Gerin, M., Georges, A., Delarge, J. and Willems, J. Pharmacological Properties of the New Potent Diuretic Torasemide in Rats and Dogs. Drug Res. 35(II), n° 10: 1520-1526, 1985.
2. Kramp, R.A. and Lenoir, R. Distal permeability to urate and effects of benzofuran derivatives in the rat kidney. Am. J. Physiol. 228, n° 3:875-883, 1975.

ROLE OF CENTRAL GABAERGIC SYSTEM ON RAT DIURESIS

P. MALMBERG-AIELLO, M. DE DONATIS, A. GALLI & A. BARTOLINI

Department of Preclinical and Clinical Pharmacology
University of Florence, Viale G.B. Morgagni 65, 50134 Firenze, Italy

INTRODUCTION

Baclofen (β-p-chlorophenyl-GABA) is considered the prototype of GABA receptor B agonists (1). Recently we have reported that baclofen induces diuresis (2); thus it seemed worthwhile to investigate the mechanism by which the stimulation of GABA B receptors increases urine output.

MATERIALS AND METHODS

160 male Wistar rats (180-250 g) were used. Diuresis was measured by placing non-starved rats in individual metabolic cages generally at 01.00 p.m. During urine collection, rats were deprived of food and water. While volumes of excreted urine were measured 0.5; 1.0; 1.5; 2.0; 2.5 and 3.0 hr following drug administration, urine osmolality and Na^+ and K^+ concentrations were determined on the whole 3-hr sample.

The following drugs were used: (±), (-) and (+)baclofen HCl, a generous gift from Ciba Geigy; furosemide "Lasix" (Hoechst AG); arginine vasopressin (Sigma) and aminooxy acetic acid - AOAA (Sigma). Drug solutions were freshly prepared prior to injection, using saline as the solvent.

Intracerebroventricular (i.c.v.) injections were performed following a light ether anesthesia.

RESULTS

As shown in Table 1, baclofen diuresis is stereospecific, (-)baclofen alone being in fact active. This is in agreement with the hypothesis that baclofen diuresis is mediated by GABA B receptors. Moreover, diuresis is dose-dependent and obtained with concentrations which have no myorelaxing

Table 1. Effect of some GABAergic drugs compared with furosemide on 3-hr diuresis in Wistar rats.

Treatment	n.of rats	%Variation±S.E. from own control Volume	Osmolality	Na^+	K^+
(±)baclofen HCl 0.05 mg/kg i.p.	8	- 25±21	- 2±15	- 1	-11
(±)baclofen HCl 1.0 mg/kg i.p.	8	+ 87±39*	-50± 9*	-65	-52
(±)baclofen HCl 2.5 mg/kg i.p.	3	+157±48**			
(±)baclofen HCl 4.0 mg/kg i.p.	23	+509±54**	-62± 4*	-71±6	-69±4
(-)baclofen HCl 2.5 mg/kg i.p.	5	+571±71**	-60± 4*		
(+)baclofen HCl 2.5 mg/kg i.p.	6	- 22±27	+13±11		
AOAA 25 mg/kg i.p.	5	+158±79*		-70±18	-69±7
Furosemide 5 mg/kg i.p.	4	+978±87***	-36± 3*	-60	-78

*P<0.05, **P<0.01,***P<0.001

effect. The diuretic action of baclofen and of the GABAtransaminase inhibitor, aminooxy acetic acid (AOAA), is mainly exerted on the free water production. As a matter of fact, the decrease in osmolality as a result of the increase in urine output is much more pronounced in baclofen and AOAA than in furosemide-treated rats.

Fig. 1 shows that the diuretic effect of baclofen takes place in the central nervous system, in fact, while 0.05 mg/kg (Table 1), roughly corresponding to 10 μg/rat, have no effect i.p., 5 μg/rat (Fig. 1) increase 3-hr diuresis by 253% if injected directly into the brain ventricles. On the other hand, as expected, furosemide at the equimolecular dose (6.5 μg/rat i.c.v.) does not change urine excretion.

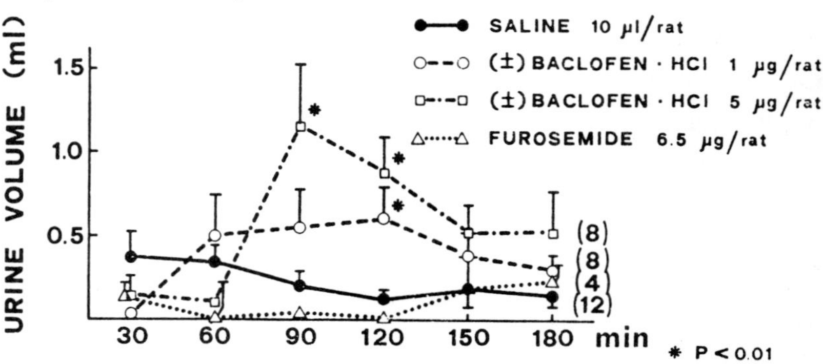

Fig. 1. Effect of i.c.v. (±)baclofen HCl and furosemide on Wistar rat diuresis. Vertical lines give S.E.M.; in brackets number of animals.

Table 2. Comparison between (±)baclofen HCl and furosemide cumulative effects (3 hr) on urine volume, osmolality and Na^+ and K^+ contents (mEq/l) in Wistar rats treated either with saline or Arg-vasopressin (ADH).

Treatment	Dose/kg	Route	n.	ml	mOsm	Na^+	K^+
Saline Saline	5 ml 5 ml	s.c. i.p.	26	0.9±0.2	690±95	111±16	233±29
						P<0.001	P<0.05
ADH Saline	10 μg 5 ml	s.c. i.p.	10	1.7±0.4	730±52	240± 5	144±26
Saline Baclofen	5 ml 4 mg	s.c. i.p.	10	3.7±0.5	390±53	81±12	94±16
				P<0.05	P<0.05	P<0.001	
ADH Baclofen	10 μg 4 mg	s.c. i.p.	6	1.6±0.5	655±15	253± 1	94± 2
Saline Furosemide	5 ml 5 mg	s.c. i.p.	6	7.0±0.7	308±17	118± 4	46± 2
ADH Furosemide	10 μg 5 mg	s.c. i.p.	6	7.8±0.5	334± 2	140± 3	46± 3

Simultaneously-injected ADH prevents baclofen but not furosemide diuretic effects (Table 2), which would suggest that baclofen diuresis occurs centrally through the inhibition of ADH secretion. It is worthwhile noting that ADH (10 μg/kg s.c.) by itself augments urine output slightly, although not statistically significantly. This is probably due to the ADH-induced increase in blood pressure. Moreover, as expected, ADH raises urine Na^+ and osmolality. (Table 2).

Our results taken as a whole support the involvement of central GABA B receptors in water balance.

ACKNOWLEDGEMENT

Supported by Italian Ministry of Education.

REFERENCES

1. Bowery, N.G., Doble, A., Hill, D.R., Hudson, A.L., Shaw, J.S. and Turnbull, M.J. Br.J.Pharmac. 67: 444P-445P, 1979.
2. Bartolini, A., Bartolini, R., Biscini, A., Giotti, A.and Malmberg, P. Br.J.Pharmac. 72: 156P-157P, 1981.

XIV. DIURETICS IN RENAL INVESTIGATION

USE OF DIURETICS TO INVESTIGATE RENAL FUNCTION.

E. BARTOLI

Istituto di Patologia Medica, University of Sassari, viale San Pietro 12, 07100 Sassari, Italy.

INTRODUCTION

Diuretics interfere with specific transport system in ways which are useful both therapeutically and in studying renal function. Thus, renal function tests have been developed in vivo in humans based on known properties of these drugs. Carbonic anydrase inhibitors were extensively used to individuate the mechanism of tubular bicarbonate reabsorption (1). The proximal tubular (PT) function has been investigated with osmotic diuretics: the results of mannitol diuresis allowed the reconstruction of distal tubular (DT) events and the identification of TcH_2O, which reflects the ability of collecting ducts (CD) to abstract solute free water from tubular fluid (2). The agents acting on the aldosterone-sensitive segment of the DT and of intracortical CDs have been extensively used to study the distal acidification process and the mechanisms of potassium wasting (3). More recently, the property of furosemide (F) to deliver saturating amounts of cations to DT has been exploited to measure the maximal distal hydrogen ion secretion (4). However, these tests investigate the function of single segments or properties of the renal tubule. In humans a method capable of yielding affidable estimates of overall and segmental renal function is needed. This had been attempted by studying renal function during maximal water diuresis (MWD): assuming that in the absence of ADH no significant amount of water is reabsorbed distally, urine flow rate ($\dot{V}$) reflects the flow escaping proximal reabsorption, calculated in fractional terms as $1 - \frac{\dot{V}}{GFR}$. Solute reabsorption without solvent along the distal segments generates distilled water, which is excreted into the urine and calculated as CH_2O, the free water clearance, which is the equivalent volume of isotonic plasma from which the solutes were reclaimed. Fractional distal reabsorption is the ratio between CH_2O and $\dot{V}$.

Some author substitute this fraction with $CH_2O/(CH_2O+2CNa)$, where CNa is the clearance of Na. Although the former expression reflects the overall Na absorption, the latter only that of Na and chloride (hence, the necessity of using 2CNa), the difference between the two formulas is numerically trivial. Fig. 1 depicts above the events of diluting ability test and Table 1 reports the data we obtained with this test. This technique allows to separately calculate PT from DT reabsorption. However, fractional proximal reabsorption (FPR) seems clearly in excess of that measured directly by micropunture. This may be due to the fact that $\bar{V}$ underestimates proximal delivery, since solvent is reabsorbed along the distal nephron even in the absence of ADH. This phenomenon, clearly demonstrated in dogs (5), was held responsible for the excretion of concentrated urines in diabetes insipidous treated with diuretics (6,7). Thus, the entity of the free-water-back diffusion (CH_2O-BD) dictates at the same time the inaccuracy of FPR reabsorption, which is overestimated, and of DT reabsorption (which is underestimated). In addition, since the water lost is solute-free, it affects both the numerator and the denominator of the fraction used to calculate fractional DT reabsorption. Thus, CH_2O-BD introduces potentially large and unrecognized sources of error in the calculations. Finally, the technique does not distinguish between salt reabsorption by the ascending limb of Henle's loop (HL) and that by DT, two segments with different transport systems, properties and response to diuretics. The above criticisms are the main reasons that fostered the development of the distal blockade technique (9): it assumes that the simultaneous administration of F (or ethacrynic acid) and hydrochlorothiazide (HCT) practically abolishes all Na (and, consequently, water) reabsorption along HL and DT. Under these circumstances, the solute and solvent excretion represents that escaping the PT. This method has been extensively applied to man and animals, representing the only way to assess proximal reabsorption in vivo independent of micropuncture techniques. Our own results (8) show (Table 1) close agreement with micropuncture data. FPR, calculated as $1 - \frac{\bar{V}f}{GFR}$, where $\bar{V}f$ is $\bar{V}$ measured during distal blockade, represents 66% of GFR, a value in close agreement with that obtained by micropuncture at the end of the proximal tubule in rats. Micropuncture data obtained from early DT samples in MWD, which minimizes water reabsorption prior to the DT sampling site, are also in close agreement with these estimates in man . Since the technique of DT-block only gave information on the PT we developed a new technique, based on the properties of loop diuretics, which allows the measurement of PT transport, of Na reabsorption by HL, by DT, and of water back-diffusion across CDs in one single experimental setting.

THEORY

The major source of error in the MWD test is represented by the unknown CH_2O-BD. This flow is abstracted in part from DT according to the formula: Distal $CH_2O\text{-BD} = Lp \cdot \Delta\pi$, where Lp is the hydraulic conductivity of DT epithelium in the absence of ADH, $\Delta\pi$ is the effective osmotic pressure gradient between the isotonic peritubular interstitium and the hypotonic tubular fluid. During F, which abolishes salt reabsorption by HL, $\Delta\pi$ is nil at the early DT, and equals $Posm \cdot \frac{CH2O\text{-}DT}{\dot{V}f}$ at the end of DT; $\dot{V}f$ is the inflow rate to DT. Since CH_2O-DT represents a small fraction of $\dot{V}f$, the average gradient is very small and CH_2O-BD is minimal during F along DT. Normally $\Delta\pi$ is large across CDs, due to the high osmolarity of the interstitium, perhaps twice that of plasma during MWD. During F, $\Delta\pi$ falls to a minimum value corresponding to that present at the end of DT, as the diuretic inhibits solute accumulation within the medullary and papillary interstitium while their hypertonicity is quickly washed out by vasa recta. Therefore, the gradient falls approximately to less than 10% of that present during MWD, and CH_2O-BD falls in proportion. The CH_2O-BD not reabsorbed is entirely recovered in the urine excreted. Hence, the difference between $\dot{V}$ and $\dot{V}f$, (measured during the peak effect of F), contains CH_2O-BD: $\dot{V}f - \dot{V} \geq CH_2O\text{-BD}$. This difference really equals CH_2O-BD only if $\dot{V}f$ equals the inflow to the DT nephron, i.e., the flow escaping FPR. Inhibition of PT reabsorption by F has been demonstrated with doses higher than those achieved with the present technique (10), during recollection-microperfusion experiments with artificial perfusates, which we showed to be affected by systematic errors (11). It was also reported during generous fluid infusions in the attempt to avoid volume contraction (12). In studies with careful

Table 1. Results in Normals.

	MWD	F+HCT	MWD+F
GFR ml/min	103±16	114	128±35
$\dot{V}$	19±7	-	-
$\dot{V}f$	-	34	36±13
CH2O-T	15±6	-	32±12
CH2O-HL	-	-	19±10
CH2O-DT	-	-	13±6
CH2O-BD	-	-	17±10
CH2O	15±6	5	13±6
Uosm mOsm/Kg	60±27	237	179±36
UNa mEq/L	19±16	129	80±20
CNa ml/min	3±5		27±12
FPR	0.81	0.66	0.64
N	14	10	14

The data reported are mean± standard errors measured during maximal water diuresis before (MWD) and during furosemide (MWD+F). F+HCT indicates the group of 10 subjects studied during distal blockade. Except for GFR, all flows are expressed in $ml \cdot min^{-1} \cdot GFR^{-1} x100$. FPR is the fractional proximal reabsorption. U refers to urine. N is the number of subjects. For the meaning of the other symbols see text.

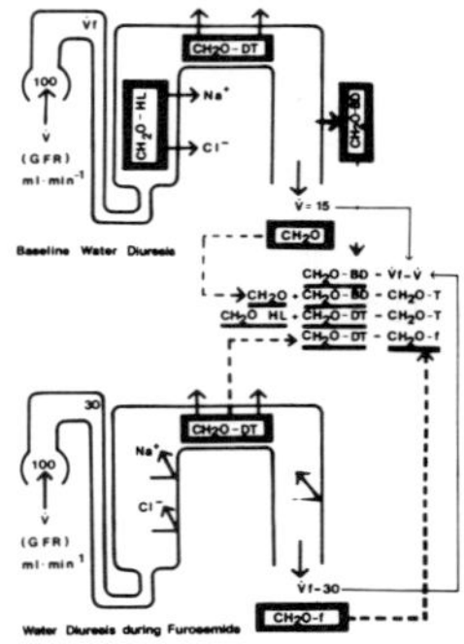

Fig. 1. The nephron on top is during MWD, at the bottom during MWD+F. The rectangles labeled with the symbols corresponding to the volumes of solute-free water (CH2O) generated are inside, those reabsorbed are outside the lumen. The formulas for calculating reabsorption by single segments link the necessary values measured in both conditions(top and bottom). For further explanations and meaning of symbols see text.

maintenance infusions, F did not change FPR, which closely matched that measured at the early DT during F and during MWD, as well as the $\dot{V}f$ of final urines (13). In dogs the fraction of filtered Na and water excreted with up to 100 mg/Kg F was constant, averaged 38% of GFR, and was accompanied by the attainment of nearly isotonic tubular fluid at the early DT sampling site, which became isotonic upon the addition of HCT (14). This also confirms that F abolishes HL reabsorption (15), and that the lack of complete isotonicity is due to reabsorption between the end of the HL and the sampling site. In other words, it is due to the formation of CH_2O-DT, which is suppressed by the HCT. This evidence supports the assumption that $\dot{V}f$ closely approximates DT delivery, and that $\dot{V}f - \dot{V}$ approximates CH_2O-BD. Adding CH_2O-BD to CH_2O measured during MWD before F, yields the total amount of solute-free water (CH_2O-T) generated by the diluting system: $CH_2O\text{-T} = CH_2O + CH_2O\text{-BD}$. In turn,

CH_2O-T is made of two components, that generated by the HL, CH_2O-HL, and that due to the DT, CH_2O-DT. Hence, CH_2O-T = CH_2O-HL+CH_2O-DT. During F only CH_2O-DT is formed and excreted quantitatively, since no water is lost by back diffusion. Therefore, CH_2O-f = CH_2O-DT, where f indicates furosemide. Finally, CH_2O-HL = CH_2O-T - CH_2O-f. With these sample formulas reabsorption by each segment of the human nephron can be measured independently, with an experimental setting that requires clearance periods during MWD before and during the peak effect of F (17).

RESULTS

The results obtained with this technique are summarized in Table 1. They indicate that FPR averages 65% of GFR. Of the total amount of free water formed, 65 to 75% is due to HL, 25 to 35% to DT. The back-diffusion, CH_2O-BD, is roughly equivalent to the urine flow rate during MWD, approximately 15% of GFR. The data obtained in Bartter syndrome, fasting diuresis, liver cirrhosis and chronic renal failure have been previously published (16-18).

DISCUSSION

The technique gives data which are reproducible and capable of indicating the defect in Na reabsorption in several clinical conditions. Two criticisms can be raised against its accuracy. Firstly, any volume lost by back-diffusion across the descending limb of HL, will be computed as CH_2O-BD and will contribute to increase the calculated CH_2O-T, while in fact it represents delivery from the PT. Direct measurements of this volume range from nil to 15% of proximal delivery (19,20). Secondly, the large rise in Na concentration occurring at the early DT during F may facilitate Na reabsorption and yield spuriously high values for CH_2O-DT. However, experiments performed with HCT given either before or after F failed to show any enhancement of HCT-inhibitable distal reabsorption when the loop diuretic preceded HCT administration (8). In conclusion, we developed a new renal function test, based on known pharmacologic properties of F, which allows an improved dissection of segmental reabsorption of the human nephron. This technique has given useful informations in a number of clinical conditions and can be applied to extensively investigate renal function in man.

AKNOWLEDGEMENTS

Supported by a grant from Ministero Pubblica Istruzione, Rome, Italy.

REFERENCES

1. Rector F.C.Jr., Carter N.W., Seldin D.W. J.Clin.Invest. 44, 278,1966.
2. Zak G.A., Brun C., Smith H.W., J.Clin.Invest. 33, 1064-1074,1954.
3. Hulter H.N., Lich J.L., Glynn R.D., Sebastian A. J.Lab.Clin.Med. 95, 637-653,1980.
4. Rastogi S., Bayliss J.M., Nascimento L., Arruda J.A.L. Kidney Intern. 28, 801-807,1985.
5. Berliner R.W., Levinsky N.G., Davidson D.G., Eden M. Am.J.Med. 27, 730-744,1958.
6. Bartoli E., Molaschi M., Viara A., Milanese U. Rass.Fisiopat.Clin. e Ter. 40: 305-343,1968.
7. Earley L.E., Orloff J. J.Clin.Invest. 41: 1988,1962.
8. Faedda R., Branca G.F., Serra G., Satta A., Bartoli E. International Meeting on Diuretics, Sorrento May 26-30, 1986.
9. Earley L.E., Martino J.A., Friedler R.M., J.Clin.Invest. 45: 1668-1684,1966.
10. Morgan T., Tadoko M., Martin D., Berliner R.W., Am.J.Physiol. 218: 292-297,1970.
11. Bartoli E., Earley L.E., Kidney Intern. 3: 142-150,1973.
12. Brenner B.M., Keimowitz R.I., Wright F.S., Berliner R.W. J.Clin.Invest. 48: 290-300,1969.
13. Tucker B.J., Blantz R.C. Kidney Intern. 26: 112-121,1984.
14. Clapp J.R., Robinson R.R. Am.J.Physiol. 215: 228-235,1968.
15. Burg M., Stoner L., Cardinal J., Green N. Am.J.Physiol. 225: 119-124, 1973.
16. Bartoli E., Satta A., Faedda R., Olmeo N.A., Soggia G., Branca G.F. J.Clin.Pharmacol. 23: 56-64,1983.
17. Zoccali C., Bartoli E., Curatola G., Maggiore Q. Nephron 32: 140-148, 1982.
18. Satta A., Faedda R., Olmeo N.A., Soggia G., Branca G.F., Bartoli E. Renal Physiol. 7: 283-292,1984.
19. Marsh D.J., Solomon S. Am.J.Physiol. 208: 1119-1128,1965.
20. De Rouffignac C., Morel F. J.Clin.Invest. 48: 474-486,1969.

THE SIGNIFICANCE OF THE MACULA DENSA MECHANISM FOR RENIN RELEASE.

J. F. BUGGE AND F. KIIL

Institute for Experimental Medical Research, University of Oslo, Ullevaal Hospital, Oslo, Norway.

The increase in renin release during renal arterial constriction (RAC) or ureteral occlusion (UO), has been attributed to reduced NaCl delivery to the macula densa and to autoregulatory vasodilation. The reduced NaCl excretion during RAC, can be restored to control values by expanding the plasma volume. This procedure reduces renin release (1), presumably because of increased NaCl delivery to the macula densa. According to this interpretation, one would expect no reduction in renin release if the plasma volume was expanded during UO.

Ethacrynic acid (ECA) inhibits reabsorption of NaCl in the thick ascending limb of Henle's loop (2, 3) and , hence, increases the delivery of NaCl to the macula densa. Despite the increased delivery, renin release is increased (4). ECA may stimulate renin release by inducing autoregulatory vasodilation (4) and / or by inhibiting NaCl reabsorption at the macula densa. To test this hypothesis, ECA was administrated during plasma volume expansion. Complete autoregulatory vasodilation was induced by RAC or UO.

The experiments were performed on anesthetized dogs with denervated kidneys. Renin avtivity was measured by radio immuno assay and renin release calculated as the product of veno arterial concentration difference and renal plasma flow. Each animal served as its own control, and all interventions were compared by a Friedman's test for multiple comparisons.

In six dogs the renal arterial pressure was reduced to 50 mmHg by RAC. This reduced sodium excretion from 14 ± 3 to 3 ± 1 $\mu mol \cdot min^{-1}$, and increased renin release from 1.4 ± 0.5 to 29 ± 5 μg AI$\cdot min^{-1}$. After expanding plasma volume by 25% with a modified Ringer's solution, sodium excretion increased to 70 ± 21 $\mu mol \cdot min^{-1}$, and renin release was reduced by 50% to 14 ± 4 μg AI$\cdot min^{-1}$. There was no change in renal blood flow (RBF). Subsequent administration of ECA raised renin release to values before expansion (35 ± 11 μg AI$\cdot min^{-1}$), despite a further increase in sodium excretion to 550 ± 120 $\mu mol \cdot min^{-1}$. Release of RAC increased RBF 80% above control. Constriction of the renal artery demonstrated that autoregulation of RBF was still abolished. Sodium excretion increased greatly to 2500 ± 200 μmol·min^{-1}, and renin release decreased to 21 ± 8 μg AI· min $^{-1}$.

In six other dogs, the ureter was occluded, raising the ureter pressure to 97 ± 4 mmHg at a renal arterial pressure of 123 ± 5 mmHg. The glomerular filtration rate was not significantly different from zero. Renin release increased from 1.0 ± 0.5 to 28 ± 5 μg AI·min^{-1}. Plasma volume expansion did not change RBF, and there was no change in renin release. Subsequent ECA administration did not significantly change renin release or any other parameter. Release of UO increased RBF by 60% and constriction of the renal artery showed abolished autoregulation of RBF. Renin release decreased slightly from 30 ± 5 to 22 ± 7 μg AI·min^{-1}.

Renin release during the two experimental conditions are summarized in Fig. 1.

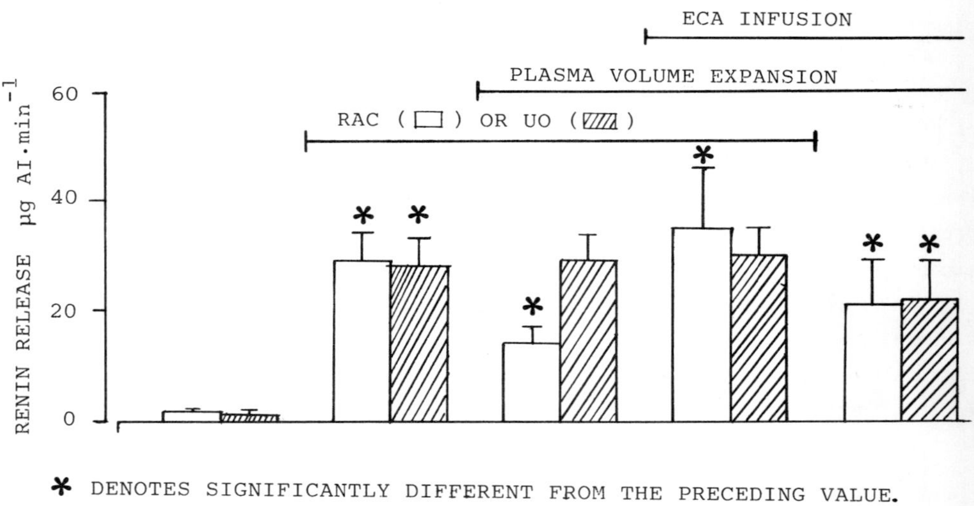

FIGURE 1.

We conclude that increased NaCl delivery to the macula densa inhibits renin release even during autoregulatory vasodilation. This inhibitory effect is cancelled by ECA, presumably by diminishing NaCl reabsorption at the macula densa.

The lack of effect of ECA during UO, signifies that ECA exerts no effect on renin release when autoregulatory vasodilation is already complete and the NaCl delivery to the macula densa is stopped. Thus ECA exerts no direct stimulatory effect on the renin producing cells.

REFERENCES

1. Vikse, A. and Kiil, F. Renal physiol 8: 169-178, 1985.
2. Lie, M. J Oslo City Hosp 26: 29-44, 1976.
3. Burg, M. B. Kidney Int 9: 189-197, 1976
4. Eide, I., Løyning, E., Langaard, Ø. and Kiil, F. Kidney Int 8: 158-165, 1975.

FUROSEMIDE I.V. TEST TO CHECK DISTAL ACIDIFICATION. NORMAL VALUES IN ADULTS

R. SARACHO, A. VALLO*, J. MORAN, J. BIDEA, J. MONTENEGRO, R.MUÑIZ, I.LAMPREABE

NEPHROLOGY AND PEDIATRICS* SERVICES, HOSPITAL DE CRUCES, BILBAO, SPAIN

INTRODUCTION

Furosemide (F) increases urinary acidification mediated, at least, by the increase of distal Na delivery. It is possible that other mechanisms also play a significant role. The test of F administration by I.V. route has been described for Distal Renal Tubular Acidosis (DTRA) diagnosis and classification, but there are few publications where normal values have been reported. In this paper we study the results of this test in 22 healthy adults.

MATERIALS AND METHODS

22 normal adults (mean age = 30 yr and ratio F/M = 1) in standard not controlled diet were submited to the following protocol. At first, basal urine and blood samples were taken. Then F was inyected by I.V. route in one dose of 1 mg/Kg. Four urine samples were collected by spontaneous voiding after 30, 60 , 120 and 180 min. At last (180 min.) a second blood sample was taken. Biochemical parameters were measured in blood : Na, K, Cl, CO_3H^-, pH, Creatinine (Cr), Plasma Renin Activity (PRA) and Plasma Aldosterone (PA). Urine Cr, Na, K and Cl were determined on Beckman analyzers and urine pH on pH-meter. Tritatable Acidity (TA) was measured by automatic titration and Urinary Ammonium (UA) with commercial kits using modified Berteloh's reaction. Fractional excretions were calculated using Cr Clearance and values of UA and AT were displayed as μEq/min. and μEq/dl = μEq/100 ml/min of C_{cr}. The maximal value of four urine samples was chosen to calculate the mean and distribution of UA and AT. Net Acid Excertion was calculared by AT plus UA. Comparison between biochemical values pre-F and post-F was done by Student's t for paired data. Results are given as mean $\pm$ S.E.M. Correlation studies were done using Pearson's r for linear, hyperbolic and reciprocal fits.

RESULTS

Plasma values

There was a significant increase PRA and PA. A positive regression was found between the basal Fractional Excretion of Na (FENa) and the following parameters: basal PRA, (r =.72, p =.00016, hyperbolic fit); basal PA (r =.55, p =.008, reciprocal); post-F PRA (r =.58, p =.005, hyperbolic). There was a more important decrease in Cl than in Na and K. (See TABLE 1).

TABLE 1. PLASMA VALUES

	BASAL	POST-F(180 min.)	STUDENT't	
ARP(ng/ml/hr)	.96 ± .16	4.06 ± .65	5.98	$p<.00001$
PA (pg/ml)	89 ± 10	221 ± 24	7.16	$p<.00001$
Cl (mEq/l)	104 ± .58	97 ± .77	-11.4	$p<.00001$
K (mEq/l)	4.14 ± .09	3.9 ± .06	-2.01	$p= .0575$
Na (mEq/l)	138 ± .48	134 ± .58	-6.81	$p<.00001$

Urine values

The most striking change was noted in urine pH (pH_u): An increase from 5.88 ± .1 (basal) to 6.2 ± .11 (sample of 30 min.) was seen initially, but in the following urine samples there was a progressive decrease. Therefore, minimal pH_u was attained at 120 min. in 64% of cases and at 180 min. in 36%. Maximal Fractional Excretion of Na (FENa), Cl (FECl) and K (FEK) were seen in urine sample taken at 30 min. and a progressive return from basal levels was observed afterwards. However maximal UA and TA were observed in samples collected between 60 and 120 min. See figure 1 and table 2.

TABLE 2. URINE VALUES

			RANGE	SIGNIF.RESPECT BASAL
MINIMUM	pH	4.56±.1	4.2-5.1	$p<.00001$
MAXIMAL	UA(μEq/min)	42.78±2.6	22.4-69.9	$p<.00001$
"	UA(μEq/dl)	39.37±2.9	22.8-64.5	$p=.0005$
"	TA(μEq/min)	28.42±2.8	13.7-65.5	$p<.00001$
"	TA(μEq/dl)	24.15±2.25	12.9-49.5	$p<.0001$
"	UA+TA(μEq/min)	69.51±3.8	46.2-100.8	$p<.0004$
"	UA+TA(μEq/dl)	60.75±3.1	39.0-87.7	$p=.0001$
"	FEK %	40±3.5	20.3-76.9	$p<.00001$

DISCUSSION

We believe that the most important effect of F in urinary acidification is the decrease in pH_u. There are no publications where such low values have been reported in humans. The effect on UA was less marked; the increase was only two-fold basal values. We observed an initial increase in pH_u in the first 30 min. This may be due to inhibitory effect of F on carbonic anhydrase (1). It is thought that F increases urinary acidification by a higher luminal electronegativity produced by an increase of distal Na delivery (2). We have found a temporal dissociation between the minimum pH_u (120-180 min) and the peaks of FENa, FEK and FECl (30 min) (Figure 1). Besides, there is no statistical correlation between pH_u and FE of ions, as other authors have reported (3). There are many theories that may explain this phenomenon. One of them is based in the possibility that the decrease in pH_u reflects acidification by the medullary collecting duct, a segment in which hydrogen secretion is independent of Na but is favoured by PA (4). It is possible that the increase in PA, produced by Na depletion, mediated by F, may play a role in the acidification of this segment. However, our results are inssuficients to clear up this point. Probably, there are several mechanisms that influence urinary acidification in this test. We believe that this study report reference values which may be useful for DRTA diagnosis and classification because it is the unique acidification test that provides stimulus on PA secretion.

REFERENCES

1. Rastogi, S.P., Crawford, C., Wheeler, R., Flanigan, W., Arruda, J.A.L. J. Lab.Clin.Med. 104:271-282,1984.
2. J.Rodriguez-Soriano, A.Vallo, G.Castillo, R.oliveros. Nephron 32:308-313 (1982)
3. Rastogi, S.P., Bayliss, J.M., Nascimento, L., Arruda, J.A.L. Kidney Int. 28:801-807,1985
4. Laski, M.E., Kurtzman, N.A. J.Clin.Invest. 72:2050-2059,1983

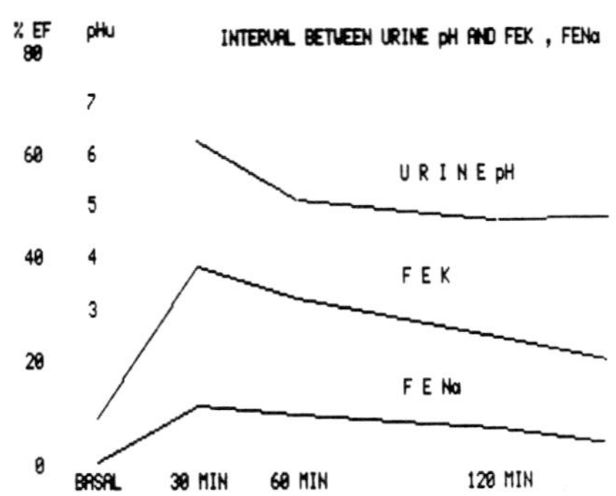

FIGURE 1

TUBULAR FUNCTION IN BARTTER's SYNDROME AND CHANGES INDUCED BY CHRONIC CONVERTING ENZYME BLOCKADE.

Dorhout Mees, E.J., Boer W.H. and Hené, R.J. Department of Nephrology and Hypertension, University Hospital, Catharijnesingel 101, 3511 GV, Utrecht, the Netherlands.

INTRODUCTION

Patients with Bartter's syndrome (BS) present several paradoxical features. Inability of the kidney to conserve K is probably the result of a defective NaCl conservation in the nephron proximal to the K secreting site (1). The localisation of the NaCl reabsorption defect has not been exactly defined. Although some studies suggested the proximal tubule (1,2) later reports pointed to the diluting segments. In patients with BS minimal urine osmolality is increased and maximal free water clearance (CH_2O) is decreased. Thus a defect in chloride reabsorption, expressed as a low ratio of CH_2O to distal delivery was proposed (3).

If there is such a distal defect, there must be a compensatory elevation of proximal reabsorption. We have therefore investigated 5 patients with BS using lithium as a proximal marker (4) and compared the results with traditional estimates of segmental tubular function derived from free water clearance. In addition we repeated these experiments in the same patients after chronic treatment with the converting enzyme inhibitor enalapril.

PATIENTS AND METHODS

Five patients with BS (aged 23-61 years) were investigated; 3 men and 2 woman. Diuretic abuse was ruled out, and renal biopsy revealed juxtaglomerular hyperplasia in all of them. Standard clearance techniques were applied in the recumbent position during maximal water diuresis. The studies were repeated after at least 3 months of enalapril treatment, which largely corrected hypokalemia (sK $2.5 \pm 0.4 \rightarrow 4.0 \pm 0.5$ mmol/l), aldosterone levels and angiotensin sensitivity (5).

RESULTS

Table I shows the results during control condition. Normal values are given on 2 levels of NaCl intake. There is no doubt that distal tubular function was abnormal in the patients: the minimal urine osmolality was invariably higher (93 mosm/kg) than in any of the normal controls, and CH_2O was lower. Fractional distal chloride reabsorption $[FDRCl = CH_2O/(CH_2O + CCl)]$ was also below normal. However, reabsorption of lithium (FRLi) was consistently lower in all BS patients compared to normal subjects. If Li is a quantitative marker of proximal Na reabsorption, this would mean a proximal defect, which is not compatible with a distal defect.

Table I Some values during maximal water diuresis in 5 patients with BS and 8 normal subjects on a normal and low sodium diet.

	FECl	Uosm	FCH_2O	FDRCl	FPRCl	FRLi
Bartter's S	1.9 ± 0.5	93 ± 15	7.8 ± 1.1	81 ± 6	91 ± 1	60 ± 4
Normal Na	1.8 ± 0.3	64 ± 12	11.8 ± 2.3	87 ± 1	84 ± 6	68 ± 3
Low Na	0.4 ± 0.1	58 ± 8	8.8 ± 2.5	97 ± 1	87 ± 4	74 ± 7

FECl = fractional excretion of chloride, FCH_2O = fractional maximal free water clearance, FDRCl = fractional distal chloride reabsorption, FPRCl = fractional proximal chloride reabsorption, FRLi = fractional lithium reabsorption (all values in %), Uosm = minimal urine osmolality (m.osmol/kg.).

Chronic enalapril treatment induced striking changes (Table II). GFR decreased in every patient. There was a consistent further increase in minimal urine osmolality to 120 mosm/kg which was reflected in a further decrease of free water clearance by 33%. The FDRCl decreased from 81 to 70% suggesting deterioration of the preexisting reabsorption defect. The most remarkable change was seen in the CLi, which decreased to less than half the control value. Thus fractional reabsorption of Li increased from the very low value of 60% to 78% which is well above the mean for normal subjects. In a study of patients with mild hypertension we found no effect of enalapril on any of these variables (6).

Table II Effect of chronic enalapril on renal functions in patients with BS.

	Cinulin	Uosm	CH_2O	FDRCl	FPRCl	FRLi
control	105 ± 48	93 ± 15	7.9 ± 1.1	81 ± 6	91 ± 1	60 ± 4
enalapril	87 ± 34	120 ± 28	5.3 ± 1.7	70 ± 2	91 ± 1	78 ± 2

For legend see also table I. Cinulin = inulin clearance (ml/min).

DISCUSSION

If indeed Li is a quantitative marker of proximal NaCl reabsorption the results of the present study indicate that a proximal NaCl reabsorption defect is present in patients with BS. However, this cannot co-exist with a defect in distal NaCl reabsorption as is suggested by the decreased free water clearance. The concept of a defect in FDRCl (3) is based on the high minimal osmolality, from which a low CH_2O is calculated, and subnormal distal NaCl reabsorption is inferred. This high minimal urine osmolality, however, does not necessarily indicate decreased NaCl reabsorption in the diluting segment, but may also be due to increased back diffusion of generated free water in the collecting ducts. An abnormality of water permeability in the distal nephron would lead to underestimation of distal NaCl reabsorption and overestimation of FPRCl. This would explain why a proximal defect is not detected when proximal reabsorption is estimated from CH_2O.

During enalapril, GFR decreased and urine osmolality increased, resulting in a decrease in calculated distal and increase in proximal NaCl reabsorption, while FRLi increased to very high values. These changes (not observed in normals) indicate an extreme dependance of glomerular and tubular dynamics on intrarenal angiotensin, consistent with a state of hypovolemia. Further stimulation of proximal reabsorption overcoming the functional defect, would decrease distal delivery and favour osmotic equilibration in the presence of increased permeability. If however there is a chloride reabsorption defect, a low delivery would facilitate generation of a high osmotic gradient, and a lower urinary osmolality. Thus the increase in urine osmolality after enalapril is more consistent with the permeability hypothesis.

In sum we can draw the following tentative conclusions:

1. Our findings are compatible with 2 abnormalities in Bartter's syndrome: decrease in proximal reabsorption and increased distal back diffusion of water.
2. Converting enzyme blockade, while (partly) correcting hypokalemia, reveals a profound intrarenal influence of angiotensin. It does not correct but profoundly changes the abnormal tubular NaCl and water handling in Bartters syndrome resulting in aggravation of the alleged "chloride reabsorption defect".

In the absence of an animal model, clearance studies under varying conditions may ultimately reveal the pathogenesis of Bartter's syndrome.

REFERENCES

1. Bartter, F.C., Delea, C.S., Kawasaki, et al Kidney Int 6:272-280, 1974.
2. Cannon, P.J., Leeming, J.M., Sommers, et al. Medicine 47:107-131, 1968.
3. Gill, J.R. and Bartter, F.C. Am J Med 65:766-772, 1978.
4. Thomsen, K. Nephron 37:217-223, 1984.
5. Hené, R.J., Koomans, H.A., Stolpe A. v.d., et al Kidney Int. 29: 190, 1986
6. V. Schaik, B.A.M., Geyskes, G.G. and Dorhout Mees, E.J. (Unpublished)

TYPE II PSEUDOHYPOALDOSTERONISM: DIFFERENTIAL EFFECTS OF LOOP DIURETICS AND HYDROCHLOROTHIAZIDE.

G. COLUSSI, M.E. DE FERRARI, G. ROMBOLA', P. ROLANDO, M. SURIAN°, F. MALBERTI°, L. MINETTI

Renal Units, Ospedale Niguarda Ca'Granda, Milan and °Ospedale Maggiore, Lodi (Italy).

A rare syndrome of chronic, mineralocorticoid-resistant, renal hyperkalemia and hyperchloremic acidosis in the face of normal glomerular filtration rate (GFR), normal plasma aldosterone and retained sodium-reabsorbing effects of mineralocorticoids (MC) has been so far described in a limited number of patients (1-9); Schambelan, Sebastian and Rector (9) have proposed this syndrome to be defined as type II pseudohypoaldosteronism (PHA II): unlikely patients with type I PHA, wich show severe salt wastage, hypotension, increased plasma renin (PRA) and aldosterone (PA) levels, patients with PHA II mantain normal Na balance, have low PRA and are hypertensive, suggesting extracellular volume (ECV) expansion. Proposed patogenethic mecanisms of PHA II have been selective distal tubule defect for K secretion (1,3,5), abnormally increased Na reabsorption in the proximal tubule (leading to renin inhibition and hypoaldosteronism) (2), generalyzed cell membrane defect for K transport (6), and abnormally increased permeability of distal tubule cells to chloride ("chloride shunt") (9). We report herein the results of functional evaluation of renal tubule function, and of the responses to treatment with loop-acting and thiazide diuretics, in a previously described patient (8) with PHA II.

Case report and functional studies.

This female patient was first seen when she was 10 years old because of short stature (135 cm, 3rd percentile), chronic hyperkalemia and hyperchloremic acidosis with normal GFR and adrenal function. Blood pressure (110/70 mmHg) was than normal; hyperkalemia had been resistant to NaCl restriction (25 mEq/day for 4 days) and MC administration (aldosterone, 0.5 mg/day for 10 days or DOCA, 5 mg/day plus $NaHCO_3$ 5 g/day for 10 days) (8). Chronic hydrochlorothiazide therapy had brought about normalisation of plasma K (PK) and bicarbonate ($PHCO_3$) levels and of growth velocity (up to 165 cm, 55th percentile). Present studies were performed at age 20, during a 2 years period.

Control data (Table I) were obtained in different occasions after at least 7 days of thiazide withdrawl. Every time there was rapid recurrence of hyperkalemia (5.9 to 7.3 mEq/l), hyperchloremic acidosis (blood pH 7.32±0.03) with retained urine acidification capacity (min. spontaneous UpH 4.85), and hypertension; GFR was normal at 120 ml/min of creatinine clearance and daily urine 17-OH corticoids (Porter-Silber cromogens) were 5 to 9 mg/g creatinine. PRA was markedly depressed, but PA and PA/PK ratio were normal;

Table 1. Main data in the control period and during diuretic therapy.

	Control	Muzolimine		Furosemide	HCT	n.v.
		30 mg	60 mg	50 mg/day	75 mg/day	
PK+, mEq/l	6.6±0.6	5.5	5.4	5.4	4.2±0.05	4.3±0.3
PCl^-, mEq/l	109±3.4	109	101	104	99±1	98±3
$PHCO_3$, mEq/l	21±1.3	17	26	19	25±0.2	25±2
PRA (↑), ng/ml/h	0.1/0.7		1.4	0.1	5.3±9.9	2-4
PAldo (↑), ng/dl	13.3/47		38	28	18/29	5-15
$PAldo/PK^+$	2.25/6.7		7.0	5.2	4/7.5	> 3
FEK^+, %	6±3			6.3	13/25	10.4±5
BP, mmHg	140-180 / 100-120	160 / 105	180 / 95	160 / 100	120-130 / 80-85	
BW, Kg	65		65	65	62	

(↑) = upright values

fractional K clearance (FEK) was low or normal-low, despite hyperkalemia, indicating abnormal renal handling.

Na sulfate and Na bicarbonate infusion: Na_2SO_4 increased FEK from 3.7 to 44.7% (n.v. 35±6), urine titratable acidity from 63 to 142 μEq/lGFR (n.v. 292±137)and decreased urine pH from 6.3 to 5.27 (n.v. < 5.3). $NaHCO_3$ increased FEK from 5.1 to 49.7% (n.v. 49.4±16.2).

Free water clearance studies: urine flow during maximal water diuresis and furosemide administration (40 mg i.v.), a good index of proximal tubule NaCl reabsorption (10), was 38.6 ml/dlGFR (n.v. 17.6±4); total free water generation (a measure of distal nephron NaCl reabsorption) was 35.1 ml/dlGFR (n.v. 15.3±3.7); net increases of FECl and FEK after acute furosemide administration were 39.6 and 60.6% (n.v. 22.5±6.3 and 53.4±18.4%, respectively).

Diuretic therapy (Table 1): Muzolimine 15 mg b.i.d. for 15 days and 30 mg b.i.d., and furosemide 25 mg b.i.d. for 15 days, significantly reduced, but did not normalize PK, while $PHCO_3$, PRA and blood pressure (BP) all remained abnormal. Hydrochlorothiazide 75 mg/day always resulted in the normalisation of PK, acid-base parameters and BP, with a striking increase of PRA and a 3% decrease of body weight.

Comments.

Our patient had chronic, MC-resistant, renal hyperkalemia, hyperchloremic acidosis, hypertension and normal GFR as in other published cases (1-9), without any known cause of hyperkalemia. It has been suggested that this syndrome be called PHA II, though different patogenetic mechanisms might be operative in different patients. A striking feature of our (and almost all reported cases) is abnormal "spontaneous" K renal handling in the face of normal intrinsic K transport capacity, as shown by normal responses to Na sulfate and bicarbonate infusions. This observation roules out the hypothesis of a primary distal tubule defect for K secretion (1, 3,5); increased proximal tubule solute reabsorption (4) is also unlikely, in the face of the increased distal delivery of fluids and the marked increase in distal nephron NaCl reabsorption. Our data are consistent with the "chloride shunt" hypotesis (9); increased permeability of distal tubule cells to Cl would impair the generation of the electrical driving force for K secretion; Na reabsorption would also be increased because its diffusion down a favorable concentration gradient might be unopposed by the negative intratubular potential: this would result in ECV expansion and hypertension. The inability of loop diuretics to completely correct the tubular abnormality and to reduce ECV expansion (as shown by the lack of changes in body weight and PRA) suggest that the tubular abnormality lies somewhere beyond the loop of Henle, so that the chloruretic effect of these drugs might be partially counteracted. Accordingly, the selective effects of thiazides suggest that the thiazide-sensitive sites of the distal convoluted tubule might be abnormal in PHA II. Though the mechanisms of action of thiazide diuretics are still incompletely known, it would appear that they are able to directly reduce the permeability of tubule cells to Cl in those sites.

References.

1. Arnold, J.E. and Healy, J.K. Am.J.Med. 47:461-472, 1969.
2. Gordon, R.D., Geddes, R.A., Pawsey, G.K., O'Halloran, M.W.: Aust.Ann. Med. 4:287-294, 1970.
3. Spitzer, A., Edelman, C.M., Goldberg, L.D. and Henneman, P.H.: Kidney Int. 3:251-257, 1972.
4. Weinstein, S.F., Allan, D.M.E., Mendoza, S.A.: J.Pediatr. 85:355-358, 1974.
5. Brautbar, N., Levi, J., Rosler, A., Leitersdorf, E., Djaldeti, M., Epstein, M., Kleeman, C.R.: Arch.Intern.Med. 138:607-610, 1978.
6. Farfel, Z., Iaina, A., Rosenthal, T., Waks, U., Shibolet, S., Gafni, J.: Arch.Intern.Med. 138:1828-1832, 1978.
7. Lee, M.R., Ball, S.G., Thomas, T.H., Morgan, D.B.: Q.J.Med. 48:245-258, 1979.
8. Torelli, D., Rovati, C., Surian, M., De Min, A., Minetti, L.: Min. Nefr. 27:323-331, 1980.
9. Schambelan, M., Sebastian, A., Rector, F.C.: Kidney Int. 19:716-727, 1981.
10. Bartoli, E., Satta, A., Faedda, R., Olmeo, N.A., Soggia, G., Branca G.: J.Clin.Pharmacol. 23:56-64, 1983.

CLINICAL EVALUATION OF PROXIMAL TUBULE Na/FLUID REABSORPTION: LITHIUM CLEARANCE vs "VOLUME OR CHLORIDE FACTORS" DURING MAXIMAL WATER DIURESIS AND FUROSEMIDE ADMINISTRATION.

G.ROMBOLA', G.COLUSSI, M.E.DE FERRARI, M.SURIAN, F.MALBERTI, L.MINETTI.

Renal Division, Niguarda Ca'Granda Hospital, Milan Italy.

INTRODUCTION.

The clinical method for evaluating proximal tubule Na and fluid reabsorption (NaPR) consists mainly on clearance studies during maximal water diuresis; in this setting, being ADH suppressed, CH2O may be used as an index of NaCl reabsorption in the diluiting segments of the nephron; as a consequence CH2O added to Cl excretion (CH2O+CCL/GFR)(chloride factor) may reasonably represent distal delivery. An alternative method is to evaluate maximal urinary flux (V/GFR)("volume factor")(1). This theoretical background is incompletely correct as a consistent, ADH independent, water back diffusion, occurs secondary to the tubule-interstitium osmotic gradient (2); this osmotic gradient can be reduced, although not abolished, by furosemide administration (f); in this condition "volume factor" may be a more accurate index of the delivery of fluid out of the proximal tubule (2). Recently (3), Li clearance has been proposed as the most specific method for evaluating NaPR.

The aim of our study was to compare with FELi different methods for NaPR determination: chloride factor (DDCl) during maximal water diuresis, volume and chloride factors during maximal water diuresis and f administration (Vf and DDClf) in normal subjects and nephropatic pts.

SUBJECTS AND STUDY METHODOLOGY.

22 subjects were studied: 7 healthy controls (C), 7 with recurrent calcium nephrolithiasis (RCN), 5 with renal glucosuria (RG) and 3 with Fanconi syndrome (FS). Renal function as GFR of endogenous creatinine clearance, was slightly reduced in FS (GFR 40 to 60 ml/min). The evening before the study, all the subjects ingested 600 mg of Li_2CO_3; the next morning, they collected urine samples (7-8 am) and blood specimen were drawn at the same time for creatinine (4) and Li determination (flame photometry IL 943). Then, they started drinking 20 ml/kg bw of distilled water in 30 min (5). At minimum and stable urinary osmolality, three 15 min clearances were collected (maximal water diuresis clearance); 40 mg f iv were injected and after the first 5 min urines were disregarded three additional 10 min clearances were performed; at the 2nd and 5th clearances period, blood specimens were collected. All the urinary and blood samples were evaluated for: creatinine, Li, Chloride, phosphorus and osmolality (Fiske osmometer Burlington Massachusetts).

CALCULATION OF DISTAL DELIVERY: all parameters were expressed as % of GFR.
FELi = CLi/GFR °100
Chloride factor during maximal water diuresis: DDCl=(CH2O+CCl)/GFR °100
Volume factor " " " " and f: Vf=Vf/GFR °100
Chloride factor " " " " " "
DDClf=(CH2O+CCl)f/GFR °100

The theoretical back-ground of the last term is: as f (at the dosages used) completely inhibits (6) Cl reabsorption along the ascending limb of Henle's loop, CH2O during f is a minimum estimate of NaCl reabsorbed in the distal convolute tubule and subsequent segments: their sum thus represents NaCl escaping proximal reabsorption. Statistical analysis was performed by use of t paired test and simple linear correlation.

RESULTS.

Table I: Mean + SD of main parameter considerated.

	GFR ml/min	FELi B %	FELi 1 %	FELi f %	DDCl ml/dlGFR	Vf ml/dlGFR	DDClf ml/dlGFR
C (7)	111±30	19.3±4.8	19.4±5.5	28.9±9.4^	9.2±2.3¨	17.6±4	21.7±5.2°
RCN(7)	118±42	29.3±13.9	27.9±8	33.7±7.6^	12.4±4.6¨	22.1±6.4	27.1±7.9°°
RG (5)	115±38	28.5±11.9	25.7±11	35.7±7.8^	10.2±3.3¨	21.5±5.7	27.4±10
FS (3)	40±5.7	45.4±5.1	52.3±3	71.1±9.3	23.1±2	35.7±2.8	39±7.1

¨$p<0.001$ vs Vf,DDClf,FELi 1 °$p<0.001$ vs Vf °°$p<0.001$ vs Vf ^$p<0.001$ vs FELi 1

C,RCN and RG did not differ for: GFR, minimal urinary osmolality (65±12; 69±7;67±12 respectively) or maximal values after f (209±13;216±31;208±23). The three pts with FS had reduced GFR; their data were not statistically considered for the low number of cases. Li excretion was not different before water ingestion (FELiB) and during maximal water diuresis (FELi 1), but increased consistently after f administration (FELif)(tab.I); its percent increase was significantly correlated with Cl percent increase (n=22; r=0.67;$p<0.001$) but not with phosphorus percent change (n=22;r=0.32;p=NS). DDCl values were lower than the other three methods; Vf and DDClf in all the pts, showed a good correlation with FELi 1 (n=22;r=0.85;$p<0.001$-n=22;r=0.83; $p<0.001$), however Vf was lower than DDClf (22.4±7.5 vs 27.08±8.9; $p<0.001$); and FELi 1 (28.1±12.6;$p<0.001$), while DDClf and FELi 1 were not different.

DISCUSSION.

The results of our study confirm that DDCl clearly underestimates GFR post-proximal delivery (1). Vf and DDClf showed concordant results with FELi, even if Vf was less accurate especially for high values of post-proximal delivery. These data may be explained by a persistent H2O back-diffusion even during f administration; in fact maximal UOsm during f was always lower than plasma osmolality. The equivalent values of DDClf and FELi support the hypothesis than the sum of Cl excretion during maximal water diuresis and f plus CH2O (generated in the distal diluent segments) may represent a good estimation of distal delivery; in addition, this method allows to calculate Na and fluid reabsorption. Also in more distal segments of the nephron, i.e. in the ascending limb of Henle's loop (as net increment of FECl after f) and along the distal convoluted tubule (CH20 after f). As for Li excretion, micropuncture data (7) show a less relevant NaPR than estimated by FELi in our C, in addition, FELi significantly increased after f, reaching a closer estimation of NaPR to micropuncture data. FELi increases were correlated with FECl increases, but not with phosphate excretion, suggesting that this was an effect of f on Henle's loop rather than on the proximal tubule. Thus FELi may underestimate the post-proximal delivery of GFR; a similar correlation is also suggested by the good agreement of FELi with DDClf (which is expected to underestimate the distal delivery by the ADH-indipendent back-diffusion).

IN CONCLUSION DDClf seems to offer an estimation of distal delivery of GFR as good as FELi. It offers the advantage over FELi of a more exhaustive evaluation of Na reabsorption along distal segments of the nephron.

REFERENCES.

1. Danovitch, G.M., Renal Physiol. 1:56-60, 1978.
2. Bartoli, E., Satta, A., Faedda, R., Olmeo, N.A., Soggia, G., Branca,G. J.Clin.Pharmacol. 23:56-64, 1983.
3. Thomsen, K. Nephron 37:217-223, 1984.
4. Prencipe, L. Quad.Diag.Sclavo 10:266-270, 1974.
5. Lau, Y.K., Wasserstein, A., Westby,G.R., Bosanal,P., Grabie, M., Mitnick, P., Slatopolsky, E., Goldfarb, S., Agus, Z.S. Min.Electrolyte Metab. 7:237-249, 1982.
6. Burg, M., Stoner, L., Cardinal, J., Green, N. Am.J.Phisiol. 225:1,119-124, 1973.
7. Burg, M.B. In: The Kidney (Eds. B.M.Brenner and F.C.Rector jr), W.B. Saunders Company, philadelphia, 1986, pp. 145-176.

HENLE'S LOOP (HL) REABSORPTION MEASURED BY FUROSEMIDE (F).

G.F.BRANCA,R.FAEDDA, A.SATTA, G.SERRA,M.SANNA,E.BARTOLI.

Istituto di Patologia Medica,University of Sassari,Viale San Pietro 12,
07100 Sassari

INTRODUCTION

We have developed (1) and extensively applied (1,4) a new method to measure transport by each segment of the human nephron.We assumed that F,by abolishing NaCl transport of HL,wipes out the osmotic gradient between collecting duct (CD) urine and interstitium,and the abstraction of solute free water (SFW) that occurs in the absence of ADH:therefore,the urine flow during maximal water diuresis (MWD) plus F ($\dot{V}f$) represents a true measurement of delivery from proximal tubule (PT). In addition,the urine will be diluted by the distal tubule (DT) during F:therefore,the SFW excreted during F, CH2Of, is that formed by the DT, CH2O-DT. Thus,CH2Of = CH2O-DT (I).The difference between $\dot{V}$ during F ($\dot{V}f$) and that during MWD alone ($\dot{V}$) measures the volume of SFW reabsorbed in the absence of ADH,indicated as CH2O-BD. This being the part of SFW which is not excreted, the true SFW generated is that excreted (CH2O) plus that reabsorbed (CH2O-BD) : hence, CH2O-T = CH2O-BD + CH2O (II), where CH2O-T is the total SFW formed. The SFW generated by HL alone can be calculated as CH2O-HL = CH2O-T - CH2O-DT (III). For these concepts to gain a wide acceptance,it is necessary to confirm the measurements by an independent method. We devised the present experiments to compare by an independent method the results obtained by previously published technique based on MWD .

MATERIALS AND METHODS

The studies were performed on 10 healthy adult volunteers.MWD was instituted exactly as previously published (1). Inulin and F infusion were the same as in antidiuresis. The test of maximal antidiuresis (MA) was performed a few days later.At 8 a.m.,after 24 hours of fluid deprivation,a bladder catheter was inserted and an i.v. infusion of 3% NaCl solution was started at a rate of 0.07 ml/Kg/min,together with Inulin 10 mg/min, and 50 minutes later two consecutive 10 minutes clearance periods were performed. Then F was injected, 0.75 mg/Kg bolus,the infusion solution was switched from hypertonic to isotonic saline at a rate equal to $\dot{V}$. 10 min. later,two final clearance periods were performed. GFR,$\dot{V}$, Cosm, CH2O or TcH2O were calculated before and after F.Thus, each patient was studied twice,under maximal diluting and concentrating conditions.During MA it is assumed that the flow escaping PT reabsorption,the generation of CH2O-HL and CH2O-DT were the same as during MWD. However, in concentrating conditions DT is permeable to water,not allowing the maintenance of an osmotic gradient,which is dissipated by the reabsorption of the total amount of SFW generated:hence,CH2O-T is entirely reabsorbed by DT during MA and the urine attain isotonicity with the cortical interstitium. We assume that from the point where isotonicity is attained,cation exchange,without net solute absorption,occurs and the tubular fluid flow rate equals Cosm. From this volume (Cosm) TcH2O is abstracted along CD. During F, no CH2O-HL is formed and no TcH2O is abstracted,since the hypertonicity of the interstitium is abolished. Therefore, only distal reabsorption takes place:thus,CH2O-DT is formed, and it is entirely reabsorbed till isotonicity is attained. Consequently,the urine flow rate during MA before F ($\dot{V}c$) is equal to the flow escaping proximal reabsorption ($\dot{V}f$) minus the water reabsorbed (CH2O-T + TcH2O) : $\dot{V}c = \dot{V}f$ - CH2O-T - TcH2O (IV).Instead,during F: $\dot{V}cf = \dot{V}f$ - CH2O-DT (V). By combining (III),(IV) and (V), we obtain: CH2O-HL = $\dot{V}cf$ - ($\dot{V}c$ + TcH2O).Thus,we can calculate CH2O-HL, a measurement already obtained during the experiment of MWD,by a totally independent method in a different experimental setting.

RESULTS AND DISCUSSION

All data were factored by GFR and expressed as $ml \cdot min^{-1} \cdot GFR^{-1} \cdot 100$.Table 1 shows that CH2O-HL measured during MWD averaged 19.4 ± 10.4 and this was not different statistically from the mean value measured,in these same subjects,during MA,of 20.4 ± 8.0 $ml \cdot min^{-1} \cdot GFR^{-1} \cdot 100$, $P > .05$.The two independent measurements of CH2O-HL were significantly correlated,$r = 0.80$,$P < .01$.From a mathematical manipulation

TABLE 1

	MWD		TMA	
		$ml \cdot min^{-1} \cdot GFR^{-1} \cdot 100$		
$\dot{V}$	20.0±8.6	$P < 0.01$	2.4±2.8	$\dot{V}$
$\dot{V}f$	45.1±14.5	NS	28.9± 13.7	$\dot{V}cf$
Cosm	4.4±2.8	NS	4.9±4.2	Cosm
Cosmf	29.5±12.1	NS	25.4±10.6	Cosmf
CH2O-HL	19.4±10.4	NS	20.4±8.0	CH2O-HL
CH2O-DT	13.3±6.1	NS	11.0±11.2	CH2O-DT
CH2O-BD	17.1±9.7	$P < 0.01$	2.6±1.9	TcH2O
		$ml \cdot min^{-1}$		
GFR	103.0±16.0	NS	96.0±9.0	GFR
GFRf	128.0±35.0	NS	113.0±18.0	GFRf

of our equations,it can be easily demonstrated that Cosm during baseline conditions must be equal in both diluting and concentrating experiments,and that Cosmf in diluting conditions must be equal to Vcf,the urine flow rate measured in MA during F.Table 1 shows that in fact these requirements were met by the actual experimental results.This is not surprising,since we calculated that the degree of extracellular volume expansion achieved during MWD and MA should have been of the same degree. Therefore,the results obtained in the measurements of CH2O-HL by the two independent methods can be considered adequate to assess the reproducibility and accuracy of the results obtained. These is a positive correlation between CH2O-HL,a value proportional to the amount of salt deposited into the renal medullary interstitium,and TcH2O,the flow of SFW reabsorbed by the interstitium from CD,two closely related variables in the renal medulla. We conclude that the present data confirm and strengthen the accuracy and affidability of our method (1) aimed at measuring Na and H2O reabsorption by each segment of the human nephron in vivo.

REFERENCES

1. Bartoli,E.,Satta,A.,Faedda,R.,Olmeo,N.A.,Soggia,G.,Branca,G.F. J.Clin.Pharmacol. 23 : 56-64,1983
2. Satta,A.,Faedda,R.,Olmeo,N.A.,Soggia,G.,Branca,G.F.,Bartoli,E. Renal Physiol. 7:283-292,1984
3. Zoccali,C.,Bartoli,E.,Curatola,G.,Maggiore,Q.Nephron 32:140-148,1982
4. Satta,A.,Faedda,R.,Branca,G.F.,Manca,A.,Bartoli,E. First Intern.Conf. on Diuretics,Miami Beach,1984,March 5-9

XV. EFFECTS OF DIURETICS ON RENAL FUNCTION

EFFECTS OF THE NEW URICOSURIC DIURETIC BAY r 4420 ON RAT KIDNEY FUNCTION

G. Sigrist, J. Greven, B. Fuchs

Department of Pharmacology, Rheinisch Westfälische Technische Hochschule
Schneebergweg s/n, 5100 Aachen, Federal Republic of Germany

INTRODUCTION

Derivatives of imidazothiadiazol-acrylamides constitute a new class of diuretically and uricosurically active drugs. Their chemical structure is not akin to any diuretics known so far. We used the derivative BAY r 4420 to investigate the mechanisms underlying the diuretic and uricosuric effects in rats. The drug has a molecular weight of 423 g/mol and is - although supplied as a hydrochloride - of poor water solubility. The uricosuric effect is of particular interest, since most diuretics in use today are weak acids and hence competitively impair uric acid excretion; this can induce hyperuricaemia under sustained treatment.

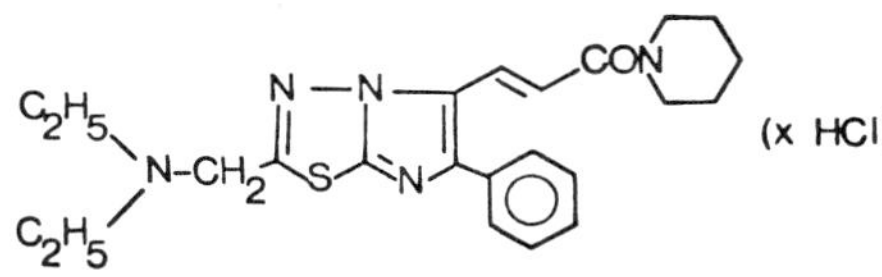

BAY r 4420

MATERIAL AND METHODS

Male Sprague-Dawley rats in different ranges of bodyweight (BW) were used. Animals were deprived of food the night before the experiment while having free access to water. They were anaesthetized with 100 mg/kg BW thiobutabarbital, tracheotomized and placed on a heating table to maintain body temperature at 37 °C. The left jugular vein was cannulated for infusion and the right carotid arteria for monitoring blood pressure and collecting blood samples. The bladder was cannulated to collect urine and the urethra was ligated. Where neccessary, additionally the left urether was cannulated to collect urine for each kidney seperatly. Physiological saline was infused in a range of 6 to 12 ml/h in clearance experiments and at 0.9 ml/h in micropuncture experiments. Sampling periods were 10 minutes and data shown here were pooled for 30 minutes before and for 10 to 40 minutes after administration of the drug.

Solutions of BAY r 4420 were prepared by dissolving the appropiate amount in physiological saline with 4 mmol/l HCl added. By successive addition of NaOH the pH was raised to 1.75 - 2.00; the solutions had to remain rather acid to avoid precipitation. Experiments were checked against a control solution of physiological saline with HCl added for the same pH. Volume administered was 5 ml/kg BW.

Urine flow and urinary excretion of Na, K, and Cl were measured; glomerular filtration rate (GFR) was determined as inulin clearance; maximum secretory tubular anion transport capacity for weak acids was determined as maximum transport capacity for paraamino hippuric acid (TM-PAH). Details for clearance and micropuncture experiments have been previously described (1,2). Renal blood flow (RBF) was measured directly by an electromagnetic flow probe around the left renal artery.

Microinjection experiments used a similar setup as the micropuncture experiments. The left kidney was exposed and superficial nephrons were punctured. Additionally urine was collected separatly for the left and right kidney. Diuresis was induced by infusion of 2 ml/h of a 5% mannitol solution. Radiolabeled ^{14}C uric acid and ^{3}H inulin were microinjected at early proximal, late proximal, and early distal puncture sites and their excretion in urine was measured. After correction for systemical recirculation (right kidney) the fractional amount of reabsorbed uric acid for different nephron segments (of the left kidney) could be determined.

RESULTS AND DISCUSSION

Clearance experiments revealed dose dependent diuretic effects after intravenous administration of 0.1 to 10 mg/kg BW and mean arterial pressure (MAP) was progressively lowered. Higher doses of 25 or even 50 mg/kg BW lead to an dramatic decrease (< 100 mmHg) in systemic blood pressure. As a consequence, GFR dropped and urine flow ceased, making it difficult to estimate renal effects properly at this doses. Maximal effects at doses of 10 mg/kg BW shew a half life time of 90 to 120 minutes. The diuretic potency of the drug is allocated between those of thiazides and loop diuretics. The table below summarizes the results of clearance and renal blood flow experiments before (upper two lines) and after administration of 10 mg/kg BW of Bay r 4420 (lower two lines).

	U-Flow µl/min·100g	E-Na µmol/min·100g	E-Cl µmol/min·100g	E-K µmol/min·100g	E-Na/E-K	MAP mmHg	GFR µl/min·100g	RBF ml/min·100g	U-Urat mg/100ml	E-Urat µg/min·100g	TM-PAH mg/min·100g
Mean	22.3	5.77	3.26	1.20	4.91	149	697	2.34	6.05	1.20	0.32
SEM	2.1	0.53	0.40	0.01	0.50	3	66	0.42	0.76	0.10	0.02
Mean	59.8	14.13	11.60	0.88	15.69	140	839	2.81	4.01	2.28	0.33
SEM	4.5	1.04	1.03	0.01	0.88	3	79	0.55	0.43	0.22	0.01
$p \leq$	0.02	0.05	0.05	0.0001	0.05	0.05	0.05	0.05	0.05	0.05	n.s.

Urine flow (U-Flow) shows a nearly threefold increase and excretion of sodium (E-Na) and chloride (E-Cl) goes parallel with urine volume. The excretion of potassium (E-K) is significantly reduced at this dose. Although mean arterial pressure (MAP) is lowered by 9 mmHg, GFR and RBF increase by more then 20%. Urine flow, salt excretion, GFR, and RBF show the same dose dependent increase, but half life time for RBF is only 10 to 15 minutes and thus much shorter as for the other effects. There is a highly significant correlation between GFR and urine flow suggesting that increased GFR is probably the major cause for the diuretic effect.

Single nephron data of micropuncture experiments support these results. They show that absolute tubular salt reabsorption (due to increased load, caused by increased GFR) is increased rather then diminished. This observation is in contrast to other diuretics which are known to exert their diuretic effect by blocking tubular salt reabsorption. Early distal sodium (40±5 mmol/l) and chloride (44±5 mmol/l) concentrations show only a slight increase (Na=47±3 mmol/l; Cl=51±2 mmol/l; not significant) which is probably due to the increased load to the tubule. Of course, minor direct effects of the drug on tubular electrolyte transport might be overlooked by these methods used. Increased absolute tubular salt reabsorption might explain the low potassium excretion observed.

The elimination of uric acid increased dose dependently in clearance experiments even at small diuretic doses, but in contrast to diuresis the uricosuric effect was still more pronounced up to the highest dose (50 mg/kg BW) tested. Experimentally lowered GFR ceased urine flow but the uricosuric effect persisted. The table above summarizes the effect on uric acid urine concentration and elimination in the last two but one columns. Simultaneously the maximal transport capacity for PAH was determined. Data in the last column of the table reveal, that the drug does not impair the secretory anion transport mechanism for weak acids in the proximal tubule. On the other hand, the diuretic and uricosuric effects of the drug are not impaired by saturating this anion transport with PAH. These results indicate that neither the drug nor relevant amounts of its metabolites are secreted by the tubular anion secretion mechanism and that there is obviously no need for this for the drug to exert its effects.

Tubular microinjection of radiolabeled uric acid at early proximal, late proximal, and early distal injection sites shows a similar increase in urine uric acid recovery from proximal injection sites by some 10% but shows unchanged recovery at distal injection sites after administration of 10 mg/kg BW of the drug. This suggests the mechanism of the uricosuric effect to be the impairment of urate reabsorption in the later part of the proximal tubule, presumably in the pars recta.

1. Greven, J., Klein, H. and Heidenreich, O., Naunyn-Schmiedebergs Arch. Pharmacol. 304:289-296 (1978)
2. Greven, J., Defrain, W., Glaser, K., Meywald, K. and Heidenreich, O., Pflügers Arch. 384:57-60 (1980)

CHARACTERIZATION OF THE RENAL AND HORMONAL EFFECTS OF THREE NOVEL ANTI-MINERALOCORTICOIDS IN VITRO AND IN VIVO

S.E. WHITEBREAD, H. HAENNI, H.P. RAMJOUE, U. JOSS, C. KRAEHENBUEHL, L. SCHENKEL, M. BIOLLAZ, J. GROB, M. DE GASPARO

Ciba-Geigy Limited, Pharmaceuticals Division, CH-4002 Basle, Switzerland

INTRODUCTION

Antimineralocorticoid compounds are widely prescribed for the treatment of essential hypertension and primary or secondary hyperaldosteronism. Spironolactone is the most commonly used drug of this type. Its administration however is limited by its anti-androgenic action.

The discovery that 9α,11α-epoxy substitution of spirolactones and other steroidal aldosterone antagonists improved their specificity at the receptor level (Joss, Kalvoda et al, in preparation) led to the synthesis of the epoxy derivatives of prorenone, mexrenone and spironolactone. Their anti-mineralocorticoid as well as their anti-androgenic, gestagenic and anti-ovulatory properties were studied in vitro and in vivo.

MATERIALS AND METHODS

Receptor binding studies using ^{3}H-aldosterone, ^{3}H-dexamethasone, ^{3}H-methyltrienolone and ^{3}H-progesterone were performed using rat kidney, rat ventral prostate or rabbit uterus cytosol by classical techniques (1). The anti-mineralocorticoid effect was measured according to Kagawa (2). The anti-androgenic effects were investigated in intact or in castrated testosterone treated male rats according to a method modified from Neumann (3). Gestagenic properties were studied following a modification of Clauberg (4). The distruption of the ovulatory cycle was assessed as described by Desaulles & Kraehenbuehl (5).

RESULTS

The introduction of the epoxy group only marginally decreased the affinity of two of the three compounds for the mineralocorticoid receptor in vitro, the exception being that of epoxymexrenone which bound roughly 15 times less than spironolactone (Table 1).

In vivo, in the adrenalectomized rat, all three epoxy-derivatives were potent aldosterone antagonists.

Table 1. Relative affinity of anti-mineralocorticoid substances in competitive binding tests

Receptor	Spironolactone	Epoxyprorenone	Epoxymexrenone	Epoxyspironolactone
Mineralocorticoid	$1.1x10^{-1}$	$1.2x10^{-1}$	$5.1x10^{-3}$	$7.5x10^{-2}$
Glucocorticoid	$1.8x10^{-3}$	$5.0x10^{-4}$	$1.8x10^{-4}$	$7.5x10^{-3}$
Androgen	$9.1x10^{-3}$	$2.4x10^{-4}$	$7.6x10^{-6}$	$1.1x10^{-5}$
Gestagen	$7.0x10^{-3}$	$8.3x10^{-3}$	$< 5x10^{-5}$	$7.4x10^{-4}$

Compared to the values in the aldosterone-treated control rats, there was a statistically significant increase in Na excretion and in the Na/K ratio. At 3 mg/kg, spironolactone and epoxyspironolactone inhibited the effect of aldosterone by 35% whereas the other antagonists induced more than 50% inhibition (Table 2).

Table 2. Effect of the drugs on the Na/K ratio in adrenalectomized rats according to Kagawa (mean $\pm$ SEM)

		1 mg/kg	3 mg/kg	10 mg/kg
Control	5.15 ± 0.15 (118)	-	-	-
Aldosterone	1.68 ± 0.04 (122)			
Spironolactone		2.26 ± 0.25 (13)	2.90 ± 0.25 (29)	4.38 ± 0.26 (40)
Epoxyprorenone		2.99 ± 0.26 (21)	4.02 ± 0.31 (9)	3.97 ± 0.34 (15)
Epoxymexrenone		2.53 ± 0.23 (12)	4.08 ± 0.26 (8)	4.11 ± 0.27 (15)
Epoxyspironolactone		2.15 ± 0.26 (9)	2.79 ± 0.27 (18)	4.35 ± 0.27 (12)

By comparison with spironolactone, the introduction of the epoxy-group significantly reduced the binding of the derivative to the androgen receptors (Table 1). A good correlation between gestagen and androgen receptor binding and the potency of the substances in vivo was observed.

Spironolactone, the reference compound, was clearly anti-androgenic, gestagenic and antiovulatory in our tests in rats and rabbits (Table 3) whereas the epoxyderivatives were either inactive or much less active than spironolactone. Epoxyprorenone, however, was as gestagenic as spironolactone.

Table 3. Endocrine-related effects of the drugs in vivo

Effect	Spirono-lactone	Epoxy-prorenone	Epoxy-mexrenone	Epoxy-spironolactone
Anti-androgenic* (prostate)	35	Ø 180	Ø 180	Ø 180
Gestagenic[b]	100	100	Ø 100	Ø 100
Ovulation[b]	50	Ø 100	Ø 100	> 100

(inactive dose, mg/kg; $^{*}ED_{30}$; $^{b}ED_{50}$)

DISCUSSION

Previous studies have suggested that the sexual endocrine side-effects of aldosterone antagonists are largely due to the high affinity of these steroids for the androgen and gestagen receptors. The introduction of a 9α,11α-epoxy group to known aldosterone antagonists decreases androgen and gestagen receptor binding both absolutely, and relative to mineralocorticoid receptor binding. The animal models used appear to be suitable for assessing the effects which cause the endocrine disorders in man upon prolonged administration of aldosterone antagonists, as illustrated by the results obtained with spironolactone. The results summarized here demonstrate that it is possible to increase the specificity of steroidal aldosterone antagonists both in vitro and in vivo.

REFERENCES

1. King, R.J.B. and Mainwaring, W.I.P. Steroid Cell Interactions. Butterworths Publ., London, 1974.
2. Kagawa, C.M. Endocrinology 67: 125-131, 1960.
3. Neumann, F. In: methods in drug evaluation (Ed. P. Montagazza and F. Piccinini) North-Holland Publ. Co., Amsterdam, 1966, pp. 548-573
4. Clauberg C. Klin. Wochenschr. 9: 2004-1005, 1930
5. Desaulles, P.F. and Kraehenbuehl, C. Acta Endocrinol. 47: 44-456, 1964

RENAL EFFESTS OF ETOZOLIN IN MAN.

R. Palla, C. Distratis, R. Cominotto, V. Panichi, G. Pozzetti, A. Bionda, M. Neri, L. Frattarelli.

Istituto di Clinica Medica II - Università di Pisa

Etozolin (E.) is an higly effective diuretic of thiazolidone group; it is well absorbed by G-I tract. E. undergoes first-pass metabolism to its 2-methilene-carboxilic acid Ozolinone wich displays a greater diuretic activity. By micropuncture studies E. site of action has been identified in the thick ascending limb of Henle's loop (1).
The present study was carried out to evaluate E. effect on solutes and water excretion and renal hemodinamics.

MATERIALS AND METHODS

The study was performed in 10 healty male volunteers. An oral tap-water load (30 ml/Kg body wt) was given over 40 min period. When the maximal steady state diuresis was achieved, water was added in order to replace the urinary and the insensible loss. A control study of 2 hrs clearance was compared to a similar period performed 4 hrs after E. administration (400 mg). Blood samples were withdrawn at the middle of each timed period and urines were collected by spontaneous voiding. Glomerular filtration rate was evaluated by creatinine clearance (Ccr) and effective renal plasma flow (ERPF) by I^{131} hippuran plasmatic clearance (2). Osmolality was determined by Knauer osmometer.
The following data were evaluated: Ccr; osmolal clearance (Cosm); free water clearance (CH2O); sodium and chloride clearance (CNa; CCl) and

fractional excretion (FENa; FECl); sodium term and chloride term: (CNa+CH2O)/Ccr; (CCl+CH2O)/Ccr (3); phosphate fractional reabsortion (FRPi); potassium and calcium excretion rate; renal blood flow (RBF) as ERPF/1-HTC, renal vascolar resistance (RVR) as Mean Blood Pressure/ERPF.

RESULTS

Ccr decreased from 149±29 ml/min to 136±43 ml/min (p=NS);

ERPF decreased from 787±230 ml/min to 625±183 ml/min (p=0.05)

RBF decreased from 1334±390 ml/min to 1055±290 ml/min (p=0.05)

RVR increased from 0.084±0.02 to 0.109±0.05 (p=0.02)

Urine flow rose from 8.7±2 ml/min to 12.4±2.3 ml/min (p=0.05)

Cosm rose from 2.98±1.1 ml/min to 4.35±1.3 ml/min (p=0.01)

CH20 decreased from 5.35±2 ml/min to 3.62±2 ml/min (p=0.02)

FENa rose from 0.48±0.1 % to 1.86±0.8 % (p=0.01)

FECl rose from 5.7±3 % TO 7.3±2 % (p=0.05)

Na term increased from 0.044±0.03 to 0.047±0.01 (p=0.05)

Cl term decreased from 0.116±0.09 to 0.098±0.035 (p=NS)

FRPi rose from 88±8 % to 94±3 % (p=NS)

Sodium excretion rate rose from 97.7±35 μEq/min to 387±238 μEq/min (p=0.01),it remained above control range during the following 12 hrs and returned to the control after 18 hrs.

Potassium excretion rate rose from 73±26 μEq/min to 97±2 μEq/min (p=0.02)

Calcium excretion rate rose from 6.7±3 μEq/min to 14.3±6 μEq/min (p=0.01) in normocalciuric subjects whereas in two hypercalciuric subjects it decreased from 15.4 μEq/min to 8.1±3 μEq/min.

DISCUSSION

E. administration in healty subjects produces a significant increase of sodium and chloride excretion, of Cosm and a reduction of CH2O; these data confirm that E. is able to inhibit sodium and chlride transport in the thick ascending limb of Henle's loop. The E. diuretic effect is still present 12 hrs after administration and disappears after 18 hrs. The increased potassium excretion, a loop's diuretic' effect, was reported to be due to the increase of distal delivery, recent data suggest an inhibition of common transport system for sodium and potassium (4). E. does not act on phosphate reabsorption whereas other loop's diuretics are able to affect phosphate reabsorption probably by changes in tubular cell methabolism (5). E. shows calciuric effect in normal subjects but it seems to reduce calcium excretion in hypercalciuric subjects; this effect, if confirmed, may be important in treatment of recurrent calcium stone-formers. The slight reduction of Ccr observed after E. is probably due to an increase in intratubular pressure (6). The significant reduction of ERPF and RBF may be mediated by hemodinamic variations (increase of RVR) but is possible that a depressed tubular hippuran secretion plays a role (7).

REFERENCES

1) Greven J., Beckers M., Defrain W., Meywald K., Heidenreich O.; Pflugers Archiv. 384: 61-64, 1980.
2) Blaufox M.D., Merril J.P.; Nephron 3: 274, 1966.
3) Danovitch G.M.; Renal Phisiol. Basel 1: 56-60, 1978.
4) Oberleithener K., Guggin W., Giebisch G.; Pflugers Archiv. 396: 27-33 1983.
5) Eknoyan G., Sawa H., Hyde S.,Wood J.M., Schwartz A., Suki W.; J. Pharmacol. Exp. Ther. 194: 614-623, 1975.
6) Burke T.J., Duchin K.L.; Kidney Int. 16: 672-680, 1975.
7) Greven J., Klein H., Heidenreich O.; Kidney Int. 13: 6 1978.

EFFECTS OF ENALAPRIL ON WATER AND SALT BALANCE AND RENAL HEMODYNAMICS.

D. RUSSO, M. ALTOMONTE, B. CIANCIARUSO, G. CONTE, G. DI MINNO°, C. ESPOSITO, G. MARTORANO, A. TESTA, A. DAL CANTON, V.E. ANDREUCCI.
Departement of Nephrology and Internal Medicine°, 2nd Faculty, Naples.

INTRODUCTION

The purpose of this study was to evaluate both the natriuretic and the renal hemodynamic effects of Enalapril (E), a new ACE-inhibitor, in hypertensive patients.

MATERIALS AND METHODS

The study was carried out in 11 inpatients with diastolic blood pressure of 100-120 mm Hg. The patients were held at constant sodium intake (90 mEq/day), and any medication was withdrawn 4 weeks before the study. When a steady sodium output was achieved, control measurements of : serum Sodium, Potassium, Aldosterone (A), PGE_2, Plasma Renin Activity (PRA), Effective Renal Plasma Flow (ERPF, as C_{PAH}), Glomerular Filtration Rate (GFR, as C_{cr}), Filtration Fraction (FF) were done.These measurements were repeated after 6 days of treatment. Blood Pressure (BP), Body Weight (BW), 24 hr urinary excretion of Sodium and Potassium ($U_{Na} \cdot V$, $U_K \cdot V$), Urine Output (V) were recorded daily throughout the study. E was administered in single oral dose (20 mg) at noon. Blood was collected at 8.00 a.m.. Serum A, PGE_2, and PRA were measured by RIA methods; Sodium and Potassium by flame photometry. Paired Student's t-test was used to compare means.

RESULTS

The effects of E on blood parameters, A, FF, GFR, and ERPF are summarized in Table 1. E induced a significant rise in serum Potassium, PRA, serum PGE_2; and a significant reduction in standing A. No changes were observed in GFR, ERPF, FF, and serum Sodium. The effects of E on BW, Mean Arterial Blood Pressure (MBP), $U_{Na} \cdot V$, $U_K \cdot V$, and V are reported in Table 2. BW, $U_{Na} \cdot V$, $U_K \cdot V$, and V were unchanged throughout the study. MBP was steadily reduced.

Table 1. Effects of Enalapril in 11 patients. Numbers are Means and (SE).

	BASALINE	TREATMENT
Serum Sodium (mEq/l)	140.6 (3.0)	141.6 (0.6)
Serum Potassium (mEq/l)	4.0 (0.6)	4.3 (0.3)°
PGE_2 (pmol/$3 \cdot 10^8$ cells)	942.4 (38.5)	1236.7 (161.3)°
GFR (ml/min)	128.0 (11.2)	126.0 (13.4)
ERPF (ml/min)	323.2 (42.7)	369.0 (29.9)
FF (%)	31.0 (0.6)	34.1 (0.3)
Supine PRA (ng/ml·hr)	0.9 (0.4)	2.5 (1.2)°°
Standing PRA (ng/ml·hr)	2.3 (0.8)	7.9 (2.9)°°
Supine A (pg/ml)	226.5 (34.7)	189.3 (20.3)
Standing A (pg/ml)	285.6 (31.5)	242.9 (24.9)°°

Table 2. Effects of Enalapril in 11 patients. Numbers are Means and (SE).

Day	Θ	1	2	3	4	5	6
MBP (mm Hg)	125.5* (1.7)	117.5* (2.4)	113.5* (4.9)	117.4* (4.7)	115.0* (4.6)	114.0* (3.7)	112.0* (3.4)
$U_{Na} \cdot V$ (mEq/24hr)	103.6 (3.4)	108.1 (6.4)	100.1 (9.6)	118.9 (9.9)	109.5 (8.7)	105.6 (6.8)	104.3 (8.1)
$U_K \cdot V$	39.9 (3.0)	39.6 (2.7)	38.9 (2.7)	42.2 (2.4)	39.9 (2.5)	43.4 (2.6)	46.6 (3.6)
V (ml/24hr)	1157.9 (103)	1311.5 (111)	1238.4 (156)	1242.0 (98)	1219.0 (74)	1223.0 (103)	1061.5 (57)
BW (Kg)	74.8 (4.2)	74.9 (4.2)	74.8 (4.1)	74.7 (4.1)	74.7 (4.1)	74.8 (4.1)	74.9 (4.1)

° $p < 0.05$ °° $p < 0.025$ * $p < 0.005$

DISCUSSION

Captopril (C) has a natriuretic effect that may cause an ECV volume depletion and account for a decrease both in ERPF and GFR (1). By this mechanism C may be responsible for functional Acute Renal Failure (1). The natriuretic effect of C has been attributed either to increased PGE_2 or decreased A secretion (2-3). In this study E causes similar changes as C in both PGE_2 and A secretion. E, however, causes no natriuresis , leaving renal hemodynamics unchanged. The reason for this difference between E and C is not apparent from our results. Pharmacodynamic studies investigating the relation of the ACE inhibitory effect of E with changes in PGE_2 , Bradikinins, and A secretion may be useful to understand why E is not natriuretic.

CONCLUSION

These results indicate that E does not cause natriuresis and volume depletion, thus leaving renal hemodynamics unchanged. This distinctive feature of E is of potential benefit by preventing ACE-dependent Acute Renal Failure.

REFERENCES

1. Andreucci, V.E. in: Acute Renal Failure (Ed. V.E. Andreucci), Martinus Nijhoff Publishing, 1984, pp 51-118.
2. Conte, G., Dal Canton, A., Maglionico, G., Di Spigno, C., Pirone, B., Russo, D., Di Minno, G., Andreucci, V.E. Proc EDTA-ERA (Eds A.M. Davison, and P.J. Guillou), Pitman Press, 1984, pp820-824.
3. Atlas, S.A., Case, D.B., Laragh, J.H. Am. J. Med. 77 (2 A),13-17, 1984.

XVI. DIURETICS AND PROSTAGLANDINS

EFFECT OF INDOMETHACIN ON THE SALURETIC ACTIVITY OF BUMETANIDE

NICOLA TESSITORE , RUGGERO PANEBIANCO and GIUSEPPE MASCHIO

Divisione di Nefrologia Medica , Università di Verona , Verona ,Italia

INTRODUCTION

Since loop diuretics increase urinary excretion of prostaglandins (PG)(1), it has been proposed that the increase in renal plasma flow (RPF),plasma renin activity(PRA) and urinary sodium (Na) excretion following these drugs is,at least in part,mediated by increased PG synthesis in the kidney. In agreement with such an hypothesis,it has been shown that inhibitors of PG synthesis,such as indomethacin (INDO) and aspirin (2),blunt the diuretic-induced increase in RPF (3),PRA (4-7)and Na excretion (4,5,7). However the latter effect is not constant in humans,since some acute studies have shown that furosemide-induced natriuresis is unaffected by PG synthesis inhibitors (6,8).

The present study was undertaken to investigate in healthy human subjects whether the diuretic effect of a single dose Bumetanide (B)(9) is altered by pharmacological inhibition of renal PG synthesis by INDO.We also tried to identify the nephron sites at which INDO might interfere with B-induced natriuresis.

PATIENTS AND METHODS

Our study included 8 healthy subjects,3females and 5 males,aged 18-45 yrs. Subjects drank 20 ml/kg of tap water over 45 minutes;after urine osmolality had reached a value less than 100 mOsm/kg water,a basal 1-hour urinary collection period was obtained;B(1 mg)was then rapidly administered i.v.,followed by 4 additional 1-hour urine collection periods;blood samples were collected at the mid-point of each collection period.Urinary losses were replaced throughout the study with oral tap water. The same protocol was then repeated in the same subjects after oral treatment with INDO (150 mg/24 h for 3 days plus 50 mg 30-60 minutes before starting the study).

GFR was evaluated as creatinine clearance;we used fractional excretion of urinary volume (V/GFR) and Na (FE Na)as indices of global renal handling of water and solutes;phosphaturia was used as an index of proximal tubule function; the delivery of solute at the diluting segment was calculated according to the formula($\frac{U_{Na + K}}{P_{Na}} + C_{H_2O}$)/GFR;fractional free water clearance divided by the delivery term ($C_{H_2O}/C_{H_2O} + C_{Cl}$)was used as an index of function of the diluting segment and fractional excretion of potassium (FE K) as an index of collecting duct function. PRA was evaluated by radioimmunoassay(RIA)for angiotensin I. Urinary PGE_2 were evaluated in the female subjects by RIA.

RESULTS

Our study shows that under basal conditions INDO did not change GFR nor urinary excretion of Na and water,while significantly decreased PRA and urinary PGE_2 excretion. Moreover INDO did not affect the total diuretic and natriuretic effect of B,while blunting the diuretic-induced increase in PRA (Table I).

Table I

	B A S A L		B U M E T A N I D E	
	CONTROL	INDO	CONTROL	INDO
GFR (ml/min)	120 ± 15	118 ± 16	112 ± 19	116 ± 15
Urine Volume (ml/min)	10.6 ± 1.4	11.1 ± 2.4	39.5 ± 4.4	48.8 ± 5.1
FE Na (%)	0.9 ± 0.2	1.0 ± 0.3	-	-
Urinary Na (mEq/3 h)	-	-	152 ± 25	163 ± 25
PRA (pmole/ml/h)	0.9 ± 0.3	0.3 ± 0.1 *	2.0 ± 0.8	0.5 ± 0.1 *
Urinary PGE_2 (ng/h)	47 ± 9	13 ± 11 *	-	-

* = $p < 0.05$ vs. control

Table II

	1st HOUR		2nd HOUR		3rd HOUR	
	CONTROL	INDO	CONTROL	INDO	CONTROL	INDO
V/GFR (%)	20 ± 3	18 ± 3	11 ± 3	17 ± 4*	7 ± 4	13 ± 3*
FE Na (%)	11 ±1.5	9 ±0.5*	5 ±1.5	6 ± 2	1 ±0.2	2 ± 0.5*
Phosphaturia (mg/h)	90 ± 20	87 ± 18	55 ± 20	65 ± 18	36 ± 9	52 ± 8*
Distal delivery (%)	17 ± 4	16 ± 4	9 ± 3	15 ± 3*	5 ± 3	10 ± 3 *
$C_{H_2O} / C_{H_2O} + C_{Cl}$ (%)	28 ± 4	25 ± 5	40 ± 10	48 ± 10	71 ± 13	72 ± 9
FE K (%)	32 ± 14	36 ± 7	21 ± 9	24 ± 6	9 ± 4	16 ± 6 *

* = $p < 0.02$ vs. control

Pretreatment with INDO changed the time course of the effect of B (Table II) . INDO blunted the diuretic and natriuretic effect of B at the peak of action and induced a more persistent effect in the latest phases of diuretic activity.INDO had no effect on the diluting segment and increased the distal delivery of solutes;the effect on phosphaturia suggests,but not prove,that a reduced reabsorption of fluid in the proximal tubule contributes to increase the delivery of solutes to the diluting segment.

DISCUSSION

In agreement with previous acute studies using furosemide (6,8),we found that inhibition of endogenous PG synthesis did not affect the total diuretic and natriuretic activity of B. However,pretreatment with INDO induced a more persistent,although modest,saluretic effect after B. Our results show that this phenomenon is the consequence of an increased delivery of fluid to the diluting segment of the nephron,consistent with an effect of PG synthesis inhibitors on the thin limb of the loop of Henle and/or the medullary segment of the ascending limb of the loop.In addition ,the data on phosphaturia suggest that a decrease in proximal tubular reabsorption of fluid may contribute to the increased distal delivery of sodium following INDO.

These tubular effects may be the result of a direct action of INDO. An alternative explanation is suggested by the finding that INDO blunts the diuretic-induced increase in PRA : it is possible that inhibition of PG synthesis reduces intrarenal vasoconstriction after B,which will lead to an increase in medullary flow and solutes wash-out and to an increase in peritubular hydrostatic pressure;those hemodynamic effects may be ultimately responsible of a decreased passive reabsorption of fluid in the medulla and in the proximal tubule,respectively.

REFERENCES

1. Olsen U.B. and Ahnefelt-Ronne I. Acta Phar.Toxicol. 38 : 219 , 1976
2. Vane J.R. Nature 38 : 231 , 1971
3. Bailie M.D.,Barbour J.A. and Hook J.B. Proc.Soc.Exp.Biol.Med. 148:1173,1976
4. Patak R.V.,Mookerjee B.K.,Bentzel C.J.,Hysert P.E.,Babej M.,Lee J.B. Prostaglandins 10 : 1649 , 1975
5. Frolich J.C.,Hollifield J.W.,Dormois J.C.,Frolich B.L.,Seybert H.,Michelakis A.M.,Oates J.A. Circ.Res. 39 : 447 , 1976
6. Weber P.C.,Scherer B.,Larsonn C. Europ.J.Pharmac. 41 : 329 ,1977
7. Kramer H.J.,Dusing R.,Stinnesbeck B.,Prior W.,Backer A.,Eden J.,Kipnowski J., Glanzer K.,Kruck F. Clin. Sci. 59 : 67 , 1980
8. Berg K.J. Europ. J. Pharmac. 11 : 117 , 1977
9. Karlander S.G.,Henning R.,Lundvall O. Europ. J. Clin.Pharmac. 6 : 220 , 1973

ROLE OF RENAL PROSTAGLANDINS IN MEDIATING THE ACTIVITY OF MUZOLIMINE IN MAN.

F.BANDIERA, P.DESSI'-FULGHERI, P.MADEDDU, F.COCCO, M.OPPES, N.GLORIOSO, M.SPANEDDA*, A.RAPPELLI.

Cattedra di Patologia Medica II, University of Sassari (Italy) and *Division of Internal Medicine, Ospedale di Ittiri (Italy).

INTRODUCTION

Renal prostaglandins are known to mediate the effects of loop diuretics (1,2). Muzolimine is a loop diuretic with a duration of action longer than furosemide. This feature makes this drug suitable for chronic antihypertensive therapy. The nonsteroidal antiinflammatory drugs block prostaglandin synthesis and their use may blunt the efficacy of many antihypertensive drugs (3). Indomethacin inhibits renal and systemic prostaglandins and has been also reported to interfere with the diuretic and natriuretic effects of muzolimine in man and rats (1,4). On the other hand, sulindac, another nonsteroidal antiinflammatory drug, is known to inhibit systemic but not renal prostaglandin synthesis (3,5). The aim of this study has been therefore to verify if the antihypertensive, diuretic and humoral effects of muzolimine in man are mediated by renal prostaglandins by comparing the effects of muzolimne alone or in association with either sulindac or indomethacin.

PATIENTS AND METHODS

The study was performed in 48 hospitalized patients (20 male and 28 female, mean age: 49$\pm$16 yrs) with mild uncomplicated essential hypertension (I-II WHO). After a 2-week wash-out period the patients were randomly allocated to one of the following one-week treatments:

1) Placebo (P); 2) Indomethacin (I) 100 mg b.i.d.; 3) Sulindac (S) 200 mg b.i.d.; 4) Muzolimine (MZ) 30 mg o.d.; 5) MZ 30 mg o.d. + I 100 mg b.i.d.; 6) MZ 30 mg o.d. + S 200 mg b.i.d.

The patients were mantained on regular sodium and potassium intake, 120 and 60 mmol per day respectively, for the duration of the study. Mean arterial pressure (MAP), heart rate, body weight, urinary volume, daily urinary sodium and potassium excretion (by flame photometry) were measured every day throughout the study. Plasma sodium and potassium were determined every other day whereas plasma creatinine, plasma renin activity (PRA) and urinary aldosterone (UA) (by RIA) were measured before and at the end of the treatment period. For statistical analysis the maximum % variation of daily urinary volume (DΔ %max) and cumulative urinary sodium balance (CuNa) were considered. Statistical comparisons were made by Student's t test for paired or umpaired data.

RESULTS

The Table summarizes the principal results obtained in the study.

TABLE

	P	I	S	MZ	MZ+I	MZ+S
MAP b	128±11	123±13	119±12	135±10	129±13	127±9
MAP a	129±10	125±10	123±15	102±19**	116±14*	97±11**
D(Δ %max)	+2±3%	-26±15%*	+3±1%	+71±15%**	+5±7%	+68±14%**
CuNa	-8±11	+87±41#	-10±23	-243±41##	-33±62	-205±37##
PRA b	1.1±0.7	3.4±2.3	3.3±1.5	2.2±1.0	3.6±2.6	2.8±2.0
PRA a	2.0±0.9	1.6±1.4**	3.0±1.9	4.0±1.8**	3.6±2.0	3.8±2.0*
UA b	11.3±4.2	11.7±4.3	10.4±3.8	9.9±3.0	12.0±3.0	10.3±4.0
UA a	12.1±2.3	7.6±2.0*	11.4±6.5	14.0±4.7*	11.5±5.1	13.0±5.0*

b = before; a = after; P = placebo; I = Indomethecin; S = Sulindac; MZ = Muzolimine. CuNa in mmol; PRA in ng/ml/h of Angiotensin I; UA in µg/24h. (* = $p < 0.05$; ** = $p < 0.01$, a vs b)(# = $p < 0.05$; ## = $p < 0.01$ vs Placebo).

Plasma creatinine did not change significantly as well as plasma sodium. Plasma potassium significantly fell by 0.7 mmol/l in the groups treated with muzolimine alone or in combination with sulindac. Heart rate did not change significantly. The positive sodium balance induced by indomethacin (see Table) was accompanied by a significant increase in body weight (from 72±7 to 73±6 Kg, $p < 0.05$) whereas the latter remained unchanged in the other groups.

DISCUSSION

Intrarenal prostaglandins are important in controlling renal sodium handling, not only as vasodilators modulating renal blood flow and glomerular filtration rate, but olso by a direct natriuretic action independent of renal vasodilatation (6). This latter effect has been variously attributed to either a direct tubular action or to an effect on water permeability by blunting the response of the distal tubule to antidiuretic hormone (7). Our results show that the antihypertensive, diuretic and humoral effects of muzolimine in man, such as the other loop diuretics, are mediated by renal prostaglandins. The lack of effect of sulindac on blood pressure and diuresis may make this agent a safer therapeutic alternative if non steroidal antiinflammatory treatment is indicated in patients with essential hypertension.

REFERENCES

1. Calò, L., Cantaro, S., Piccoli, A., Vianello, A., Borsatti, A., Bardini, R., Antonello, A. Z.Kardiol.74, Suppl.2: 157-160, 1985;
2. Patak, R.V., Mookerjee, B.K., Bentzel, C.J., Hysert, P.E., Babej, M., Lee, J.B. Prostaglandins, 10: 649-659, 1975;
3. Puddey, B., Beilin, L.J., Vandongen, R., Banks, R., Rouse, I. Clin.Sci. 69: 327-336, 1985.
4. Garthoff, B., Thomas, G. Clin.Nephrol. 19, Suppl.1: S5-S10, 1983.
5. Ciabattoni, G., Cinotti, G.A., Pierucci, A., et al. N.Engl.J.Med. 310: 279-283, 1984.
6. Lee, J.B., Patak, R.V., Mookerjee, B.K., Am.J.Med. 60: 798-816,1976.
7. Bartoli, E., Branca, G.F., Faedda, R., Olmeo, N.A., Satta, A., Soggia, G. Brit.J.Pharmacol. 76: 357-360, 1982.

CICLETANINE - AN ANTIHYPERTENSIVE DRUG WITH A POWERFUL NATRIURETIC EFFECT; ROLE OF RENAL PROSTAGLANDINS

A. HORNYCH, J. BOISSON*, J.C. GASCHARD*, E. DESCHAMPS, J. BARIETY

Hôpital Broussais, U-28 INSERM, and Hôpital Notre Dame de Bon Secours*, 75014 Paris, France

INTRODUCTION

The aim of our study was to compare, in normotensive and essential hypertensive patients, the effect of CICLETANINE*, a new furopyridine derivative with antihypertensive and diuretic properties, on renal functions and renal prostaglandin secretion.

SUBJECTS AND METHODS

Subjects :

Two groups of subjects were included : 1) 10 normotensive healthy volunteers comprising 5 men and 5 women aged 47 ± 2 years with mean arterial blood pressure of 115 ± 4/77 ± 3 mm Hg. 2) 12 essential hypertensive patients, comprised 7 men and 5 women, aged 65 ± 3 years, with mean arterial blood pressure 170 ± 6/102 ± 2 mm Hg.

Methods :

1) Clinical investigation was carried out as a double blind cross-over study with ambulatory subjects for four days: Day 1 (D 1) and D 3 were controls; on D 2 and 4, which were experimental, either placebo (P) or Cicletanine (CIC) 150 mg was given at random at 8:30 A.M. and urine was collected for 6 hours thereafter, until 14:30. Four other patients were studied in an open study with Indometacin (IND) : D 1 : control, D 2 : 150 mg CIC, D 3 : 150 mg CIC and 25 mg IND, D 4 : 25 mg IND.

2) The renal functions measured in 6 hour urine samples included diuresis (UV), natriuresis ($U_{Na}V$), chloruresis ($U_{Cl}V$), kaliuresis (U_kV) and creatinine excretion ($U_{Cr}V$). Glomerular filtration (GFR) was calculated from creatinine clearance (Technicon).

---

* Institut IPSEN, Paris

3) Urinary prostaglandins were measured after previous extraction and chromatography by radioimmunoassay according to described methodology (1). The antisera against 6-K-$F_1\alpha$, TxB_2 and $PGF_2\alpha$ were raised in our laboratory; the antiserum against PGE_2 was from the Pasteur Institute. ^{3}H-PGs were from New England Nuclear.

RESULTS

The effect of Cicletanine on renal functions in normotensive and hypertensive subjects is shown in table 1 :

TABLE 1 :

	NORMOTENSIVES		T	HYPERTENSIVES		T
	Control	Cicletanine	test P <	Control	Cicletanine	test P <
V ml/min	1.4 ± 0.2	2.5 ± 0.3	0.02	1.2 ± 0.1	1.8 ± 0.1	0.05
$U_{Na}V$ umol/min	120 ± 19	214 ± 21	0.02	118 ± 3	214 ± 31	0.005
$U_{Cl}V$ umol/min	135 ± 21	266 ± 23	0.005	128 ± 14	237 ± 34	0.005
U_KV umol/min	73 ± 7	100 ± 12	0.05	62 ± 7	75 ± 17	NS
GFR ml/min/1.73m²	128 ± 18	132 ± 11	NS	88 ± 8	96 ± 14	0.05

NS = not significant

Single dose of 150 mg Cicletanine had a significant diuretic, natriuretic and chloruretic effect in both groups of subjects but much less in essential hypertensive patients (EHP). GFR rose moderately in both groups but significantly in EHP. The effect of Cicletanine on prostaglandin excretion in normotensive and essential hypertensive patients is shown in table 2.

TABLE 2 :

	NORMOTENSIVES		T	HYPERTENSIVES		T
	Control	Cicletanine	test P	Control	Cicletanine	test P
6-K-$F_1\alpha$	122 ± 32	158 ± 44	NS	81 ± 22	118 ± 27	NS
TxB_2	229 ± 32	285 ± 37	NS	137 ± 31	247 ± 47	0,01
PGE_2	181 ± 29	183 ± 25	NS	136 ± 25	217 ± 47	NS
$PGF_2\alpha$	493 ± 61	534 ± 178	NS	403 ± 92	446 ± 88	NS

Expressed as percent changes of control value, these results show that Cicletanine stimulated renal release of prostacyclin and other PGs more strongly in hypertensive patients than in normotensive subjects.

A significant positive correlation was found between GFR on one hand and on the other, PGE_2 excretion ($P < 0.025$), $U_{TxB2}V$ ($p < 0.02$) and $U_{PGF2}\alpha V$ ($p < 0.001$) in EHP under Cicletanine but not in normotensive subjects; during the control periods, GFR was significantly correlated only with $U_{PGE2}V$ in normotensive subjects ($p < 0.05$), and with $PGF_2\alpha$ ($p < 0.02$) in EHP. $U_{Na}V$ was significantly correlated during this period only with $U_{TxB2}V$ in EHP ($r = +0.71$, $p < 0.01$) and this correlation was the same under Cicletanine. $U_{Na}V$ was also positively correlated with $U_{PGF2}\alpha V$ under CIC treatment in EHP ($p < 0.001$).

The effect of indometacin treatment with and without Cicletanine on glomerular filtration and sodium excretion in 4 essential hypertensive patients is shown in table 3 :

TABLE 3:

	CONTROL	CICLETANINE (150 mg)	CICLETANINE (150 mg) + INDOMETACIN (25 mg)	INDOMETACIN (25 mg)
GFR ml/min	72 ± 11	118 ± 40	47 ± 27	75 ± 7
$U_{Na}V$ umol/min	70 ± 33	132 ± 23	70 ± 41	51 ± 23

These data show that in EHP, GFR-enhancement by Cicletanine and the natriuretic effect are prevented by simultaneous treatment with indometacin, a cycloxygenase inhibitor.

CONCLUSION :

The new antihypertensive drug Cicletanine, at a daily dose of 150 mg, exerts a significant natriuretic effect in both normotensive and essential hypertensive subjects without causing significant kaliuresis in essential hypertensive patients. Cicletanine increases glomerular filtration in essential hypertensive patients but not in normotensive subjects. The latter effect is prostaglandin dependent.

REFERENCES :

Hornych, A., Krief, C., Bariéty, J. Prostaglandins Leukotrienes and Med. 8 : 467 - 480, 1982

EFFECTS OF MUZOLIMINE ON RENAL PROSTAGLANDIN BIOSYNTHESIS IN HEALTHY SUBJECTS.

BAUMELOU A.[1], FAUCHER C.[1], HORNYCH A.[2], DERAY G.[1], BROUARD R[1].
[1]Hopital de la Pitié. 83, bd de l' Hôpital. 75651 Paris Cedex 13.
[2]INSERM U 28. Hôpital Broussais. 96, rue Didot. 75674 Paris Cedex 14.

Muzolimine is a loop-diuretic agent. It is indicated in the treatment of edema and arterial hypertension. For the latter indication a low-dosage form of 20 mg is appropriate(1).
A stimulatory effect of loop diuretics on the renin-angiotensin- aldosterone system and on kidney prostaglandin biosynthesis has been clearly established(2,3). To our knowledge this activation has not been clearly demonstrated in man with muzolimine.
This study was undertaken to establish the effects of a low antihypertensive dose of muzolimine on the renin-angiotensin-aldosterone system and renal prostaglandins (PGs) production in relation to sodium and fluid balance.

Methods
20 mg of muzolimine were administered, once a day at 8:00 am in the morning for seven days in six healthy volunteers, 4 men and 2 women,with a mean body weight of 64.7kg . Urines were collected on the third and seventh days of treatment. Blood was drawn on the morning of the forth day before administration(D3) and on the morning of the eighth day at the end of the study(D7). The data were compared with the mean of two control periods. Water and salt diet were free. Plasma renin activity and aldosterone were measured in the upright position and determined by radioimmunoassay. Urinary PGE_2, $PGF_2\alpha$, 6keto $PGF_1\alpha$ and TXB_2 were evaluated by radioimmunoassay as previously described(4). Data are expressed as mean ± SD. Student's t-test for paired variables was used for statistical evaluation.

Results.
None of the volunteers reported any symptomatic diuretic effect. No clinical adverse effects were reported during the treatment period.
After three days of treatment we observed a significant decrease in body-weight from 64.7±6 kg to 64 ($p<0.05$). At the same time there was a significant increase in serum total protein. The increase in serum creatinine was not significant on day 3, the decrease of the creatinine clearance as well.
Blood potassium was significantly decreased on D3, without a significant increase of bicarbonates. It returned to the pretreatment level on D7. Plasma magnesium was unchanged by treatment but globular magnesium was

significantly decreased on D3 and D7 (table 1). Plasma renin activity increased from the basal value of 1.9± ng/ml/h to 4.8± on day 3 ($p<0.01$) and 3.3± on day 7($p<0.05$). Plasma aldosterone concentration increased from 77± pg/ml to 127± on day 3 and 161± on day 7($p<0.05$). The urinary elimination of PGE_2, $PGF_2 \infty$, 6keto $PGF_1 \infty$ and TXB_2 was unchanged in the six volunteers on day 3 and in five of the six on day 7. In the sixth, a very large increase of all the urinary PGs on day 7 contrasted with normal values on day 3. Contamination of the urinary sample by seminal fluid was initially anticipated. However seminal fluid does not contain TxA_2: therefore this large increase is not fully elucidated. Excluding this patient from the global analysis it appears that the urinary prostaglandin elimination is unchanged during the treatment (table 2).

Tab1 : HYDROELECTROLYTIC EFFECTS OF MUZOLIMINE 20 mg once a day IN SIX HEALTHY VOLUNTEERS.

		CONTROL DAYS	DAY 3	DAY 7	S
PROTIDEMIA	(g/l)	72.2 (±.9)	76.7 (±3)	76.2 (±5)	1 vs 3 ; 7
KALEMIA	(mmol/l)	3.74 (±.4)	3.25 (±.3)	3.73 (±.2)	1 vs 3
BICARBONATES	(mmol/l)	28.9 (±1)	27.7 (±2)	29.7 (±2)	
SERIC MG	(mmol/l)	0.84 (±.03)	0.87 (±.05)	0.81 (±.02)	
GLOBULAR MG	(mmol/l)	1.72 (±.1)	1.5 (±.2)	1.73 (±.2)	1 vs 3
CREATININEMIA	(µmol/l)	82.6 (±15)	85.7 (±20)	86.2 (±15)	1 vs 7
CREA clearance	(ml/mn/SC)	128 (±14)	120 (±12)	116 (±21)	
UR flow rate	(ml/day)	1608 (±711)	1558 (±1028)	1733 (±762)	
UR sodium	(mmol/day)	153 (±30)	120 (±53)	124 (±25)	

Discussion

At the dosage of 20 mg, muzolimine appears to have a mild natriuretic effect in the healthy volunteer. The body-weight loss observed after three days of treatment corresponds to a salt loss of 100 mmol during the first two days. These data are not in agreement with the results of Leary and co.(5). For these authors, a single dose of 20 mg of muzolimine in ten adult male volunteers did not increase significantly the mean 24 hour urinary output of fluid, chloride and sodium. In this work after a single dose of 30 mg sodium balance and fluid balance were negative, 60 mmol/day and 410 ml/day respectively. These values are very close to our own observation.

The diuretic effect of muzolimine 20 mg is supported by the significant increase in plasma renin activity and plasma aldosterone concentration. In spite of these effects we did not observe a significant increase of urinary prostaglandin elimination.

Urinary PGs (pg/mn)	control	DAY 3	DAY 7	F
PGE_2	107±25	70±18	106±36	1 NS
$PG\ F_2\alpha$	315±80	234±55	277±132	0,32 NS
$6kPGF_1\alpha$	75±30	75±39	68±31	0,02 NS
TxB_2	80±46	122±70	51±26	0,88 NS

Tab2 : EFFECTS OF MUZOLIMINE 20 MG ONCE A DAY ON PROSTAGLANDIN URINARY EXCRETION IN FIVE HEALTHY VOLUNTEERS.

The urinary elimination of prostaglandins is assumed to be the reflection of renal prostaglandin biosynthesis(6). It has been clearly established that the loop diuretics stimulate kidney prostaglandin biosynthesis(2,3). The same stimulatory effect was observed with muzolimine in the rat but after acute admininistration of very high doses (7).The absence of stimulation of PGs production in our study can receive two explanations: 1) There is an undershoot in urinary sodium flow and volume on day 3. Perhaps a stimulation of PGs production would be observed in single dose administration in man with a larger dose of muzolimine. A study of the effect of muzolimine during the first hours after administration is needed to explore this possibility. 2)It is possible that this effect of muzolimine is original in the class of loop-diuretics. Muzolimine may act directly on the peritubular membrane of the tubular cell(8). All other diuretics act upon the mucosal side of the membrane. The absence of stimulation of renal PGs could be in relation with this property.

This fact may have important clinical implication. Increased renal prostaglandin biosynthesis is generally assumed to protect against low renal blood flow during hypovolemia. Under these conditions the administration of a non steroidal antiinflammatory drug (nsaid) that inhibits the cyclooxygenase activity is prone to provoke an acute decrease in renal blood flow and glomerular filtration rate(9). In light of the absence of effect of 20 mg of muzolimine on renal PG biosynthesis further research would be needed to determine the safety of simultaneous administration of this diuretic with a non steroidal antiinflammatory drug.

References

(1)Lucsko M., Kerihuel JC., Chaignon M., Aubert PH., Guedon J.: Z. Kardiol. 74, S2, 73-76, 1985
(2) Abe K., Irokawa N., yasujima M., Seino M., Chiba S., Sakurai Y., Yoshinaga K., Saito T.: Circ. Res. 43: 254-260, 1978
(3) Attallah AA.: Prostaglandins 18, 369-373, 1979.
(4) Hornych A., Krief C., Bariéty J.: Prostaglandins, Leukotrienes and Medicine 8: 467-480, 1982.
(5)Leary WP., Reyes AJ., van der Byl K.: Z. Kardiol. 74, S2, 135-140, 1985.
(6)Frolich JC., Wilson TW., Sweetman BJ., Smigel M., Nies AJ., Carr K., Watson JT., Oates JA.: J. Clin. Invest. 55: 763-770, 1975
(7) Calo S., Cantaro S., Piccoli A., Vianello A., Borsatti A., Bardini R., Antonello A.: Z. Kardiol. 74, S2, 157-160, 1985
(8) Faedda R., Satta A., Branca GF., Contu B., Bartoli E.: Z. Kardiol. 74, S2, 166-170, 1985
(9)Dunn M., Zambarski EJ.: Kidney Internat. 18: 609-622, 1980

EFFECT OF MUZOLIMINE ON PROSTAGLANDIN E_2 SYNTHESIS AND CATABOLISM IN RAT KIDNEY.

L. CALO', S. CANTARO, A. VIANELLO, A. ANTONELLO and A. BORSATTI

Institute of Internal Medicine, Postgraduate School of Nephrology, University of Padova, 35100 Padova, Italy.

INTRODUCTION

A stimulatory effect of loop diuretics on renal prostaglandin production has been clearly estabilished (1-5) and this has been considered as one of the mechanisms of their pharmacological action. The way by wich the increase of urinary prostaglandin E_2 (PGE2) takes place is probably due both to an inhibition of PGE2 catabolism (6,7) and to a stimulation of Phospholipase A_2 (PLA2) activity in kidney tissue (8,9).

Recently we have demonstrated that Muzolimine (M) increases urinary PGE2 excretion (5). The present study was undertaken to investigate whether M is capable to modulate PGE2 production in the renal tissue.

MATERIAL AND METHODS

Experimental protocol.

10 male Sprague-Dawley rats weighting about 250 g. were used. The rats were placed in metabolic cages and, after a few days of adaptation, 5 rats were treated with a single oral dose of M (100 mg/kg); 5 rats were used as untreated controls. After a 24-hour long urine collection, the rats were killed and the kidney excised and homogenized. Tissue protein content was determined according to Lowry et al. (10).

Determination of PLA2 activity.

PLA2 assay was carried out by a radioenzymathic method according to Cosentino and Ellis (11) with some modifications. Results were expressed as pmol of arachidonic acid/min/mg protein.

Determination of PGE2 catabolic rate.

0.3 ml of PBS (0.1 M pH 7.4 containing 0.9% gelatin and 17000 cpm of ^{3}H-PGE2) were added to 0.1 ml of homogenate. The samples were incubated at 37°C for 10 minutes and then extracted twice at pH 3 with 3 volumes of ethylacetate; the organic phase was evaporated to dryness and applied to a silica gel column (100 mesh, Mallinckrodt) for PGE2 separation as previously described (12). All the chromatographic fractions were collected to calculate recovery; the mean recovery was 75%. PGE2 catabolic rate was expressed as pmol of native PGE2 catabolized/min/mg of protein.

<u>Determination of PGE2 urinary excretion.</u>

PGE2 urinary excretion was assayed according to Dray e coll. (13) and expressed in µg/mg urine creatinine.

RESULTS.

Results are summarized in the following table:

	M-treated r.	control rats	t	p
PLA2 activity	0.0279±0.0064	0.0204±0.005	2.064	ns
PGE2 catabolic rate	0.813±0.030	0.88±0.037	3.41	<0.01
PGE2 urinary excr.	7.08±3.22	0.65±0.19	4.01	<0.005

A significant inverse correlation between PGE2 catabolic rate and PGE2 urinary excretion ($r=-0.92$; $p<0.05$) was found in M-treated rats.

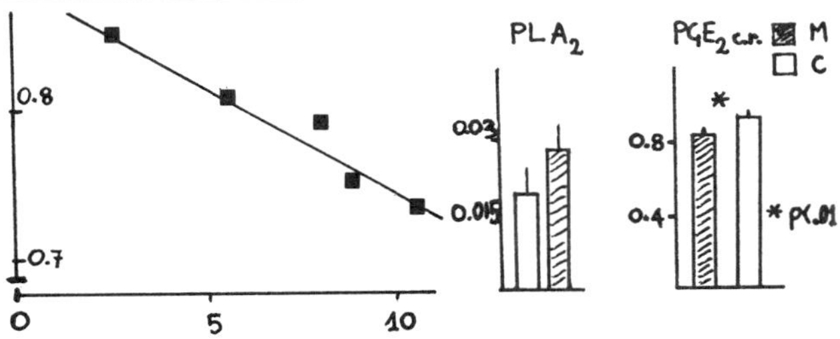

DISCUSSION.

In a previous study (5), we demonstrated that M, a new diuretic with some peculiar properties, enhances urinary PGE2 excretion in the rat and that indometacin, a known Pgs synthesis inhibitor, lowers the natriuretic effect of M, such suggesting that the saluretic property of the drug is at least partially PGs modulated.

Since PGs have no tissutal storage, but are synthetized on demand, an higher tissutal level of Pgs can result from a faster prostanoid synthesis and/or from a slower catabolic rate of the prostanoid. PLA2, an enzyme that cleaves arachidonic acid from membrane phospholipids, is considered the rate limiting step for prostanoid anabolism (14). Our data rule out the possibility that the increased urinary excretion promoted by M is due to a stimulatory effect on PLA2 activity. The lack of effect on PLA2 activity differenziates M from furosemide, of which a stimulatory effect on PLA2 activity has been reported (8,9).

Many enzymes are involved in PGs catabolism, among which 9-ketoreductase and 15-dehydrogenase are the most active ones (15). From our data, overall PGE2 catabolism seems to be significantly reduced by M and this could be sufficient to justify the increase in PGE2 urinary level found after M administration. It is quite true that a washout effect on renal prostaglandins by massive diuresis cannot be denyed "a priori", however the existence of a negative correlation between PGE2 kidney tissue catabolic rate and PGE2 urinary excretion seems to strenght the opinion of a catabolic control on PGE2 urinary levels.

In conclusion, the control of PGE2 catabolic rate seems to be the main mechanism by which M increases the urinary level of this prostanoid.

REFERENCES

1. Nascimento L. Fiallo A.J., Negron M.T., Cruz N., Ayala S.M , Baquero R., and Martinez-Maldonado M. J. Pharmacol. Exper. Ther. 210:147-151, 1979.
2. Oliw E., Anngard E. Acta Physiol. Scand. 105:367-373, 1979.
3. Patak R.W., Fadem S.Z., Rosenblatt S.G., Lipschitz M.D., Stain J.H. Am. J. Physiol. 236:F494-F500, 1979.
4. Katayama S., Attallah A.A., Stahl R.A.K., Bloch D.L., Lee J.B. Am J. Physiol. 247:F555-F561, 1984.
5. Calo' L., Cantaro S., Piccoli A., Vianello A., Borsatti A., Bardini R., Antonello A. Z. Kardiol. 74 suppl. 2:157-170, 1985.
6. Paulsrud J.R., Miller O.N. Fed. Proc. 33:590, 1977.
7. Stone K.J., Hart M. Prostaglandins 12:197-207, 1977.
8. Weber P.C., Sherer B., Larsson C. Europ. J. Pharmacol. 41:329-332, 1977.
9. Vincent J.E. In: Proc. 4th Int. Prost. Conf., Washington, D.C, p. 120.
10. Lowry O.H., Rosenbrough N.J., Farr A.C., Randall R.J. J. Biol. Chem. 193:265-275, 1951.
11. Cosentino M.J., Ellis L.C. Prostaglandins 22:309-322, 1981.
12. Calo' L., Cantaro S., Bertazzo L., Vianello A., Vido L., Borsatti A. Cancer 54: 635-637, 1984.
13. Dray F., Charbonnel B., Maclouf J. Europ. J. Clin. Invest. 5:311-318, 1975.
14. Kunze H., Vogt W. Ann. NY Acad. Sci. USA 180:123-125, 1971.
15. Sun F.F., Taylor B.M., Mc Guire J.C., Wong P.Y.K. Kidney Int. 19:760-770,1981.